A Soup for the Qan

Sir Henry Wellcome Asian Series

VOLUME 9

A Soup for the Qan

Chinese Dietary Medicine of the Mongol Era As Seen in Hu Sihui's *Yinshan Zhengyao*

Introduction, Translation, Commentary, and Chinese Text.
Second Revised and Expanded Edition

By

Paul D. Buell and Eugene N. Anderson
With an appendix by Charles Perry

BRILL

LEIDEN • BOSTON
2010

Published with financial support from the Wellcome Centre for the History of Medicine, London, UK.

On the cover:
Mute Swan and Variegated Swan, *Yinshan zhengyao*, 3, 21B (1456).

The Sir Henry Wellcome name is used under licence from the Wellcome Trust.
The volumes in this series are published with financial support from the Wellcome Trust Centre for the History of Medicine at UCL.
The peacock logo of the series was drawn by the artist Phyllida Legg.
This book is printed on acid-free paper.

Library of Congress Cataloging-in-Publication Data

Husihui.
[Yin shan cheng yao. English & Chinese]
A soup for the Qan : Chinese dietary medicine of the Mongol era as seen in Hu Sihui's Yinshan zhengyao : introduction, translation, commentary, and Chinese text / by Paul D. Buell and Eugene N. Anderson ; with an appendix by Charles Perry. -- 2nd ed., rev. and expanded.
p. ; cm. — (Sir Henry Wellcome Asian series, ISSN 1570-1484 ; v. 9)
Includes bibliographical references and index.
English and Chinese text with introduction and commentary in English.
ISBN 978-90-04-18020-8 (hardback : alk. paper)
1. Husihui. Yin shan zheng yao 2. Diet therapy—China—Early works to 1800. 3. Nutrition—China—Early works to 1800. 4. Medicine, Chinese—Early works to 1800. I. Buell, Paul D. II. Anderson, Eugene N. (Eugene Newton), 1941- III. Perry, Charles, BA. IV. Title. V. Series: Sir Henry Wellcome Asian series (Brill Academic Publishers) ; v. 9. 1570-1484
[DNLM: 1. Husihui. Yin shan cheng yao. 2. Diet Therapy. 3. Cookery. 4. Medicine, Mongolian Traditional. WZ 290]

RM217.B79 2010
615.8'54—dc22

2010027361

ISSN 1570-1484
ISBN 978 90 04 18020 8

He also said: "After us the descendants of our clan will wear gold embroidered garments, eat rich and sweet food, ride fine horses, and embrace beautiful women but they will not say that they owe all this to their fathers and elder brothers, and they will forget us and those great times."

The Maxims of Cinggis-qan as quoted by Valentine A. Riasonovsky, *Fundamental Principles of Mongol Law*, Bloomington: Indiana University, Uralic and Altaic Series, Vol. 43, 1965, 88.

We dedicate our work to the memory of two who have gone before:
Edward Schafer and Berthold Laufer

CONTENTS

PART C: APPENDICES

ACKNOWLEDGEMENTS TO THE SECOND EDITION

In addition to those listed in connection with the first edition, we would like to thank the expert readers of the text of this new edition, namely Ulrike Unschuld, of Berlin, Germany, Angelika Messner, of Kiel, Germany, and Ruth Meserve, of Bloomington, Indiana. Needless to say, in spite of their help, only the authors are responsible for any errors that remain. Dalena Pham has ably served as the research assistant for the second edition; including helping recompile a complex index. She was assisted by Kun Yang. In Berlin, Siglinde Mooney has untiringly provided secretarial support to PDB and this is most gratefully acknowledged and likewise, in Seattle, the legal assistance of attorneys David Lovik and Nicholas Juhl in helping settle thorny contractual issues with publishers. Among our colleagues, the advice and encouragement of Vivienne Lo, John Carswell, Françoise Sabban, and Judy Kolbas, also Jacqueline Newman, H. T. Huang, Sidney Mintz, David and Taiping Knechtges, Lisa Raphals, Christopher and Gala Muench and Igor de Rachewiltz are also gratefully acknowledged. Teresa Wang has continued to be of enormous help to us by supplying books from China, including tracking which ones to supply, often no easy task. Paul Unschuld has served above and beyond as series editor and we would like to thank him for his continued encouragement of our work. Without him it would never have seen the light of day. In this same connection, particular thanks go to Patricia Radder of Brill for solving a series of technical issues with our typescript and for her warm encouragement of our endeavors. Eugene Anderson has continued to be funded by the University of California at Riverside and Paul Buell would like to thank the National Endowment for the Humanities for an individual fellowship during 2006-7.

We have attempted this new edition both to update and expand our presentation and to correct many errors still found in the first edition in spite of careful editing and proofing. Also, our view of some of the material and of the Mongol world in general has changed over the years. Our work with the set of early Ming 明 fragments of a Yuan 元 encyclopedia now called the *Huihui yaofang* 回回藥方, "Muslim Medicinal Recipes," has also led to some reassessment. The influence of Arabic medicine on our dietary seems far clearer now than it once was. Despite this, we have resisted the temptation to completely redo the present book and will keep most of our new material for later. In fact, the favorable reception that our work has received since it was first published has made clear to us that we, by and large, got it right the first time. Above all, we want to make our efforts available to a larger audience than was the case for the original edition, priced too high even for large libraries.

Berlin
Christmas, 2009

ACKNOWLEDGMENTS TO THE FIRST EDITION

First, we are grateful to our families, who had to put up with a great deal of lamb and goat, among other things, in the process of kitchen testing. Secondly, we are grateful to the University of California, Riverside, for providing generous funding and facilities for research (grants and facilities to ENA), and to the Wilson Library of Western Washington University for making its excellent collection of Mongolian and Turkic materials and facilities freely available. Finally, we are grateful to a large number of friends and advisors, including Paul Unschuld, whose efforts went far beyond what is normally required of a series editor, Françoise Sabban, Francesca Bray, Christopher Muench, Dru Gladney, William Jankowiak, Nancy Peterson Walter, Jacqueline Newman, Penelope Van Esterik, Igor de Rachewiltz, Henry Schwarz, Edward Kaplan, Linda Kimball, Kathleen Tomlonovic, Wayne Richter, Edward Vajda, Angelo Anastasio, Tamsin Hekala, Olav Hekala, Ilse Cirtautas, Thomas A. P. Gwinner, Linda Vane, Penny Goode, Sabrina Wilson, Hen Sen Chin, Jeffrey MacDonald, Richard Brzustowicz, Chung Chih-hui, Phyllis Graham, Julia Fearing, Jennifer Jay, Robin Mayberry, Iris Olga Ludviksdottir, Arienne Dwyer, Judy Kolbas, Dominik Wujastyk of the Wellcome Trust, Kaori O'Connor of Kegan Paul International, and to the countless house guests who served as guinea pigs, willing, eager, and enthusiastic, to be sure, for the kitchen tests. Herbert Franke and Françoise Sabban served as the publisher's reviewers for the manuscript and we thank them for many useful suggestions. Auður Ingolfsdottir was briefly project research assistant and provided much needed help with indexing. Her replacement was Christine Buell who undertook final proofreading and helped with the index. Thanks also to Frau Holler of Munich and John Donahue of the University of California at Riverside who helped prepare the text facsimile. Special thanks goes to "Hafiz" of Microsoft Corporation for hours spent on the phone helping solve some tricky formatting problems as we pushed the parameters of Microsoft Word™ to the limit. The Department of Liberal Studies, Western Washington University (William Stoever, chair), also provided travel support for PDB to attend Paul Unschuld's important 1986 München, Federal Republic of Germany, conference on traditional medical literature. The vote of confidence is gratefully acknowledged. Needless to say, none of the above mentioned individuals or organizations are in any way responsible for any errors or misconceptions in our book, for which the authors take full responsibility.

When we began our book none of us suspected in the slightest that its realization would take most of two decades, at least a third of that time spent in solving the technical problems associated with producing the camera-ready copy required by the publishers. We did not intend to make it our "life's work," but it has turned out that way. We sincerely hope that the reading public will think that the results are worth the effort that has gone into producing them as we finally offer our too many pages in print.

Seattle
Easter, 1999

A NOTE ON TRANSCRIPTION

A simplified system has been employed to transcribe Classical Mongolian, Medieval Turkic, Persian, and Arabic except in Appendix II, reproduced as published with minor changes. Most but not all diacritic marks have been omitted including indications of vowel length. "H" has been used after consonants to indicate voicing in Classical Mongolian and Turkic. As much as possible, forms are spelled consistently and usually according to some authority, Perry for most Turkic grain foods, Doerfer for most other Turkic words. Middle Mongolian is transcribed according to the simplified system employed in Igor de Rachewiltz, *Index to the Secret History of the Mongols* (Bloomington: Indiana University Publications, Uralic and Altaic Series, Vol. 121, 1972), except that "š" is used consistently where appropriate. All Chinese is transcribed according to the Pinyin system except for reconstructed forms and bibliographical entries originally using Wade-Giles transcription. For Japanese the Hepburn system has been used. Western European languages are spelled normally but Russian and most other languages written in the Cyrillic Script have largely been transcribed according to systems employed in United States Government publications except that front and back vocalization is shown by umlauting in the transcription of Khalkha Mongolian. Those knowing the relevant languages will have no difficulty in restoring the original forms. Throughout the text, reconstructions from Chinese transcriptions made by the present authors are marked with "*," except in Appendix II where the asterisk indicates reconstructed proto-Turkic forms. Reconstructions made by others are not so marked but the source of the reconstruction is indicated in each case.

A SOUP FOR THE *QAN*: CHINESE DIETARY MEDICINE OF THE MONGOL ERA AS SEEN IN HU SIHUI'S *YINSHAN ZHENGYAO*

Part A

* * *

Background and Analysis

INTRODUCTION

In Xanadu did Kublai Khan
A stately pleasure dome decree...

Coleridge, in his vision of this romantic garden, sees himself as eating divine food:

And close your eyes in holy dread,
for he on honeydew hath fed
and drunk the milk of paradise.

In fact, Kublai Khan (more correctly Qubilai-qan) did indeed eat honey and milk, but mostly he ate sheep. His grandfather, Cinggis-qan, had first invaded China in the early thirteenth century. His uncle, Ögödei completed the conquest of the north by crushing Jin 金 in 1234. In 1260 Qubilai himself came to power and in 1266 built a new winter capital at what is now Beijing, alternating between it and his old princely residence, after 1263 his summer capital of Shangdu 上都, Coleridge's Xanadu, on the cool fringes of the steppe. By 1276 Qubilai's Mongols had conquered all China and established the Yuan 元 Dynasty.

Amazingly enough, we have an excellent record of the haute cuisine of this court. In 1330 there was presented to the emperor a dietary manual, the *Yinshan zhengyao* 飲膳正要 (*YSZY*), or "Proper and Essential[1] Things for the Emperor's Food and Drink." This book was written by Hu Sihui 忽思慧, who had been an imperial dietary physi-

[1] The translation of *zhengyao* in the title is somewhat uncertain. *Zheng* is taken here as a noun but could just as easily be an adjective, in which case the title should be understood as "Proper Essentials for the Emperor's Food and Drink," also "The Most Important Things for the Emperor's Food and Drink." We prefer the translation "Proper and Essential Things for the Emperor's Food and Drink" since it is expressive of the two very distinct types of material contained within the text: canonical prescriptions for life and health taken from various classics (the *zheng*); and court delicacies, essential (*yao*) from the point of view of the Mongols and their followers. We are indebted to Igor de Rachewiltz (unpublished letters of 28 January and 6 February, 1992, to PDB) for discussing alternative translations of the title with us.

cian under several short-lived descendants of Qubilai in the early 1300s. Although his name appears purely Chinese,[2] Hu himself, if he was not a foreigner, must have come from a culturally mixed background. He quite likely came from a bilingual, Chinese and Turkic family resident in the former Xixia 西夏 domains of northwest China, perhaps from what is now Ningxia 寧夏 Province.[3] His work reflects the cuisine of the era in some detail, also long-term Chinese assimilation of foreign foods and foodways, and a considerable "future shock" due to conquest and rule of China by foreigners, with only limited interest in China and Chinese culture. Since Hu's primary interest and charge was the medical aspect of nutrition, always a central focus in the Chinese world, much of the book is an account of the medical values of foods and recipes, in terms of Medieval Chinese nutritional therapy.

Hu's dietary is thus a rich source for the study of many areas of the complex cultural history of Medieval Eurasia, one that lends itself well to the investigations of the "New History." This school has developed in response to the realization that study of the societies and civilizations of the past can no longer focus merely upon political

[2] Hu's apparently Chinese name proves nothing in and of itself since many non-Chinese took Chinese names in Yuan times in what is seen by Ch'en Yüan 陳垣 in *Western and Central Asians in China under the Mongols*, Monumenta Serica Monograph XV, Trans. by Ch'ien Hsing-hai and L. Carrington Goodrich, (Los Angeles, 1966), 226-41, as an on-going process of Sinicization. Ch'en himself lists Hu Sihui as one of the foreigners writing books in Chinese during Yuan times (1966: 305). Igor de Rachewiltz suggests that Hu's seemingly Chinese name may not be Chinese but a transcription of Turkic Qusqi (unpublished letter of 26 September, 1991, to PDB).

[3] Two facts are clear about Hu from a simple reading of his book: One is that his Chinese education was good and thorough (his Classical Chinese is excellent); and that he must have grown up in or near China, or at least in a highly Sinicized environment to identify so strongly with Chinese culture. The other is that his Turkic, and to some extent Mongol culture, was natural to him, more than simple exposure to the court environment of the era would have accounted for. The many Turkic words and expressions in the *YSZY* are absolutely germane to the text, are used correctly, and exhibit a dialectical consistency. Hu's Turkic language is East Turkistani and very close to Modern Uighur with forms such as *tutum ash, um ash, sajhimur*. He must have spoken a Turkic language, probably Uighur, as a first or a second language; and he must have grown up in a culture where Chinese and Turkic, and for that matter Mongolian, cultural elements existed side-by-side and interacted freely. This can only have been in one of the highly mixed societies of the Sino-Mongolian borderlands. Many *YSZY* recipes have a clear connection with the modern Hui 回 cooking of Ningxia. This connection is best understood if we assume that *YSZY* foodways and modern Ningxia cooking have common roots and that Hu Sihui, a native of the area, drew upon them.

events, or other great and obvious achievements of a time. Historians must also take into consideration more mundane areas of human life, perhaps less obvious, but none the less vital for understanding what actually happened. The French *Annales* school (named after the journal of the same name founded by Marc Bloch and Lucien Febvre) has taken the initiative in this area. Leading exponents, such as the late Fernand Braudel,[4] have placed at the center of their considerations neglected topics once at the periphery of historical studies, with brilliant results.[5] These topics include kinship. Bloch, for example, was one of the first historians to fuse anthropological study of kinship with medieval studies, which had revolutionary impact upon his field. Annalists are also concerned with man and environment, the realities of production and trade, the evolution of prices, the nature of transport, individual perceptions of space and time, the focus of Braudel's later work,[6] and food and food production.

This last area is of particular concern to the "New History," since food and food production are the most immediate of all the material underpinnings of life. Bound up within it are also man's conceptualization of food and food products, as sources of nutrition, and as medicine. Here, interests of the "New History" coincide with those of historians of medicine, of ideas, in the broadest sense, and of anthropologists, always concerned about food and the social realities and interactions which it reflects.

Food and foodways are sensitive barometers of material and social conditions. They reveal change in process and cultural interactions which may be studied through archaeology, art, linguistics, and the philological examination of texts. Textual evidence is of particular usefulness for those cultures with long written traditions since it permits detailed study of food, food production, and foodways over the long term. Cultural changes taking place far too slowly or too subtly to draw much notice from contemporaries can be charted and explored. Also revealed are periods of sharp departure from the past, in

---

[4] See in particular Fernand Braudel, *The Mediterranean and the Mediterranean World in the Age of Philip II*, Trans. by Sian Reynolds (New York, 1973).

[5] See, as the most outstanding recent example of the "new history," Fernand Braudel, *Civilization and Capitalism: 15-18th. Centuries*, vols. 1-3, Trans. and Revised by Sian Reynolds (New York, 1979-84).

[6] See Fernand Braudel, *The Identity of France*, vols. 1-2, Trans. by Sian Reynolds (New York, 1988-90).

which the shock of the new is obvious. This is the case in the *YSCY*, above all on account of its association with the Mongols.

The Mongols consciously sought, once their movement had taken root, to create a universal world empire. By 1330, this dream had faded politically in bitter wars of succession among Cinggis-qan's descendants, but pretensions of cultural universality persisted. One manifestation is the eclecticism of the *YSCY*. It incorporates foods from all the realms conquered or even affected by the Mongols and seems a deliberate attempt to represent the Mongolian world order in visible, tangible, edible form. A dignitary receiving hospitality at a Yuan feast could be served dishes from Baghdad, Kashmir, and China, as well as Mongolian game and Manchurian wildfowl. Hu interprets the dietary and nutritional values of foods served more or less in Chinese terms. In some places he simply copies out the appropriate sections of Chinese medical classics. None the less, some of his medical recipes appear to include traditional Mongolian medicinals and some are straight borrowings from Middle Eastern medicine. Even some of his "Chinese" prescriptions are clearly adapted with Middle Eastern medicine in mind. Hu was also strongly influenced by West Asian and Mongol perceptions of health and of the human place in the cosmos. This was the cuisine of a world empire, one standing at the crossroads of the many different cultures finding expression within it: Mongol, Turkic, South and West Asian, Chinese.

But while Hu's cuisine and the medical traditions used in its interpretation have been constructed with the universalist aims of the Mongol court in China in mind, the end result is also expressive of particular economic realities and value choices on the part of the Mongols and those closest to them. Many Mongols, for example, including many coming to court, still lived the traditional way of life in the fourteenth century and were dependent upon traditional foods and modes of food production. Through them, and through nostalgia even the most culturally assimilated Mongols felt for the common Mongol past, traditional Mongol foods and foodways continued to exert a strong influence. Yet while this was the case, the Yuan court was no longer dependent upon herding, hunting, and gathering for its food, although those serving the court continued to engage in these practices at its behest. It could literally call on the entire continent of Asia for foods and medicines. The exotic was, as a consequence, often freely available. Coupled with this fact, the Mongols were also self-consciously eclectic and eager to try new things, perhaps to appear cosmopolitan and impress others.

The Mongol court was thus bound by tradition, but was relatively free of narrow economic and social determinants. It provides us with a fascinating study in cultural history. By observing the Mongol court elite of the time at their table, in good health and in bad, we can reach a new understanding of what actually determines specific cultural repertoires.

Yuan court cuisine as reflected in the *YSZY* rests upon a foundation of Central Asian pastoralism. The sheep is paramount. Most main dishes are based on its meat or broth. Literally all parts were used: head, and feet, skin and intestines, bones, and tail.[7] Wild game meats also loom large, as do the meats of other herd animals. Only the pig, the principal animal of Chinese diet, is virtually absent from the *YSZY*. If, among other products of pastoralism, dairy products are somewhat neglected in the book, it may be because most were such everyday fare that Hu did not need to mention them. Some accommodation to Chinese norms may be evident in this area as well.

Grains and dry legumes were important but they are, in most cases, used as additives, in raw or processed form, in mutton-based soups and stews. Fresh vegetable foods are rather few and far between, as they were on the steppe. Most are those which could be grown successfully in the cold, dry northwest. Many are gathered foods rather than cultivated ones, daily usage of the ordinary folk of the steppe. Some are used consciously with their medicinal values in mind. Nothing is more revealing of the deeply Mongol roots of the court. China did not "conquer her conquerors"; indeed, the conquerors did not even abandon wild roots and herbs for the succulent fruits and specially cultivated vegetable delicacies of Chinese traditional elite taste. Where the Tang 唐 court sent for lichees from the far south, the Yuan court sent for mushrooms and eleagnus fruits from the cold high steppe lands.

Medical influences in the *YSCY* include the particular problems of Chinese and Mongols of the age. The book is, of course, overwhelmingly concerned with the nutritional aspects of health, and thus most of the directions fall into a few categories. Most important is the value of the foods in maintaining and regulating *qi* 氣 (vital essence, finest

---

[7] Stefán Adalsteinsson, in his "Importance of sheep in early Icelandic agriculture," in Gerald F. Bigelow, ed., *The Norse of the North Atlantic*, Acta Archaeologica 61 (Kobenhavn, 1991): 285-91, provides detailed information about how medieval and early modern Icelanders used virtually all products of the sheep except the hooves. Mongol uses were comparable except that they did use the hooves, or at least the feet.

matter). Strict instructions given about avoiding contaminated, rotten or suspect foods alternate with ideas drawn from the logic of cosmology: magical lore, folk beliefs, and accumulated wisdom from millennia of misguided searches for immortality and long-lasting youth. Some suggestions are now recognized as being based on empirically-observed vitamin and mineral contents of foods, mixed with Mongolian and other cosmological ideas. There is little apparent structure: Hu simply listed ways he thought that diet could strengthen the body and make it last longer, and ways he thought diet could endanger health. Specific therapies and logically consistent theories were not part of his plan.

Cultural roots explain more than ecology in this case, for even the most stringent ecological determinants of Yuan cuisine were mediated by cultural tradition. It included new traditions developed since the establishment of an empire, peculiar to post-conquest Mongols and to the cultures of those associated with them in power. Although the emperor and his establishment went through the motions of annual transhumance between winter and summer capitals until the end, by 1330 most of the court elite had grown up in the sedentary luxury of Qanbaliq (Beijing) and of other cities, rather than beside a mountain stream in the Mongolian pasture lands. Most court Mongols, as a consequence, knew dried mutton, wild currants, and Amur river sturgeons as things appearing on a table; not foods they had to gather or catch and prepare for themselves.

Cultural background was greatly complicated by court internationalism. Mongols were a small minority. Most of the middle and lower echelons of the court were comprised of various Turks, Chinese, Koreans, Russians, and other ethnic groups. Turkic noodle dishes, Chinese fish and chicken recipes, and Tibetan tsampa were part of a collective culinary heritage. It also included substantial borrowings from Iran and Mesopotamia due in large part to the conquest of Baghdad by Qubilai's younger brother Hüle'ü and the relations which his descendants continued to maintain with China. We should not be surprised to find the first recipe in the *YSZY* to be an adapted Baghdadi dish. It was all in the family. Only in medical matters do cultural traditions become heavily determinative, for here Hu tends to follow, rather uncritically, the received wisdom in Chinese, Muslim, and Mongol medical circles of the time.

In short, cultural background could be interpreted in many ways and could allow the court to draw on almost anything eaten in Asia. In a court which recruited people as far away as France and Italy, almost any imaginable food could be part of someone's cultural background.

The *YSZY* reflects the cuisine of the sophisticated court of a world empire. Feasts were lavish, and the Mongols did everything they could to impress visitors, as we know from accounts such as those of Marco Polo and William of Rubruck. Food was used, deliberately, as a way of showing power, generosity, and wealth. It was thus an implement of statesmanship. As in most societies, feasts were used to cement alliances, celebrate important events, reward friends, overawe enemies, and lubricate politics in general.

We believe that the international flavor of the *YSZY* reflects the deliberate construction of a cuisine to reflect the scope of the empire. Foods and foodways from all parts of the Mongol realm were brought together to show Mongol power.

Finally, Hu was writing as court nutritionist, and the book has a major medical function. He was trying not only to codify recipes, but to improve the health of the court. Thus, the *YSZY* is a nutritional manual, reflecting the food beliefs of the time. It is a rather heterogeneous one. Chinese classical medical lore and folk beliefs are mixed with Mongol and west Asian practices. This leads to inconsistencies and even contradictions. It also leads to the incorporation of some magical lore that cannot have had much real-world benefit for the Mongol elite. Nonetheless, Hu's advice is generally sound. At worst, he seems to have lived up to the old medical truism, "First, do no harm." At best, he counseled moderation in eating and drinking, avoidance of spoiled food, and a balanced diet providing protein, minerals, and vitamins.

CHAPTER ONE

HISTORICAL AND CULTURAL CONTEXT

I. *YINSHAN ZHENGYAO*: TEXT AND AUTHOR

In its present form, the *YSZY* is an illustrated dietary manual and cookbook in three *juan* 卷 (chapters). There are many modern printed editions and also at least two manuscript versions.[1] Without exception all are based upon the 1456 Ming edition used for the present translation in its Sibu congkan xubian 四部叢刊續編 reprint. This edition is a reproduction of a Yuan original that now survives only in fragments.[2]

The best modern edition of the *YSZY* remains that of Li Chunfang 李春方.[3] Li provides a full text and notes, and a modern Chinese

---

[1] These are located in Japanese libraries and were not available for examination. See Ishida Mikinosuke, "*Inzenseiyō* ni tsuite," *Shisen* 15 (1959): 40–58.

[2] These fragments, along with a new reproduction of the 1456 edition, have been published as *Yinshan zhengyao san juan fu yuan ke Yinshan zhengyao can juan* 飲膳正要三卷 附元刻飲膳正要殘卷 in the collection Zhongguo gudai banhua congkan 中國古代版畫叢刊二編, series 1, by the Shanghai guji chubanshe 上海古籍出版社 (Shanghai, 1994). That little or nothing was changed in making the 1456 edition is clear from a comparison of surviving Yuan pages with their equivalents in the Ming edition (contents are identical other than more detailed Yuan illustrations). Also, according to Herbert Franke (unpublished letter of 29 April, 1986 to PDB), Yuan printing practices are evident in a number of places. For example, in both the author's and Yu Ji's prefaces to the Ming edition a new line is begun "whenever the emperor or an imperial ancestor or a term relating to the emperor occurs..." This practice, he goes on, "... is compatible with a Yuan print, but not with a Ming one. It would be unusual to respect the imperial rules of typography of a former dynasty unless the later edition is a retraced newly cut block print of an earlier—in this case, Yuan edition." I would like to thank to Prof. Franke for sharing his insights on the history of the *YSZY*.

[3] We are grateful to Teresa Wang for bringing the Li edition to our attention. By and large Li's interpretations agree with our own. But there are two areas of significant disagreement: Botanical and zoological identification of some *YSZY materia dietica et medica* and interpretation of non–Chinese terminology. Most of the differences in botanical and zoological identification are due to obsolete terminology and classification systems in use in the PRC when Li wrote his book and typographical errors and misspellings. None of these differences is serious. Li also differs in a few

translation (Hu Sihui. *Yinshan zhengyao*, ed. Li Chunfang. Zhongguo pengren guji congkan 中國烹飪古記叢刊. Beijing: Zhongguo shangye chubanshe 中國商業出版社, 1988). Another modern edition, edited by Liu Yushu 劉玉樹 (Hu Sihui. *Yinshan zhengyao*, ed. Liu Yushu. Beijing: Renmin weisheng chubanshe 人民衛生出版社, 1986), is largely based upon the defective 1934 Shanghai edition of the Commercial Press edited by Wang Yunwu 王 雲五 (Hu Sihui. *Yinshan zhengyao yi ce* 飲膳正要一册, ed. Wang Yunwu. Shanghai: Zhongguo shangye chubanshe, 1934) and is a far less useful. The original Wang edition was republished in 1971 in Taibei by the Commercial Press in its popular Renren wenku 人人文庫 series (Hu Sihui. *Yinshan zhengyao yi ce* 飲膳正要一册, ed. Wang Yunwu 王雲 五. Renren wenku. Taibei: Zhongguo shangye chubanshe, 1971). Since the first

---

species and sub–species identifications. Identification of plants and animals mentioned in early Chinese sources is always difficult. Traditional Chinese botanical and zoological terminology is ambiguous and precise equation of Chinese and Western nomenclature is not always possible. A *huanggua* 黃瓜, "yellow melon," for example, is a cucumber in much of China but a zucchini on Taiwan. Li generally chooses to follow the standard reference works, which reflect modern, all–China usage, and to make broad, generic identifications within a greater context of Chinese cultural tradition. We usually do so as well but opt for species and sub–species most common in the north, or in Mongolia, when a choice must be made between similar plants or between closely related species, carefully following the valuable evidence provided by *YSZY* illustrations. In most cases our differences with Li are trivial. In others the present authors and Li take radically different points of view reflecting radically different assumptions regarding the *YSZY* and the foods and food sources described in it. Li, for example, seeing the *YSZY* as a more Chinese document than we do, translates the rather vague Chinese term we translate as "acorn" as "kumquat." The term does mean that in the south but not in the north whose usage the *YSZY* overwhelmingly reflects. Kumquats would in any case be quite out of place in this section of the text. There are other serious misidentifications in Li's edition. Li, for example, calls the unidentified "Muslim green" azurite. "Muslim green" is a term for azurite, but the *YSZY's* "Muslim green" is clearly a plant, possibly mint. It is unfortunately not illustrated. In a few cases, identifications are highly uncertain and Li's guess is as good as ours. We can do no more than justify our choices. Caution is always necessary since Hu Sihui and his collaborators were never as precise in their terminology as their modern interpreters would like. Thus we have identified many *YSZY* names to the genus or even the family (only), where Li gives a particular species.

Otherwise, our main differences with Li come in regard to Mongol, Turkic, Iranian, and other names, words, titles, and phrases. Here we have the benefit of better available reference works, and have taken the liberty to differ (usually silently) with Li on these matters. This should in no way be taken as a criticism. Li's edition is excellent, important and valuable, and we welcome it. It adds to the growing body of research on an important text. The last word has yet to be said, and Li and others will no doubt find much to add to our own efforts.

edition of this book several new editions have appeared (Hu Sihui. *Yinshan zhengyao* 飲膳正要. Beijing: Zhongyi jingdian wenku 中醫經典文庫, 2009; Hu Sihui. *Yinshan zhengyao xin pian* 飲膳正要新編, ed. Jiang Runxiang 江潤祥 (Y. C. Kong). Hong Kong: The Chinese University Press, 2004; and Hu Sihui. *Yinshan zhengyao, Zhonghua yi ji jingdian zhushi* 飲膳正要，中華醫籍經典注釋. Beijing: Nei menggu kexue jishu chubanshe 内蒙古科學技術出版社, 2002. Of these, the Jiang Runxiang edition, which contains annotations by botanist Hu Xiuying 胡秀英, is the most valuable. It largely follows our own work.

Other than our present translation, and Li's Modern Chinese version, there are two other full translations of the text, into Mongolian, by Kököluu (Huhelu 胡和祿), as *Idege umdagan–u jhingkini tobchi* ("The Essential Short History of Food and Drink"),Hailar: Inner Mongolian People's Press, 1982, and into Japanese by Jin Shilin 金世 琳 (Hu Sihui. *Yakuzen no genten, Inzenseiyō* 藥膳の原典，飲膳 正要. Trans. from the Chinese by Jin Shilin. Tōkyō: Yasaka shobō 八坡書房, 1993).[4] Portions of *juan* 2 (on foods to treat disease, pages 27b–41b in the 1456 edition) have been translated into German by Thomas Gwinner in his *Essen und Trinken*: *die klassische Kochbuchliteratur Chinas* (Heidelberger Schriften zur Ostasiankunde 11), Frankfurt: Haag + Herchen, 1988: 81–108; and selections from *juan* 1 and 2 into Japanese by Nakamura Shōhachi 中村璋八 and Satō Tatsuzen 佐藤達全 in their *Shokkei* 食經, Tōkyō: Meitoku shuppansha 明德出版社, 1978: 41–141.

Contents are as follows: *Juan* 1, the shortest (pages 1a–50b in the 1456 edition), contains prefaces and other introductory materials (1a–6b),[5] a general table of contents (7a–12b), and short biographies of sages Fuxi 伏羲, Shennong 神農, and Huangdi 皇帝 (13a–13b). There follows sections on "Nurturing Life and Avoiding Things to Be Shunned" (14b–17b), "Food Avoidances during Pregnancy" (18a–20b), "Avoidances for a Wet Nurse" (21a–22b), and for postpartum women (23a–b),[6] and "Things to Avoid and Shun when Drinking Liquor" (24a–25b) (a topic of particular interest to the Mongols with their well–known proclivities in this area). The most important part of the *juan* follows, ninety–five recipes for "Strange Delicacies of Combined

[4] We are indebted to Françoise Sabban for bringing this new translation to our attention. See the review by Ohase Ariki in *Vesta*, No. 16 (July, 1993): 49.

[5] Most of this material is translated in full in Paul U. Unschuld, *Medicine in China: A History of Pharmaceutics* (Berkeley, 1986): 213 ff.

[6] Partially translated in Unschuld, 1986: 217.

Flavors" (26a–50b). Most, as we shall see, are of Middle Eastern inspiration if not origin and there is Middle Eastern influence present in other sections of this chapter as well, including the material on wet nurses.

Juan 2 (1a–52a) begins with recipes for fifty–seven drinks and liquid foods ("Various Hot Beverages and Concentrates") (1a–11b), and some "Doses and Foods[7] of the Beneficent[8] Immortals" in many forms (12a–20a). Next is a detailed description of "What Is Advantageous for the Four Seasons" (20b–24a), a listing of the negative results from over–indulgence in any of the five flavors and general ways to avoid them (25b–26b), sixty–one "Foods that Cure the Various Illnesses" (27b–41b), "Food Avoidance when Taking Medicines" (42a–43b), properties making certain foods dangerous to eat (44a–45b),[9] "Foodstuffs which Mutually Conflict" (46a–48b), foods containing poisons and how to process them (49a–50b), and dangerous "Animal Transformations" (51a–52a). *Juan* 3 is an illustrated catalog of the *materia dietica* of the entire work (1a–59a) under 221 headings.[10]

Not including introductory materials and the table of contents (1a–12b), which is roughly eight percent of the entire book, material in the *YSZY* falls into one of three general categories: 1) Recipes, 2) the listing of various *materia dietica*, and 3) "erratic blocks"[11] of material

---

[7] Donald Harper in a letter of 13 January, 1997 (to PDB), suggests the translation "dietetics" for our "doses and foods." This is also possible but we prefer "doses and foods" to avoid any possibility of overtranslation. It is not entirely certain that the Medieval Chinese possessed a concept of dietetics similar to our own.

[8] In Chinese the term translated beneficent here, *shen* 神, is properly a kind of god but which, in contrast to *gui* 鬼, is a good spirit, thus the translation here. "Divine immortals" would be an alternative but would not confer the idea that the spiritual power in question is for the good, not evil.

[9] Partially translated in Unschuld, 1986: 218.

[10] Compare the listing of the *YSZY*'s contents in Unschuld, 1986: 216–18.

[11] On this concept as it relates to Arabic medical and dietary texts, see Manfred Ullmann, *Islamic Medicine* (Edinburgh, 1978), 24. By "erratic blocks" Ullmann means extraneous, heterogeneous textual elements that are plugged into another text often without regard to context or the fact that such materials may even contradict information included elsewhere. In the Arabic world such elements were often apt quotations and selections from classics of Greek medicine, on occasion from bad translations. In addition to obvious examples such as the "Doses of the Immortals," a patchwork of quotations from various Daoist macrobiotic classics, much of *juan* 3 also appears to be comprised of such "erratic blocks." The *materia dietica* discussed often has very little to do with the rest of the book. We would suspect that the various sections on "prohibitions" include a substantial amount of such materials as well, some of it, as will be shown, from non-Chinese origins. Some of the sources for these and other sections have been identified by Li in Li, 1988.

from various sources scattered throughout the text. Of these, recipes are the most important and the nucleus of the text with a total of 219 headings. The three main groups of recipes are: 1) The 95 recipes for "Strange Delicacies of Combined Flavors" (1, 26a–50b), 2) the 57 "Various Hot Beverages and Concentrates" (2, 1a–11b), 3) the 61 "Foods that Cure the Various Illnesses" (2, 27b–41b). There are also six Daoist recipes included among the "Doses and Foods of the Beneficent Immortals," including the recipe for the "Spirit Pillow" (2, 12a–13b; 18a–19b). Recipes constitute about one–third of the *YSZY*. Nearly all are original, although not the Daoist material.

The second homogenous body of material is the listing of *materia dietica* in *juan* 3 (1a–59a). The 221 main headings list about two–thirds of all primary *materia dietica* mentioned anywhere in the *YSZY* (compare the listing in Appendix I, following the translated text). This section comprises nearly 38 percent of the text and like most such material is based upon information found in classical texts, here combined with empirical data and facts specific to the Mongol court.

The smallest section of the text, about 21 percent, is comprised of the miscellaneous texts, "erratic blocks," constituted by the "avoidances" (1, 14b–25b; 2, 25b–26b; 2, 42a–52a), the biographies of the "Three Sages" (1, 13a–13b), the "Doses and Foods of the Beneficent Immortals" (2, 14a–17b, 20a), and "What is Advantageous for the four Seasons" (20b–24a). Much of these materials was drawn from canonical texts such as the *Yellow Emperor's Inner Canon*.

The completed work was presented to the Mongol emperor Tuγ–temür (r. 1328–1332) on the third day of the third month of the third year of Tianli 天裡, *i.e.*, in the late spring of 1330. In his preface to the *YSZY*,[12] Yuan scholar and official Yu Ji 虞集 calls its author Hu Sihui senior [court] dietary physician (*shan taiyi* 膳太醫) under the control of one Chang 常 Buralgi[13] and says that his work was the culmination of efforts reaching back to Qubilai's time (1,1a). Hu's

[12] See the complete translation of this preface in the text below. Compare Unschuld, 1986: 215–6. On Yu Ji, see Magnus Michael Kriegeskorte, "Yu Ji (1272–1348), Ein Literaten–Beamter unter der Mongolenherrschaft" (Inaugural–Dissertation, zur Erlangung der Doktorwürde, vorgelegt der Philosophischen Fakultät der Rheinischen Friederich–Wilhelms–Universität zu Bonn, 1984).

[13] Chang Buralgi was the son of Chang Yaozhu 常咬住, a chief officer of the Mongol emperor's table, and came from an old North Chinese aristocratic family long associated with the Mongols. Buralgi most likely inherited his post from his father. (We are grateful to Herbert Franke for his help in identifying Chang Buralgi and his family.)

own preface (1, 3a–4b) adds that he was first appointed to office during the Yenyou 延佑 period (1314–20).

The *YSZY* is thus a product of the time of greatest Mongolian power and cultural influence in China, the decades immediately following the final subjugation of Song 宋 (1279). During these years Mongol rule over China was still unquestioned and the interests and tastes of the Mongol court were taken seriously and even imitated. Outside of China, much of the Old World was influenced, if not directly ruled, by Mongolian successor states. A Mongol world order thus persisted. Political, economic and cultural interchanges promoted by Mongolian universality continued in spite of the antagonisms of the successor states, in the case of Mongol East Asia, increasingly using the seas.

The *YSZY* reflects these facts, as well as the unique fourteenth century court environment of Mongol China which produced it. It also reflects a broader process of political and cultural amalgamation through which the Mongolian world order had taken shape.

II. The Rise of Mongolian Empire

At the end of the twelfth century several charismatic Mongol leaders, including the young Temüjin,[14] founded chiefdoms. They soon began to compete with one another for dominion over other Mongols. By 1206 only one remained, Temüjin's Mongqol. The others had been defeated and destroyed, and survivors enslaved or forced to flee Mongolia. In that year, as a symbol of his success and the new state of affairs in the steppe, Temüjin took the imperial title Cinggis–qan ("Universal *Qan*"). Even before this event his movement had begun to spread outside Mongolia, with raids on neighboring Tangut and Jin domains.

Although small scale, early raids achieved unanticipated success. The Jin dynasty proved unable to resist the Mongols successfully. It had been weakened by protracted wars with Southern Song, and civil strife.[15] By 1207 much of what is now Inner Mongolia, with its large

---

[14] See Paul Ratchnevsky, *Cinggis–khan, sein Leben und Wirken*, Münchener ostasiatische Studien 32 (Wiesbaden, 1983) and Paul D. Buell, "The Role of the Sino–Mongolian Frontier Zone in the Rise of Cinggis–qan," in *Studies on Mongolia, Proceedings of the First North American Conference on Mongolian Studies*, ed. Henry Schwarz (Bellingham, 1979), 63–76.

[15] On Jin see M. V. Vorob'yev, *Chzhurchzheni i gosudarstvo tszin'* (Moskva, 1975).

sedentary, as well as pastoral nomad population (Khitan, Turkic), had come under Mongolian control. In 1211, using this conquest as a base, the Mongols launched a general assault. By 1214 it had taken them to the walls of the Jin main capital of Zhongdu 中都, which they besieged unsuccessfully.

Simultaneous with a growing Mongol involvement in the China borderlands, and in China, a slow movement west began. It was at first directed against survivors of the chiefdoms which had once opposed Cinggis–qan. It soon turned against isolated Mongolian and Turkic groups of southern Siberia (the "Forest Peoples"), which had previously escaped Mongol notice. Contacts with the sedentary powers of Turkistan followed. In 1209 the Uighurs submitted to Mongol armies under Jebe and Sübe'edei as they crossed Uighur territories in hot pursuit of defeated enemies. Later that same year Jebe and Sübe'edei, operating still further west, unexpectedly encountered the *Xwarazm–shah.*[16] The battle was indecisive and tacitly ignored by both sides, anxious to develop better trade relations. Trade was then of greater interest to the Mongols than further expansion.[17]

Two fortuitous events led to a more systematic process of empire building. The first was the Jin court's unexpected and sudden abandonment of its capital, Zhongdu, in 1215. This was in violation of an agreement with the Mongols. By 1215 the Mongols had acquired substantial local allies. These were Khitan and Chinese warlords with a vested interest in the expansion of their own power through further Mongol invasions. They called in local Mongol armies and together with them assaulted and took Zhongdu. Jin control north of the Yellow River crumbled.[18] Another fortuitous incident led to even greater conquests in the west. In 1218, the Xwarezmian governor of Otrar, acting with or without the sanction of the *shah*, ordered the massacre of visiting Muslim merchants under the protection of the Mongols. The Mongols, affronted at this serious breach of the diplomatic conventions of the era reacted with a massive invasion of Western Turkis-

[16] On these events and the collision with the *Xwarazm–shah,* see Paul D. Buell, "Early Mongol Expansion in Western Siberia and Turkestan (1207–1219): A Reconstruction," *Central Asiatic Journal* XXXVI (1992): 1–2: 1–32.

[17] Early Mongol relations with the Muslim world are described in Xiao Qiching, *Xiyuren yu yuanchu zhengzhi* (Taibei, 1966).

[18] See Paul D. Buell, "Tribe, *Qan* and *Ulus* in Early Mongol China: some Prolegomena to Yüan history," (Ph.D. dissertation, University of Washington, 1977), 60ff.

tan (1219). This invasion entirely destroyed the Xwarezmian Empire in just a few years.[19]

By 1223 Mongol armies under Jebe and Sübe'edei had appeared in Russia. The slow movement of Joci's *ulus*[20] west had already begun although it was not to reach its final destination on the Volga until the early 1230s. In 1227, the year of Cinggis–qan's death, another component was added to the Mongolian empire with the final conquest of Tangut domains (Xixia).

Uncontrolled expansion continued under *Qan* Ögödei (r. 1229–1241). He inherited from his father not only the powerful confederation of tribes that was the foundation of Mongolian power but a large part of the surrounding sedentary world as well. To rule this empire, the new *qan* turned more and more to bureaucratic methods. This led to the emergence of a formal government, paralleling tribal control based upon the steppe.[21]

The new Mongolian empire united three distinct cultural spheres: The first sphere, heartland of the empire, embraced Mongolia. It also included areas adjacent to the Mongolian steppe and more distant pastures, anywhere Mongol power reached and found suitable for a mounted, pastoral way of life. The second focused on China, more or less corresponding to the China of today, less the southwest, Tibet, and Turkistan. This sphere had the outward appearance of cultural and historical unity, but blended into non–Chinese reality locally. Early modern China was more a matter of cultural and sometimes political identification and choice, than of a strict ethnic unity. The Mongols controlled only the north in *qan* Ögödei's time (1229-1241), an area of

---

[19] The best account is W. Barthold, *Turkestan down to the Mongol Invasion*, translated by Mrs. T. Minorsky, 4th. edn. (London, 1977), 393–427. On the Xwarezmian Empire see Z. M. Buniyatov, *Gosudarstvo Khorezmshakhov–anushteginidov* (Moskva, 1986).

[20] An *ulus* was a nomadic patrimony comprised of traditional rights of control largely over people and sometimes, but less frequently, over territories (the institution became "territorialized" over time). Each of the Mongol princes, sons of Cinggis–qan, was given his own personal holdings with which to form an *ulus*, and out of these patrimonies the later successor qanates grew. The Mongolian empire as a whole was also an *ulus*, a "great" or "original" *ulus* (Middle Mongolian: *yeke Mongqol ulus*). On the institution of the *ulus* see Buell, 1977.

[21] On the development of bureaucratic institutions under Ögödei see Buell, 1977: 82ff. On the tribal side of the Mongolian regime see also Paul D. Buell, "Kalmyk Tanggaci People: Thoughts on the Mechanics and Impact of Mongol Expansion," *Mongolian Studies* VI (1980): 41–59. The later development of Mongolian empire under the last *qan*, Möngke (1251-59), is reviewed in Thomas T. Allsen, *Mongol Imperialism* (Berkeley, 1987).

great cultural diversity, and one long accustomed to foreign rule. The third sphere was that part of the Muslim World directly controlled by the Mongols, namely the Islamic communities of Turkistan, Northern Iran, portions of the Caucasus region, and the Pontic Steppe. Like China, the Muslim World extended far beyond the zone of Mongol control, south into Iran, the Arabian Peninsula, India and Southeast Asia, Central and East Africa, and west through Iraq, Syria, Palestine, and Egypt towards a distant vanishing point in Portugal and Spain, where portions of Iberia, along with adjacent West African domains, remained under local Muslim control in the thirteenth century. Islamic communities were also found sprinkled in China, particularly along the southeast China coast, with distant links to the Persian Gulf. Muslim society was even more diverse than Chinese, but unified by the common religion and cultural traditions of Islam.[22]

Each of the three spheres received separate governments as "provinces" of a Mongolian world empire. The nomadic domains of Mongolia, ruled directly by the Mongol emperor, became the *yeke qol*, "great pivot," the inner province of empire. This was where the *qan* and his closest retainers nomadized, where he maintained his capital, the new city of Qaraqorum. Appended to it was a province (*el/il*) of occupied (North) China, administered from the former Jin capital of Zhongdu. Two other provinces shared control over the Mongol domains in the south and west. One was based in Beshbaliq and governed culturally and religiously mixed Turkistan. The other in Tus administered almost exclusively Muslim Iranian–speaking areas.[23] The Mongols were now secure in their rule and had achieved a political integration of their heterogeneous and diverse domains. Cultural integration proved more difficult, but the Mongols strongly encouraged the mutual assimilation of the cultures coming under their rule

[22] It should be made clear in this context that the culture of Islam, by this period, was no longer just the culture of Arabia, although this was still the basis of traditional Islamic religion, but represented the entire assimilated legacy of the classical worlds and pre–Islamic Middle East as well. The Muslim World, although more disparate geographically, and strongly multi–cultural, represented, no less than China, and in no ways inferior, a "great tradition" of world cultural development of the profoundest implications. As an introduction to achievement and intermediating role of the Islamic world see John R. Hayes, ed., *The Genius of Arab Civilization, Source of Renaissance*, 2nd. edn. (Cambridge, 1983).

[23] See the discussion in Buell, 1977: *loc. cit.*, and in Buell, 1980.

and themselves set an example as willing cultural intermediaries, new roles for once rude conquerors.[24]

III. MONGOLS AS CULTURAL INTERMEDIARIES

The Mongols are usually viewed in highly negative terms, due to the great wave of destruction which the establishment of their empire touched off. They also suffer from a strongly biased press. Most of our sources reflect the perspective of the conquered, rather than of the conqueror. They tend to exaggerate the ill effects of Mongol conquest and rule. As a result, positive Mongol contributions are less often recognized.

In fact, Mongol rule resulted in important innovations in government, in military organization, in technology, in taxation, and even in weights and measures[25] nearly everywhere they ruled. Most important, the *pax mongolica* of the thirteenth and fourteenth centuries opened Asia to Europe,[26] to a lesser extent Europe to Asia (*e.g.*, the journeys of Rabban Sauma).[27] It resulted in an unparalleled cultural

---

[24] Since we first wrote these words more than a decade ago there has been a major rethinking of the role of the Mongols thanks largely to the efforts of Jack Weatherford who has popularized the Mongols in a way that they have never been popularized before. See Jack Weatherford, *Cinggis-qan and the Making of the Modern World* (New York, 2004).

[25] On this last area see Matsui Dai, "Unification of Weights and Measures by the Mongol Empire as Seen in the Uigur and Mongol Documents," in Desmond Durkin-Meisterernst, Simone-Christiane Raschmann, Jens Wilkens, Marianne Yaldiz and Peter Zieme, eds., *Turfan Revisisted, The First Century of Research into the Arts and Cultures of the Silk Road*, Berlin, 2004, 197-202. The Mongols also sought to unify calendars, and attempted to establish a universal dating system beginning with the coronation of Cinggis-qan in 1206. See, as an introduction, Benno van Dalen, "Islamic Astronomical Tables in China: The Sources for the Huihui li," in S.M. Razaullah Ansari, editor, *History of Oriental Astronomy. Proceedings of the Joint Discussion-17 at the 23rd General Assembly of the International Astronomical Union, organised by the Commission 41 (History of Astronomy), Held in Kyoto, August 25-26, 1997* (Dordrecht, 2002), 19-31, and Benno van Dalen, "Islamic and Chinese Astronomy under the Mongols: a Little-Known Case of Transmission," in Yvonne Dold-Samplonius, Joseph W. Dauben, Menso Folkerts and Benno van Dalen, eds., *From China to Paris: 2000 Years Transmission of Mathematical Ideas* (Stuttgart 2002), 327-356.

[26] See J. R. S. Phillips, *The Medieval Expansion of Europe* (Oxford, 1988).

[27] See Morris Rossabi, *Voyager from Xanadu: Rabban Sauma and the First Journey from China to the West* (Tokyo, 1992) and E. A. Wallis Budge, *The Monks of Kublai Khan Emperor of China* (London, 1928).

exchange. One has only to think of the *Travels of Marco Polo* to realize how profound the influence was.

There are many reasons why Mongol rule had the impact that it did. One was the sheer magnitude of the Mongolian achievement. Mongols were able to unite more of the earth's surface under a contiguous political authority than has any other empire, before or since, and were relatively effective in ruling it. The writ of *qan* Möngke, for example, at the time of his death, after another impulse of Mongol expansion, was recognized in nearly all of Russia, in Seljuq Anatolia, in Iraq, Iran, Afghanistan, parts of northern India, Siberia, Mongolia, Tibet, Manchuria, North China, Southwest China, and parts of Vietnam.

Under such conditions, international trade moved far more easily under Mongol protection than it had in centuries. A steady flow of embassies from all parts of the world brought the greatest possible variety of goods, ideas, and people to Qaraqorum. There Mongol rubbed elbows with Turks, Chinese, Tibetans, Xwarezmians, Iranians, Armenians, Russians, and even a Fleming (William of Rubruck), and a Frenchman.[28] The Mongol rulers eagerly heard what each had to offer and selected the best, cultural and institutional,[29] for closer examination and possible use.

Sheer size promoted cultural exchanges, as did the juxtaposition of representatives of once isolated cultures. Mongol openness to new ideas was important as well. But there were also other, more subtle forces at work. One was demographic reality. There were too few Mongols, perhaps 1.5 millions in 1200,[30] to rule such a vast empire. Cooperation with representatives of other cultures, including the cultures of the conquered sedentary areas, was necessary and unavoidable. The Mongols themselves lacked the expertise required to administer, rather than pillage large subject agricultural populations.

---

[28] The great fountain of beverages that was a centerpiece of *qan* Möngke's court was designed by the Parisian goldsmith William Buchier. See William of Rubruck in Anastasius van den Wyngaert, ed., *Sinica Franciscana*, vol. I: *Itinera et Relationes Fratrum Minorum Saec. XIII et XIV* (Quaracchi–Firenze, 1929), 276–7. See also Leonardo Olschki, *Guillaume Boucher, a French Artist at the Court of the Khans* (New York, 1969).

[29] On the interaction between Mongolian, Chinese and other institutions in the emergence of Mongol China see Buell, 1977.

[30] On the size of Mongolia's population in the early 13th century see N. Ts. Munkuyev, "Zametki o Drevnikh Mongolakh," In *Tataro–Mongoly v Azii i Evrope: Sbornik Statey*, ed. S. L. Tikhvinskiy (Moskva, 1970), 352–81.

Because of these considerations, the Mongols were willing to utilize manpower from all parts of the civilized world in mixed administrations. One, headed by a Khitan from China, and staffed by other Khitans and Chinese, as well as by local people, governed Muslim Bokhara for several decades.[31] In China itself various Xwarezmians and other western Muslims controlled much of the administration and introduced Iranian–style tax–farming.[32] Later the Venetian Marco Polo made his contributions.

Such administrations helped stretch Mongol power and provided the experienced manpower the Mongols lacked. An international imperial bureaucracy loyal to the Mongols, and not to local interests, from which it was largely isolated, resulted. This bureaucracy shared common values and had common vested interests. The exchange of administrative techniques among its members promoted institutional uniformity while exposure to the culture of the court and of other centers of Mongol power actively encouraged cultural assimilation. An imperial elite that was highly mixed culturally emerged. Since the Mongols themselves, particularly in the West, became increasingly Turkicized as their empire embraced more and more Turks, and the proportion of Mongols diminished, this elite became Turkicized as well.

IV. The Successor States

The pattern of rich social, political, and cultural interaction encouraged during the era of unified Mongolian empire persisted, even broadened, under the successor states: In China, Chagatay dominions, Russia, Iran, and even, to some extent, in Siberia. A Mongol cultural and spiritual unity was preserved long after political association had broken down irreparably.[33] For Mongol China, the nature of the political compromise made by Qubilai to come to power and its relationship with the Il–qanate Iran played a most important role.

Qubilai was the last Mongolian ruler of China born on the steppe (in 1215) and fully cognizant of the old Mongolian way of life. He

---

[31] See Paul D. Buell, "Sino–Khitan Administration in Mongol Bukhara," *Journal of Asian History* XIII (1979): 2: 121–51.

[32] On the role of Mahmud Yalawanci, a Xwarezmian long in effective charge of the Mongol administration in China, see Buell, 1977: 82ff.

[33] See Wladyslaw Kotwicz, "Les Mongols, promoteurs de l'idée de paix universelle au début du XIIIe siècle, " *Rocznik Orientalistyczny* 16 (1950): 428–34.

grew to maturity in a culturally diverse world empire which took for granted Mongolia's political superiority and integrative relationships with North China, and the Islamic World. Thus, although based in China, and forced to accommodate himself to Chinese culture and traditions as the foundations for his rule there, Qubilai still gravitated towards the steppe. His traveling court not only spent as much time as possible on the fringes of the Mongolian plateau, but for his entire life Qubilai maintained the trappings of Mongolian universality, to which he claimed legitimate succession. Because of this, he tolerated and even identified with the multi–cultural values of the old imperial elite. He also by and large maintained the system, even Sinicized, supported and staffed by this same imperial elite.

Qubilai, for example, as a symbol of his authority,[34] and of his "Mongolness," even after the reorganization of his government in the

---

[34] The elite status of Qubilai's guard (*Kesikten*) emerges clearly from Marco Polo's descriptions:

a) But know that the Great Kaan, to maintain his grand state, has himself guarded by 12,000 horsemen; and they are called Quesitau, which means in French, "knight loyal to the grand overlord." And he does not do so out of any uncertainty he feels before anyone, but for his great exaltation. And the 12,000 men have four captains; for each is captain of 3,000 men, and these 3,000 take up position in the palace of the overlord for three days and three nights. And they eat and drink at the same place. And later they leave, and another 3,000 come and guards for the same period of time. And later they leave and the others appear so that there are guarding the great Kaan 3,000 horsemen at all times. And they are called Questiaus, as has been said, up to 12,000. And subsequently the shift begins again and it goes thus for the entire year. (M. G. Pauthier, ed., *Le Livre de Marco Polo* (Genève, 1978), 277–9).

b) But know truly that the Great Kaan has appointed 12,000 of his men who have the name Quesitan, as I have said to you before. And on each of these 12,000 has been bestowed thirteen robes all different the one from the other. That is to say, that all 12,000 are of one color, and then another 12,000 of another so that the robes are different from the one from the other in thirteen manners of colors. And the robes are adorned with stones and pearls and with other noble things very richly and of very great value. Simultaneously the Great Kaan bestows with each robe on each of the 12,000, which is thirteen times during a year, a very beautiful chain belt of gold and of great value. And also [he bestows] a pair of boots of camut, which is bourgal [camel leather], very skillfully worked with silver thread, so that, when they are wearing this clothing, they appear like a king, each of them. And it is established which robe they should wear during each of thirteen festivals. And the grand overlord too has thirteen robes similar to those of his barons; that is, in color, but these are more noble and more rich

Chinese mold to satisfy his Chinese allies,[35] maintained the imperial bodyguard establishment of the *qan* of empire. This was simultaneously a military organization, the nucleus of the emperor's own armies, the *yeke qol*, "great pivot," of imperial armies; a select association of the elite of empire; and a personal service establishment. From it were chosen not only important officers of state, but also the immediate attendants of Qubilai and of his successors. Hu Sihui, author of the *YSZY*, was among them and was almost certainly a member of this bodyguard establishment.[36]

> and of much greater value. Thus all this requires such treasure that they may scarcely count or number it; so that he can always dress in the same color as his barons which are [as if his] companions. (Pauthier, 1978: 297–8. Brackets mark textual additions by Pauthier).

On the imperial bodyguard establishment of the Mongol emperors of China see also Hsiao Ch'i–ch'ing [Xiao Qiching], *The Military Establishment of the Yuan Dynasty* (Cambridge, 1978), 33–50 and *passim*.

[35] For a description of Yuan government in Chinese terms see D. M. Farquhar, *The Government of China under Mongolian Rule, A Reference Guide*, Münchener ostastasiatische Studien 53 (Stuttgart, 1990). See also his "Structure and Function in the Yüan Imperial Government," in J. D. Langlois, Jr., ed., *China under Mongol Rule* (Princeton, 1981), 25–55.

[36] By Hu's time much of the personal service establishment of the Mongol emperor of China, while remaining, at the level of the court, institutionally part of the bodyguard establishment, had been reorganized as part of a Chinese–style Xuanhui yuan 宣徽院, "Bureau for Imperial Household Provisions." Its *Yuan shi* description clearly shows its origin in the bodyguard of the Mongol emperors:

> The Xuanhui yuan, rank 3A, has charge of supplying the emperor's food. All things connected with various substances such as grains, meat, liquors, and vegetables, all business connected with banquets for imperial relatives and guests and provisions of the various princes and bodyguard and of the *ger–ün ke'ü* [hereditary household slaves] and the *chaifa* 差法 [allotments] to be received by Mongolian myriarchs and chiliarchs are all under the control of the Xuanhui yuan. The herding of [imperial] herds, yearly provision of fodder and feed, establishment of prices for sheep and cattle, recovery and return of various *buralgi* matters, and the three administrators: Shangshi ju 尚食局, "Administrator Presenting Food to the Emperor," the Shangyao ju 尚藥局, "Administration Presenting Drugs to the Emperor," and the Shangyun ju 尚醞局, "Administration Presenting Fermented Beverages to the Emperor," are under its control. As for all the internal and external offices under its control, they choose the people they wish to use (*Yuan shi*, Zhonghui shuju edition, 87, 2200).

Noteworthy among other offices under the Xuanhui yuan was a Chinese–style Office of the Chief Physician (Taiyi yuan 太醫院), rank 2A, charged with preparing and presenting "the emperor's medicinal substances" and all "subordinate medical functions" (*Yüan shi* 88, 2220). Under its control was a Guanghui si 廣惠司, charged with

One principal source of foreign influence for Qubilai's China and its link with a larger Mongolian world order, and with a distant west, was Mongol Iran. Connections were maintained almost to the end, by sea when land links failed. The association was based in dynastic affiliation. Both Qubilai and Hüle'ü, founder of the Iranian Il–qanate were sons of Tolui–noyan, as was the last Mongol *qan*, Möngke. Qubilai's China and Mongol Iran also had common enemies, the House of Ögödei and his allies. The Il–qanate was also willing to recognize Qubilai and his successors as the "Great Kaans," pretenders to a now defunct Mongolian empire. The close political alliance was cemented by frequent embassies, including one headed by Marco Polo, and continued exchanges of personnel.[37]

Through these cherished connections China and the Islamic heartland carried on an active exchange of cultural goods of every sort. One product, on the Chinese side, was the *Huihui yaofang* 回回藥方 [*HHYF*], "Muslim Medicinal Recipes," based on various Persian, Arabic and possibly Uighur sources, most now lost. Four *juan* now survive in the Chinese National Library in Beijing. This work is

---

"preparing and presenting Muslim (Huihui 回回) drugs and preparations to the emperor in order to treat members of the bodyguard and poor people in the capital" (*Yuan shi* 88, 2221). The association of the two offices was certainly no accident, as can be seen from substantial Muslim and Western influence upon the *YSZY* itself. For a late Yuan unofficial listing of the various subordinate agencies of the Xuanhui yuan see also Tao Zongyi, *Zhuogeng lu* (Taibei, 1970), 21, 307–8. The *Zhuogeng lu* version of Xuanhui yuan organization includes a "Sugar Office" (Shatang ju 砂糖局), not mentioned above.

The word *buralgi* (*buralki*) is discussed by Paul Pelliot, *Notes on Marco Polo* (Paris, 1959–73), I, 112–4, and by G. Doerfer, *Türkische und mongolische Elemente im Neupersischen* (Wiesbaden, 1963–75), I, 213–5. Its original meaning of the word was lost property left behind when the *ordo* (tent palace) of the *qan* and associated elements moved to a new site. The word is probably a Mongolian pronunciation of Turkic *bulargi*, "pertaining to what is, what exists, is found," although there is dispute about the etymology. *Buralgi* was placed in the charge of a *bularquchi*, who by the early fourteenth century did a great deal more than clean up the imperial campsite and had become the primary administrator of the *ordo*–court as a whole. On the *bularquci* in the Yuan period see Buell, 1977: 192–3. See also Pelliot, *loc. cit.*, Doerfer, *loc. cit.* Other officers in the emperor's household establishment with old Mongolian titles included the *bawurci,* "table manager" (see Doerfer, 1963–75: I, 202–5), the *ide'eci,* "imperial waiter" (Doerfer, 1963–75: I, 188–9), and the *dara[sun]ci,* "dispenser of liquor" (Doerfer, 1963–75: I, 326–7). On the similar bodyguard officers, often there with Turkic titles, of the Il–qans see the excellent and detailed discussion in Ismail Hakkı Uzunçarsılı, *Osmanlı devleti teskilâtina medhal* (Ankara, 1970), 188ff.

[37] See Thomas T. Allsen, *Culture and Conquest in Mongol Eurasia* (Cambridge, 2001)

unique in its subject matter, and is unparalleled in providing Arabic script as well as Chinese forms of the names of herbs used and even of Muslim and other authorities cited, including Galen. Directly relevant to the discussion here, there is considerable dietary lore in the text.[38]

Mongol China contributed early gunpowder technology,[39] printing, medical theory and even translations of specific texts,[40] and Chinese style landscape painting, transmitted through Turkey, to the Renaissance West.[41] Less beneficially, the idea of paper money also went to

[38] There are now two editions of this important work, both providing facsimiles of the original manuscript. The first was published privately in Hong Kong by Jiang Runxiang 江潤祥 (Y.C. Kong), along with the results of initial research on the text by an international team of scholars. See Kong, Y.C., et al., *Huihui yaofang* 回回藥方 (Hong Kong, 1996). The second, with an accompanying volume of notes, is Song Xian 宋峴, *Huihui yaofang kaoshi* 回回藥方考釋, two volumes (Beijing, 1999). We are endebted to Igor de Rachewiltz for providing us with a copy of the important edition Kong edition, primarily used here as it is easier to read. We are impressed by the many similarities of content between the *HHYF* and the *YSZY* including herbs used, some terminology, and even linguistic forms but the former is more unassimilated in its content than the *YSZY* with much that is purely Arabic medicine in it. Nonetheless, a conscious effort has been made there too to seek an accommodation with Chinese and other medical traditions, including the Mongols' own and possibly Tibetan medicine. See Paul D. Buell, "Food, Medicine and the Silk Road: The Mongol-era Exchanges," *Silk Road*, V, II (winter 2007), 22-35; Paul D. Buell, "How did Persian and other western Medical Knowledge Move East, and Chinese West? A Look at the Role of Rashīd al-Dīn and others," *Asian Medicine, Tradition and Modernity*, 3.2 (2008), 278-94; and Paul D. Buell, "Tibetans, Mongols and Cultural Fusion," in Anna Akasoy, Charles Burnett und Ronit Yoeli-Tlalim, eds., *Islam and Tibet, Interactions along the Musk Route* (Aldershot, Hants, 2010) forthcoming. A complete translation of the *HHYF* has now been completed by Paul D. Buell with the support of the National Endowment for the Humanities.

[39] See Joseph Needham, Ho Ping–yü, Lu Gwei–djen, and Wang Ling, *Science and Civilization in China,* vol. 5: *Chemistry and Chemical Technology,* part VII: *Military Technology; The Gunpowder Epic* (Cambridge, 1986), 41ff and *passim.*

[40] See Haneda Kōichi 羽田亨一, Perushia goshaku 『Wang shuhe mai jue』 no Chūkokugenhon ni tsuite ベルシア語釋『王叔和脈訣』の中國語原本 について, Ajia·afurika gengobunkakenkyū アヅア·フりカ言語文化研究 *Journal of Asian and African Studies*, 48/49 (1995), 719-726, J. Rall, "Zur persischen Übersetzung eines *Mo–chüeh*, eines chinesischen medizinischen Textes," *Oriens Extremus* 7 (1960): 2: 152–7, and T. T. Allsen, 2001, 141-160. The *Tanksūk-nāmah* of 1313 which contains the Wang Shuhe text along with excerpts from others is now being investigated in detail by Vivienne Lo and her team.

[41] On Chinese influence on Renaissance painting see Bernard Berenson, *Essays in the Study of Sienese Painting* (New York, 1918); Gustave Soulier, *Les influences orientales dans le peinture toscane* (Paris, 1924); I. V. Pouzyna, *La Chine, l'Italie et les débuts de la Renaissance*, Paris: les Editions d'Art et d'Histoire, 1935; Jurgis Baltrusaitis, *Le Moyen Age fantastique, Antiquités et exotismes dans l'art gothique* (Paris,

Iran, with devastating results for the Il–qanate economy.[42] Given this environment, and the political and cultural background to Mongol rule in China, it is perhaps to be expected that the *YSZY* too is a product of broad cultural exchange. For the historian of food and foodways, the *YSZY* provides evidence of two related areas of change. First, its recipes represent the culmination of a millennium and a half of cultural influence from the Middle East. This influence was above all in the form of food plants and spices. It was associated in Chinese tradition, often incorrectly, with the name of the Han 漢 dynasty explorer and diplomat Zhang Qian 張騫.[43] Also involved were food processing technology, *e.g.*, finely milled wheat, and recipes: Breads, bread foods, noodles of every sort, foods later much developed by the Chinese themselves. In this respect, the *YSZY* may provide earlier evidence for mass biological and associated cultural interchange rivaling those exchanges which took place between the Old and the New World after Columbus.[44]

On the other hand, the *YSZY* is also of a time and of a place. It clearly expresses the cultural values of the Mongol elite of the fourteenth century, the cultural realities of the era, and the shock that exotic Mongol court environment presented to China, and to the Chinese. Each of the cultural spheres of the then Mongolian world order finds expression within; with Mongol interests culturally dominant, as they were politically dominant within the Mongol world order. To understand how Chinese, Mongolian and Middle Eastern influences combined into a whole in our source it is necessary first to characterize

---

1955). On Chinese influence (and actual Chinese paintings) in Iran see O. Grabar, "The Visual Arts, 1050–1350," in J. A. Boyle, ed., The *Cambridge History of Iran,* vol. 5: *The Saljuq and Mongol Periods* (Cambridge, 1968), 626–58 (see 652–7); J. M. Rogers, ed., *The Topkapi Saray Museum*: *The Albums and Illustrated Manuscripts* (Boston, 1986), 114–56; Jill Sanchia Cowen, *Kalila wa Dimna*: *An Animal Allegory of the Mongol Court* (New York and Oxford, 1989); and E. J. Grube and Eleanor Sims, eds., *Between China and Iran* (London, 1985). There is now a large literature on the topic.

42 See Berthold Spuler, *Die Mongolen in Iran*, 3rd. edn. (Berlin, 1968), 88ff and *passim*; J. A. Boyle, "Dynastic and political history of the Il–Khans," in J. A. Boyle, 1968: 303–421 (see 374ff).

43 See B. Laufer, *Sino–Iranica, Chinese Contributions to the History of Civilization in Ancient Iran*, Field Museum of Natural History Publication 201, Anthropological Series Vol. XV, 3 (Chicago, 1919).

44 On this see Alfred W. Crosby, Jr., *The Columbian Exchange, Biological and Cultural Consequences of 1492*, Contributions in American Studies 2 (Westport, 1972).

each society involved, with special reference to food and foodways. We begin with Mongolia.

V. Cultural Spheres of The Mongolian World Order

Steppes of Mongolia[45]

The Mongolian Way of Life

Traditional life on the Mongolian steppe was extremely harsh, environmentally and socially. It was only possible at all through a well thought–out strategy of life, and of resource use developed over the centuries involving near constant movement. Prior to the establishment of Mongolian empire this strategy centered about Mongolian variations of nomadic pastoralism, the herding of sheep, some goats, and occasionally cattle from horseback.[46]

Two types of seasonal movement were involved. The most common was transhumance. It required alternation between low–lying winter pastures and mountain summer pastures, with as much of the year as possible being spent at high altitude. In areas where convenient mountain pastures were lacking movement was circular with even greater distances covered, largely at the same altitude. Such pastoralism was often carried on in conjunction with the flowing of a seasonal river.

Almost constant movement was necessary because sheep (and goats in particular) tend to overgraze and destroy pastures. Herds were also large, exhausting even good pastures quickly. A minimum of 60–100 sheep, a higher number of goats, in areas where goats replaced

---

[45] This section is largely based upon the forthcoming Paul D. Buell and Angelo Anastasio volume "Mongols and the outside world." See also B. Vladimirtsov, *Le Regime Social des Mongols*, translated from the Russian by Michel Carsow (Paris, 1948); D. Gongor, *Khalkh Tovchoon*, vols. 1–2 (Ulaanbaatar, 1970–1978); A. M. Khazanov, *Nomads and the Outside World*, Cambridge Studies in Social Anthropology 44 (London, 1984), 15–84; and Tim Ingold in his *Hunters, Pastoralists and Ranchers*, Cambridge Studies in Social Anthropology 28 (Cambridge, 1980).

[46] In a few very arid areas the horse was replaced by the camel. Reindeer were also herded on the fringes of the steppe, by ancestors of the modern Tsaatan. On the key issue of horse domestication and on the horse in a larger, Eurasian context see Paul D. Buell, Timothy May and Dave Ramey, "Greek and Chinese Horse Medicine: *Déjà Vu* All Over Again," *Sudhoffs Archiv*, Band 94 (2010), forthcoming. See now also John Travis, "Trail of Mare's Milk Leads to First Tamed Horses," *Science* 322 (2008): 368-69.

sheep, was necessary to support each member of a traditional Mongolian household. This was due to low herd productivity and the need for substantial livestock insurance in the face of potential enormous losses. Failure to move on meant herd losses, hunger, and ultimate starvation for Mongol herdsmen. This was because overgrazing could destroy, for the short or the long term, the normally low biological capacities of Mongolian pastures, which had to be used over and over again, sometimes twice in the same year.

Since movement was nearly continual and good pastures few and far between in an arid land, the horse was a vital necessity. Without the horse to move himself, his family and retainers, and the goods of his household and camp, a Mongol could not keep pace with the voracious appetites of his nomadic capital. In addition, the horse was vital for herding itself since only on horseback could a few Mongols watch hundreds and thousands of animals, divided into separate herds by type. The superior mobility of the horse also allowed physical contacts between often distant groups and individuals in lightly populated Mongolia. It was also vital for raiding, war, and hunting. The life of the Mongol was thus not possible without the horse. It was the centerpiece of Mongolian life and also a central focus of Mongolian cultural expression.

Pastoralism supervised from horseback completely dominated the life of Mongolia until the most recent times, probably involving 90–95 percent or more of the population at any one time.[47] But it is a mistake to think of the Mongol solely in terms of his pastoralism. Pastoralism, although making the Mongol potentially protein–rich compared to North Chinese farmers, for example, could not alone provide a balanced diet. In addition, its products were highly seasonal and highly subject to destruction or catastrophe.

Although milk, and milk products, for example, were available in abundance in the autumn, when there was also much meat from reducing the herds to prepare for winter, the opposite was true during difficult late winter, early spring conditions. This was before the new grass had begun to grow. It was also the time of lambing by weakened

[47] Pastoralism remains very important for the Mongols today but the coming of the railways and world markets, and even Mongolian industry, has now made an urban way of life possible for many although this has been accompanied by major cultural changes among the Mongols, including the loss of much of the traditional Mongolian way of life. On this see Paul D. Buell, and Ngan Le, "Globalization in Mongolia: Blessing or Curse," in H. G. Schwarz, ed., *Mongolian Culture and Society in the Age of Globalization* (Bellingham, 2006), 27-66.

ewes, the majority of winter and early spring herds, with no milk or flesh to spare. Animals could be slaughtered, but were unlikely to produce much usable meat. To do so would also severely damage the future prospects of the herd. It was possible to dry curds, milk, cheese, and even meat for later use, when it was abundant, but finding space to store such foods and long–term storage without deterioration was always a problem. Limited supplies of such foods would in any case have been exhausted by late winter.

Since few imported foodstuffs were available due to the remoteness of Mongolia and problems of transport, the Mongol had no choice but to supplement the products of his pastoralism with foods assembled through hunting and gathering. This was particularly true during those periods when the products of animal husbandry were either in short supply, or unavailable. Both activities were as a consequence far more important for Mongolian life and livelihood than scant references in the sources would lead us to believe.

Another side to Mongolian hunting and gathering was the presence of significant survivals of a hunter–gatherer way of life among the Mongols themselves and the existence of groups on or near the steppe for which hunting–gathering was a primary focus, *e.g.*, the ancestors of today's Khamnighan. In addition, the nearest neighbors of the Mongols to the west, north, and east were nearly all hunter–gatherers. It may even be argued that some steppe groups started out as hunter–gatherers themselves, and only moved into the steppe to become full pastoralists after a long and complicated social evolution.[48]

These facts mean that we must accept a blurring of our view of the pastoralist culture of the Mongolian steppe. There was no generalized pattern of pastoralism, merely a continuum of herding possibilities to further shade matters. Individual Mongolian societies grouped at one end or the other. At one extreme were pure reindeer herders, with strong hunting–gathering traditions. At the other were most Mongols, more or less pure mounted pastoralists, classic sheep–herders, with less developed hunter–gatherer traditions and even contacts with the sedentary world. Such contacts would allow them to ignore certain realities of steppe existence, either on account of trade, the products of pillage or of sedentary tribute. In every case a specific strategy of survival had been worked out to suit specific local conditions and specific social relationships.

---

[48] The "Forest Peoples" (including the ancestors of the steppe Oyrat and Kirghiz), mentioned in the *Secret History*, seem to have included such groups, to cite but one example.

Traditional Mongolian Society

Social relationships themselves were strongly conditioned by economic realities. Under normal conditions, centralized control and highly developed political hierarchies were out of the question. This is because the required centralization of power, resources, and people conflicted with the needs of an efficient pastoralism according to which groups and even individuals lived in isolation most of the year. Only during the winter months could normally dispersed herding units camp together for a brief time. Stored foods were relatively abundant, perhaps including harvests from planted crops in more favored areas. Fresh meat was available as animals continued to be cut out from the herds. Much nourishing grass still lay under protective covers of snow. The snow also provided abundant moisture. By very early spring the large camps had already begun to split up as herders moved out in small groups to prepare for lambing. By late spring, most groups were already well into the mountains, completely dispersed as they moved towards rich summer pastures. In the desert, large camps were possible only under still more limited conditions. Only in contact situations, and during empire building, which permitted the utilization of other–people's resources, could this basic reality of Mongolian life, the need for maximum dispersal, be ignored.

Under such conditions, economic considerations were paramount and the interests of the small herding units (*ayil*) that were best suited to Mongolian conditions. What higher level organization did exist was based upon real or fictional bonds of kinship. This also determined most social relationships.[49] In twelfth century Mongolia, each social unit usually had connection with some *oboq*, or extended kinship group, tracing descent to a maximal common ancestor, usually a convenient fiction. Within the *oboq*, descent was traced through a lineage (*uruq*), descended from a recent, historical common ancestor.

Membership in such groups was vitally important because the *oboq* and its lineages controlled access to pasturage, owned by groups, and never by individuals. An individual with no recognized kinship connections within a greater Mongolian society had no right to use herding resources, and thereby no right to survive. Among Mongolian kinship groups, certain lineages and families even had the right to provide political, military, and religious leaders, as an hereditary privilege.

[49] The situation, of course, was altogether different in a contact situation. On this Buell, 1977, 1980.

Mongolia's traditional kinship system thus played an important stabilizing role, in the face of a seeming anarchy in most other areas of Mongolian life. It provided agreed–upon patterns for the use of scarce resources, including vital pasturage, and higher level social organization through a recognized hereditary leadership. Kinship also offered a strong sense of regional and national identity, through descent of *oboq* from even more distant common ancestors, *e.g.*, Gray Wolf and Beautiful Doe, ancestors of all Mongols, in a way that conflicted little with the needs of pastoralism. Kinship also provided an important basis for the mutual support of groups and for social solidarity. It was a mechanism for smoothing the impact of a harsh environment and softening otherwise continued competition of groups and individuals for survival, and for the scarce resources permitting survival.

Also serving this purpose were traditions of social support governing the relationships of individuals not especially connected by close kinship. One such tradition was a highly developed "Gastfreundschaft" not unlike that of the ancient Germanic world where hospitality had to be offered even to an enemy, *e.g.*, by Hunding to Siegmund. One Mongolian example is when Dobu[n]–mergen demands and receives a very good share of a buck killed by Uriangqan strangers, as recorded in the *Secret History*:

> After that, when Dobun–mergen one day when to hunt on Toqocaq Rise, he encountered Uriangqadai people in the forest. They had killed a three–year–old deer and were cooking its ribs and intestines. When Dobun–mergen spoke he said: "Please give me [some meat] as the share of meat due another [*nökör sirolqa ke'ejü'ü*]." Taking [only] half a breast side of the meat with the lungs, and the hide, they gave all [the rest of the] three–year–old deer's meat to Dobun–mergen.[50]

This same tradition was also one underpinning for the great feasts later sponsored by the Mongolian *qan* of empire and post–empire days as described by Marco Polo:

> And when the Great Kaan has his table for any formal court occasion he sits thus; for his table is considerably higher than the others. He sits positioned to the north so that his face is directed south and his primary wife sits next to him on his left side. And on his right side, a little lower, his sons sit; and his nephews, his relations, those who are of the imperial line. And they are so low that their heads are at the level of the feet of the grand lord. And after that the other barons sit at tables still lower. And the same thing is true for the women; for all the wives of the sons

[50] Chapters 12–3. All *Secret History* translations are from the text published by Louis Ligeti as *Histoire Secrète des Mongols,* Monumenta Linguae Mongolicae Collecta I (Budapest, 1971).

of the overlord and of his nephews and of his other relations sit on his left side, but lower. And next sit all the other women of the barons and of the knights, still lower; for each sits in his place as ordained by the overlord. And the tables are [arranged] in such a manner that the grand lord can see them all, from one head to the other, such as there are in such very great numbers. And outside of this hall there are more than 40,000 persons; for many people come bearing many presents for the overlord. And these are people from foreign countries who bear foreign things.

And in a certain place in this hall where the Great Kaan has his table, there is a pot of fine gold which contains easily as much wine as a large cask. And at each corner of this great pot there is a similar smaller one so that the wine from the great pot goes into the smaller ones which surround it, likewise full of good beverages [made from] very fine spices of great quality.[51]And the wine is drawn from there with handleless

---

[51] Compare Rubruck's description (in Wyngaert, 1929: 276–7) of *qan* Möngke's fountain of beverages:

> Mangu himself has a great court at Caracarum near the walls of the town. It is closed off by a brick wall, just as priories of monks [are closed off] among us. There is a large palace there in which Mangu holds his drinking parties twice a year, once around Easter when he passes by there, and once in the summer when he returns. And the second drinking party is the greater since on that occasion there convene at his court all the nobles from anywhere as far away as two months' journey. And on that occasion he bestows attire and favors and shows his great glory. There are there many other houses, long as barns, in which are stored his food provisions and treasures.
>
> At the entrance of this great palace, because it would be unseemly to introduce skins with milk and other drinks, master William of Paris made for him a great silver tree, at the roots of which are four silver lions each having a channel spurting out white mare's milk. And four pipes are led into the tree leading up to the summit of the tree and the tops of the pipes are bent back downwards and over each of them is a gilded serpent, the tails of which envelop the trunk of the tree. And from one of these pipes pours forth wine, from another *caracosmos*, that is, clarified mare's milk, from another *boal*, that is, a honey drink, and from another rice beer, called *terracina*. And for each drink there has been prepared at the foot of the tree its own silver vessel for receiving the drink, between the four pipes. At the very top master William has made an angel holding a trumpet and below in the tree he made a crypt in which a person can hide. And a channel ascends through the middle of the heart of that tree as far as the angel. At first master William made a bellows but it did not provide enough wind. Outside the palace there is a room in which the drinks are stored and there stand there officers ready to pour them whenever they hear the angel trumpeting. And the tree has silver branches and leaves and fruits.
>
> Therefore, whenever there is need of drink, the master of the waiters calls to the angel to sound the trumpet. Whereupon, the one who is hidden in the crypt,

> bowls of fine gold which are easily so large that there would be enough for ten persons to drink. And one of these bowls is set between every two persons as well as two other small drinking goblets with handles, so that each gets wine from the bowl placed between the two. And the same arrangement holds for the women. You should know that these bowls and goblets are worth a great treasure; for the Kaan has such a great quantity of such dishes and other things of gold and silver such as no one would dare claim; and no one would believe unless they have seen.
>
> And know that those who serve the Great Kaan with food and beverages are various great barons. And their mouths are covered, likewise their nostrils, with beautiful napkins of gold and silk in order that their breath, nor their odor, enters neither into the food nor into the beverages of the great lord. And when the grand lord would drink all the instruments, of which there are a great quantity there of every manner, begin to sound. And when he takes his cup in hand, all the barons, and all of those who are present, kneel down and give indication of great humility. And then the great lord drinks and each time that he drinks it is done just as you have heard.[52]
>
> Concerning the foods I will say nothing since each of you must believe that there is there an abundance of every manner.[53]

Through such feasts, whose at times elaborate and highly acculturated dishes find reflection in the *YSZY*, the good things of life were shared, with great pomp and ceremony and elaborate food ritual, as a social obligation of power.[54] Food ritual was also a part of the simpler repasts of individuals and of families,[55] whose meals duplicated, on a

---

> hearing this, blows strongly into the channel leading to the angel, and the angel puts the trumpet to its mouth and the trumpet sounds extremely loudly. Whereupon, the officers in the room, hearing this, each of them pours out his drink in the appropriate channel and the pipes pour them from above and below into the vessels prepared for that purpose, and thereupon the waiters draw them and bear them through the palace to the men and women.

[52] On Mongol drinking ritual see Rubruck in Wyngaert, 1929: 175–6; the *Zhuogeng lu*, 21, 314; and F. W. Mote, "Yüan and Ming," in K. C. Chang, ed., *Food in Chinese Culture* (New Haven and London, 1977), 195–257 (206–7).

[53] Pauthier, 1978: 279–82.

[54] Also playing a role in such feasts was, no doubt, a magical reaffirmation of ownership and control on the part of the ruler, since to eat his food meant to accept his special position. Here Mongolian and Chinese customs were remarkably the same. On the Altaic side, see the discussion in S. Ye. Tolybekov, *Kochevoye obshchestvo Kazakhov, v XVII–nachale XX veka, politiko–ekonomicheskiy analiz* (Alma–ata, 1971), 120–25.

[55] For a description of similar Turkic food rituals see Ellsworth Huntington, *The Pulse of Asia* (Boston and New York, 1907), 117–21.

smaller scale, the vast public sharings of food sponsored by Mongolian rulers.

Traditional Mongolian Foods[56]

Thanks to the *YSZY*, and a few other contemporary and near–contemporary sources, we have a good idea of what the foods of the Mongolian court elite were like in the late thirteenth and early fourteenth centuries. But what of earlier times? What did the steppe Mongols of the late twelfth century eat? Also, do the foodways of the *YSZY* represent a sudden acculturation, an abrupt change, or are they the product of a gradual evolution taking place simultaneously with the emergence of Mongolian empire, and of a post–empire political, social and cultural environment.

There is not a lot of information available to tell us what the Mongols ate when they still lived primarily on the steppe and first began their conquests. It is clear from early travelers' accounts and the few mentions of food in early Mongolian sources such as the *Secret History of the Mongols* that the earliest Mongolian food was by and large what would be expected in a pastoralist culture. That is to say, it placed a heavy reliance upon products of animals herded, supplemented by what else could be acquired from the environment with a varying amount of effort, depending upon need, the season, and convenience. Our sources also make clear that Mongolian foodways rapidly became more sophisticated as expansion continued.

The most important food sources for the early Mongols were the sheep making up the largest part of their herds. Sheep produced milk, sheep's butter and cheese, other fermented products, and occasionally meat, when the animals could be spared. Almost all parts of the animal were used.[57] Horses produced, above all, milk and kumiss. They

---

[56] Part of the material here is also summarized in Paul D. Buell, "Pleasing the Palate of the *Qan*: Changing Foodways of the Imperial Mongols," *Mongolian Studies* XIII (1990): 57–81. We are indebted to the late Angelo Anastasio for sharing materials on Mongolian foods and foodways collected by him over the years with us.

[57] The various products of the sheep and how they are used by the Mongols are discussed in detail in Damrinbazar, *et. al.*, *Mongolyn ideen tovchoo* (Ulaanbaatar, 1991), 10ff, 38–63. See also Adalsteinsson, 1991. Adalsteinsson points out in his article that sheep's milk is an excellent source of Vitamin C. Icelanders have been known to subsist entirely on sheep's milk, other sheep dairy products, and dried fish, with little ill effect. Scurvy was known in Medieval and recent Iceland only in coastal areas where sheep's milk was not commonly available and where fish was almost the entire means of subsistence.

also produced a high caloric meat, and blood.[58] Goat products[59] were similar to those of the sheep; and those of cattle are well known.[60] Also important domestic animals, where they could be kept, were camels, *sarlag* (a cross between cattle and the yak), and reindeer.[61]

In addition, the Mongols hunted most wild animals of the steppe on a regular basis, including beasts as lowly as the marmot (*tarbaqan*), which figures in the *YSZY*, and even small birds.[62] They also fished, although the importance of fishing varied greatly from group to group. Grain was eaten, usually as a booty or trade food, although there was some agriculture among the twelfth century Mongols, mostly in Western Mongolia,[63] not as a regular part of the steppe diet of the time. Wild vegetables, fruits and berries, and fungi also played a part in early Mongolian diet, as available, probably a major one.

---

[58] On these and other Mongolian horse foods see John Masson Smith Jr., "Mongol Campaign Rations: Milk, Marmots and Blood?," in *Turks, Hungarians and Kipchaps: A Festschrift in Honor of Tibor Halasi–Kun,* ed. Pierre Oberling (Washington, DC, 1984), 223–228; and Damrinbazar, 1991: 12–3, 71–2, and *passim*.

[59] See Damrinbazar 1991: 11–2, 72–3, and *passim*.

[60] See Damrinbazar 1991: 8–10, 64–70, and *passim*. William of Rubruck (Wyngaert, 1929: 179) contains the following description of Mongol processing of cow's milk:

> They first extract the butter from cow's milk and boil it until it is perfectly decocted and subsequently they store it in rams' paunches which they keep for that purpose. And they do not put salt into the butter which nevertheless does not putrefy on account of the great degree to which it has been decocted. And they keep it for the winter. The buttermilk which remains after the butter [has been removed] they allow to become sour, as sharp as it can be. And they boil that and it is coagulated by the boiling. And that coagulated buttermilk they dry in the sun, and it is thereby made hard, just like the slag of iron, and they store the dried buttermilk in sacks for the winter. During the winter when they lack for milk, they place this bitter coagulated milk, which they call *grut*, in a hide bag and pour on top hot water and they shake the bag strongly until the coagulated milk is dissolved in water which is made totally acid by this. And this water they drink in place of milk. They take the greatest care lest they drink pure water.

[61] On their use as sources of milk see Damrinbazar, 1991: 8 and *passim*.

[62] Damrinbazar (Damrinbazar, 1991: 120ff) lists the following wild animals as common sources of wild meats: Deer, reindeer, elk, antelopes, wild sheep, wild and mountain goats, wild camels, kulan and other wild asses, the wolf, the lynx, the snow leopard, the leopard, the bear, wild swine, hares, *tarbaqan*, badgers, bustards, geese, snipe, the lammergeyer, pheasants, quail, partridge, cranes, duck, and swans. See also below in the text.

[63] On agriculture, hunting and fishing in twelfth and thirteenth century Mongolia see Iwamura Shinobu, *Mongoru shakai keizai shi no kenkyū* (Kyōto, 1968), 29–93.

When Cinggis–qan's mother, Hö'elün–eke was abandoned on the pastures with her young children and a few retainers, after the poisoning of her husband Yesügei by the Tatars, it was just such foods that allowed their survival. In this plight she and her brood were forced to consume such normally despised foods, or so the *Secret History* would have us believe, as wild apples (*ölirsün*), probably *Malus pallasiana*, bird cherries (*moyilsun*; *Prunus padus*), various roots including garden burnet root (*südün*; *Sanguisorba officinalis*) and cinquefoil root, (*cicigina*; *Potentilla anserina*),[64] scarlet lily bulbs (*ja'uqasun*; *Lilium concolor*), wild garlic (*qaliyarsun*; *Allium victorialis*), wild onions (*manggirsun*; *Allium senescens*), garlic [*i.e.*, Chinese] chives (*Allium tuberosum*; *qoqosun*) as well as some small, "misshapen" *jebüge* (*Salmo lenok*) and *qadara* (*Salmo thymallus*) fish:

> The Tayyici'ut elder and young brothers, set out on trek, leaving behind on the pasture grounds Hö'elün–üjin [Lady Hö'elün], the widow, and the little children, the mother and the children:
>
> Hö'elün–üjin, being born a wise woman,
> when she nourished her little children,
> attaching firmly her *boqta* [high Mongolian hat],
> tying up her robe tightly,
> she went running upstream and downstream the Onon,
> She went collecting the wild apples and the bird cherries,
> day and night she nourished their throats.
> Mother Üjin, born with courage,
> when she nourished her children favored by ancestral power [*sutan*],
> taking cypress sticks,
> she nourished them digging up garden burnet and cinquefoil roots.
>
> Mother Üjin's
>
> children, nourished with wild garlic and wild onions,
> managed to grow up to become *qans*.
> The children of the proper Üjin–mother,
> nourished with scarlet lily [bulbs],
> became wise, well–behaved children.
>
> The beautiful Üjin's
> proper children,
> nourished with garlic chives and wild onions,
> became ancestral figures with posterities [*qoyira'ut sayit*].
> Ending their lives by becoming hero–ancestral figures [*eres sayit*],
> Bold and brave ones they would seem to have been made.

---

64 The term *cicigina* may refer to both *P. anserina* and to the Mongolian jujube, *Zizyphus vulgaris* var. *spinosus* (in the *YSZY*, for example). The latter, however, has an inedible root and *cicigina* here must be *P. anserina*.

Agreeing with one another to nourish their mother,
stationing their mother on the banks of the Onon,
making bent fish hooks together,
they went fishing with hooks for miserable fish.
Bending a fish hook from a needle,
they were fishing with hooks for *jebüge* and *qadara*.
Weaving together nets and weirs,
they were fishing out little fry.

But they nourished to satisfaction their mother.[65]

Mongol consumption of a wide range of plant foods is also strongly confirmed by recent ethnographic surveys. The following are some Mongol gathered plant foods listed by B. Rinchen.[66] Botanical identifications are as provided by Rinchen, corrected in a few cases:

1. Cereals:[67]

(generally)

seed of *Artemisia anethifolia*; "a sagebrush (wormwood)"
seed of *Convolvulus gortschakovii*; "morning glory"
seed of *Agriophyllus arenarium* or *A. gobicum*
seed of *Polygonum alpinum*; "smartweed (knotweed)"
seed of *Artemisia pectina*

(Locally)

seed of *Artemisia scoparia*; "sagebrush"
seed of *Artemisia annua*; "sagebrush"
seed of *Kalidium foliatum* or *K. gracile*
seed of *Artemisia xerophytica*; "sagebrush"
seed of *Psammochloa villosa*
seed of *Elymus giganteus*; "ryegrass/wild rye"
seed of *Polygonum sibiricum*; "smartweed"
seed of *Corispermum mongolicum*

---

[65] *Secret History*, chapters 74–5. We are indebted to Igor de Rachewiltz for help in identifying these plants and animals (unpublished letter of 19 October, 1990 to PDB). See also BNMAU shinzhlekh ukhaany akademi, *Ulsyn ner tom'yoony komissyn medee*, no 89–90 (Ulaanbaatar, 1973); and *no 96–7* (Ulaanbaatar, 1974); and B. Rinchen, *Mongol ard ulsyn ugsaatny sudlal, khelniy shinzhleliyn atlas*, vols. 1–2 (Ulaanbaatar, 1979). See now also U. Ligaa, *Mongol orny ashigt urgamal*, vol. 1 (Ulaanbaatar, 1978).

[66] Rinchen, 1979.

[67] Most of these plants are described and illustrated in *Üretü urgamal-un jirugtu toli* (Kököqota, 1976).

2. Fruits and Berries

(generally)

Vaccinium vitisidaea; "huckleberry"
Amygdalus mongolica or *A. penduncul*ata; "wild almond"
fruit of *Fragaria orientalis*
Padus asiatica [should be *Prunus padus*]; "wild cherry"
"hips of roses;" *Rosa acicularis* or *R. davurica*
Vaccinium uliginosum; "huckleberry"
Grossularia [=*Ribes*] *acicularis*; "gooseberry"
Ribes rubrum; "red currant"
Ribes nigrum; "black currant"
Malus [=*Pyrus*] *pallasiana*; "crab apple"
fruit of *Hippophae rhamnoides*

(locally)

fruit of *Crataegus sanguinea*; "a hawthorn"
Ribes altissimum; "currant"
Rubus sachalinensis; "blackberry or raspberry"
Prnus armeniaca sibirica; "wild apricot"
fruit of "saltworts" *Nitraria Roborowskii*, or *N. sibirica*
fruit of *Oxycoccus microcarpus*
fruit of *Sorbus sibirica*; "mountain ash"
Elaeagnus angustifolia; "Russian olive"

3. Mushrooms

Psalliota [=Agaricus] arvensis
Psalliota [=Agaricus] campestris

4. Onion Family

Allium lineare or *A. odorum* [=*A. tuberosum*]; "garlic chive"
A. prostratum, or *A. senescens*; "wild onion"
A. altaicum
A. victorialis; "wild garlic"
A. mongolicum
A. schoenoprasum; "common chive"
A. anisopodium
A. fischeri

5. Nuts

Pinus sibirica; "pine [nuts]"

6. Spices

Carum buriaticum; "Buriyat caraway"
Schizonepeta annua

7. Substitutes for Tea

(generally)

Chamaenerion angustifolium
Paeonia anomala; "herbaceous peony"

(locally)

Populus tremula; "aspen"
Spiraea media; "meadowsweet"
Betula gmelinii; "birch"
Bergenia crassifolia
Serratula cardunculus
Dasiphora fruticosa
Lagopsis supina
Geranium pseudosibiricum; "geranium"

8. Starchy Foods

(generally)

Butomus umbellatus
root of *Potentilla anserina*; "cinquefoil/silverweed"
Rumex undulatum, *R. altaicum,* and *R. compactum*; "docks"
Cirsium esculentum; "thistle"
rhizome of *Polygonum viviparum*; "a smartweed"
root of *Sanguisorba officinalis*; "garden burnet"
Asparagus dahuricum
Lilium tenuifolium
Phragmites communis; "common reed"

(locally)

Phlomis tuberosa
Sinomorium songaricum
Agropyron repens; "quackgrass"
Lilium martagon; "tiger lily"
Typha laxmanni; "cattail"
Polygonum divaricatum; "smartweed"
Sphallerocarpus gracilis

9. Sweetener

Glycyrrhiza uralensis; "liquorice root"

10. Greens

Rheum nanum; "dwarf rhubarb"
Heracleum dissectum
Polygonum aviculare; "smartweed"
Rumex acetosa; "sourdock/French sorrel"
Urtica angustifolia; "nettle"
Cynanchum sibiricum[68]

The preferred diet was fermented milk products, supplemented by wild meats and, on special occasions, or when there was abundance, meat from domestic animals. Horse meat was especially liked. Among these foods highly nutritional, although slightly alcoholic, kumiss[69]

---

[68] See Rinchen, 1979: 93–141. This list may be compared with (Inner Mongolian) gathered vegetable, fruits and berries listed and discussed in Damrinbazar, 1991: 149ff. They include: wild leeks, a variety of onions, nettles, *Cynanchum*, Chinese yams, lily bulbs and seeds, *Chenopodium*, *Sonchus brachyotus*, the persimmon, *Pteridium*, *Hemerocallis minor*, *Senecio campestris*, mushrooms, *Suaeda* spp, dock, *Imperata cylindrica*, wild Chinese flower pepper, ephedra, wild cabbage, wild celery, *Cistanche deserticola*, *Rheum Franzenbachii*, *Pugionium cornutum*, *Ulmus pumilla*, *Agriophyllum arenarium*, apples, mulberry fruits, red currants, hawthorn fruits, gooseberries, pears, bird cherries, acorns, chestnuts, apricots, pinenuts, wild grapes, wild jujubes, elm fruits, wild rose hips, walnuts, fruit of *Hippophae rhamnoides*, nitraria fruits, *Securinega suffruticosa* fruits, and oleaster fruits.

[69] On kumiss (and camel kumiss, Turkic *shubat*, plus those made from many other milks) see *Kumys Shubat* (Almaty, 1979). See also [Ya.] Tsevel, *Mongolyn tsagaan idee*, Studia Ethnographica I, 6 (Ulaanbaatar, 1959). William of Rubruck (in Wyngaert, 1929: 177–8) provides the following account of Mongol kumiss–making:

> *Cosmos*, that is, mares' milk, is made in this manner: they extend a long rope over the ground attached to two posts and to that cord they tie the foals of the mares they want to milk around the tenth hour. Thereby the mothers stand near their foals and allow themselves to be milked peacefully. And if any is somewhat ungovernable, a man then takes the foal, puts it to the mare, and allows it to suck a little. The foal is then withdrawn and the milker takes its place.
>
> And when a great quantity of milk has thus been collected, milk which is as sweet as cow's milk, while it is fresh, they pour it into a great hide bag or sack and they begin to shake it with a piece of wood made for that purpose. It is as large as a man's head farther in and hollow below. And as they shake it very quickly, it begins to boil just like new wine and to sour like things fermenting. And they shake that until they remove the butter.

was the favorite of the Mongolian elite and was the food associated with the greatest social prestige. Mongol emperors preferred to live on it during the summer, when the mare's milk from which it was made was most abundant, and most often did.

Cooking of meat was generally either by roasting or by boiling in a cauldron. In which case, almost all parts of an animal, including the bones, were used. The aim was to produce a thick and nutritious broth, believed to contain the very essence, the soul,[70] of its animal source. Other foods could be added to the broth, including dried fermented milk products as well as grain, or wild seeds as substitutes, where available, or even wild vegetables, fruits, and berries. The result was a *šülen*, a "soup," the honorific word for "food" in the *Secret History*.[71]

> They then taste it and when it is moderately bitter, they drink it. It bites the tongue like a harsh wine while it is being drunk. And after a person ceases to drink, there remains a flavor on the tongue of almond milk. And it provides a great deal of internal human joys and it even intoxicates weak heads. It provokes urine a great deal.

[70] On traditional Turkic and Mongolian religion see Jean–Paul Roux, *La religion des Turcs et des Mongols* (Paris, 1984), and specifically on the Mongols of the imperial period N. Pallisen, *Die alte Religion des mongolischen Volkes während der Herrschaft der Tschingisiden*, Micro Bibliotheca Anthropos 7 (Posieux, Freiburg, 1953). On Mongol concepts of the soul resident in the bone and marrow of an animal see the discussion in Roux, 1984: 160ff.

[71] *Šülen* is carefully distinguished in the *Secret History* from a simple "drink" [*umdan*] as in the following passage from chapter 124 dealing with the functions of the *qan*'s bodyguard, members of which also prepared his food:

> When [Temüjin] had become Cinggis–qahan, Ögölei–cerbi, the younger brother of Bo'orcu, put on a quiver [*i.e.*, became a member of the *qan*'s bodyguard]. Qaci'un–toqura'un put on a quiver. Jetei and Doqolqu–cerbi, the two brothers, put on a quiver. When Önggür, Söyiketü–cerbi and Qada'andaldurqan, the three of them, spoke, saying:
>
> Let us not allow [your] morning drink
> [*umdan*] to be too little,
> let us not allow [your] evening drink
> to be neglected,
>
> they became stewards [*bawurcin*]. When Degei spoke, saying:
>
> Making a wether of two years into *šülen*,
> let me not allow it to be too little in the morning.
> Let me not be late with it at night.
> Having [your] spotted sheep herded,
> let me fill a cart [with them].
> Having [your] yellow sheep herded,
> let me fill up a pen [with them].

The practice of consuming virtually all parts of an animal was above all a reflection of frequent food shortages on the steppe. It also accorded with the dictates of a conservation–oriented Mongolian traditional religion which stressed taking no more from nature than was absolutely needed and the insult to the local spirits ("lords of the lands and waters") from an unnecessary waste. Mongol informants of John of Plano Carpini justified this tradition by assigning it to the authority of Cinggis–qan himself:

> And while Cyngis was returning from that county [of the Tatars] he lacked foodstuffs and they [the Mongols] suffered from great hunger. And on that occasion it happened that they found the fresh entrails of a beast. They took them and cooked them, discarding only the dung. And bearing them before Cyngis can, he ate the entrails with his men. And from this it was ordained by him that they should throw away neither blood, nor entrails nor nothing else from a beast which they eat, excepting the dung. [72]

Carpini also informs us that:

> It is considered a great sin among them if anything is allowed to be wasted either from food or drink. Thus they do not allow bones to be given to dogs unless the marrow has first been extracted.[73]

Mongolian foods are well represented in the following short quotations from observers of the Mongols during the first years of empire:

1. [1220s] The land of the Tatars [Mongols] has abundant water and grass and is suitable for sheep and horses. Their way of life is only a matter of drinking mare's milk to assuage hunger and thirst. As a rule, the milk of one mare is enough to satisfy three persons. When they are on campaigns or at home they drink only mare's milk, or they can slaughter sheep for provisions. Within the Tatar nation, whoever has one horse must have six or seven sheep. This means that if one has a hundred horses, they must have a sheep herd of 600 or 700. If they go campaigning in China, and their mutton provisions are exhausted, they shoot hares, deer, and wild pigs as their food. Thus when they encamp an army of several myriads, they do not light cooking fires [*i.e.*, every

---

> I have been gluttonous and bad.
> Having [your] sheep herded,
> let me eat their rectums,
>
> Degei caused the sheep to be herded.

Šülen is also mentioned in chapters 192, 214, 229, 279, and 280, nearly always in connection with duties of members of the bodyguard.

[72] C. Raymond Beazley, ed., *The Texts and Versions of John de Plano Carpini and William de Rubruquis* (Nendeln/Liechtenstein, 1967), 57.

[73] Beazley, 1967: 52.

man fends for himself]. Recently they have taken inhabitants of China as slaves. These slaves must eat rice to be satiated. For this reason they [the Tatars] seize rice and wheat and cook and eat congee in their stockades. There are also one or two places in the Tatar land which produce black panicled millet.[74] They also cook that and make a substitute congee. [75]

2. [1230s] Their food is meat and not grain. Animals captured in hunting are the hare, deer, wild pigs, the marmot, wild sheep ([Textual note:] One can make soup spoons from its vertebra), the dseiren antelope [*Procapra gutturosa*] (The back is yellow. The tail is large like a fan), wild horses (like an ass in form) [*Equus przewalskii*], and fish from rivers and springs (they can be obtained when the land is frost covered). The animal normally raised to be eaten is the sheep. The ox is second. They do not slaughter horses unless it is a major feast or assembly. Meat is almost always roasted. Only rarely is it cooked in a pot. One cuts off a piece of meat and eats. Afterwards the meat is given to others to eat. (During the more than one month that I, Ting 霆, was in the steppe, I did not see the Tatars kill an ox to eat.)[76]

3. [1240s] Furthermore, they are the most unclean and filthy in their eating. They use neither table cloths nor napkins, nor do they have bread [to use as a plate], or pay any attention to it, and scorn to eat it. They have not vegetables or even legumes; and nothing other than meat to eat, and they eat so little meat that other peoples could scarcely live from it. And further they eat all kinds of meats except for that of the mule, which is sterile, and this they do disgracefully and rapaciously. They lick their greasy fingers and wipe them dry on their boots. The great ones are wont to have little cloths with which they wipe their fingers carefully. They do not wash their hands before eating, nor their dishes afterwards; and if perchance they wash them in meat broth, they put the dish they have washed back into the pot along with the meat. Otherwise they do not wash pots or spoons or utensils of any kind. They like horse meat more than any other meat. They even eat rats and dogs and dine on cats with great pleasure. They drink wine with great pleasure whenever they have it. They get drunk every day on the mare's milk which they call kaumous, just as others get drunk on strong wine. And when they celebrate holidays and the festivals of their forefathers, they spend their time in singing, or rather shrieking, and in drinking bouts; and as long as such drinking bouts last, they attend to no business and dispatch no envoys. This is what the brothers of the Order of Preaching Monks, sent to the Mongols by the Pope and staying in their

---

[74] This should in theory be a "black" variety of *Panicum miliaceum*.

[75] Chao Hung, *Mengda beilu*, in Wang Guowei, ed., *Menggu shiliao si zhong* (Taibei, 1962), 447.

[76] Peng Daya 彭大雅, *Heida shilüe* 黑韃事略, in Wang, 1962: 475–6. The textual notes are by Xu Ting 徐霆, who also visited the steppe, and has added extensive comments to Peng's basic text.

> camp, experienced continuously for six days. They eat human meat like lions; devouring it roasted on the fire and soaked with grease. And whenever they take someone contrary or hostile to themselves, they come together in one place to eat him in vengeance for the rebellion raised against them. They avidly suck his blood just like hellish vampires.[77]

These simple Mongolian foodways soon changed along directions already suggested in the accounts above. Note, for example, evidence for the growing role of grain foods in the Mongolian diet in the first quotation. There is a reference to wine in the last. Wine seems to have been totally unknown to most twelfth century Mongols[78] but by the time of Simon de Saint–Quentin was part of an unfortunately growing range of alcoholic beverages available to the Mongols.

John of Plano Carpini, writing in the late 1240s confirms the increasingly important role of flour in Mongolian diet:

> Their food consists of anything they can eat. They eat dogs, wolves, foxes, and horses, and, in necessity, human flesh. Thus when they were fighting against a certain Chinese city where the emperor himself lived, they laid siege to it for so long a time that they were entirely out of supplies. And since they did not have anything to eat at all, they then took one in each ten men to eat. They even eat the water which comes out of mares giving birth to foals. Indeed, we even saw them eating lice. We also saw them eating mice.[79]
>
> They drink mare's milk in the greatest possible quantities if they have it. They also drink the milk of ewes, she goats, cows, and camels. They do not have wine, beer, and mead, unless it is given to them or sent from other peoples. During the winter, unless they are rich, they do not have mare's milk. They cook millet in water and make it so thin that they drink rather than eat it. And each of them drinks a small cup full or two in the morning and they eat nothing more during the day. In the evening a portion of meats is given to each and they drink the broth from the meats. During the summer, however, when they have sufficient

[77] Simon de Saint–Quentin, *Histoire des Tatares*, ed. Jean Richard (Paris, 1965), 40–1. Note that a number of lines of the passage given above are excerpts from the travelogue of John of Plano Carpini. Simon and his brothers have added additional detail from the hearsay of other eyewitnesses to Mongol daily life, including some dubious claims of cannibalism of enemies.

[78] See the *Yuanshi*, 118, 2924 (biography of Alaquš–digit–quri). The *jiu* 酒 in question must have been grape wine, known to have been produced in those days in Inner Mongolia probably by the Önggüt or some other Turkic people resident in the area. See Buell, 1977: 253.

[79] Beazley, 1967: 52.

> mare's milk, they rarely eat meats unless these are per chance given them, or when they have taken some beast in the hunt, or some bird.[80]

From this type of usage, involving only a little flour, the jump to a *tsampa*, to simple hearth breads,[81] or even to the steamed or boiled buns of the type found widely throughout China, the Middle East, and Central Asia was not a great one and soon made. In any case, the prevalence of foods of this type in the recipes of the *YSZY* is no accident. They had already become completely Mongolian.

The other clearly defined post–empire change in Mongol dietary patterns, improved access to more, and to a greater variety of alcoholic beverages, was less fortunate for those Mongols who could afford to drink them. The new beers, wines, and distilled liquors were often far more potent than what the Mongols had hitherto been used to. Even kumiss, little dangerous to health when used in moderation, seems to have become a problem as it became more and more prevalent, too prevalent, as time passed.

Other liquors, including low proof distillates, were freely and generally available no later than the time of *qan* Ögödei, as witnessed by that ruler's famous fountain producing wine, mead (boal), and rice beer, as well as (qara–)kumiss.[82] Since most of these new alcoholic

---

[80] Beazley, 1967: 52.

[81] This transition from flour thickened broth to *tsampa* seems already to have been made by the time of William of Rubruck, who was in Mongolia only a few years after John of Plano Carpini:

> ...And we found him [Möngke] with a few members of his household drinking liquid *tam*, that is a food made from dough, for the comfort of his head. (Wyngaert, 1929: 267).

Elsewhere he also notes:

> ...And thus our food was millet with butter, or dough cooked in water with butter, or sour milk and unleavened bread cooked in the dung of oxen or of horses. (Wyngaert: 271–2).

[82] The making of *qara–kumiss* is described by William of Rubruck as follows:

> They likewise make *caracosmos*, that is, black *cosmos*, for the use of the great lords, as follows: The milk of mares does not coagulate. The rule is that the milk of no animal in the stomach of whose young rennet is not found coagulates. Rennet is not found in the stomachs of foals so mares' milk does not coagulate. They thus shake the milk so that everything which is dense in it properly moves to the bottom, just like lees of wine, and that which is pure remains on top and is as if a milk whey or just as white must. The lees are very white and are given to the servants and they greatly promote sleep. The lords drink the clear liquid, and

beverages could easily be stored, unlike kumiss, normally available only in quantity during the early summer and thus drunk throughout the year, over–consumption now became a perennial, and no longer just a seasonal problem. Unfortunately too for the Mongols, the appearance of their empire coincided with the first broad use of distilled brandies and whiskies.[83] Large numbers of Mongols, who had never been exposed to such temptations in the past, or such powerful intoxicants, succumbed, including *qan* Ögödei himself.[84]

China

Utterly different from the steppe was the world of China which the Mongols invaded, and ultimately (1279) conquered. China was a region of unparalleled economic, social and cultural achievement coupled with political division and military weakness, especially in the south. Just prior to the Mongolian invasions the combined populations of north and south had reached an early modern high of at least 120,000,000 to 130,000,000, and perhaps as many as 150,000,000, if marginal areas including Tangut domains are included.[85] Of this total, some 53,500,000 are estimated to have lived in Jin domains, a region then nearly as developed as the south.[86]

Most of the world's largest cities were located in China, its economy was the most sophisticated in the world with trade links as far away as East Africa since Chinese maritime expansion into the South Seas, Indian Ocean, and beyond anticipated the Age of Exploration by several centuries. China also led the world in technology. It already, to give but a few examples, had access to gunpowder weapons, including

---

it is certainly a very agreeable drink and of good efficaciousness. (Wyngaert, 1929: 178).

[83] On the history of distilling in East Asia see Joseph Needham, Ho Ping–yü and Lu Gwei–djen, *Science and Civilization in China,* vol. 5: *Chemistry and Chemical Technology,* part IV: *Spagyrical Discovery and Invention: Apparatus, Theories and Gifts* (Cambridge, 1980), 55–162.

[84] See now Thomas T. Allsen, "Ögedei and Alcohol," *Mongolian Studies*, XXIX (2007), 3-12.

[85] See Ho Ping–ti, "An Estimate of the Total Population of Sung–Chin China," in *Études Song in memoriam Étienne Balázc*, ed. Françoise Aubin (Paris, 1970), 3–53. Ho's figures understate the total population of the era since they rely upon official figures of numbers of tax–paying households, less than the total number of households. They also do not include Tangut Xixia, which may have been densely populated during the period to which Ho's figures refer.

[86] Vorob'yev, 1975: 147ff.

hand guns,[87] mechanical clocks,[88] the compass, the sternpost rudder, watertight compartments in ships,[89] printing, and sophisticated building techniques and even building codes. The latter provided imperial standards which guaranteed excellent and environmentally well–adapted buildings in a bureaucratic move far ahead of the rest of the world.[90] Coal was already widely used as a fuel in the treeless north, as Marco Polo noted, and in the eleventh century Chinese production of steel reached a level not exceeded by Industrial–Revolution Britain until well into the nineteenth century. The north continued to produce large amounts of cast iron and steel, even in the thirteenth century.[91] No less an accomplishment were successful use of paper money and some very modern vehicles of long–distance commercial exchange. China's agriculture[92] was also a world leader. South Chinese rice fields[93] probably produced a higher yield per acre than fields in any other part of the world, even intensively cultivated gardens of the Muslim west. It was not only from rice, since a sophisticated complex of food production was involved, using the same fields. The high yields and variety of Chinese food production, particularly in the south, were above all a reflection of experience garnered by the Chinese farmer over the millennia.[94] Borrowings from a variety of other

---

[87] On the history of gunpowder weapons see now Joseph Needham *et al.*, 1986.

[88] See Joseph Needham, and Wang Ling, *Science and Civilization in China,* vol. 4: *Physics and Physical Technology,* part II: *Mechanical Engineering* (Cambridge, 1965), 435–532. For a divergent view see also David S. Landes, *Revolution in Time, Clocks and the Making of the Modern World* (Cambridge, 1983).

[89] On China's early achievements in maritime technology and exploration see, as an introduction, Joseph Needham, Wang Ling and Lu Gwei–djen, *Science and Civilization in China,* vol. 4, *Physics and Physical Technology,* part III: *Civil Engineering and Nautics* (Cambridge, 1971). See also J. V. G. Mills, trans., *Ma Huan Ying–yai sheng–lan*: *"The Overall Survey of the Ocean's Shores,"* Hakluyt Society Extra Series No. XLII (Cambridge, 1970).

[90] Else Glahn, "Chinese Building Standards in the 12th century," *Scientific American* 244 (1988): 5: 162–73.

[91] See the groundbreaking article by Robert Hartwell, "A Cycle of Economic Change in Imperial China: Coal and Iron in Northeast China, 750–1350," *Journal of the Economic and Social History of the Orient* X (1967): 1: 102–59.

[92] As an introduction, see Francesca Bray, *Science and Civilization in China,* vol. 6: *Biology and Biological Technology,* part II: *Agriculture* (Cambridge, 1984) and Hsu Cho–yun, *Han Agriculture*, ed. by Jack L. Dull (Seattle, 1980).

[93] See Francesca Bray, *The Rice Economies, Technology and Development in Asian Societies* (Oxford, 1986).

[94] The discussion here summarizes E. N. Anderson, *The Food of China* (New Haven, 1988). The most important source is Kenneth Ruddle, and Zhong Gongfu, *Integrated Agriculture-aquaculture in South China: The Dike-pond System of the Zhu-*

cultures, including Siberian and Central Asian were also of key importance.

Agriculture had begun in China by 8000 BC, when foxtail millet was grown along the Wei 渭 and probably in the Huanghe 黃河 river valley.[95] Broomcorn (panic) millet[96] soon followed, by 6000-6500 BC. Rice is first documented from the Yangze 楊子 Valley, where it was domesticated by around 8000 BC[97] and was common by 5000 BC. By that time agriculture was probably also practiced along the Central Yangze.[98] The Wei/Huanghe and Yangze areas continued to be the primary focuses of Chinese agriculture, but astonishing recent finds have revealed that the northern marches were far more important than previously thought. Agricultural settlements, based on millet, have been found in south Manchuria and Inner Mongolia, extending

---

jiang Delta (Cambridge, 1988). See also Robert Marks, *Tigers, Rice, Silk and Silt* (New York, 1998).

95 See Chang Kwang-chih, "China on the Eve of the Historical Period," In *The Cambridge History of Ancient China*, eds. Michael Loewe and Edward Shaughnessy (Cambridge, 1999), 37-73; Liu Li, *The Chinese Neolithic* (Cambridge, 2004); and Laurent Sagart, Roger Blench, and Alicia Sanchez-Mazas, eds, *The Peopling of East Asia: Putting Together Archaeology, Linguistics and Genetics* (London, 2005).

96 See Peter Bellwood, "Examining the Farming/Language Dispersal Hyothesis in the East Asian Context," In Laurent Sagart, Roger Blench, and Alicia Sanchez-Mazas, eds, 2005: 17-30. The world's oldest cultivated panicled millet or *proso* (*Panicum miliaceum*) is from Greece, 6000–5000 BC. See Ho Ping–ti, *The Cradle of the East* (Hong Kong and Chicago, 1975), 240. It first appeared in China in the late Neolithic or early civilized period and assumed particular importance under the Zhou whose legendary ancestor was Houji 后稷, "Emperor *Proso,*" or even "Emperor Foxtail Millet," since the use of the term is uncertain. Coming from a drier, cooler area than the Shang heartland they conquered, the Zhou may have regarded millet as "their" crop. Both glutinous and non–glutinous millets are mentioned in their songs, and later Zhou texts also notice the glutinous as an important brewing grain. It has continued to be. *Proso* grows farther north and under drier conditions than other "millets," *i.e.*, small–grained grass crops. It is most popular on the fringes of Inner Asia and remains predominately a crop of the Chinese north. On the early history of millet in China see Chang Te–tzu, "The origins and early cultures of cereal grains and food legumes," in David N. Keightley, ed., *The Origins of Chinese Civilization* (Berkeley, 1983), 65–94.

97 See Chang, 1999; Jiang Leping, and Liu Li, "New Evidence for the Origins of Sedentism and Rice Domestication in the Lower Yangzi River, China." *Antiquity* 80 (2006): 355-361; Liu, 2004; and Richard S. MacNeish and Jane G. Libby, *Origins of Rice Agriculture: The Preliminary Report of the Sino-American Jiangxi (PRC) Project SAJOR* (El Paso, 1995).

98 See Chang, 1999. On the different zones of botanical development in ancient China see also Li Hui–lin, "The Domestication of Plants in China: Ecogeographical Considerations," in Keightley, 1983: 21–63.

back in time almost to the dawn of East Asian agriculture.[99] This culture may have given China the soybean sometime in the late second millennium.[100] Pigs were domesticated by 6000 BC.[101] An astonishing recent find shows that noodles were common by 2000 BC.[102]

It is important to stress the almost complete isolation of early Chinese agriculture from developments in west Asia. The deserts of Xinjiang proved a formidable barrier. They kept the millets, rice, chicken, and pig complex found in East Asia separated from an early west Asian agriculture based upon wheat, barley, and the goat. Although this complex had already reached Afghanistan by 5000 BC, Xinjiang, by way of contrast, does not seem to have reached the Neolithic till 3000 BC or slightly before.[103] There is some evidence of early contacts through the Siberian steppes, forests, and taiga. Panic millet is early in Europe, common by 5500 BC in the Linearbandkeramik and

---

[99] An Zhimin, "Archaeological Research on Neolithic China," *Current Anthropology* 29 (1988): 5: 753–59. At Hongshan 紅山 in Manchuria, a large town with impressive sculpture has been found, and may date as early as the fourth millennium BC. The site reveals a culture as impressive as any in East Asia at the time. The people of Hongshan were almost certainly not Chinese. They may have been related to the ancestors of modern Koreans in view of early agricultural developments now found elsewhere in the Korean peninsula and the likelihood, based upon present evidence, that the Koreans are indigenous to Korea and not intrusive invaders. See Sarah Milledge Nelson, *The Archaeology of Korea* (Cambridge, 1993). It now appears that the non–Chinese north must be taken very seriously as a homeland for East Asian agricultural development, but see also Gina L. Barnes, *China, Korea, and Japan: The Rise of Civilization in East Asia* (London, 1993), 108ff, and passim.

[100] See Ho: 1975, and Ho: 1988. See also Chang, 1983: 65–94 (see pages 80–1 in particular). Nothing is more characteristic of China than soybeans, yet the soybean was clearly a latecomer to Chinese civilization. It was not known until well into the Zhou Dynasty, when it first appears as an item received from the "Rong 戎 Barbarians" in the northwest (Ho, 1975). Wild soybeans (*Glycine max.* var. *ussuriensis*) are native to this area and points southwest, along the hills behind Beijing. They are also widely scattered throughout northeast and north China, but usually in weedy situations where they are likely to be weeds or hybrids with the cultivated crop.

[101] Jing Yuan, and Rowan K. Flad, "Pig Domestication in Ancient China," *Antiquity* 76 (2002): 724-732.

[102] Lu Houyuan, Yang Xiaoyan, Ye Maolin, Liu Kam-Biu, Xia Zhengkai, Ren Xiaoyan, Cai Linhai, Wu Naiqin, Liu Tung-Sheng, "Millet Noodles in Late Neolithic China," *Nature* 437 (2005): 967.

[103] Liu, 2004 and An, 1988. Neolithic culture or not, this does not seem to have prevented the arrival of the sheep and goat from the Middle East in China, the first probably preceeding the second, although this is debated. See now Yuan Jing and Rod Campbell, "Recent Archaeometric Research on 'the Origins of Chinese Civilisation,'" *Antiquity* 83 (2009): 96-109.

other cultures,[104] and probably spread from China, though independent domestication cannot be ruled out. The Tripolye Culture of the Ukraine (ca. 4500–4000 BC) introduced painted pottery much like that of earlier Neolithic China while pointed–bottom unpainted vessels may have spread through Siberia from the east, but no equivalent "western–looking" traits reached China until the goat, an unmistakably west Asian animal, arrived by 2800 BC.[105]

The ancestors of the later Altaic peoples would have been involved in mediating any exchanges that did occur. They were placed at the midpoint, and their radiation probably went along with the spread of Neolithic and later Bronze–age patterns of adaptation in high Asia. China's earliest dynasties parallel the development of bronze cultures in Central Asia and Siberia.[106] Shang 商 tombs, for instance, look much like those of the steppes while early Lena valley bronzes appear to incorporate *taotie* 饕餮 –like decorations. Wheat and barley had by this time reached China and begun their rapid rise to pre–eminence there. Very possibly they came via Siberia, although an oasis route across Xinjiang is also possible.[107]

From the Zhou 周 Dynasty on interactions between Chinese and the peoples of Central Asia and Siberia increased considerably but cultural lines were also drawn with increasing rigidity.[108] From the end of the Zhou date the first detailed descriptions of steppe nomads and seminomads, peoples described as sharply different from Chinese. In fact groups like the Xiongnu 匈奴 practiced a great deal of agriculture and had large settlements.[109] Many were "nomadic" only by contrast with the sedentary Chinese. But, as the latter realized the full potential of their fertile soils and relatively beneficent climate, they pulled ahead demographically and economically. Mongolia also suf-

---

[104] Bellwood 2005: 21.

[105] An, 1988.

[106] The only general study is William Watson, *Cultural Frontiers in Ancient East Asia* (Edinburgh, 1971). See also A. P. Okladnikov, *Yakutia before Its Incorporation into the Russian State*, Anthropology of the North, Translations from Russian Sources 8, ed. Henry N. Michael (Montreal and London, 1970).

[107] See Chang, 1983: 77–9.

[108] See in particular Owen Lattimore, *Inner Asian Frontiers of China* (Boston, 1962), 255 ff. Early relations of China with the north are the subject of a monograph by Jaroslav Prusek, *Chinese Statelets and the Northern Barbarians,* 1400–300 BC (Dordrecht, 1971).

[109] For a survey of early permanent settlements in what is now the Mongolian People's Republic see D. Majdar, *Mongolyn khot tosgony gurvan zurag (ert, dundad üye, XX zuuny ekh)* (Ulaanbaatar, 1970).

fers from severe wind erosion which renders most agricultural land unsuited for that purpose after only a few years' use.

The steppe and northern peoples retained considerable strength, however, partly because of their superiority in horses. Horses were raised with difficulty in China, but were available in quantity and quality on the steppe.[110] Their contact with west and south Asia also allowed them to benefit from any new military or economic developments there. The Mongols, for example, perfected the technique of using new Chinese weapons against the West, including gunpowder, and new Western ones, such as counterweighted trebuchets,[111] against China.

China's first green revolution took place under Qin 秦 and Han.[112] Late Zhou developments such as the moldboard plow and other efficient farm machines found their potential realized as the emperors invoked policies that benefited agriculture and food production. Flour milling, learned from the Western world, released the potential of wheat and oilseeds. Grapes, alfalfa and possibly other Western crops arrived.[113] More important were the first agricultural manuals and extension services, agricultural administration, the "ever–normal granary," and government research and development involving such

[110] Wild claims have been made regarding the very early domestication of the horse but any date before 3000 BC is suspect and then riding came only much later. There was also more than one domestication. See the discussion in Buell, May and Ramey, forthcoming, and in Carles Vilá, Jennifer A. Leonard, Anders Götherström, Stefan Marklund, Kaj Sandberg, Kerstin Lidén, Robert K. Wayne, and Hans Ellegren, "Widespread Origins of Domestic Horse Lineages," *Science* 291 (2001): 474-477. See now also, for a slightly earlier date for horses as a milk source, certainly one of the earliest uses, Travis, 2008.

[111] If counter-weighted trebuchets were, in fact, a Western invention. See John Masson Smith, Jr., "High Living and Heartbreak on the Road to Baghdad," in Linda Komaroff, ed., *Beyond the Legacy of Genghis Khan* (Brill, 2006), 111-134 (124ff).

[112] See Anderson, 1988: 36ff.

[113] The following west Asian contributions to Chinese agriculture are listed in Laufer (1919): Alfalfa, grapes, the pistachio, the walnut, the pomegranate, sesame and flax, coriander, the cucumber, the (western) chive, bulb onion and shallot, safflower, jasmine, henna, the balsam–poplar, manna, asafoetida, galbanum, oak–galls, indigo, black pepper, sugar, myrobalans, "golden peaches," mustard, the date palm, spinach, sugar beets, lettuce, ricinus, the almond, the fig, the olive, cassia pods, carob, the narcissus, the balm of gilead, the watermelon, fenugreek, nux–vomica, the carrot and various aromatics including spikenard, storax, myrrh, putchuck and styrax benjoin. Most of these had long been in China by the time the *YSZY* was written, others, *e.g.*, watermelon, were recent introductions. See now also Hu Shiu-ying, *Food Plants of China* (Hong Kong, 2005).

modern concepts as controlled case studies.[114] An ideology of "agriculture (as) the basis of the state" led to imperial ceremonies and local rites to glorify it. North Chinese agriculture rose to high levels of intensification, primarily because of government policy and the existence of an enormous urban market.

During the following dynasties, Central Asian influence became strong in China. The (Toba) Wei 魏 Dynasty, the most powerful and dynamic of the many successor regimes to Han, was ruled by a Mongol–Turkic (Xianbei 鮮卑) ruling house. Central and south Asian foods, ideas and medicines flowed into China.[115] Tang, also, was ruled by a family with some Altaic (Turkic) forebears. Overland contact with Altaic and Iranian peoples was the most important external communication. Indian and Central Asian monks, first appearing in the late Han, if not earlier, brought Buddhism and its food and medical traditions to China. Sea traffic was not neglected although at first usually not in Chinese ships and Canton, among other Chinese cities, had a large Irano–Arabic colony, from which came not only ordinary foods but even luxuries, including sugar.[116]

An important document for early Tang food and health is the *Qianjin bei ji fang* 千金備急方, "Recipes for Emergency Use Worth a Thousand in Gold," of Sun Simiao 孫思邈 first published in 654.[117] This work draws heavily on earlier writings, particulary of Tao Hongjing 陶宏景 (456-536). Despite these borrowings, Sun incorporates a great deal of west Asian lore, gleaned from Buddhist medical missionaries and writings most of whom came from Central Asia and beyond. Sun (like Tao) already employs the western humoral heating/cooling medical system, prominent in the *YSZY*, but he sees it as a somewhat exotic idea, to be added to the more traditional and familiar ideas of "five phases" and *qi* dynamics. Sun's book began a tradition of nutritional medicine, of which the *YSZY* is a later representative.

---

[114] On all this, see as an introduction Bray, 1984, and Hsu, 1980.

[115] See as an introduction Laufer, 1919, and Edward H. Schafer, *The Golden Peaches of Samarkand* (Berkeley, 1963). It is anticipated that F. Sabban will deal with this subject in her forthcoming translation of the *Qimin yaoshu*, a text which has some early descriptions of wheat flour foods from the West. See also below in chapter 2.

[116] On the many western contributions to life in Medieval China see, as an introduction, Schafer 1963; and Laufer, 1919.

[117] Our comments here are based on unpublished work by Yi Sumei (Yi Sumei, translator, *Recipes Worth a Thousand Gold*, n.d.). On the general history of Chinese food see also Hu, 2005, and Frederick Simoons, *Food in China* (Boca Raton, FL, 1991)

The main route remained overland. Everything from spinach to fenugreek was moving across the Silk Road.[118] North Chinese food was becoming strikingly Westernized. Wheat technology was almost entirely Near Eastern.[119] Foods now thoroughly Sinicized, like the *shaobing* 燒餅, were then still very obviously intrusive; Persians sold ancestral *shaobing*, small versions of their traditional *nan*, in the streets of Changan 長安. Dairy products were abundant. Yogurt was a regional marker, indeed a stereotype, for north China[120] and a whole milk technology grew up, enormously complex and important through

---

[118] See Laufer, 1919.

[119] Wheat seems to have come to China in the late Neolithic Period or at the beginning of civilized times, around 2000 BC. China lacks more primitive forms and the only wheat known there (except for rare curiosities) is bread wheat, a complex hybrid that is the hexaploid result of millennia of interbreeding species of *Triticum* and *Aegilops*. It first appeared only after farming had become highly developed and sophisticated in the Neolithic Near East. Like the Near East, a great variety of both primitive and modern forms occurs in the western Turkistan and Afghanistan, where cultivation may go back at least 7000 years. Since these areas transmitted wheat to China, the coming of wheat to China must have been much delayed if we are to account for the paucity of Chinese varieties. The primary reason was probably the deserts of Turkistan and Chinese resistance to wheat cultivation due to its established culture of millets. Predynastic finds are rare, if indeed they are not contaminated samples. Shang Dynasty texts mention wheat/barley (confused in Chinese terminology), and by Zhou it was a major crop. But its great importance in China, where it is now the second most important crop, dates from the Han Dynasty, when superior milling technology was introduced from Central Asia. The wheat grain, "berry" in agricultural jargon, though it is not a berry, is very hard. North China's varieties in particular are typically relatively hard wheats. Thus, unlike millet, it cannot be cooked into a gruel or mush, and cooking it into any state of edibility requires much water and fuel, both scarce in North China. Milling into flour was necessary if wheat was to be at all important, and the coming of efficient, economical milling allowed its spread. Even so, wheat did not displace millet from first place in the north until long after Han. Early Tang still was a millet culture; late Tang writings speak of millet and wheat as both important, but wheat somewhat a luxury. The Song "green revolution" seems to have led wheat to its final victory, but millet remained important. By the time of the *YSZY*, wheat may have been dominant over millet, but this is by no means clear. Note that the *YSZY* gives far more importance to millet in the listings of *juan* 3, although not in the recipe sections. Wheat was being grown in rotation with millet (wheat in winter, millet in summer) in the southern parts of North China, where the climate was favorable. Sorghum and the minor grains were, then as now, grown on land too poor for wheat, or, in some cases, as summer rotation crops. After this time, its cultivation continued to expand. On wheat in China see, as an introduction, the relevant discussions in Ho, 1975; Bray, 1984; and Sterling Wortman, ed., *Plant Studies in the People's Republic of China* (Washington, DC, 1975).

[120] Anderson, 1988: 50ff.

Tang, Song, and Yuan. This has been described in detail by Sabban[121] in one of the finest articles ever written on Chinese food production or consumption. The food of the Tang elite of Changan was simple and included much grilled meat and processed milk. Likewise, the food of high Central Asia included much grain. An observer would not have seen anything close to the differences so often emphasized in nineteenth and twentieth century accounts.

Recipes also show similarity. The *YSZY* was not the only, nor the first, Chinese source to feature recipes that draw on Central Asia. The *Qimin yaoshu* 齊民要書 of *circa* 550 already reflected the many Western influences that had come in with the Wei Dynasty and even earlier. Tang poems and stores reflect a real idealization of Iranian and other Western influences.[122] In Yuan, naturally enough, there was a minor boom in western recipes (*e.g.*, in addition to those in the *YSZY*, the "Muslim" recipes in the late–fourteenth–century collection *Jujia biyong shilei* 居家比用事類 [*JJBYSL*]).[123] On the other hand, east and south China remained relatively free of such influences. Ni Zan 倪瓚 (1301–74) shows little Central Asian influence in his recipes in his *Yunlintang yinshi zhidu ji* 雲林堂飲食制度, which reflects foodways very close to what one would find today in eastern China. Nor do Marco Polo's observations in Hangzhou 杭州 indicate any heavy Central Asian influence there.

What we see, over time, is a pattern in which Central Asian influences waxed and waned in north China. During times of strong influence from westward, such as Yuan, Central and West Asian foodways became more widespread and elaborate. During periods of Chinese strength and Central Asian weakness, the opposite occurred. Thus, the contrast between northwest and southeast is still obvious and pronounced in China. Today as in Yuan, one finds more lamb, more elaborate breadstuffs, more fried dumplings and so on in the former, and more fish, pork, rice and vegetables in the latter. Today, also, the food of the Turkic peoples of Xinjiang is much closer to Afghan and other

121 See Françoise Sabban, "Un savoir–faire oublié: le travail du lait en Chine ancienne," *Zibun: Memoirs of the Research Institute for Humanistic Studies* No. 21 (1986): 31–65 (henceforth Sabban, 1986a).

122 See Schafer, 1963.

123 These recipes are translated in Paul D. Buell, "Mongol Empire and Turkicization: the Evidence of Food and Foodways," in Reuven Amitai–Preiss and David Morgan, eds., *The Mongol Empire and its Legacy* (Amsterdam, 1999): 200–23. On the *JJBYSL* see the discussion in Nakamura and Satō, 1978: 26ff.

Central Asian foodways than to Chinese foodways.[124] The Mongols of Inner Mongolia preserve old ways self–consciously, often as a political statement. The court food described in the *YSZY* represents a peak of westward influence, but not a sudden intrusion of a totally new cuisine.

Song and the conquest dynasties brought changes. The Song center of gravity was well southeast of China's earlier centers. This was true even with the capital at Kaifeng 開封, and of course much more so in Southern Song. The old stereotypes persisted at first, with northwesterners typed as eaters of wheat and mutton, southeasterners as people of rice and fish.[125] Rice and fish won out as the Song economy shifted and Song territory contracted. Moreover, the expansion of seafaring and the arrival of high–yield quick–growing rice and bean varieties gave Southeast China and its foods and enormous boost.[126] With other technological innovations, these things produced a second green revolution. Golas and Huang point out that it was not a very rapid process, but neither is the green revolution of our own times.[127]

Going hand–in–hand with this green revolution of quantity was a great qualitative change in Chinese foodways due to an increasingly thorough exploration of the food and seasoning resources of the south itself, witnessed by an explosion of information about the plants of the

---

[124] We are indebted to personal communications (to ENA) from Dru Gladney, William Jankowiak, and Nancy Peterson Walter on modern West Chinese foods. For a sampling of recent recipes see: Chen Rui 陳銳, *Xibei caixi qutan* 西北菜肴趣談 (Lanzhou 蘭州, 1985).

[125] See Stephen P. West, "Cilia, Scale and Bristle: the Consumption of Fish and Shellfish in the Eastern Capital of the Northern Sung," *Harvard Journal of Asiatic Studies* 47 (1987): 2: 595–634.

[126] See Peter J. Golas, "Rural China in the Song," *Journal of Asian Studies* 39 (1980): 2: 291–325; Ho Ping–ti, "Early Ripening Rice in China history," *Economic History Review* 9 (1956–7): 2: 200–18; and Philip C. C. Huang, *The Peasant Family and Rural Development in the Yangzi Delta, 1350–1988* (Stanford, 1990).

[127] Golas, 1980; Huang, 1990. See now the more tempered view presented in Li Bozhong. "Was There a 'Fourteenth-Century Turning Point?'," In Paul Jakov Smith and Richard von Glahn, eds., *The Song-Yuan-Ming Transition in Chinese History*, (Cambridge, MA: 2003), 135-175. Li sees the culmination of China's second green revolution only in Ming times but admits that the effects were already being felt in Song times in the Yangtse Delta, which was, after all, the economic powerhouse of the country. See also Richard Von Glahn, "Towns and Temples: Urban Growth and Decline in the Yangzi Delta, 1100-1400," In Smith and von Glahn, eds., 2003: 176-211.

south in the Chinese herbal literature of the time,[128] and increasing availability and range of the exotics brought by Chinese merchants and others from the Southseas and beyond. This revolution is witnessed by a variety of botanical and other works including Zhao Rugua's 趙汝适 *Zhufan zhi* 諸番志,[129] Zhou Qufei's 周去棐 important *Lingwai daida* 嶺外代答,[130] and later by the *YSZY* itself, produced by a court with its own overseas connections.

Chinese food as we know it today owes much of its complexity to Song, and even Jin. An economic boom, the rise of the Middle Class, the growth of national and international trade, and an ideology of refinement and subtlety combined to take Chinese food to new heights of gourmet pleasure. The variety of foods, for example, freely available on the Chinese market, in all but the most poverty stricken parts of China, was far beyond anything hitherto achieved, anywhere in the world. This food was produced not only by agriculture and livestock–raising, but also by highly developed fisheries, by the hunting of wild animals, and even overseas trade. Thanks to a most sophisticated and efficient internal exchange system Chinese food markets, such as those in the former Song capital of Hangzhou, described here, utterly amazed foreign observers such as the Venetian Marco Polo who speaks (in this the version of the text) of no less than ten major markets, along with innumerable others, large and well served by streets, thoroughfares, and bridges, thronged by an abundant populace (he speaks of 40,000–50,000 on market days) and frequented by merchants from all the countries near and far to China and offering every possible variety of raw and processed foodstuff. He mentions in particular a great deal of wild game meats (principally deer and fowl), a full range of meats from domestic animals, a profusion of delicate fresh fish, every kind of vegetable and of fresh and dried fruits, and liquors. Such an abundance there was, he goes on, that local people could eat meat and fish at the same meal, something unheard of in the

[128] The foundation for this was laid in the first regional *Bencao* 本草, Ji Han's 嵇含, *Nanfang caomu zhuang* 南方草木狀. See Li Hui–lin, *Nan–fang ts'ao–mu chuang, A Fourth Century Flora of Southeast Asia* (Hong Kong, 1979).

[129] See Zhao Rugua 趙汝适, *Zhufan zhi jiaozhu* 註番志校注, Feng Chengjun 馮承鈞, Taibei: The Commercial Press, 1967 (1940). See also Friedrich Hirth and W. W. Rockhill, trans., *Chau Ju–Kua: His Work on the Chinese and Arab Trade in the twelfth and thirteenth centuries, entitled Chu–fan–chï* (Chicago, 1966).

[130] See Almut Netolitzky, *Das Ling–wai tai–ta von Chou Ch'ü–fei, eine Landeskunde Südchinas aus dem 12. Jahrhundert*, Münchener ostasiatische Studien 21 (Wiesbaden, 1977).

Europe of the time where fresh (as opposed to preserved) fish was a rare delicacy, directly the opposite of China.[131]

Distinctive regional traditions of cooking had also already become well established by Song.[132] The first true restaurants also appeared. They too were quite unlike anything found in the Western World, as this reaction of Marco Polo makes clear:

> And in proximity to the city there is a great lake which is a good 30 miles around. And all around this lake there are many very fine palaces and very beautiful and rich mansions, belonging to the elite of the city. And there are many abbeys and churches of the idolaters. There are two islands in the middle of this lake and on each of them is a fine and very rich palace looking like the palace of an emperor. And whenever any one from the city wishes to hold some kind of great festival, they would do it in this palace; for they find there prepared silver, and instruments, and everything which they would have at their disposal. And the king provided it to honor his people; and it would be common to all, whoever should hold a festival.[133]

In another version of the text, Marco Polo goes on to speak of a hundred different celebrations going on at once, all accommodated and fed in different parts of the same facility without any interfering with the other.[134] The West Lake is still famous for its restaurants and cuisines.[135]

The following are some examples of the types of recipes served in them in the thirteenth and fourteenth centuries, as recorded by Yuan and early Ming artist and art critic (and food connoisseur) Ni Zan:[136]

---

[131] Henry Yule and Henri Cordier, *The Book of Ser Marco Polo, the Venetian*, vols. 1–2 (Amsterdam, 1975), II: 201–2.

[132] Anderson, 1988: 57ff.

[133] Pauthier, 1978: 495–6. For more information about the many Hangzhou restaurants and specialty foods of the era see also Jacques Gernet, *Daily Life in China on the Eve of the Mongol Invasion*, 1250–1276, Trans. from the French by H. M. Wright (London, 1962), 133ff. See also Michael Freeman, "Sung," in K. C. Chang, 1977: 141–76 and Anderson, 1988.

[134] Yule and Cordier, 1975: II: 187.

[135] For a Ming dynasty celebration of the West Lake and its rich cultural tradition see Tian Rucheng, *Xihu youlan zhiyu* (Shanghai, 1958).

[136] These samples (from pages 34, 27, 28) are from Teresa Wang and Eugene N. Anderson, "Ni Tsan and His 'Cloud Forest Hall Collection of Rules for Drinking and Eating'." *Petits Propos Culinaire,* 60 (1998): 24–41. See now the revised translation in Eugene N. Anderson, Teresa Wang, and Victor Mair, "Ni Zan, *Cloud Forest Hall Collection of Rules for Drinking and Eating,*" in *Hawai'i Reader in Traditional Chinese Culture*, eds. Victor Mair, Nancy Steinhardt and Paul R. Goldin (Honolulu, HI, 2005), 444-455.

Cooking Carp (Recipe #27)

Cut into chunks. Cook in a mix of half water and half wine. Grind peeled and sliced fresh ginger. Mix with flower pepper. Grind again. Gently mix with wine till liquid. Then first add a little soy sauce, then put the fish in the pan. Bring to boil thrice. Then add the ginger–pepper mix. When it boils again, take it out.

Honeyed Stuffed Crabs (Recipe #4)

Cook in salted water. When the color begins to change (to red), take out. Break up the crab and extract the meat from claws and legs. Cut this into small pieces and stuff into the shell. Combine egg with a small amount of honey and mix with meat in shell. Spread some fat on the egg. Steam until the egg has just solidified. Do not overcook. For eating, it can be dipped into ground orange peel and vinegar.

Cooking Wonton (Recipe #7)

Chop the meat finely. Add riced bamboo shoots or wild–rice shoots, [Chinese] chives, or *Basella rubra* tips. Use flower pepper and a bit of apricot kernel paste. Wrap. The skins should start out thick and small when cut out. Then flour them and roll them out. (When stuffed) put into fully boiling water. Stir; do not cover. When they float up, take them out, stirring no longer. Do not use Chinese cardamom in the filling, except to warm the *qi*.[137]

---

[137] The "riced bamboo" is "bamboo shoots (cut up like) grains." Another typically Chinese cookbook of the era is Jia Ming's賈銘 *Yinshi Xuzhi* 飲食須知 (Beijing, 1988), from 1368. Jia Ming was a minor official of Yuan and moderately educated. Living to a purported 106, he was asked by the first emperor of Ming to write down his secrets of longevity. This he did, and they consist mostly of recommendations about food, water and cooking fires (see Mote, 1977: 227–34). Like the *YSZY*, his book is full of recommendations for moderation and of specific taboos on particular combinations: food with food, food with particular behavior, food with particular climate or weather, *etc*. These were loosely grounded in the *yin–yang* 陰陽 and Five Phases system, but, like the *YSZY*'s rules, seem to be a mass of empirical and magical lore somewhat extended and loosely held together by the logic of Chinese medicine. The framework is the same, but the specific content is different: The recommendations and counter indications are not the same as the *YSZY*'s. Also, Jia Ming is much more concerned with water quality (he lived in Zhejiang, where the water was more polluted). His fascination with fires is unique as far as we know. Many pages are devoted to recommending particular fires or firewoods for particular purposes, a bizarre lore not found in the *YSZY* although the Arabic dietary literature, e.g., the cook book of Ibn Sayyar al-Warraq, does know the tradition of associating different humoral properties with different woods for cooking. See Nawal Nasrallah, *Annals of the Caliphs' Kitchens: Ibn Sayyār al-Warrāq's Tenth Century Baghdadi Cookbook* (Leiden, 2007). Nonetheless, we suspect that Jia's recommendations are more often magical than related to actual heat or flavor or even the humoral properties of fires. In any case, Jia's long tables of foodstuffs cover most common Chinese Foods, including a

Another scholar's book of nutritional medicine and refined recipes similart to that of Ni Zan was written by Lin Hong 林洪 (fl. mid-thirteenth century). Like Ni, he also promoted a highly refined cuisine. Based on delicate vegetables, this cuisine could accommodate delicate meats and fish, but—except for an odd stew of wildcat—few more robust meats, though mutton and venison did make it in. Lin Hong warns against certain food combinations, just as the *YSZY* does, and also against the mysterious "wind worm" and other medical problems avoidable through careful eating. Many other cookbooks and food books are known from this period.[138]

The sophisticated Chinese economy of the era, the basis of the cuisine revolution of Song, and reflected in surviving Chinese cookbooks, seemed poised to break through to capitalism and modernity. This it did not do, at least in part because of increasingly autocratic rule and conservative social attitudes (fostered, among other things, by Neoconfucianism); but no one interfered with good eating, and Chinese cuisine grew on when the "sprouts of capitalism" wilted in a veritable food revolution the effects of which persist unto the present day.

The Muslim World

The last of the three cultural and geographical spheres united by the Mongolian empire was the Muslim World.[139] This world was similar to China in many respects: It was also sophisticated, both technologically[140] and culturally, was possessed of great cities and a complicated trade network and economic system, including a highly productive agriculture. There was a Muslim as well as Chinese agricultural revolution,[141] although the Muslim agricultural system had a different

---

vast number not in the *YSZY*. Not surprisingly, he does not mention specifically Near Eastern items like almond, pistachio and most of the spices. No rosewater, saffron, mastic or asafoetida in his Zhejiang!

[138] On Lin see Françoise Sabban, "La diète parfaite d'un lettré retiré sous les Song du Sud," *Études chinoises* XVI (1997): 7-57.

[139] The interpretations given here are strongly influenced by Thomas F. Glick, *Islamic and Christian Spain in the Early Middle Ages* (Princeton, 1979), and the essays in Hayes, 1983. See also Ernest Gellner, *Muslim Society* (Cambridge, 1981).

[140] See, as an introduction to the growing field of the history of Islamic science and technology, Seyyid Hossein Nasr, *Islamic Science, an Illustrated History* (Westerham, 1976).

[141] See, as an introduction, A. M. Watson, *Agricultural Innovation in the Early Islamic World: The Diffusion of Crops and Farming Techniques, 700–1100* (Cam-

foundation than the Chinese. Even more than China, the Muslim West was a world in which bourgeois culture grew and flourished. There were significant differences, other than the obvious ones of culture and of religion, as well.

One was the recognized and accepted cultural diversity of the Muslim World. China was in practice multi–cultural and multi–religious, but in theory monolithic, *i.e.*, Chinese and Confucian, although there was some disagreement from period to period about precisely what these categories entailed. The Muslim World, in contrast, although unified by the framework of Islam, was so diverse that even a fiction of monolithic culture and tradition could not be maintained. There was fundamental division, for example, between the three major cultural groups of Western Islam: Arabs, Iranians, and Turks; leaving aside the complications of India or of points farther east. There were also the strong cultural divisions between those groups which were direct inheritors of Hellenistic culture, principally converts and their descendants living in regions once part of the Roman Empire, and those whose roots lay outside the Roman frontier. Their Hellenism was, as a consequence, indirect. The latter included most Iranians, the Arabs themselves, and the Turks, although Seljuq and Ottoman Turks ultimately came to center their geographical power upon formerly Roman Anatolia.

In addition, even though the Muslim World was the community of Islam, Islam was by no means the only accepted religion practiced so that there never existed in the Muslim World even the theoretical ideological conformity claimed in China by the Confucians. "Peoples of the Book" included a large and healthy Jewish community spread throughout the Islamic world.[142] There were Christian minorities in the West, particularly in Spain, also in Seljuq Anatolia and in Syria. Later Zoroastrians in Iran, and even some Buddhists were recognized as communities under this category.[143]

This cultural diversity, accepted as a fact of life in the Middle East, and in the Muslim World generally, meant an easier acceptance of

bridge, 1983). See also the same author's earlier article "The Arab Agricultural Revolution and Its diffusion, 711–1100," *Journal of Economic History* 34 (1974): 8–35 and more recently his "A Medieval Green Revolution: New Crops and Farming Techniques in the Early Islamic World," in *The Islamic Middle East, 700–900*, ed. A. L. Udovitch (Princeton, 1981), 29–58.

[142] On this community and its culture, as seen from Cairo, see S. D. Goitein, *A Mediterranean Society*, vols. 1–5 (Berkeley, 1967–1988).

[143] See the article "Ahl al–kitab" in H. A. R. Gibb and J. H. Kramers, eds., *Shorter Encyclopaedia of Islam* (Leiden and London, 1961), 16–7.

outsiders such as the Mongols, and the Turks before them. Religious assimilation was expected, but not total acculturation. There was, in any case, no single pattern of acculturation applicable to all.

Thus Mongol conquest was a physical shock for the Muslim World, with the destruction and dislocation it caused. But once converted to Islam, the Mongols became just one more cultural group of the Muslim World. Accommodation with the Mongols in fact began long before conversion and there were few if any groups in Muslim society actively seeking to isolate them culturally. No movement in the Muslim World was comparable to so–called Song loyalism, in which thousands of the south Chinese elite often refused to acknowledge even the existence of the Mongol Yuan Dynasty. Likewise nothing was fully comparable in the Muslim world to endless Chinese disputes over *zhengtong* 正統, the orthodox succession of dynasties, although there was considerable discussion as to exactly who had the right to be caliph, an argument that the Mongols made their own contribution to through a definitive conquest of Baghdad and their ending of the main ʻAbbasid line.

But in China, still, Conquest dynasties of non–Chinese origin were excluded wherever possible. This is a tendency which persists to this day, and which has routinely given later historians difficulty in dealing with the Mongols and their role in Chinese history.

A second significant difference between the Muslim world as it was encountered by the Mongols and China involved attitudes towards the state, society and the good life, including food and the joys that eating and cuisine represented. The state was then generally weak in the Muslim West and then, as in many periods of Muslim history, individual loyalties seldom extended much beyond the walls of a single city, or even a community within it. Family and household, on the other hand, were the central focus of life with the world of religion, and the religious experience providing, for males, the only potential distraction.

In many areas, most noticeably Spain, Muslim society, no matter how public the actions of many of its members, was turned inward. This fact finds reflection, among other things, in the typical Muslim house of the Mediterranean World, with is blank, white outside walls enclosing a lush garden interior, the realm of the family, of relaxation and of individual pleasures. Among them was, for the elite at least, a lavish array of fine foods: Fine breads, sweet drinks, pastries and confections, and many exotic dishes, highly spiced and well prepared.

How could we expect anything less from the people who first popularized refined sugar?

In China, on the other hand, no matter how private the individual, even as a retired scholar, public and other larger social interests dominated. Ideology emphasized service to a usually strong state, and to society, and public not private action. Life in Ancient, Medieval and Early Modern China was turned outward with great emphasis upon the symbolic importance of the acts of the individual within an interconnected and interactive society and cosmos. Even so basic an activity as eating was caught up in such considerations, all the more so if eating was public and ritualistic. There was nothing in Islamic culture equivalent to the great, minutely planned ritual feasts described in Zhou dynasty texts, nor were individual Islamic foods loaded with so much ideological content, or even the power resident in *qi*. A feast might be a political act in Medieval Islam, even an expression of religion (during Ramadan, for example), but the pleasure of it was still one primary justification.

Although a full history of the foods of Middle Eastern, and of the associated Irano–Turkic world of Oasis Turkistan remains to be written, what is known indicates clearly that traditions are very old. Most of the characteristic foodways of the area were already fully developed more than ten thousand years ago (after the domestication of wheat and barley), and perhaps before that. Early Middle Eastern food was based on wheat, barley, sheep and goats, in about that order. Chickpeas and several other legumes (vetch and broad bean, and probably fenugreek) were soon added. So were olive, apple, pear, date, grape, and other tree crops.[144] Pigs, independently domesticated at about the same time in China, and cattle appeared by or before 6000 BC. A wide range of vegetables and minor crops has accumulated over time, whose origins have been forgotten. These included common onions and garlic, known in the Middle East before the dawn of civilization[145] and widely disseminated from there, including to China, at an early date.

By the time civilization began around 3000 BC staples in Egypt and Mesopotamia were bread, beans and milk products, in some places supplemented with substantial amounts of tree crops, principally dates in the hot desert oases. Bread was preferably made from wheat.

[144] See Jack Harlan, *Crops & Man* (Madison, 1975) and Daniel Zohary and Maria Hopf, *Domestication of Plants in the Old World* (Cambridge, 1988).

[145] Zohary and Hopf, 1988.

This is the only grain with the right kind of gluten[146] for leavened bread. Other grains have little gluten or a less "glutinous" form of this protein, and cannot retain many of the bubbles that make bread rise. But wheat is a sensitive crop. It requires a temperate climate and fertile salt–free soil. The poor in marginal areas (hot, dry, cold, wet, saline or alkaline) had to be content with other grains. Leavening with yeast not only raises bread, it also destroys much or most of the phytic acid in the grain husk. This acid forms tight compounds with many nutrients, rendering them unavailable for digestion, and thus greatly lowers the nutritional value of unleavened bread. In most areas of the Middle East leavened bread was thus a matter of life and death, not just a convenience.

Oil was derived from a variety of oilseeds, later, as processing technology improved, from the olive. In most cultures, the earliest oils were melted animal fats, including sheep's tail fat, which continues to be a preferred source of oil in parts of Iran, for example. In recent times, there have been two "quality oils" recognized in the Middle East: olive oil, wherever the olive can be grown, and sesame oil, the "quality oil" of the *YSZY*. Sesame oil was first used in India and appeared in the Middle East rather late, perhaps after 1000 BC.[147] It reached China not much later, perhaps in Han times.[148]

---

[146] Gluten, a special protein molecule, has the property of forming long strings when wet. Relatively abundant in wheat, it forms the tight mesh of strands that traps carbon dioxide gas, allowing bread to rise. A specific form of gluten, originally derived from a race of goat-face grass (*Aegilops squarrosa*) growing in the southwest Caspian Sea region, was bred into wheat about 6000 BC, producing bread wheat. This gluten has an amazing property: it permits the dough to be made into long thin strings, networks, twists, and sheets thin enough to read through. (This was the test of good strudel dough, and some Chinese wrapping doughs are almost as thin.) Other grains do not have it in significant amounts. ("Glutinous" rice, better called "sticky rice," has a form of the starch amylose that becomes sticky when cooking.) To develop gluten, flour is made into dough. The gluten develops after about twenty minutes in the wet dough. During this time, the dough can be kneaded, mixed and stretched. Gluten, like other proteins, makes up a higher percentage of hard red wheats than of soft white wheats. Therefore the former are preferred for bread, which needs to have a good deal of gluten to hold the bases that lets it rise, while the latter are preferred for delicate products like cakes. Pasta requires the most gluten–rich flour of all, durum. Gluten is an "incomplete" protein, not containing all the amino acids necessary in the human diet. However, other proteins in the wheat grain do contain them all.

[147] Zohary and Hopf, 1988: 126.

[148] It should be noted that Chinese sesame oil is quite different from Middle Eastern since the Chinese toasted the seeds, giving a richer, dark colored oil, strongly tasting of sesame.

The existence of fermented beverages is very old in the Middle East. The standard baking and brewing yeast, *Saccharomyces cerevisiae,* finds its natural home on grape skins, and was only secondarily applied to beer and bread.[149] Presumably, bread was earlier leavened with sourdough starters instead of this yeast. The same process of yeast fermentation, so vital to good bread, was early put to work to create alcohol. As a result, beer and wine, including date wine, were consumed in large quantities in all the ancient civilizations of the area. A quite different fermentation, less often stressed but far more important nutritionally, was lactic acid fermentation. This allowed preservation of milk in the forms of yogurt, kefir, kishk (dried yogurt and/or similar dried products, the *qimaq* of the *YSZY*), strained yogurt (labni, *etc.*), and cheese. Lactic acid fermentation was also used to preserve chopped meat in the form of salami and similar sausages.

The diet of the ordinary peasant in the early Middle East, as in remote parts of Iran and Central Asia today, was bread, leavened or not, yogurt or cheese, and whatever wild or cultivated greens and herbs were available, including onion and garlic. In many areas, such as Egypt, beans made up much of the diet and provided crucial protein. Meat was a luxury, but was rarely absent from the festive board of even the poor, for herding and hunting were much more important than in China's metropolitan provinces. In the great riverine civilizations, meat was often very scarce. Fish provided a substitute.

No difference between West Asia and China has been of greater importance than the prevalence of processed grain foods in the former. Gluten, particularly that of bread wheat (*Triticum aestivum*), not only permits leavening of bread, it also makes easy the production of thin, tough sheets, suitable for wrapping food as dumplings or for cutting and cooking as phyllo dough, noodles, and pastas of all kinds. West Asia also grew protein–rich "hard wheat," *Triticum durum*,[150] for its specialized pastas. Most of these seem to date back at least to Greek Classical times and may be older. Only phyllo is a relatively recent Turkic innovation, although one based upon older precedents. It is hard to imagine Arab cooking without *sanbusak,* the filled dough–wrapped dumpling that probably inspired the *piräk* (boreks), *jiaozi* 餃子, and possibly the *manta* that we find in the *YSZY*. Surely, in the Near East, land of flatbreads often filled like sandwiches, cooks must

[149] See now Patrick E. McGovern, *Ancient Wine, the Search for the Origins of Viniculture* (Princeton and Oxford, 2003).

[150] See the discussion of this important Islamic crop in Watson, 1983: 20–3.

have realized early that one could create many things from dough sheets.

The food of the early Middle Eastern civilizations, then, was wheat bread, also barley bread, dairy products, beans, oil crops, fruit, vegetables, beer, meat, and wine, in about that order of importance. The diet of the ordinary person varied considerably from place to place. Bulghur was probably still used as much as bread in the areas to which wheats are native. Beans were much more important in Egypt than in Mesopotamia. Dates and milk seem to have comprised virtually the sole food in some desert oases. India had its own crops, as well as Middle Eastern and Southeast Asian staples, and very early plant–immigrants from Africa, such as sorghum, millets, and watermelon.

To improve on a sometimes bland diet, herbs and some spices in the Near East, and spices in India, became exceedingly important. Most, if not all, of them appear to have been used first for medicinal or nutritional reasons, and only later become integral to culinary art. Thus fenugreek, for example, was an important food in some areas around Mesopotamia, declining to spice status.[151] Apiaceous fruits like caraway, cumin, fennel, and dill "seeds" were used for their carminative and digestive effects, desirable indeed to control flatulence in a diet with a high percentage of beans. Herbs like oregano and tarragon were used for medicinal values. Even lettuce may have been cultivated first as a medicinal herb. The wild form is too bitter for a staple vegetable; the Romans believed that wild lettuce induced sleep, probably because of its milky, opium–like sap.

In the late Persian Empire and early Islamic period, a considerable growth in agriculture took place. Irrigation greatly expanded and its sophistication improved. At least in the Diyala plain and neighboring areas of Mesopotamia, irrigation seems to have reached its apogee in the terminal Sassanian period, reviving to almost or quite as high a point during the 'Abbasid Period, and declining thereafter due to wars that wiped out the works and allowed waterlogging and salt buildup.[152] In the early Islamic period, many crops from Southeast Asia and India came via the connection from Western India to the Gulf and Arabian Sea states. Rice and sugar became widespread, while eggplants, coconuts, mangoes, lemons, limes, taro, cotton, and the like flourished. Watermelons and sorghum from Africa, expanded their

---

[151] Zohary and Hopf, 1988: 110.

[152] Robert McCormick Adams, *Land Behind Baghdad* (Chicago, 1965).

range and even entered China.[153] Thus although the Mongol conquerors of the mid–thirteenth century found a system already in decline from its great days,[154] the Middle East was still a major agricultural power and a brilliantly innovative source of foods and food technologies. These they naturally adopted and disseminated.

With the rise of the great empires, culinary arts reached a high pitch.[155] Dishes often combined wheat products, vegetables, meat and fruit, with spices and herbs added. These added local refinements to pre–existing local dietary differences, producing a range of separate cuisines.[156] From all of this, it is easy to separate out the specific source of the *YSZY's* main Near Eastern component: Mesopotamia and the Persian region. This is the specific area where wheat, chickpeas, meat, and pastas form the basis of dishes; where light spicing with cinnamon, apiaceous "seeds," vinegar and onions is the rule where minced lamb is basic to cuisine, and often used in stuffings; and where tree crops are relatively unimportant. Farther north into Turkey lie the lands of bulghur, fruits, and heavy consumption of vegetables; farther south into Arabia lie lands of heavier spicing, different grain mix, and dates. Westward, the Levant and Egypt used more legumes and tree crops. From sheer proximity and from the course of trade and conquest routes, as well as from historic connections,[157] we would expect to find the Yuan court closest to the Persia–Baghdad axis and this is exactly what we do find.

The most striking difference between *YSZY* and Irano–Mesopotamian cooking is the vastly greater importance of dairy products in the latter but this difference may be more apparent than real. The Mongol elite, and many of their courtiers, consumed vast amounts

---

[153] Watson, 1981, 1983. One suspects that, as with irrigation, Watson's "green revolution" began in pre–Islamic times. He gives little credit to pre–Islamic cultures, and gives suspiciously late dates for several introductions from south Asia.

[154] See Watson, 1983.

[155] See Ann Gunter, "The Art of Eating and Drinking in Ancient Iran," *Asian Art* 1 (1988): 2: 7–52.

[156] See, *e.g.*, Alice Bezjian, *The Complete Armenian Cookbook* (Fair Lawn, 1983); Arto der Haroutunian, *Middle Eastern Cookery* (London, 1982); Julia Najor, *Babylonian Cuisine* (New York, 1981); Claudia Roden, *The New Book of Middle Eastern Food* (New York, 2000); Clifford Wright, *A Mediterranean Feast*: *The Story of the Birth of the Celebrated Cuisines of the Mediterranean from the Merchants of Venice to the Barbary Corsairs, with More than 500 Recipes* (New York, 1999); M. Rodinson, A. J. Arberry and Charles Perry, *Medieval Arab Cookery* (Totnes, Devon, 2001); and Charles Perry, *A Baghdad Cookery Book* (Totnes, Devon, 2006).

[157] See, as an introduction, Schafer, 1963 and Laufer, 1919.

of dairy products (as William of Rubruck, Marco Polo, and Song loyalist poet Wang Yuanliang 汪元量, see below, all attest). Sabban reminds us that milk products were important even to north Chinese at the time.[158] The popularity of dairy products may in fact have been so obvious to Hu Sihui that he saw little need to say much about it. Hu may also have been unaware of the food value of dairy products or found difficulty in evaluating them in terms of Chinese food theory. Another more pronounced difference between the cuisine of the *YSZY* and that of Medieval Iraq is the absence in the former of the marvels of Medieval Arab–Persian cooking: the rich stews of fruit and meat, the huge pies, the dishes with ten or twelve spices, the complicated pasta dishes, the subtleties of all kinds. Hu and the Mongols seem to have found simplicity more healthy and appealing. The only really complex dishes are the Indian ones and the bizarre and unclassifiable *Qurim* [Feast] "Bonnets," which has Arabo–Persian analogs and is as close as Hu comes to the high art of that cuisine.

Many new elements also came in from outside, both with the expansion of Middle Eastern horizons due to the conquests of Islam, and the appearance of major new invaders, mainly Turkic.[159] Turks in fact dominated Middle Eastern life in the years immediately preceding the appearance of the Mongols and expanded their influence greatly in the years after Mongol rule, thanks to political dislocations occasioned by Mongol conquest itself and the many new Turkic groups arriving along with the conquerors.[160]

Seljuq[161] and Mamluk Turks, like the Umayyads and 'Abbasids before them, although remaining true to older indigenous traditions,

[158] See Sabban 1986a. See also Anderson, 1988 and Paul Wheatley, "A Note on the Extension of Milking Practices into Southeast Asia during the First Millennium AD," *Anthropos* 60 (1965): 577–90.

[159] While most general contributions of Turks to Middle Eastern foodways are the product of Ottoman times, except in those areas directly occupied by Turks, the fifteenth century cookbook *Kitab al–Tabakhah* includes at least two purely Turkic dishes, *tutmaj* (the *Tutum ash* of the *YSZY*) and *salma*, "a coin–shaped Turkish soup noodle." See Charles Perry, "Kitāb al-ṭibākha: A Fifteenth Century Cookbook," in *Medieval Arabic Cookery*, Maxime Rodinson, A. J. Arberry, and Charles Perry, editors, Blackawton, 2001), 467–475. For a recent Turkish view of Turkic contributions to Middle Eastern Foodways see Vural Yighit, "Türk–Islam kültürürün, gıda bilim ve teknolojisinin gelismesine katkıları," *Proceedings of the II. International Congress on the History of Turkish and Islamic Science and Technology*, vols. 1–3 (Istanbul, 1986), I, 183–95. See also Paul D. Buell, 1999.

[160] See the discussion in Buell, *op. cit.*

[161] On the history of the Seljuqs see Claude Cahen, *Pre–Ottoman Turkey*, Trans. from the French by J. Jones–Williams (London, 1968).

encouraged the development of cosmopolitan court cultures. They included uniform traditions of cuisine which the Turks spread throughout the Middle East. This development culminated in the generalized Middle Eastern foodways of the late Middle Ages as described from the cookbooks of the era by Peter Heine and others.[162] Their principal characteristics are as follows:

---

[162] On Medieval Arabic and Turkic cooking see, as an introduction, the following:

a) Peter Heine, *Kulinarische Studien, Untersuchungen zur Kochkunst im arabisch–islamischen Mittelalter, mit Rezepten* (Wiesbaden, 1988).
b) ———, *Weinstudien, Untersuchungen zu Anbau, Produktion und Konsum des Weins im arabisch–islamischen Mittelalter* (Wiesbaden, 1982).
c) M. M. Ahsan, *Social Life under the Abbasids*, Arab Background Series, ed. N. A. Ziadeh (London and New York, 1979), 76–164 on food.
d) A. J. Arberry, "A Bagdad cookery book," in *Islamic Culture* 13 (1939): 21–47, 184–214.
e) Bernard Rosenberger, "Les pâtes dans le monde musulman," *Medievales* 16–7 (1989): 77–98.
f) M. Rodinson, "Recherches sur les documents arabes relatifs à la cusine," *Revue des Etudes Islamiques* 17 (1949): 95–165.
g) M. Rodinson, A.J. Arberry and Charles Perry, 2001.
h) Charles Perry, 2006.
i) Necip Usta, *Türk Mutfak Sanati* (Isbanbul, 1999).
j) Leman Cilizoğlu Eryılmaz, *Türk Mutfağından Seçme Yemekler* (Istanbul, 2000).

On modern Middle Eastern cooking see also, in addition to cookbooks already cited above:

a) Tess Mallos, *The Complete Middle East Cookbook* (Sydney, 1979).
b) Ahmad–Chabir Ahmadov, *Azarbajchan Kulinarijasy* (Baku, 1986).
c) A. Bagdasarov, A. Vanukevich, and T. Khudaishukurov, *Turkmenskaya Kulinariya* (Ashkhabad, 1981).
d) *Kazakhskaya Kukhnya* (Almaty, 1981).
e) Arif Tursunov, and Karim Makhmudov, *Uzbekskiye Blyuda* (Tashkent, 1982).
f) Ayla Esen Algar, *The Complete Book of Turkish Cooking* (London, 1985).
g) ———, *Classical Turkish Cooking, Traditional Turkish Food for the American Kitchen* (New York, 1991).
h) Najmieh Batmanglij, *Food of Life. A Book of Ancient Persian and Modern Iranian Cooking and Ceremonies* (Washington, DC, 1990).
i) Elisabeth Rozin, *Ethnic Cuisine, the Flavor Principle Cookbook* (Lexington, 1983).
j) Nawal Nasrallah. *Delights from the Garden of Eden: A Cookbook and a History of Iraqi Cuisine* (author, 2003).

See also the appendix II, "Grain Foods of the early Turks" by Charles Perry in this volume and Silvano Serventi and Françoise Sabban. *Pasta: The Story of a Universal*

1. Extensive use of leavened and unleavened wheat products; with wheat in many cases finely milled into a high quality flour to make very fine and thin doughs; great preference for noodles of various shapes and forms. Whoever invented pasta, the Medieval Arabs were some of its greatest proponents. Hard wheat preferred, especially in pilafs and soups, for couscous, pasta, stuffings. Another grain diffused by the Arabs was sorghum.[163]

2. Extensive use of bean additives; to give body to dishes, and purees made by soaking, trimming, *i.e.*, removal of legume skins, and crushing chickpeas, *e.g.*, in hummus, lentils, mung beans, and other legumes.

3. Great preference for toppings, sauces and stuffings of nuts; including almonds, walnuts, hazelnuts, and pistachios. Also widely used were pine nuts. Nut oils, for example, walnut oil, were used to flavor. The resin of the wild pistachio tree, *Pistacia lentiscus*, was processed into mastic.

4. Use of characteristic vegetables and fruits: Swiss chard and spinach leaf,[164] grape leaf, coriander leaf, parsley, water cress, melilot, mint, purslane, colocasia,[165] globe artichokes, okra, taro, eggplant, carrots, leeks, gourd, asparagus, the radish, tarragon, chicory, beets, turnips, lettuce, pomegranates, red currants, unripe grapes, apples, olives, bananas, and plantains,[166] the coconut (far south),[167] the Hami melon and watermelon,[168] and a great variety of other cucurbits (especially in Turkic–speaking areas), often in the form of a puree (*e.g.*, like *baba ghannouj*). The Persians propagated sour sumac fruit and various sour species of citrus, including the sour

---

Food (New York, 2002).

[163] See Watson, 1983: 9–14. See appendix II by Charles Perry. Perry sees the popularity of many of these grain foods among cosmopolitan Arab cooks as a sign of an on–going Turkicization which later culminated in the new international Middle Eastern cuisine of Ottoman times. See C. Perry, "Three Medieval Arabic Cook Books" (manuscript).

[164] See Watson, 1983: 62–5.

[165] See Watson, 1983: 66–9.

[166] See Watson, 1983: 51–4.

[167] See Watson, 1983: 55–7.

[168] See Watson, 1983: 58–61.

orange (*Citrus aurantium*), the Lemon (*C. limon*), the Lime (*C. aurantifolia*), and the Shaddock (*C. grandis*).[169] Persian, especially northern Persian cooking is unique in the world in its fondness for sour tastes. In many cases vegetables and fruits came as prepared sauces and purees, these including orange blossom and rose water.

5. Extensive use of rice pilafs, particularly among the Turks.[170] Rice dishes were mostly based upon Asiatic rice, extensively propagated by the Arabs.[171] Among the Iraqi Arabs, rice was most often served as a sweet, also in rice puddings.

6. Syrups and sweetmeat puddings (*halwa*); wide use of sugar in various forms, also pastries, candies, jams, a wide range of fruit, and other sweet drinks.[172]

7. Extensive use of yogurt to flavor; also ghee, vinegar, and various cheeses. Other important spices: allspice, asafoetida, basil, bay leaf, black pepper, cardamom, carob, cassia, cinnamon, cloves, coriander seeds, cumin, black cumin, dill, limes, fennel, thyme, clove, fenugreek, nard, garlic, garlic chives, nutmeg, caraway, oregano, rosemary, saffron, salep, sesame seeds, tamarind, troumis (dried and prepared *Lupinus luteus*), and turmeric. Although these were apparently already

---

[169] See Watson, 1983: 42–50.

[170] The association with the Turks may not be accidental. Charles Perry, for example, notes in a letter of 2 January, 1994, to PDB that pilafs appear late and then only in the eastern Arabic world in the thirteenth century cookbooks *Kitab al–At'imah al–Mu'tada* and *Kitab al–Wulsa ila al–Habib*. Since pilafs are not mentioned in the tenth century *Kitab al–Takibh*, and were unknown in Muslim West until much later (there are no pilafs in the two thirteenth century Spanish Arabic cookbooks) he postulates that the pilaf was an eastern Arabic, "post–tenth century innovation." Thus the era in which pilafs first became part of mainstream Middle Eastern cooking is conspicuously the very era when the Turks first appeared and became dominant. Is the pilaf just one more example of the Central Asian love of boiled foods and the influence of this tradition beyond the steppe? See Rodinson, Arberry and Perry, 2001.

[171] See Watson, 1983: 15–9.

[172] As an excellent introduction to the history of sugar and sweets, and how they have changed the world, see Sidney W. Mintz, *Sweetness and Power: The Place of Sugar in Modern History* (New York, 1985). On Arab diffusion of sugar cane growing and processing technology see also Watson, 1983: 24–30 and for China Sucheta Mazumdar, *Sugar and Society in China: Peasants, Technology, and the World Market* (Cambridge, 1998).

on the way out, a great love of rotted condiments. These included *budhaj*, a rotted barley or barley–wheat flour; *murri*, usually prepared from *budhaj* with the addition of spices including "broken carob, fennel stems, citron leaves, pine nuts and pith of bitter orange wood along with a number of spices;"[173] *bunn*, also made with *budhaj*, to which flour of rotted bread and spices is added; and *kamakh* made in various ways with long fermented milk.[174]

8. Sesame oil the preferred cooking oil in all parts of the Middle East; olive oil in areas where it grows. Rendered fat of sheep's tail widely used in most parts of the Middle East, particularly in Iranian and Turkic areas.
9. Lamb as preferred meat; also chicken, beef, fish, and goat. Meat often served with a bean or other puree or covered by a sauce.

The following are some typical examples of the foods (main dishes, including a stuffed fish, a sauce, a relish, and a sweet) of the thirteenth century, and of earlier periods, as described in Medieval Arabic cookbooks largely reflecting Iraqi traditions. Note the close similarity of recipe #1 and several others to *YSZY* recipes and cooking methods that are closely parallel if not identical to some of those found in the Chinese source:

1. *Safarjaliya*

Cut fat meat into small, thin slices and cook in dissolved sheep's tail fat (remove the sediment). Flavor with salt (a *dirham*), finely–ground coriander (two *dirham*), cinnamon bark, and a pinch of mastic. Add water. When nearly done add seasoned, minced meat kebabs. Cook meat in broth. Take large–size, ripe bitter quinces, peel and remove the seeds. Cut into medium–size pieces and add on top of the cooked meat. Pound other quinces in a mortar and extract the juice. Strain and add. Add wine vinegar (5 *dirham*), and sweet almonds (10 *dirham*), finely chopped and soaked in

[173] Charles Perry, "Medieval Near Eastern rotted condiments," paper prepared for the Oxford Symposium 1987: Taste. After experimentation, Perry found traditionally prepared *murri* to be essentially identical to soy sauce. *Murri* was also prepared by adding additional flour to *budhaj*. See Heine, 1988: 55.

[174] See Perry, 1987.

water. Use saffron as a food coloring. Wipe sides of pan clean and settle over a slow fire.

2. *Mudaqqaqat Hamida*

Thinly slice and mince red meat finely. Season with coriander, black pepper, cinnamon, and mastic. Combine with chickpeas and onion and form into large meat balls. Brown meat balls in dissolved sheep's tail fat. Add water to cover meat balls along with two or three cut–up onions. When done skim oil from surface. Sprinkle with a small amount of lemon or grape juice or a combination of both. Sumach or pomegranate juice may also be used. Rub pan with dry mint. Add a small amount of mastic, black pepper, and cinnamon. Wine vinegar may also be sprinkled over the top and saffron added as food coloring. Spray pan lightly with rose water. Wipe sides clean and heat for an hour over a slow fire.[175]

3. *Tharida Shamiyya*

Use lamb, chicken or the meat of some other fowl. Cut into moderate–sized pieces and clean. Remove innards from chicken or the meat of some other fowl and put meat into a clean pot. Add mushrooms soaked overnight along with the water used to soak them. As a substitute for the mushrooms cook honey dark and add water from vegetables preserved in vinegar (*ma'kamikh*). Add mushrooms or honey–vegetable water mixture to pot, along with chickpeas and salt. Cook. Add fresh rue, various kinds of leek, and fresh cilantro to the pot (together not more than 1 *uqiyya*). When cooked, add as seasoning: dried ground coriander, star anise, caraway seed, and black pepper. Add bread chunks and place cooked meat on top.[176]

4. *Buraniya*

Cut fat meat into small pieces. Season with a dash of salt and ground coriander and fry in dissolved sheep's tail fat from which

---

[175] Both of the above examples from A. J. Arberry, 1939: 189–91. Both are from the Arabic food category *nashif*, in which the end product is usually a pilaf or "dry soup." See also Rodinson, Arberry and Perry, 2001.

[176] Heine, 1988: 116. The recipe is from the *Kitab al–Tabikh wa–islah al–aghdhiyat al–ma'qulat* of Muhammad al–Muzaffar b. Nasr b. Sayyar al–Warraq. This is possibly the earliest surviving Arabic cookbook. On the dating see Heine, 1988: 14–15. See now also the detailed discussions in Nasrallah, 2007.

the sediment has been removed. Fry until fragrant and brown. Season with cilantro and cinnamon bark and cover with water. Skim and boil down to one–half. Add several onion halves, salt (1 *dirham*), and finely ground coriander (2 *dirham*), cumin seed, cinnamon, black pepper, and mastic. Season and mince red meat, form into small meatballs and add. Take whole eggplant, remove stalk, make holes with knife and fry with whole onions in sesame oil or dissolved tail. *Murri* may be added to flavor meat when cooked. Use pinch of saffron as a food coloring. Layer fried eggplant on top of meat. Sprinkle with finely–ground coriander and cinnamon and spray with rose water. Wipe sides of serving pan clean and leave for an hour over a slow fire to settle.

5. *Dinariya*

Cut fat meat into small, thin slices and fry lightly in dissolved tail seasoned with salt (1 *dirham*) and finely–ground coriander. Add cinnamon bark and cilantro and cover with water. Skim. Add cut–up peeled onion. Season and mince red meat finely. Form meat into cakes the size and shape of dinar coins and add. Peel large carrots and cut into dinar shapes. Add along with boiled eggs cut into dinar shapes. Fry some egg slices in sesame oil before adding. When cooked, season with finelyground mastic, black pepper, and cumin seed. Sprinkle with mixture of old *murri* (10 *dirham*) and vinegar (3 *dirham*). Add cinnamon (half a *dirham*). Wipe sides of serving pan clean and leave for an hour over a slow fire to settle.[177]

6. Stuffed Fish

Prepare and carefully skin, as large a fish as possible, without damaging the head, fins, tail or the skin itself. Bone fish meat and chop up finely. Season with salt and herbs and continue chopping into a fine marrow. Cover with egg and add sugar and honey. Season with the required quantities of: nard, cloves, cinnamon, ginger, black pepper, cumin, and caraway seed. Also add water from vegetables preserved in vinegar and oil. Add chopped rue and cilantro and add with shelled almonds and sesame seeds. Combine ingredients fully and stuff fish. Sew up any especially large fish prior to baking. Turn fish while baking. Eat with a sauce.[178]

---

[177] Recipes from Arberry, 1939: 191–2, 194–5.

[178] Heine, 1988: 123. The recipe is also from al–Warraq.

7. *Na'na' Mukhallal*

Wash large mint leaves, dry in the shape and sprinkle with aromatic herbs. Celery leaves and peeled garlic are optional. Ferment in a glass bottle covered with a good vinegar and color with a pinch of saffron. Use when the sharpness of the vinegar has been absorbed by the mint.

8. *Isfanakh Mutajjan*

Cut off the lower roots and wash spinach. Dry after boiling lightly in salted water. Fry spinach in refined sesame oil until fragrant. Add chopped garlic. Season by sprinkling with finely–ground cumin, coriander, and cinnamon.

9. *Khabis al–Lauz*

Dissolve sugar (3 *ratl*) in rose water (2 *uqiya*). When the sugar begins to harden add peeled, ground sweet almonds (1 *ratl*). Stir. When ready coat with finely ground sugar. Flour (2 *ratl*) may also be added to the sugar.[179]

Another aspect of Medieval Arabic cuisine, breads and breadmaking is described in detail by M. M. Ahsan. He records an incredible variety of breads made from millet, rice, barley, or wheat, although wheat bread was preferred and recommended by Muslim physicians. The two main varieties of bread were *al–khubz al–huwwara* and *al–khubz al–khashkar*, the former made from a fine white flour and the latter from coarse, whole grains. Then as now, people preferred the quality and texture of the white bread. Milling was done at home by women in rural areas but by commercial mills in the cities. Most baking was also done commercially, even of dough kneaded at home. Bread came in all shapes and sizes, sometimes in a bulbous loaf, more often as a kind of waffle or a flatbread. Extremely thin, wide breads baked in a *tannur* were known as *awraq al–riqaq*, "flat bread leaves," or simply *riqaq*. Breads could be prepared plain or stuffed with honey, sugar, ground or whole almonds, mastic or other flavors and sweets. *Khushknanaj*, for example, a bread of Persian origin, was made from white flour into which sesame oil was worked, and was stuffed with ground almonds and a scented sugar, combined using rose water. *Akras Mukallala* was a loaf bread made from dough combining flour and a scented paste of ground pistachios and a syrup. After baking loaves were glazed with scented sugar dissolved in water. *Khubz al–*

[179] Recipes from Arberry, 1939: 205–6, 210.

Abazir was made from dried dates, shelled sesame seeds, roasted poppies, rose water, and either almonds or pistachios. Another special kind of bread was glazed with borax (*bawraq*) specially imported from Lake Van in Armenia for the purpose. Some popular breads were named after their inventors or the baker who first baked them.[180]

Judging from the above examples, by no means exhaustive of even the major categories of the Arabic cooking of the time, the range, complexity and quality of foods available in the Medieval Arabic world was impressive even by the most jaded modern standards. The Near and Middle East also seems to have been as diverse then as now. Indeed, the *YSZY* recipes show Near Eastern food in a quite modern form. Recipe #2 is still common in north Iraq and neighboring areas. The recipes for lamb marinated in saffron and rosewater and then broiled are recognizably Arab. Several other recipes can be linked with modern recipes characteristic of various parts of the region. There is every reason to believe that they were linked with the same parts in Mongol times. Near Eastern local foodways differ greatly from place to place, due to differences in ecology and history.

Also an impressive feature of medieval Near Eastern foodways is the degree to which Bagdhadi and other Islamic cooks and aficionados of the ‘Abbasid and post–‘Abbasid world sought to communicate their skills to the outside world in what has to be the world's first fully–developed cookbook literature[181] beginning with the *Kitab al–Tabikh wa islah al–aghdhiyat al–ma‘qulat* of Muhammad al–Muzaffar b. Nasr b. Sayyar al–Warraq, dating to the tenth century and including the most important *Kitab wasf al–At‘imah al–Mu‘tadah*, later re–edited by Muhammad b. al–Hasan b. Muhammad b. ‘Abd al–Karim al–Katib al–Baghdadi as the *Kitab al–Tabikh*, the basis, in a further abridgment, of the Daud al–Chelebi text translated by A. J. Arberry as "A Baghdad Cookery Book."[182] Two examples from the *Kitab al–Tabikh wa islah al–aghdhiyat al–ma‘qulat* are cited above along with several examples from the Daud al–Chelebi text.

---

[180] See M. M. Ahsan, 1979: 87–9.

[181] This, of course, is not to deny the importance of Greek and Roman traditions represented by Athenaeus and Apicius respectively and other authors whose works have not survived. See as an introduction John Edwards, *The Roman Cookery of Apicius, Trans. and Adapted for the Modern Kitchen* (London, 1984). We also now know that the Medieval Iraqis built upon traditions stretching back to the Bronze Age. See the discussion in Peter James and Nick Thorpe, *Ancient Inventions* (New York, 1994).

[182] See Charles Perry, "Three Medieval Arabic Cook Books."

In these books recipes, not food lore, are the direct focuses, with sufficient information provided so that foods described can be prepared more or less from the descriptions given alone, provided that one has a basic knowledge of the cooking traditions which the recipes represent. Arabic cookbooks also provide considerable information about cooking techniques, kitchens and kitchen implements, about individual foodstuffs, and in many cases, about the medicinal properties of foods. Some, like the *YSZY*, even provide specific recipes for medicinal foods designed to cure this or that condition.[183]

There is nothing like this in China prior to the *YSZY* and Ni Zan's *Yunlintang yinshi zhidu ji*, at least no such reliably dated work has survived. We do have occasional recipes and even short collections of recipes, books of food anecdotes, lists of famous dishes (but no recipes), short description of how to cook with this or that ingredient, and even detailed expositions of dietary and sometimes cooking principles.[184] But, if we may judge by the materials translated by Gwinner,[185] real cookbooks, that is, specialized texts devoted more or less entirely to recipes, ingredients, cooking techniques, and to food lore as an organized and focused whole, did not emerge in China until the fourteenth century and cannot be said even to have been a popular genre, in spite of Chinese interests in this area, until early Qing 清 times, at the earliest. The Muslim world, on the other hand possessed real cookbooks at least four centuries before China with the late twelfth, early thirteenth century, *i.e.*, the period just before Mongol conquest, and the linking of East and West, a period of particular interest in literature of this type.[186]

Chronologically therefore, the cookbook as we know it today was clearly an Arab invention and while the Chinese equivalents may have

---

[183] The most prominent early Arabic cookbook to include medicinal recipes is the *Wusla ila l–habib fi wasfi l–tayyibati wa–l–tib*, of Kamal ad–Din b. al–Adim, extensively studied by M. Rodinson in Rodinson, 1949: 117ff. See also the discussion in Perry, "Three Medieval Arab Cook Books." Al–Warraq, includes a section on "the beneficial and harmful properties of various foods" See Ahsan, 1979: 77. A work devoted entirely to the theme of food and medicine is Mahmud ibn Ilyas al–Shirazi's *Tuhfat al–Hukama*. See the discussion in Cyril Elgood, A *Medical History of Persia and the Eastern Caliphate*, revised edition (Amsterdam, 1979), 312–13. Ibn Ilyas was a confident of Rashid al–Din, the great minister of the Il–qans. On Arabic dietary medicine proper see the discussion in Ullmann, 1978: 97–106.

[184] But this is not to say that the Chinese had no well developed tradition of dietary medicine. See the discussions in the next chapter.

[185] Gwinner, 1988.

[186] See Heine, 1988: 14–6.

been independently derived, and the cookbook thus independently invented in China, it is highly suspicious that cookbooks begin to appear in numbers there just after the establishment of the Mongol empire, suggesting a West–East diffusion of at least the idea of the cookbook. That more than the idea may have been involved is, however, clear from detailed comparison of the content of slightly earlier or contemporary Arab cookbooks with the *YSZY*.

There are many reasons why such cookbooks should first appear in the Islamic World, then be transmitted east, to China. First of all, as indicated earlier, was the highly developed interest of the Islamic World in good eating for its own sake. Secondly, there was the important factor of receptivity of Islamic society to a developed cuisine and to cookbooks describing it in the period just prior to Mongol conquest. Finally, there was the matter of the cultural interchanges represented by the early cookbooks. China was certainly willing to take up new recipes from abroad, but not openly. The Muslim World was openly multi–cultural and cultural interchange was fundamental to its existence and a way of life. The surviving Medieval Islamic cookbooks are one clear witness.

CHAPTER TWO

ANALYSIS OF THE TEXT

I. Introduction

We have shown in Chapter 1 that the Mongol world order, including qanate China, was supranational in character. Mongols dominated politically, and to some extent socially, but were very few in number and thinly spread. As a consequence they were hardly in a position to force others to become Mongol, or to impose more than superficial conformity with important Mongol customs. Mongol conquerors were exposed to, and welcomed the influence of, other cultures as long as they could continue to perceive themselves as Mongols.[1]

Food and cuisine were no exceptions. Mongols were willing to try new foods and dishes, with lavish and conspicuous public consumption to promote their new role as would-be rulers of the world. Many of the new foods even gained their ultimate acceptance, but the conquerors remained remarkably true to their own traditions as well.

The *YSZY* is unmistakable proof of the power and stamina of Mongolian food preferences. The work is in Chinese and embodies a framework of Chinese medical and dietary theory within which Chinese, Mongolian, Turkic, and Turko–Islamic elements freely coexist. Yet it is not the dietary's overriding Chinese theory and culture which

---

[1] The following incident from the travelogue of William of Rubruck makes very clear just how important identity was for Medieval Mongols (see Wyngaert, 1929: 205):

> Thus as a consequence going towards Baatu due east, we arrived at the Ethilia [Volga] on the third day and when I saw the waters of that river I wondered from where in the north so much water descended. Before leaving Sartach, the above mentioned Coiac said to us, along with many other secretaries of the court: "Do not say that our lord is a Christian, for he is not a Christian but a Moal." For this is because the name Christian seems to them to be the name of some people, and they have such a pride that although perhaps believing something of Christ, they are nonetheless unwilling to be called Christians, desiring their own name, that is, Moal, to be exalted above all other names.

provides the unifying element. It is rather, in Sabban's words, "des goûts mongols,"[2] the "Mongol tastes," which dominate the work from beginning to end, no matter how Chinese it may appear on the surface. The *YSZY* is in its essence a Mongolian document, but this is not to say that the Mongol foods or culture of the fourteenth century *YSZY* represent purely ancestral usage. A great deal had changed since the days of Cinggis–qan.

At the time the *YSZY* was written, the Mongol elite had left the steppe behind for more than 100 years. New political and social alliances had been made. There had been new compromises with the sedentary world, including China, so that local Mongolian rule could continue after the collapse of empire in regionally–based successor qanates. In forming these qanates Mongols had collaborated closely with representatives of many other cultures. It may even be argued that, in addition to broader accommodations within a greater world order, the Mongols had only been able to come to power in China through close alliances forged with the various ethnic groups and regional communities of the culturally diverse north.

These alliances continued to be important even after the establishment of Yuan. The Mongols, for example, continued to recruit northerners by preference among their Chinese subjects. They continued to base their power in the north even after the conquest of Song in 1276, and continued to regard the north as the most important, if not richest, part of their East Asian domains. They even discriminated legally against southerners, barred in theory from holding most high offices.[3]

---

[2] Françoise Sabban evaluates the *YSZY* as follows: "Média au service des détenteurs du pouvoir, ces Mongols à peine sinisés, encore imprégnés des odeurs de la steppe, le traité de Hu Sihui apparait comme une traduction dans le langage de la cuisine chinoise des appétits et des goûts mongols." See page 42 of her excellent study "Cuisine à la cour de l'empereur de Chine: les aspects culinaires du *Yinshan Zhengyao* de Hu Sihui," *Medievales* 5 (November, 1983): 32–56. Our evaluation agrees with hers with the significant difference that we also see a Turkicization as well as Sinicization of *YSZY* recipes, and a translation into the conventions of Muslim as well as Chinese cuisine. Sabban's French–language article has appeared in an English version as "Court Cuisine in Fourteenth–Century Imperial China: Some Culinary Aspects of Hu Sihui's *Yinshan Zhengyao*," *Food and Foodways* I (1986): 161–96. (Henceforth Sabban, 1986b.)

[3] In the Yuan political/judicial hierarchy of the fourteenth century, Mongols and their West Asian allies (*semu ren* 色目人) ranked first, followed by north Chinese (including assimilated members of non–Chinese groups such as Khitan and Jürched) and southerners, with the former enjoying far more rights. The classic study of this

The northern orientation of the Yuan court was thus political reality. It had its profound influence upon the political history of the dynasty, and upon the Mongols themselves. It also strongly colored Mongol perceptions of China. It was the culture of the north, for example, which came to signify Chinese culture for the conquerors. Since this culture was anything but purely Chinese in the fourteenth century, there is much in the *YSZY* which seems highly assimilated, in addition to the purely non–Chinese influences present there.

North China was probably less than 80% Chinese ethnically in the fourteenth century,[4] and many of these Chinese participated in quite

---

hierarchy remains Meng Siming 蒙思明, *Yuandai shehui jieji zhidu* 元代社會階級制度 (Hong Kong, 1967).

[4] It is extremely difficult to estimate the ratio of Chinese to non–Chinese in North China during the fourteenth century. Available Yuan dynasty statistics are incomplete and fail to provide an ethnic breakdown. Vorob'yev (1975: 295), using better Jin dynasty figures, has estimated that 87% of the population of Jin domains was "Chinese" at the beginning of the twelfth century, 10% Jürched, 1% Bohai 渤海, 2% Khitan. He gives no figures for other non–Chinese groups inhabiting Jin domains, known to have been together perhaps as numerous as the Khitan. They included Turkic–speakers, other "Hui 回," Tanguts living outside of Xixia 西夏, and other small but still distinct cultural groups. All have apparently been lumped by him with the "Chinese" whose numbers must be adjusted accordingly. Any estimate of the ethnic breakdown for North China as a whole must also take into account the population of Xixia, a large percentage of which was Tangut, in addition to smaller numbers of other non–Chinese groups including Turkic–speakers and other "Hui." At best the Chinese were a bare majority in this small but relatively populous state, judging from the archaeological remains of the period. Thus substantially less than 87% of North China's total population was Chinese *circa* 1200, probably less than 85%, the actual figure depending upon how large the total population of Xixia was at the time. In 1330 the total population of the North was almost certainly smaller than it was in 1200, among other things due to the damage inflicted by the Mongol conquest itself. The percentage of non–Chinese was also higher, both due to the entry of new groups, including the Mongols, and the Turks and others they brought along with them, and differential proportions of demographic loss for Chinese versus non–Chinese groups. The Mongols actively promoted pastoralism within their early conquests at the expense of agriculture. They favored the tribal groups which were their closest allies over the local Chinese who almost certainly suffered heavier losses during the establishment of Mongolian rule in the north. A general recession of Chinese settlement in the north particularly noticeable in the Sino–Mongolian borderlands was one result. Although Qubilai, more dependent upon China and the Chinese, looked more favorably upon his Chinese subjects, Yuan policy continued to favor non–Chinese groups in the North, the Jürched, for one example. Only their Sinicized elite had been destroyed by the Mongols, not the masses of Jürched still living more or less in the traditional way as the strength of the Manchus two centuries later makes clear. In addition, most of the tribal groups probably had reproduction rates considerably higher than village and urban Chinese

divergent local cultures. Some of them had strong non–Chinese roots going back centuries. The degree of Turkicization of North China since the early Middle Ages in particular remains unassessed but must have been substantial.

The proportion of Chinese to non–Chinese was greatest in the old cultural heartland of the north, along the Wei 渭 and Yellow Rivers, and in Shandong 山東. It decreased rapidly as one went west and north. Northeast China, centered around what is now Beijing 北京, for example, where the Mongol court spent most of the year, was perhaps half Chinese at best. It was an area which had, in any case, become thoroughly accustomed to foreign rule and influence thanks to a succession of steppe conquerors and local non–Chinese rulers from late Zhou times on.[5] Present in the north were various Tungus groups, such as the Jürched, and Bohai, surviving Tanguts, and tribal Khitan increasingly assimilated to Mongolian and Tungus–speaking neighbors, and "Hui," North China's Muslim community. By the fourteenth century the latter included many new arrivals from points west. The key Turkic communities of the North had also received much new blood during the Yuan period, and thus considerable cultural influence from without.

---

and were more likely to have recovered sooner demographically for any lingering effects of Mongol conquest and, given favorable conditions, to have rapidly increased in numbers. For these reasons the non–Chinese population of North China was likely to have been considerably higher proportionally in 1330 than it was in 1200, although absolute numbers may have been about the same. The figure given here seems a reasonable guess.

[5] A full history of the complex cultural interactions which have characterized North China since the dawn of recorded history are beyond the scope of this study. However, one source (from 1296) cited by Rall brings home the degree of mutual assimilation of all North Chinese cultures of the fourteenth century quite forcefully. In it the zhongshu sheng 中書省 complains of disorder in a Beijing market called *Bazaer* 八匝兒, Y *patsarʐ̩*, Persian *bäzär*, English bazaar, making clear from the types of disorder, and activities, mentioned that the market was in every respects just that, an oriental bazaar. See Jutta Rall, *Die vier grossen Medizinschulen der Mongolenzeit*, Münchener ostasiatische Studien 7 (Wiesbaden, 1970), 24. The example points of the error of thinking of North China, under the Mongols, or in any period, as too narrowly Chinese in culture. Chinese culture has been as assimilative as any other and has also had to redefine itself constantly. The Yuan period is simply one era in which this redefinition was particularly striking. All reconstructions marked Y, L and E, standing for Yuan, Late Middle and Early Middle Chinese, are from Edwin G. Pulleyblank, *Lexicon of Reconstructed Chinese, in Early Middle Chinese, Late Middle Chinese, and Early Mandarin* (Vancouver, 1991).

There were three distinct groups of Turks in China or in nearby border–lands in the fourteenth century. Most important were the Islamized and Sinicized oasis and Inner Mongolian Turks, principally the Uighur[6] but also included the largely Christian Önggüd.[7] There groups were so similar in culture that they are often confused in our sources.[8] Scarcely less important were representatives of other Turkic groups present in China with still strong pastoral nomadic traditions. These were principally the largely Kipchaq–speaking Turkic guards[9] of the Mongol *qan* of China, guards so politically important during the last half century of Mongol rule in China.[10] These Turks were far less influenced by Islam and Middle Eastern culture, or by China, but were increasingly in touch with larger patterns of Eurasian cultural development through their association with the Mongol court. More marginal but still influential due to long–term historical interaction with the Mongols and common cultural experience were the more primitive, culturally unassimilated Turkic groups, ancestors of today's Al-

---

[6] On the Uighurs in Yuan times see T. T. Allsen, "The Yuan Dynasty and the Uighurs of Turfan in the 13th. century," in M. Rossabi, ed., *China Among Equals* (Berkeley, 1983), 243–80. See also Igor de Rachewiltz, "Turks in China under the Mongols: a Preliminary Investigation of Turco–Mongol relations in the 13th. and 14th. Centuries," in the same volume, 281–310. On the culture of one Eastern Turkistan Uighur community in a somewhat earlier period see also A. von Gabain, *Das Leben im uighurischen Königreich von Qocho (850–1250)*, Veröffentlichungen der Societas Uralo–altaica 6, vols. 1–2 (Wiesbaden, 1973).

[7] See P. Pelliot, *Recherches sur les chrétiens de l'Asie centrale et d'Extrême–orient* (Paris, 1973).

[8] The term Uighur is often used indiscriminately in Yuan era texts to refer to members of both groups, pointing up the difficulty contemporaries had in distinguishing between them. Rabban Sauma, for example, is called an Uighur in some texts, although there is every indication that he was an Önggüd. See Pelliot, *op. cit.*: 242ff. See also Paul D. Buell's biography of Chinqai in Igor de Rachewiltz, Chan Hok–lam, Hsiao Ch'i–ch'ing, and Peter W. Geier, editors, *In the Service of the Khan, Eminent Personalities of the Early Mongol–Yuan Period (1200–1300)* (Wiesbaden, 1993), 95–111, and Paul D. Buell, "Chinqai (ca. 1169–1252): Architect of Mongolian Empire," in *Opuscula Altaica, Essays Presented in Honor of Henry Schwarz*, Studies on East Asia 19, eds. Edward H. Kaplan and Donald W. Whisenhunt (Bellingham, 1994), 168–86.

[9] On the Kipchaq (Qangli) and other foreign guards of the Mongol *qan* of China see, as an introduction, Hsiao Ch'i–ch'ing, *The Military Establishment of the Yuan Dynasty* (Cambridge and London, 1978), 92 ff.

[10] See de Rachewiltz, 1983, and J. W. Dardess, *Conquerors and Confucians, Aspects of Political Change in Late Yuan China* (New York, 1973).

tay Turks and Soyot, among others, positioned at the outermost limits of Yuan authority.

Mongol contacts with all of these Turkic groups were of relatively long standing. They substantially predated the era of Mongol Empire, when contacts were enhanced and broadened. Turks had controlled the steppe before the Mongols. As the latter emerged as a nation they took over not only elements of Turkic pastoral nomadic material culture (*e.g.*, clothing, housing, the outfittings of pastoralism, and probably a good part of their foodways), but intellectual and spiritual elements as well. The Mongolian language, for example, is replete with words and expressions derived from Turkic. Mongolian folklore and religion are also heavily influenced by Turkic traditions. During the earliest days of Mongolian Empire Turks taught the Mongols how to write and helped them govern.[11] More recently, Turks, as the one group well represented in all parts of the Mongolian world order, had come to be key links between its various Mongols, and also intermediaries between Mongols and a greater Turkic and Islamic world beyond. Sinicized groups such as the Uighurs also helped introduce Chinese culture to the Mongols, more willing to borrow it through their Turkic cousins than directly. Turks, after all, unlike the Chinese, spoke languages closely related to Mongolian and were pastoral nomads or descendants of pastoral nomads, with values similar to those of the Mongols.

Mongol fascination with all things Turkic finds its expression in the *YSZY* in the text's many purely Turkic dishes (**ishkänä*,[12] **shoyla*

---

[11] Note, however, significantly, that the fourteenth century Mongolian word for *shaobing* 燒餅, "roast bun," was *ütmek*, from Turkic *ötmek*, rather than the Chinese. See Antoine Mostaert, *Le matériel mongol du Houa I I Iu de Houng–Ou (1389)*, Melanges Chinois et Bouddhiques 18, ed. Igor de Rachewiltz and Anthony Schönbaum (Bruxelles, 1977), 109. This same source, although reflecting the late fourteenth century usage of the Eastern Mongols, reveals other Middle Eastern borrowings for foods as well including *arbus*, "watermelon," from the Persian *xarbuze*, "melon," *badinqa*, "eggplant," from Persian *badenjan*, and *üdzüm*, "grape," from the Turkic *üzüm*.

[12] The Chinese for the title of recipe 33 (1, 36B), a topping for the Iranian bread, called for in the recipe, is *weixiang* 圍像, Y *ujsjaŋ*, we think from the *ishkänä* known in Iranian sources. On the word see G. Doerfer, 1963–75: IV, 261. This word appears to be perfectly good Turkic in which case the *ish–* or *esh–* means "one of a pair, companion." The similarity to the Western *companatium*, "food eaten with bread," is striking. Note the much–assimilated, modern Iranian recipe for *ehkeneh*, here an "onion soup," in Batmanglij, 1990: 33.

toyym[13]), above all Turkic and Turkicized bread and grain foods (*pirӓk, tutam ash, um ash, *chuqmin*[14]), integral parts of Mongolian court cuisine. It also finds expression in many Mongolian recipes Muslimized almost certainly through the agency of Turks. A large part had increasingly become bearers of Islamic Iranian and Arabic culture, as well as their own, by the thirteenth and fourteenth centuries and a principal source of Muslim influence for the *YSZY* as a whole.

One example, among many, of such a Turkicized and Muslimized *YSZY* recipe is #32 in *juan* 1 (36b), "Roast Wolf Soup." Hu Sihui freely admits in his introduction to the recipe that it has been modified, in this case largely through the addition of Muslim spices used by Medieval Turkic cooks.

The presence of so many diverse cultural groups in North China, their mutual assimilation to one another, sometimes in interactions extending over a thousand years or more, and the clear impact of the many Chinese and non–Chinese local cultures of North China upon the Mongols and their court culture and cuisine, makes precise definition of the various cultural layers of the *YSZY* at times difficult. A particular problem is distinguishing Chinese from non–Chinese traditions that are similar due to mutual borrowings and use of the same foods for the same purposes.

Mutton and dairy products, for example, were both important in the northwestern Chinese diet of the time. The mutton dishes of the *YSZY* may not always reflect Central Asian influence and the use of dairy products there seems on the surface to be more typical of north Chinese than steppe norms. Sabban, for example, in her superb study of

---

[13] Franke (Franke, 1970: 9) prefers to read the first character of the name of recipe #44 (1, 39b), 搠, as *chuo*, rather than the expected *shuo* (搠 is not in Pulleyblank but 朔 is Y ʂwaw). Either way, *shuolo* 搠羅 (perhaps Y *ʂwawlɔ)* or *cholo* represents something quite close of Modern Uighur *šoyla*, "a very thick porridge consisting mostly of rice, fat, carrots and meat" (Schwarz, 1992: 523). The second word, Chinese *tuoyin* 脫因, Y *t^hɔjin*, is clearly related to *toyyim*, a word not in the Schwarz dictionary but in Modern Kazakh meaning "abundance," "profusion," "satiation," a derivative of *toy*, "feast." Note that the food is specifically labeled as Uighur.

[14] The Chinese is *zhengbing* 䭪餅, "*zheng* cakes," or "*zheng* bread," with a rare character for *zheng*. The reading for both characters might have been *tʂiŋpiŋ* during Yuan. The description (in recipe #93; 1, 49b) makes it extremely likely that what is known in Mahmud of Kashgar's dictionary as *chuqmin*, steamed "in a special pot," is meant. As Perry suggests, the *+min* of *chuqmin* may be from Chinese *mian* 麪. It could be a very old borrowing, from E *mɛn^h*. The word does not seem to occur outside Central Asia. See also Appendix II.

the *YSZY*, gives statistics on how often these ingredients figure in the book. Dairy products figure in only 12 of the 95 full–scale recipes in *juan* 1, as opposed to 72 that include mutton, and a few others that include minor sheep products.[15]

Since Sabban's list concentrates on the assimilated exotic recipes of *juan* 1, it fails to take into consideration fermented milks listed elsewhere, many by their Central Asian names, *e.g.*, *qatiq*. Independent evidence also indicates that most fermented milk products were consumed directly by Mongols and Turks as preferred foods, not as ingredients in other foods, and were available in abundance during feasts.[16] Even in the *YSZY*, dairy foods are more evident than they would be in modern China.

Also complicating the problem of determining cultural influences present in the *YSZY* is the influence there of cultural groups which were numerically insignificant but which, through a close association with the court, exercised an inordinate influence. We have already mentioned the Turkic guards of the *qan*. Their members must have been the source of northern Turkic vocabulary and foodways that is a minor tradition in the *YSZY*, but is represented none the less, *e.g.*, in the typically steppe–Turkic sausage and tripe recipes of *juan* 1. See particularly recipes #57 and #72, a classic **qazi*[17] and *qarta*, two popular varieties of Turkic "sausage," respectively. Another small but influential group was comprised of Tibetans and associated Kashmi-

---

[15] Sabban, 1986b: 171.

[16] The Sung loyalist Wang Yuanliang 汪元量, an eyewitness to Mongol feasting at Qubilai's court as an unwilling participant, specifically mentions in his account the prominent serving of kumiss. Other foods mentioned by him are: "tender" scallions (*jiu* 韭), onions, served together on an engraved platter, horse meat and roasted mutton, congee to wash it down with, a ruby–red grape wine, diced chicken (*tianji* 天雞), steamed and roasted venison, bear meat, quail, and pheasant. See Wang Yuanliang, *Shuiyun ji* 水雲集, Wulin wangzhe yishu edition 武林往哲遺著, 7b–8a.

[17] The Chinese transcription for **qazi* in this recipe (1, 43a) is *qianzi* 簽子, Y *tshjɛmtsz̧*, usually referring to a flat, bamboo tally, also a bamboo slip, which makes no sense here. This must be a foreign word and, although the fit is not perfect, the phonological similarity to Turkic *qezi* cannot be an accident. The recipe, in any case, does describe the making of such a Turkic sausage. On the preparation of *qezi* or *qazi* from sheep intestines in Mongol times see Doerfer, 1963–75: III, 359–60. For the modern Kazakhs see also Dosymbek Qatran, *Qazaqtyng Dasturli As-tagham Madeniyeti* (Almaty, 2002), 30-44. For the Kazakhs, *qazy* is, by definition, from the horse and secondarily from camels, but it is also made in the modern Turkic world from sheep intestines, as here.

ris.[18] They must be the source of the two *YSZY* recipes which are specifically from the area of north India and south Tibet (#3 and #49). In addition, Rashīd al-Dīn specifically associates Tibetan doctors with the dietary regimen of the Mongol court in China.[19]

In the following pages we will examine in detail Mongol, Turkic, and other cultural influences at work in the *YSZY*, including evaluation of key Chinese contributions: the medical framework of the whole and a pervading Chinese culinary influence. In the final section of this chapter we will examine *YSZY* foods in their broader social context, with particular reference to the social, political and cultural message which the foods and medical lore of the text are intended to convey. We begin our survey with the Mongolian elements of the text.

II. Analysis

"Des Goûts Mongols:" the Persistence of the Steppe

Mongolian culture finds expression in the *YSZY* in Mongolian foods, medicines,[20] terminology, and cooking traditions found there, in the ideological orientation and framework of the text, and in its specific mix of traditions. Like the qanate of China itself, the *YSZY* is neither Chinese, nor Mongolian, nor, for that matter, Middle Eastern. The Chinese base of the Mongol East Asian qanate is implicitly acknowledged. The opening passages of the dietary, for example, in spite non–

---

[18] On Tibetans at the Yuan court see Herbert Franke, "Tibetans in Yuan China," in John D. Langlois, Jr., ed., *China under Mongol Rule* (Princeton, 1981), 296–328. See also Paul D. Buell, "Tibetans, Mongols and Cultural Fusion," *Islam and Tibet, Interactions along the Musk Route* (Aldershot, Hants, forthcoming).

[19] See Christopher I. Beckwith, "Tibetan Science at the Court of the Great Khans," *Journal of the Tibet Society*, 7 (1987), 5-11 (6-7). The individuals involved were the associates, Mongolian *nöker*, of the noted Tibetan dignitary Sga A-gnyan Dam-pa (1230-1303), well known in Chinese and non-Chinese sources.

[20] We are indebted to our colleague Tamsin Hekala for pointing out that the garden burnet and cinquefoil used by Hö'elün in maintaining herself and her children under difficult conditions are not only widely–used foods but have medicinal properties as well and may have been used by Hö'elün with just these properties in mind to heal as well as feed. Burnet, for example, is used in treating dysentery, is a vermifuge, and applied externally is good for burns and various skin diseases. See Lily M. Perry and Judith Metzger, *Medicinal Plants of East and Southeast Asia, Attributed Properties and Uses* (Cambridge and London, 1980), 347.

Chinese content so abundant elsewhere, appeal strongly to Chinese tradition by calling upon the three patron saints of Chinese herbal medicine, the Yellow Emperor, Fuxi 伏羲, and Shennong 神農, but elsewhere the *YSZY* primarily expresses an institutional and cultural compromise between almost all the various groups represented at the Mongol court. Intentional violence is done to the sensitivities of none. Mongolian political institutions were similar: free combinations of Mongolian, Chinese, Turkic, and Middle Eastern ideas. A veneer of standardizing Chinese terminology and apparent Sinicization was carefully maintained to mask an often quite un–Chinese reality.

It may even be argued that the many *YSZY* recipes, Mongolian in essence, but cooked with Muslim spices and additions, sometimes in a Chinese way, are artificial and the result of a conscious attempt on the part of the Mongols to create a new international cuisine, one with something for everyone. In this respect the banquet soups of *juan* 1 may parallel *qan* Qubilai's attempt, in another realm, to create a universal alphabet with his aPhags–pa Script. The foods, medicines and advice of the *YSZY* are thus an eloquent political and ideological statement, expressing simultaneously the supranational character of the Yuan court, its power, and the world–conquering, world–ruling spirit of its rulers, the Mongols.

In this latter connection the Mongol imperial table followed the grand tradition of court foods in Eurasia in setting a huge, splendid, festive board on which everything from swans to venison found their place. It was laden with many kinds of meat, notably including the most spectacular and exotic species available. Fancy drinks were served in golden fountains. There were visually dazzling displays of color and edible sculpture. It also boasted many rare delicacies of magically restorative and potency–inducing efficacy. The *qan*, like other Emperors, had to impress the world with the manifold ways in which they could obtain, increase, and display their personal powers. In this regard, the medical lore of the *YSZY* is inseparable from its food lore. Like the taste and color of the food, its medical values made a statement about the great and increasing power of the sovereign. This power was sexual, social, muscular, and financial all at once. It was also cosmological. The medical rules of the *YSZY* are an inseparable component of the cosmic order. The empire and, above all, its rulers had to function in accordance with this order.

In Mongol traditional thought, as in Chinese, power was ultimately a unity. He who controlled the sources of power controlled its uses and manifestations. Power came from Heaven, from food, from the lineage, and from knowledge. It manifested itself in the engendering of sons, in riding and shooting, in conquering and ruling. To what extent the various kinds of power were regarded as one in actual practice, and to what extent they remained distinct but interdependent, is a question awaiting further research. In the *YSZY*, this is not an issue. We simply observe how food is manipulated there to increase or restore physical power, and to demonstrate and validate political power.

This brief discussion owes much to Michel Foucault,[21] and to Pierre Bourdieu,[22] but more to field experiences among many East Asian communities, where a feast is a social message and the choice of dishes is carefully contrived to send that message. They are the "words" of that discourse. With Elster[23] we hold that the conspicuous display of power is more deliberate, more complex, and more subtly constructed than Foucault and Bourdieu allow. The *qan* did not simply invoke food to show that they were better than others. Nor did they hold power simply to dominate and oppress. They wanted food that was not only splendid but also genuinely tasty within their ancient traditions, and genuinely healthy according to the best medical standards of the time.

They were sophisticated enough rulers to realize that they had to build up the state and manage its ideology deliberately. The men who ate Hu's cuisine were the same men who succeeded in taming the Yellow River for the first and only time in pre–industrial history, who oversaw the revival, and, perhaps, the cynical manipulation of Neoconfucianism as a validating ideology, and who patronized skilled persons of every religious and ethnic background in a display of tolerance far ahead of its time. They were shrewd and dynamic men who created, quite consciously, an imperial order that would do what they wanted. It did not prevent their fall, a mere 38 years after Hu's book was written. The wonder is that they succeeded so spectacularly for so long.

Still, in more mundane terms, for all the assimilation that the text expresses as part of the Mongol attempt to create a cuisine to please almost anyone and express the power and magnificence of the Mongol

---

[21] Michel Foucault, *The History of Sexuality,* vol. 1: *An Introduction* (New York, 1978).

[22] Pierre Boudieu, *La Distinction* (Paris, 1979).

[23] Jon Elster, "Snobs," *London Review of Books*, 5–18 November 1981: 10–2, and *Sour Grapes* (Cambridge, 1983).

court at the same time, there remains a recognizable and substantial substratum of everyday Mongolian culture. The *YSZY* is replete with specifically Mongolian *materia dietica*, preferred types of foods, *e.g.*, organ meats, a taste shared with Turks, specific Mongolian recipes, and terminology. There also appears to have been a conscious effort to use traditional Mongolian foods with their medicinal values in mind, judging from the uses to which these foods are put today, and from a few suggestions in the sources indicating that present conceptions of medicinal value of foods may have a high antiquity among the Mongols.[24] A key Mongolian organizational element of the *YSZY* may be the division of the recipes into three main groups, two of which reflect the two main divisions of food found in the *Secret History*, *i.e.*, *šülen*, "soups," and *umdan*, "drinks." The vast majority of recipes have been cooked to suit the "Mongol taste," whatever the ideological interests of the cooks.

Mongolian Words and Phrases of the YSZY

Perhaps the most conspicuously Mongolian elements in the *YSZY* are the text's 23 Mongolian words and phrases. These words, like other foreign terminology in the *YSZY* must be reconstructed from their Chinese transcriptions. The transcriptions are in most cases inexact, either due to mishearing, mistransmission[25] or even misunderstanding[26] of the original words themselves, or due to the inability of the

[24] William of Rubruck, for example, records, in a passage already quoted above, that he found *qan* Möngke eating tsampa "for comforting his head." See Wyngaert, 1929: 267.

[25] Perhaps the most glaring example of the mistransmission of Mongolian words in Mongol–era Chinese sources is miswriting of Sübe'edei–ba'adur's name by some authorities resulting in two separate biographies in the *Yuan shi* 元史, one under Subutai 速不台, a poor transcription of his name which gets the vocalization wrong, the other under Xuebutai 雪不台. There are other, similar examples.

[26] Most often this takes place when a foreign word is identified with another word which sounds like it in the host language and assimilated to it. Thus Old Norse *gata*, "street," has become "gate" in some English usage, *e.g.*, Newgate and Highgate, whose names having nothing to do with "gates" but recall the commercial streets active in Anglo–Saxon times which gave them their names. Sometimes the misunderstanding may result from an intentional misuse by native speakers, for example, in tabu usages which may alter, sometimes greatly, the sound of a word to prevent some undesired reaction on the part of the spirits. This is probably the reason why Tolui is written Toli, a Turkicized form, in some sources, or for that matter why Cila'un, a son of Muqali, is called Taš in some sources. Both names mean "stone," the one in Mongolian, the other in Turkic.

phonologically much simplified North Chinese dialects of the era to represent many foreign words, particularly Turkic and Mongolian, with their complex consonantal clusters and many diphthongs.[27] In some cases, transcriptions have been simplified to provide transcriptions which, although phonologically inexact, attempt to render meaning as well as sound, for a more popular Chinese consumption. This seems to have been the case with many of the *YSZY*'s Turkic noodle dishes in particular. Uighur **chöp*,[28] for example, a single syllable, is

[27] The problem was not unique to Chinese. One example which continues to haunt us is Arabic Genghiz khan. The situation has been complicated for our understanding of the Chinese of the early fourteenth century because China was in a linguistic transition during the time leading to the emergence of what Pulleyblank (1991), for example, sees as a definitive Early Mandarin *circa* 1360 (Y), specifically the dialect of Beijing, as reflected in the rhyming aPhags-pa script *Menggu ziyun* 蒙古字韻 and in the somewhat later *Zhongyuan yinsun* 中原音韻, also rhyming but designed to help authors of *qu* 曲, the verse form in use in the drama of the time. Unfortunately, Pulleyblank's reconstructions, although still useful here, look more towards the Ming period and fail to take into consideration the very large foreign populations in Beijing *circa* 1330, and what linguistic impact their languages had on the Chinese of the time, beyond literati culture, the focus of the second dictionary mentioned above, and a court accent that may have been different than the pure Beijing accent of the period *per se*. Also an issue is that many Chinese forms in the *YSZY* may have been intermediated by Uighurs who played a dominant cultural role in Mongol China and whose pronunciation of Chinese characters was extremely conservative, even retaining some Late Middle Chinese elements (L). See as an introduction Shōgaito Masahiro, "How Were Chinese Characters Read in Uighur?, in Desmond Durkin-Meisterernst, Simone-Christiane Raschmann, Jens Wilkens, Marianne Yaldiz and Peter Zieme, eds, *Turfan Revisisted, The First Century of Research into the Arts and Cultures of the Silk Road* (Berlin, 2004), 321-24. Because of these and other issues, including those affecting the languages from which the Chinese forms were taken, we have avoided relying upon purely linguistic criteria in our reconstructions below of Mongolian, Turkic, and other foreign vocabulary found in Chinese transcriptions in the *YSZY* and have looked not only at phonological similarities of the Chinese and reconstructed forms but also upon the internal evidence provided by the *YSZY* itself. This internal evidence includes Chinese names for plants and animals, when they are provided to translate foreign terms, illustrations, textual comments, and in a many cases the meanings of the characters chosen to transliterate a foreign term as well as their phonological content. Where appropriate there has also been comparison with other Mongol–era sources, which include many of the same Mongolian, Turkic, and other terms found in the *YSZY* in Chinese transcription, and with more recent usage. Because the evidence is not always clear and some Chinese transcriptions appear particularly defective, some proposed reconstructions are as a consequence very tentative.

[28] On *chöp* see also Appendix II.

written as two in the *YSZY*, *choufen* 搊粉.[29] In this case the first syllable, which means "rolled by hand," is indicative of the elaborate process by which such noodles were made[30] in Turkistan and points farther west, while the second syllable not only represents the "p," which did exist as a final consonant in the early Mandarin of the time, but tells Chinese readers that this is a "noodle," a *fen*. Likewise the *shuihua* 水滑[31] of the text not only renders, inexactly, Turkic **salma*, another noodle, but also by using the characters "water–polished" to represent the sound tells readers something very important about how *salma* are made, namely their "polishing" in water. The second syllable, "hua," is also not so inexact when we consider that it, roughly, attempts not only to represent the "ma" of the last syllable of *salma*, but also the "l" of the first which in most Turkic dialects would be partially assimilated to the "ma." The "hua," with its falling or fourth tone also may render the Turkic accent of the final syllable.[32] Examples could be multiplied. They are found in many other sources besides the *YSZY*.[33] In fact such things are almost universal when one language borrows from another and attempts to fit foreign words not only into existing phonological but also conceptual systems.

The various Mongolian words found in the *YSZY* have been divided here according to usage. The 11 plant and animal names of List A below comprise 10 of traditional cultural significance to the Mongols, along with a plant and a name, *šaqimur*, recently borrowed from Persia by way of the Turks (*shajhimur*). This is the "rape turnip," the swollen root of *Brassica rapa*, as opposed to the common turnip *B. napus*. The 9 terms in List B are mostly names of recipes but the list also significantly includes 4 words referring to varieties of kumiss,

---

[29] Y *tʂʰəwfun*, L *tʂʰəwfjyn*. In Early Middle Chinese (E), the language of early Tang, the resemblance is even closer, i.e., *tʂʰuwpun*, and this form although only known from the relatively late *YSZY*, may be a very old transcription made by the Uighurs to represent a favorite food and used among them.

[30] See Algar, 1985: 250ff. Turkish noodles, also *börek* shells, must be rolled out flat, then rolled up again, sliced and the sliced dough placed flat and rolled out again, sometimes many times.

[31] Y *ʂujxwa*, L *ʂyjxɦwa:t*.

[32] The spelling here is from the Arabic recipe books. This noodle is almost certainly not Uighur.

[33] One example, found throughout Mongol–era documents in China, is the writing of Cinggis–qan's name as Chengjisihan 成吉思汗, the "*Qan* who has fulfilled an omen." Other transcriptions would have been far more accurate phonologically but might not make the same ideological point.

one generalized word for cooking fat or grease, **tosu[n]*,[34] also, in compounds, a term for fresh or for boiled butter, *e.g.*, *sini tosu[n]*, or *sira tosu[n]*. List C includes Mongolian words for cooking platter and bucket and the key cultural term **qurim*,[35] a Mongolian ritual feast, in this case used in the name of a recipe. The areas of Mongolian cultural interest are quite clear from the lists, reproducing terms clearly intended to be evocative of the Mongolian past. When we agree with their interpretations, items adequately discussed by Lao and Franke are left unannotated, here and below:[36]

A. Mongolian names for Plants and Animals:

abarqu "Siberian sturgeon," *Huso dauricus*
alaq qun, "immature swan"
cicigina, "jujube" (error for *cibuqan*?)[37]
ja'uqasu[n], "lily root"
**möög*, *Tricholoma mongolicum*[38]

---

[34] The Chinese transcription (37B) is relatively straightforward, *tusu* 土蘇, Y *tʰu-su*, and it is made clear from the context that butter or some other cooking oil is meant. **Tosu* was easily missed by Lao and Franke since this term occurs only once in the middle of a recipe.

[35] **Qurim* is written *helian* 荷蓮, Y *xɔljɛn*, "lotus," in the highly elaborate and unique recipe #90 (1, 49A) but this meaning makes little sense in the context of "bonnets" and the word must be a transcription. Middle Mongolian *qurim* is in fact relatively well known and occurs in both the *Secret History*, as a noun, in chapters 67, 131, 275; as *qurimla–* in chapters 50, 57, 67, 117, 130, 185, 240ff, 279; and in the *Huayi yiyu* (see Mostaert, 1977: 92). The word is a deverbal noun derivative of *quri–*, "meet together, assemble," and is thus related to the reciprocal action form of *quri–*, *qurilta–*, "assemble together, hold a *qurilta*." The *qurim* is best understood as the ritual feast accompanying a *qurilta*.

[36] Below we draw heavily upon their work. See Lao Yan–shuan, "Notes on non–Chinese terms in the Yuan imperial dietary compendium *Yin–shan Cheng–yao*," *The Bulletin of the Institute of History and Philology, Academia Sinica* XXXIX (Oct. 1969): 399–416; and Herbert Franke, "Additional notes on non–Chinese terms in the Yuan imperial dietary compendium *Yin–shan Cheng–yao*," *Zentralasiatische Studien* IV (1970): 7–16. Mongolian botanical and zoological names are, unless otherwise indicated, from Mongolian Terminological Commission reports already cited above.

[37] This is the word used in the *Huayi yiyu* 華夷譯語 for the jujube, see Mostaert, 1977: 46.

[38] On the Mongolian or perhaps Siberian origins of this word see R. Gordon Wasson, *Soma, Divine Mushroom of Immortality*, Ethno–mycological Studies I ([New York], 1968), 170–1. Although the appearance of this loan may have pre-dated the Mongols, the popularity of the word during and after their time is conspicuous.

**qaralaq qun*, “lesser golden–headed swan”," or or “tundra swan,” *Cygnus columbianus* [39]
qilam “Chinese sturgeon,” *Acipenser sinensis*
šaqimur (Mo. from Tu.), “rape turnip”
tabilqa, “spiraea,” *Spiraea media*
tarbaqa[n], “*tarbaqan* marmot,” *Marmota bobak*
yeke siraqun qun, “golden–headed swan,” “whooper swan,” *Cygnus Cygnus cygnus*

B. Names of Dishes, Raw or Processed Foods

airaq, in the *YSZY*, “camel kumiss”
borbi[n], “Achilles tendon of sheep”
**caqa’an*, “white [*i.e.*, boiled] kumiss”[40]
cige’en, “kumiss”
**jasa’a*, “mountain oysters” [of a ram?][41]

---

[39] Lao and Franke follow F. W. Cleaves’ reconstruction of *chulugehun* 出魯哥渾, Y *tʂʰylɔkɔxun*, as *cürge qun*, “*cürge* swan,” although *cürge* refers to a species of grebe (Khalkha *chörkh nugas*, genus *Colymbus*) and not to a swan. The modern Mongolian name for *Cygnus columbianus* is *xarlag xun* and in our view the *chulugehun* of the text is a somewhat defective transcription of an equivalent Middle Mongolian *qarlaq qun*. This is one example of how a strictly philological reconstruction of Mongolian and other terms in Yuan–era transcription can lead to error and misunderstanding. Such transcriptions are rarely as consistent as the burden placed on them by philological analysis would lead us to believe. The identification of this swan is from the illustration and description (3, 21B). What is shown is most certainly not a grebe or any related bird.

[40] There is some uncertainty about the reading of the second character which appears in the text (3, 9b) to be the character *wu* 兀, but also has what looks like the remnant of an upper, parallel stroke suggesting that it is in fact *Yuan* 元, and not *wu*. The spacing of the characters at this point also suggests that something has been left out. If we assume a damaged original printing block and read *chuangyuan* 窗元, or Y *tʂhwaŋɥen,* this would seem to correspond, although not exactly, to Middle Mongolian *caqa’an*, Khalkha *cagaan*, “boiled kumiss.”

[41] This word occurs as part of the title of recipe #73 (1, 46a), where the transcription is somewhat problematical. The name of this recipe, *zhazhaer* 煠牒兒probably Y *tʂatʂarr̹,* literally translates as “fried” *zhaer*, and the recipe does indeed call for frying or scalding in this case. In addition, the first “*zha*” is dropped when ingredients are listed, indicating that Hu Sihui, or his editor at least, took the first *zha* separately, in the sense “fried.” Despite this evidence we believe that the word is to be read *zhazhaer*, for Middle Mongolian *jasa’a*, Khalkha *zasaa*, with the “er” being an effort to represent the final “a” after the glottal stop, and that the first *zha* has been dropped by mistake, by someone not realizing that this word is Mongolian, in the ingredients section. In any case, the recipe is clearly a Mongolian one for “mountain oysters”

**jingtei*, "heavy, weighty"[42]
miqan–u kö[n]lesün, "meat sweat"
qongqor, "chestnut–colored kumiss"
**tosu[n]*, "fat," "grease;" "butter"

C. Other

**qurim*, "feast," "common ritual meal"
**tabaq* (Mo. from Ar.?), "platter"[43]
**telir*, "basket for feeding an animal" (used as a measure for water)[44]

Mongolian materia dietetica et medica

As can be seen from the above examples, the range of Mongolian vocabulary in the *YSZY* is relatively small. But this cannot be taken to mean that the range of Mongolian *materia dietetica et medica* in the text is also small. The majority occur under Chinese rather than Mongolian names. They must include most, but certainly not all, of the wild plant and animal foods.

The interest of the medieval Mongols in hunting is well known and was noticed by a number of authorities including Marco Polo in his descriptions of the annual migrations of the Mongol court between Qanbaliq and the Inner Mongolian highland:

(described unmistakably) and the close phonological similarity of the Mongolian word for animal "testicle" to the Chinese name for the dish cannot be coincidental.

[42] This word was also missed by Lao and Franke but the text's *jingdai* 經帶, Y *kiŋtaj*, appears to be a relatively close transcription of the Mongolian in recipe #38 (1, 38a), and not just a Chinese description of the shape of the strips of meat and mushroom. The meaning seems to be that the "noodles" in question are "real," *i.e.*, are substantial food.

[43] The *tieba* 鐵芭, Y *tʰjɛpa,* of recipe #80 (1, 47a) is Khalkha *tabag*, "plate, dish, platter, tray," Middle Mongolian *tabaq*. This word is probably a borrowing from Arabic (*tabaq*, a "tray," etc., related to the verb "to cook").

[44] The *tieluo* 鐵絡 , Y *thjɛlaw* or *thjɛlɔ*, of recipes #49 (1, 41a) and 94 (1, 50a) is apparently the rare Mongolian word represented by Classical Mongolian *telir*, which in the compound *telir sebeg* means "basket for feeding animals." See Ferdinand D. Lessing, ed., *Mongolian–English Dictionary*, corrected reprinting (Bloomington, 1973), 798. The word does not seem to survive in modern Khalkha. Note that in this case the transcription, "iron bucket," seems to provide some hint of the meaning of the original Mongolian word. In view of the lack of further information about the word *telir* this identification must be considered highly tentative.

Throughout these three months, that is to say, December, January, and February, when the lord resides in his capital city, it has been established that, up to a distance of 40 days' journey from the capital, people must hunt and fowl and send [to court] such as they take of large beasts. This is to be taken to mean such things as wild boars, hinds, deer, stags, lions, bears, and other manner of great wild beasts and also fowl. And he [the Great Kaan] gets the greater part of everything.[45]

Also know that the grand lord has very [well–]trained leopards which are all good at hunting and at taking beasts. There are also a grand quantity of trained wolves, all of which take beasts and are very good for hunting. He has again many great lions, much greater than those of Babylon, and they are very beautiful in color and in coat; for they are all striped lengthwise, of black, of vermilion, and of white. And they are trained so as to take wild boars, and [wild] cattle, and bears, and wild asses, and stags, and other grand and fierce beasts.[46]

And there are also a great multitude of eagles which are all trained to take wolves, and foxes, and deer, and roe deer; for they catch them in great numbers.[47]

And when the overlord thus remains in his capital for those three months that I have named for you above, that is, December, and January, and February, he so departs from the city the first day of March and goes towards the south up to the Ocean Sea, a two days' journey away. He keeps with him a good ten–thousand falconers and takes a good 500 gyrfalcons, and other manners of peregrine falcons and sakers in grand abundance, and a very great number of goshawks to fowl in the rivers. But one should not understand that he would keep all of them with himself in one place; to the contrary, they are divided up here and there, a hundred to two hundred at a time, and more, just as he sees fit. And at all times they are fowling; and the greater part of their catch thus belongs to their grand lord.[48]

---

[45] Pauthier, 1978: 298–9.
[46] Pauthier, 1978: 299–301.
[47] Pauthier, 1978: 301.
[48] Pauthier, 1978: 303–5.

And the grand lord goes on four elephants, upon which has been made a very beautiful chamber of woodwork which is, inside, entirely covered by sheets in beaten gold; and the outside is covered by lion skins. And he keeps at all times with himself there a dozen of the best gyrfalcons that he has. And there are with him also many barons who keep him company. And some times when they are going along, the lord, in his chamber, and [he] talking to his barons, who also travel around him very close on horseback, they say to him: sire, there are cranes! And he immediately has his chamber uncovered and sees them; and he takes whatever gyrfalcon pleases him and releases it to hunt and often it takes them and kills them before him, so he has a great deal of pleasure and joy, although always in his chamber reposing in his bed; and likewise all the barons which are thus around him [have a great deal of pleasure and joy].[49]

And when it has so happened that he finds himself in a place which is Cacciar Modun, his tents can be found pitched there, and those of his sons, and of his barons, and of his armies, and of them there are a good ten–thousand beautiful and rich... And the lord remains thus in that place until it is spring. And during all this time he does nothing else but fowl in the area, on the lakes, and on the rivers, of which there are a great many there, and some beautiful areas where there are cranes and swans and every other manner of birds. And all the other people around him never cease to hunt and to fowl. And they bring home for him each day a great quantity of venison and of birds of every manner in abundance... And if I may tell you something else; namely that no person, whoever he might be, dares to keep any bird for the pleasure of his fowling, nor dogs to hunt, for 20 days' journey from that place. Although in all other parts each may maintain such as he would. And again, that in all the lands of the lord no one dares, however daring he might be, or who he might be, to take any of four manner of beasts: that is, the hare, stag, roe deer, and hind. That is during the months of March to October.[50]

---

[49] Pauthier, 1978: 308.
[50] Pauthier, 1978: 308, 310.

Marco Polo mentions the following Mongolian game animals: wild boars, hinds, roe deer, deer, stags, lions, bears, wild cattle, wild asses, wolves, foxes, hares, and various water–fowl including cranes, and swans. The *YSZY* lists them too, or their equivalents. It also lists many other wild animal foods as well, including wild fish. Some must be Chinese. Bear paws, for example, are hardly Mongolian, even if Mongols certainly did eat bear meat. Most of the fish, if identified correctly, are south Chinese varieties and hardly traditional Mongolian foods.[51] The rare and now extinct Yangtse River dolphin is also unlikely to have been a Mongolian food, nor the Chinese and other species of rhinoceroses mentioned in *juan* 3. But most of the *YSZY* wild animal foods listed below, 5 out of 42 under their proper Mongolian names, must have been hunted and eaten primarily by Mongols, although the Mongols doubtless shared their taste for wild animal foods with Turks and other former nomads resident at court as well. Entries marked in bold are, as far as can be determined, first described or are first assigned medical properties by Hu Sihui. Some, *e.g.*, the *tarbaqan* marmot, are frequently mentioned in later *bencao*; some, those marked with an †, only in the *YSZY*:

Abarqu [Siberian Sturgeon] **meat and fat**
Badger [*Meles meles*] **Meat**
Bear [*Ursus arctos* or *Selenarctos thibetanus*] Meat and Fat
†**Black–headed Crane** [black–necked crane, *Grus nigricollis*] **Meat**
Black–Tailed Gazelle [*Procapra gutturosa*] **Meat**
Blue Sheep [*Pseudois nayaur*] **Meat**
†**Common Pintail Duck Meat**
Common Quail [*Coturnix coturnix*] Meat
†**Eurasian Curlew Meat** [*shuizha* 水札, ***Numenius arquata***]
Fox [*Vulpes vulpes*] Meat
Great Bustard [*Otis tarda*] **Meat**
Hare [*Lepus tolai* or *L. mandschuricus*] Meat and Liver
†**[Immature] Mute Swan**, [*Cygnus olor*] **Meat**
†**"Iranian Crane"** [the common crane, *Grus grus*?] **Meat**
†**Kulan** [*Equus hemionus*] **Meat**
†**"Mountain Pheasant"** [Probably the Hazel Hen, *Bonasia bonasus*] **Meat**

[51] Although, according to William of Rubruck, the Mongols knew and ate carp (Wyngaert, 1929: 260).

Muntjac Deer [*Muntiacus reevesi*] Venison
Musk Deer [*Moschus moschiferus*] Venison
Otter [*Lutra lutra*] Meat and Liver
Pere David's Deer [*Elaphurus davidianus*] Venison
Pheasant [*Phasianus colchicus*] Meat
†****Qaralaq Qun*** [Lesser Golden–Headed Swan] **Meat**
Qilam [Chinese Sturgeon] **meat and fat**
Red Deer [*Cervus elaphus xanthopygus*] Venison
River Deer [*Hydropotes inermis*] Venison
[Siberian] Tiger [*Panthera tigris altaica*] Meat
Sika Deer [*Cervus nippon*] Venison and Fat
Snow Leopard [*Panthera uncia*] **Meat**
Tarbaqa[n] [Marmot] **Meat**
†**Tufted Duck** [*Anas fuligula*] **Meat**
Weasel [*Mustela sibirica*] **Meat**
†**"White Crane"** [Siberian Crane, *Grus leucogeranus*] **Meat**
†**White Gazelle** [*Procapra picticaudata*] **Meat**
Wildcat [*Felis bengalensis*, also possibly *Felis euptylura*, also *F. manul* or *F. margarita*] Meat
Wild Boar [*Sus scrofa*] Meat
Wild Camel [*Camelus bactrianus*] Meat and Hump
Wild Goose [probably *Anser albifrons albifrons*, in Mongolia also *A. indicus*] Meat, Grease, and Fat
Wild Horse [*Equus przewalskii*] Meat
Wild Sheep [*Ovis sp*. probably *O. ammon*?] Meat
Wolf [*Canis lupus*] **Meat**
Yeke siraqun qun [Golden–Headed Swan] **Meat**

Also mostly Mongolian are the following foods produced by the domestic animals herded by Mongols, although Turks also avidly consumed fermented milk products as, apparently, did the North Chinese of the era (Sabban, 1986a):

Borbi[n] [Achilles Tendon of Sheep]
Camel Meat and Fat
**Caqa'an* [White] Kumiss
Cige'en [Fermented Mare's Milk]
Cooked Sheep's Marrow
Cow's Milk, Butter, Cream, Cheese, and Curds
Fermented Camel's Milk
"Five Internal Organs of a Sheep"

Horse Meat, Heart, Liver, Stomach and Intestines
Jasa'a [Mountain Oysters of a ram?]
Meat of the Rear Hoof of a Sheep
Qongqor
Sheep's Bitter Bowel, Blood, Brain, Head, Breast, Lungs, Fat, Loins,
Spine, Stomach, Tail, Tendons, Thorax, Tongue, Kidney, White [Blood Irrigating] Bowel [rectum and lower colon?], and Tripe
Sheep's Milk Cream

Mongolian plant foods in the *YSZY* are far more difficult to identify but must certainly include those listed below, although the oleaster fruits and nuts were shared with the Chinese and others. Many were probably eaten not only as food but as medicine since the Mongols already appear to have begun to assign healing properties to certain gathered and cultivated foods. The associated lore has, unfortunately, only been systematized recently[52] and we cannot say with certainty how old much of the tradition is. Despite this lack of evidence, it seems likely that one reason for Mongol persistence in eating their traditional gathered plant foods, and probably some animal foods as well,[53] was not just cultural conservatism, but their perceived medicinal properties. Plants apparently new to the Chinese herbal tradition are shown below in bold:

Acorns [in Mongolia *Quercus* spp]

---

52 See, for example, properties assigned gathered plant foods in Damrinbazar, 1991: 149ff, and *passim*. We have only begun to study the history of Mongolian folk medicine in part because so few texts have been published.

53 The *YSZY* is unusual, although not unique in Chinese tradition, in the degree to which the meats and other parts of specific animals, a great many of them, are assigned medicinal properties. Much of this tradition must have been Mongolian, the majority of the animals mentioned certainly were of more interest to the Mongols than to the Chinese, and some even have Mongolian or Turkic names, but other influences may have been at work as well, including Arabic. Of particular interest in this regard is the *Manafi' al-ḥayawan*, "usefulness of animals," a Persian "translation" prepared in Ilqanate times based upon an earlier text by Ibn Bakhtīshū (died 1058). The *Manafi' al-ḥayawan*, completed at the end of the thirteenth century, is a general work on animals but includes detailed material on the usefulness of animal (and human) organs for treating various diseases. Among other things, although an Arabo-Iranian work, it shows substantial influence of Chinese art on its illustrations, pointing up a possible connection with Qubilai's China. See the detailed discussion of this work in Linda Komaroff and Stefano Carboni, eds. *The Legacy of Genghis Khan, Courtly Art and Culture in Western Asia, 1256-1353*, New York, 2002), 244.

Bracken
Cattail [*Typha latifolia*] Rhizome
Chestnuts [*Castanea mollissima*]
Junzi 菌子 [Fungi] [*Agaricus* spp]
Crab Apples [probably *Malus pallasiana* rather than the Chinese *M. pumila]*
Lily [*Lilium concolor*] Root
***Möög Mushroom**
Nettle [*Urtica* spp including *U. angustifolia*] **Leaf**
Oleaster fruits
Pine nuts[54]
Red Currants ["Northern Schisandra"] [*Ribes rubrum*]
Reed [*Phragmites communis*] Rhizome Juice
Russian Olive Fruits [*Elaeagnus* spp including *Elaeagnus angustifolia* and possibly *E. pungens*]
Smartweed and Smartweed Shoots [in Mongolia probably *Polygonum aviculare*]
Sonchus spp greens
Tianhua 天花 **Fungus** [unidentified, Kitamura calls this *Pleurotus Ostreatus*, the oyster mushroom][55]
Tabilqa [*"Spiraea"*]
Walnuts

Other Mongolian plant foods may be subsumed under Chinese generic names. Mongols gathered many varieties of *Allium*, pears, and cherries. *Trapa* fruits, wild hazelnuts, wild vetches, water celery, and even wild Chinese flower pepper are also found in Mongolia.

Thus there is a surprisingly large and recognizable Mongolian substratum of *materia dietetica et medica* in the *YSZY* indicating a more considerable persistence of Mongolian foodways in the *YSZY* than

[54] Pine nuts were an extremely popular food with the Mongols according to the Persian historian Juvaini, who refers to the nut of the Siberian pine (*Pinus cembra*), *qusuq*, as their "dessert." See 'Ala–ad–din' Ata–Malik Juvaini, *The History of the World–Conqueror*, trans. by J. A. Boyle, vols. 1–2 (Manchester, 1958), I, 21. The usage of the *YSZY* almost certainly reflects the Mongolian preference, although we have every reason to assume that pine nuts were known to and consumed by Chinese as well. In China nuts consumed were likely not from *P. cembra* but from a locally more common *P. koraiensis* or *P. bungeana* or other *P.* spp.

[55] On this fungus see Kitamura Shirō, "*Inzenseiyō* no shokubutsu," *Acta Phytotax. Geobot*. 24 (1969): 65–76 (72).

might otherwise be expected. The number and range of Mongolian recipes is additional confirmation.

Mongolian Recipes

The *YSZY*'s Mongolian recipes fall into two categories: 1) relatively unassimilated, traditional recipes using more or less traditional ingredients; 2) recipes cooked with the "Mongol tastes" in mind, and with ingredients preferred by the Mongols. They have been substantially improved by added spices and improved cooking techniques and in many cases have been made to resemble other traditional foods of Eurasia, in particular those of the Irano–Mesopotamian region. None the less, Mongolian origins remain in most cases unmistakable. Recipe #2, for example, is very similar if not identical to an Irano–Mesopotamian *qarisa* but when compared with a recipe for the real thing in the *JJBYSL* (13, 19b), its origins as a soup, cauldron–cooked in the Mongol style, with whatever was available added as a thickener, remains clear.

Examples of purely Mongolian recipes in the *YSZY* include #62, "Salt Stomach," #80, "Willow Steamed Lamb," #94, "*Borbi[n]* Soup," #95, "*Miqan–u kö[n]lesün*," #190, a kind of tsampa, and #191, "Cheese Flour." None is very sophisticated and none calls for spicing beyond basic ingredients.

Examples of the second, culturally assimilated, Mongolian recipes are far more numerous and constitute the majority of all *YSZY* recipes. They include recipes of the following kinds:

1. The mutton/large cardamom[56] *šülen* (soups, stews and "dry soups,") of *juan* 1 (recipes #1–6, 8–27 and 29);

[56] In the text the tsaoko cardamom (*Amomum tsao–ko*), a general term there for "large" cardamoms. They have large (1–3 cm) fruits with thick shells and intensely aromatic seeds. In cooking, one fruit will flavor a whole stew, for example in "sand pot" cooking. There is considerable confusion regarding cardamoms in East Asia literature. See, for example, the discussion in the *Bencao gangmu* 本草綱目 (*BCGM*), vols. 1–2 (Hong Kong, 1979), I, 14, 26ff, where Li Shizhen 李時珍 correctly distinguishes between large, *caoguo* 草果 and small, *doukou* 豆蔻 cardamoms, but also reproduces a great deal of obsolete traditional lore as well, confusing the issue. A basic distinction is to be made between small, true cardamom, *Elettaria cardamomum*, and a whole class of larger, darker, more camphor–flavored cardamoms of the genus *Amomum*, called for here.

Amomum fruits, "large" and "brown cardamoms" of commerce, occur in several species in China. Many were known and distinguished, at least in south China, by

2. Most other *YSZY* recipes in which boiling of one or more ingredients is the primary form of preparation;

3. Most roasted, broiled, and fried dishes (including #73, although the recipe is an assimilated one, and #78, with the particularly Mongolian touch of roasting the fowl inside a sheep's stomach);

4. Most recipes calling for blood[57] or organ meats;

Medieval times. See Edward Schafer, *The Vermilion Bird, T'ang Images of the South* (Berkeley, 1967), 193–4. Hu Sihui's beloved *caoguo* is properly *A. tsao–ko*, but we suspect several species are conflated here. *A. compactum* (*sens. lat.*) and *A. globosum* (if they are indeed distinct) are good probabilities.

Another of these cardamoms is *shusha* 縮砂 (=*shushami* 縮砂米), "grain–of–paradise," mentioned in the *YSZY*. It is identified as *A. xanthioides* in Stuart. See G. Stuart, *Chinese Materia Medica* (Shanghai, 1911), 36–9. This is very possibly too exact. *A. villosum* is another name often given for this plant, *e.g.*, in the *ZYDZD* (1623). There this *Amomum* sp. is called by its alternative name *sharen* 沙仁, "sand kernel." On the terminological confusion, see I. H. Burkill, *A Dictionary of Economic Products of the Malay Peninsula* (Gainesville, 1966), 137; Stuart 1911: 38–9.

True cardamom is known in China as *bai doukou* 白豆蔻, "white nutmeg." It is already well described in the *Nanfang caomu zhuang* 南方草木狀 (Li, 1979: 38–9; the illustration is not from the original text and is not very accurate) but rarely occurs in Chinese cooking and in the *YSZY* is only called for twice (for example, 2, 6a–b).

Cardamoms are carminative and digestive, and in China are held to be warming and strengthening, especially true cardamom, but, in folk practice observed by ENA, the large ones also. These are regularly used in Chinese health cookery, in protein–rich tonic soups like those of the *YSZY*, and may be found sold for that purpose in Oriental markets. They also figure importantly in Indian and Southeast Asian cooking. A Western notion that they are merely inferior substitutes for true cardamom is incorrect. In Asia, they are considered separate spices with different names and uses.

For an excellent sixteenth century discussion of cardamom, what the ancient and modern authors thought about them, and the trade at the time, see Garcia da Orta, *Colóquios dos simples e drogas da índia*, vols. 1–2 (Lisboa, 1987), II, 173–91. The original edition of da Orta's work was published in 1563 in Goa.

[57] One major influence on West Asian cuisine has been the Judeo–Islamic tradition of food taboos. Blood, and sometimes such blood–rich organs as lung and liver, are avoided. Thus such recipes as #77, "Red Strips," in which sheep's blood is combined with flour to make a kind of noodle, would be unthinkable in the Near East since the seventh and eighth centuries. However, noodles and dumplings using blood as a nutritive binder are common in central Europe, specifically in German–influenced cuisines, today. One example of such a food is Icelandic *slátur*, prepared from oats, sugar, raisins, sheep's fat, and sheep's blood. Probably a relationship across the steppes, perhaps extending into central Europe, is involved. Islam also forbids not only pigs but also other animals banned in *Leviticus* and *Deuteronomy*. Thus, such items as

5. Any recipe in which bone plays a conspicuous part (*e.g.*, #162–3);

6. Any recipes not already included in the above categories featuring some Mongolian traditional food, especially gathered vegetable foods;

7. Many but certainly not all of the recipes in which cow's milk, butter, cheese, curds, or any other dairy product plays a role (*e.g.*, #214).

Of these 7 categories, the first, with a total of 27 similar *YSZY* dishes, 12.3% of all recipes (219), is the most important. It is the single most important recipe category in the *YSZY*. In these recipes, a variety of ingredients, some processed foods, *e.g.*, noodles, sheep's liver sauce, cheese *etc*., others raw, are added to a base mutton/large cardamom broth. The fundamental flavor is in seven cases improved with lesser galangal and once with cinnamon.

More than half of the recipes (15) are thickened during the primary stage of preparation with chickpeas which have been skinned and pulverized,[58] in one case with fenugreek seeds. To add still more body to these dishes, additional chickpeas (3 times), rice (6 times, 3 times together with double applications of chickpeas), barley (1 time), and oleaster fruits (1 time) are added later in some recipes, resulting in a more of less solid dish.

Others are semi–solid or at least a thick liquid. Altogether at least 7 of the 27 recipes (#1–4, 6, 8, 22 above) are for dry soups or pilafs, assuming that the rice is boiled for several minutes before it is put into the cooking pot, as is done today in modern Afghan cooking, for example. Seven more (#13, 18–21, 24, 27) are very thick stews, 1 is a spicy bread–stuffing (#7). Twelve are thick but more or less liquid "soups" (#5, 9–12, 14–17, 23, 25–26).

But all these variations in the final texture of the cooked dish are in fact relatively insignificant. What is important is that the flavor base for all 27 recipes (mutton cooked with large cardamom) is the same,

wolf, otter, bear, donkey, and badger represent a strictly Central and East Asian presence in the *YSZY*.

[58] Note that this is the typical way of cooking with chickpeas in the Muslim world, even until this day. Removal of the skins is also characteristic of Middle Eastern use of chickpeas. According to Heine, (1988: 69), chickpeas were added to dishes to even out flavors, absorb them, and provide otherwise lacking consistency, as is clearly the case here.

that all are boiled and stewed, and that the range of additional ingredients is small. In the 27 recipes vinegar is called for no less than 17 times, onions, leeks, or chives 16 times, ginger in various forms 12 times, sheep organ meats 10 times, usually various organ meats together in the same recipe, black pepper 9 times, coriander leaves 6 times and "sheep's liver sauce" 5 and probably 6 times. The 27 recipes are clearly a flavor, texture and foodstuff complex, one that is clearly and unmistakably an expression of "des goûts mongols," and was so perceived by other peoples of Central Asia as late as the Moghul Empire.[59]

Such foods perpetuate the ancient Mongolian tradition of food as a boiled pot (*šülen*) of whatever was available. It preferably comprised mutton, possibly very poor cuts, or bones for broth, if mutton was unavailable, some grain or legume as a thickener, some spice or herb to give flavor, principally onions or garlic, and some vegetable or fruit to make up for the thin broth, and provide at least some nutritional content. Other similar flavor, texture and foodstuff complexes may be identified among the other six categories of by and large assimilated Mongolian recipes, underscoring the persistence and dominance of Mongolian cultural interests in the foods and medicines of the *YSZY*.

Turko–Islamic Influences

But if recipes such as the 27 *šülen* analyzed above speak eloquently for the Mongolness of the *YSZY*, they also make clear the degree to which the food culture there is indebted to the Islamic World and to

---

[59] A sixteenth century court etiquette book from the Moghul court (the *Ain-i-Akhbari*) includes the following "Mongolian" recipe called, significantly, a *shölen*:

1 lb meat	1/2 oz fresh ginger
1/4 lb dried chickpeas	1 tsp minced garlic
2 tsp salt	1 tsp pepper
1 cup rice	1 tsp cinnamon
2 oz butter	1 tsp cardamom
half an onion	1/8 tsp clove

Bring the meat to the boil in 5 cups of water with the salt; skim, add the chickpeas and cook for 1 1/2 hours, then add the rice and cook for another 1/2 hour, stirring from time to time and adding water as needed to keep a porridgy consistency. The onion and garlic would be fried with the spices and stirred in toward the end.

See Charles Perry, "A Mongolian Dish," *Petits Propos Culinaire* 19 (March, 1985): 53–5. Note the great similarity of this dish to the mutton/cardamom *šülen* of the *YSZY*.

China. Boiling mutton with whatever was available, trade grains, wild seeds, roots, vegetables, *etc.*, may be an old Mongolian idea, but the spicing, cooking methods, and most of the additional ingredients of the dishes discussed above, are not. Cooking mutton with fenugreek seeds, or cinnamon, for example, adding skinned and pulverized chickpeas to thicken the broth, its careful straining, even most of the noodles mentioned, are Turko–Islamic refinements, not Mongolian ideas. As is the case with the Mongolian culture of the *YSZY*, Turko–Islamic influences in the dietary can be seen through terminology, predominantly Turkic, through individual *materia dietetica et medica*, most common Muslim, although obviously known to and used by Turks, and in the recipes sections.

Terminology

There are a total of 49 Turkic, Persian and Arabic words and phrases in the *YSZY*, the Turkic including Turkicized words from other languages. Most were recent borrowings at the time that the *YSZY* was written, but some, *e.g.*, *zhira*, "cumin," and the various words for asafoetida, already had a long history. They are included below for the sake of completeness and because they were still considered foreign words at the time the *YSZY* was written. This is in part because Hu Sihui still uses the foreign transcriptions even when Chinese equivalents were available. See also the relevant discussions of these words by Lao and Franke:

A. Spices, Raw Foods:

angwa (Pr.), asafoetida[60]
anjudan (Ar. from Pr. *anguzhad*), "asafoetida root"[61]
badam (Pr.) "almond"
chugundur (Pr.) "sugar beet"
ka'fur (Ar.) camphor
hulba[t] (Ar.) "fenugreek"
kasni (Pr.) "asafoetida"
mäskä (Tu.) "refined liquid butter"

[60] See Laufer, 1919: 361.

[61] The Chinese *wenzhan* 穩展 is much closer to the Arabic derivative than the Persian original. See the discussion of these words in Laufer, 1919: 361.

mastajhi (Tu. from Ar.) “mastic”[62]
nabat (Pr.) “cane sugar”
pistä (Pr.) “pistachio nut”
**qamh* (Ar.) “durum, hard wheat”[63]

---

[62] This is a heavily palatalized, Turkic form of Arabic *mastaki. Mastajhi* or *Mastiki*, from Greek *mastikh*, is made from the resin of *Pistacia lentiscus*. It is most often used in powdered form in modern Middle Eastern cooking to remove unwanted flavors from meats, but is also a spice, particularly in breads, in its own right, as is apparently the case here. The application in this recipe is typical of Middle Eastern usage of both the past and the present. On Chinese early references to *mastiki* see Laufer, 1919: 252–3.

[63] In *juan* 3 (2b) *heximi* 河西米, Y *xɔsimi*, L *xɦasiajmjiaj*, literally “Tangut grain,” is said to the be “hardest of all grains.” This must be durum or “hard” wheat, Arabic *qamh*, a word which appears to be reproduced, somewhat defectively, unless we assume that the "xi" is an attempt to reproduce the guttural sounds of the original word, by the Chinese transcription. It can also be taken to mean that this kind of wheat was first grown in the Hexi or Tangut/eastern Uighur area, something not unexpected if durum was introduced from the West via the Silk Route. This may be another example of how characters of *YSZY* transcriptions of foreign words often are more than simple phonological renderings and also carry meaning. In a letter of 7 June, 1993 to PDB, Françoise Sabban raises a number of objections to this identification, “meme si cela est séduisant...” Briefly she argues that the generic *mi* is always applied to rice and millet but never to wheat, a fact which must have been well known to Hu Sihui, well grounded as he was in Chinese culture, that the cultivation of durum wheat in China is not confirmed by other sources and is in fact entirely unknown outside of the possible *YSZY* references, and that durum wheat is very slow cooking as whole grains and would be an unlikely ingredient in recipe #48, for example, where cooking is entirely by boiling. Prof. Sabban's points, as always, are carefully considered and we respond in detail to them here due to the potential importance of the *YSZY* references in the history of pasta:

1. While it is true that any person well–educated in the Chinese language and in Chinese culture such as Hu Sihui would have been aware of the standard usage of *mi* in reference to rice or millet, and not to wheat, the term *heximi* may not have been his invention. It may have originated in the culturally mixed environment of the China frontier where traditional linguistic distinctions were not so well drawn and taken over unchanged by Hu, linguistically accurate or not. In addition, if *heximi* is a transcription of Arabic *qamh*, the character *mi*, “rice or millet grain,” was chosen more for its phonetic than semantic value. *Mi* is not confined in usage just to “rice and millet.” Job's Tears and Pearl barley can also be *mi* and a careful search of the sources will no doubt turn up many other examples as well.

2. It is not true that the cultivation of durum wheat is otherwise unattested in China. Buck encountered durum as a well established, traditional crop in early 20th century China, for example. See John Lossing Buck, *Land Utilization in China* (Chicago, 1937). But Hu nowhere says that the grain was

qatiq (Tu.) "dried sour milk"[64]
qima (Tu.) "chopped meat (as noodle stuffing)"
shajhimur (Tu. from Ar. *shaljam*) "rape turnip"
**suqsur* (Tu. from Mo.?) "common pintail," *Anas acuta*[65]

---

cultivated in China. He merely says that it "comes from Hexi" (3, 2b), in complete contrast to another Western import, the chickpea, which he characterizes as grown here and there in China (by Muslims). Hu's *heximi*, while it might have been grown locally, is also quite possibly an exotic import from Turkistan or farther afield known under a local name that refers to its point of appearance, not point of origin. Hu's Hexi, in any case, as is abundantly clear from his use of the term to describe what is known indubitably as an "Uighur" dish from other sources (his "Tangut Lungs," recipe #55, the "West of the River Lungs" from the *JJBYSL*, 13, 19a–b), is not just the old Tangut domains but includes associated portions of Turkistan just to the west. Thus, Hu neither claims that the grain is grown in China, nor does he directly associate it with China. At best he associates it with China borderlands that were not very Chinese in the Mongol era. The history of durum wheat cultivation in China may as a consequence be largely irrelevant in this context, the exotic uses of the Mongol court.

3. The point about durum wheat grains being slow cooking is well taken. None the less, there is no indication in the recipe in question (#48) how long the cooking is to be; it could easily be overnight or longer, given the Mongol propensity for boiling the essence out of foods. Second, *YSZY* recipes leave out important details. What was really involved, for example, in the "scouring" of the durum grains called for in the recipe? Was the scouring done after boiling and intended to remove the hard outer covering of the wheat grains and facilitate cooking? The cooking called for in the recipe might not be so unreasonable even for durum if we knew all the details.

4. *Heximi* is specifically referred to as the "hardest of all grains." Such "hardness," while characteristic of durum wheat and the origin of its name, is not so readily applicable to either millet or rice, both of which are relatively easily milled, especially after a light soaking. Why does Hu make such a point about the "hardness" of *heximi* unless he is referring to something quite beyond the Chinese experience, *e.g.*, durum? It is this reference to the particular hardness of the grain, coupled with what appears to be an attempt to transcribe an Arabic word for durum in its Chinese name that leads us to conclude that *heximi* is durum, although in the *YSZY* it is little more than an exotic import. We agree with Sabban that there is little evidence for the widespread use or cultivation of durum wheat in the China of the era.

[64] This is Franke's guess but in our view he is quite correct. See Franke, 1970: 11. On *qatiq* see Doerfer, 1963–75: III, 374–5.

[65] On this word see Franke, 1970. The form here, *susu* 速速 (3, 26a), Y *susu*, apparently to be understood as **su(q)su(r)*, is clearly akin to the Modern Uighur form *suqsur*. It is unclear whether or not Khalkha *soqsor*, as in *sogsor nugas* for *Anas acu-*

*_surqyl_ (Tu.), ["grayish, whitish one"] "immature mute swan"[66]
*_süttigen_, (No. Tu.: "having a basis in milk"), here "Mongolian tea"[67]
za'faran (Ar.) "saffron"
zhira (Pr.) "cumin"

B. Names of Dishes (bread and grain foods discussed in Appendix II by Perry are shown in bold):

*_Achchiq_ (Tu.), "Sour"[68]
arajhi (Tu. from Ar.), "distilled liquor"

_ta,_ unmistakably the duck shown in the illustration (a female), is a loan word from a Turkic language or the reverse. If the word is originally Mongolian, this is still another example of Hu Sihui's Turkic lapses.

66 The reconstruction is hypothetical. The illustration (3, 21b) shows a non–descript swan which could be _Cygnus olor_, here, correctly, called the "swan that does not sound," although lacking the distinctive black head marking. If it is _Cygnus olor_ it is probably an immature one, although the head marking is not always distinctive. We suggest, for that reason, that _suerqila_ 速兒乞剌, Y _sur̯kʰila_, must represent something close to Modern Kazakh _surqyl_, "gray, grayish one" or "having become whitened, lost color" (variants in Kazakh include _surghylt_ and _surlau_)" and here refers to the immature _Cygnus olor_, or possibly other immature _Cygnus_ spp. The usage would thus be similar to Kazakh _kögildirlik_, "bluish, greenish," referring to a swan chick or fledgling. The Khalkha name for _Cygnus olor_ is said to be _al–süül_, "red tail," but this swan does not have a red tail and some other bird may be meant, probably a stork. The first part of the Chinese transcription, _suerqila_, could be a Middle Mongolian _se'ül_ but such an interpretation does not explain the _qila_. The Turkic derivation seems more likely.

67 This term (2, 10b) is obviously a transcription. The _su_ 酥, Y _su_, is probably Turkic _süt_, milk, but the rest of the transcription, e.g., _qian_ 簽, Y _tsʰjɛm_, is uncertain. We conjecture that the original was something similar to Kazakh _süttigen_, "having a basis in milk," with the middle syllable devoiced as it would be today, yielding a form relatively close to the transcription. Here again the characters chosen to represent the non–Chinese sounds of the word often give a suggestion of meaning as well as phonology. _Suyou_ 酥油, or in the transcription, _su_, is liquid butter in the _YSZY_. This appears to be one of the earliest references to what later became known as "Mongolian tea" in Central Asia and would seem to indicate, if our Turkic reconstruction is correct, that the Mongols borrowed the practice from some Turkic group.

68 The Chinese is _acai_ 阿菜, Y _ɔtsʰaj_, a fairly good transcription of Uighur _achchiq_, even closer to the modern Kazakh form _ashchy_. The recipe, #14 (1, 30b), with the lesser galangal, the Sheep's Liver Sauce, kidneys and mushrooms would probably be very sour in fact.

****boza*** (Tu.) "beer," "brandy?"[69]
****chöp*** (Tu.) "noodles"[70]
**Chöppün* [or *chöp bün*] (Tu.) "Noodle Soup"[71]
****chuqmin*** (Tu.) "bread steamed in a pot"
**Chizig* (Tu.) "dish made from sheep's tail fat and flour"[72]
**Ishkänä* (Tu.) "broth into which bread is crumbled, food taken with bread"
**jis kebabi* (Tu from Pr.) "kebabs," piece of meat roasted on a skewer[73]
**Jüzmä* (Tu.) a flat pancake noodle filled with onions and meat[74]
**manta* (Tu. from *mamata*?) "stuffed bread, breaded meat"[75]

---

[69] The text's *bozao* 撥糟 (3, 6b), Y *pɔtsaw*, is given as an alternative to *sürma*, a brandy in the *YSZY*. *Boza*, by contrast, is without question a beer (usually fermented from millet) rather than a brandy so that the equation of *sürma* and *boza*, in the *YSZY* at least, is not entirely correct. See the discussion of *boza* in Appendix II and in Doerfer, 1963–75: II, 337–41.

[70] The Chinese (1, 30a, 31b) is *choufen* 搊紛, Y *tʂʰəwfun*. On the semantics of the Chinese name for this noodle see above. See also the next note.

[71] A *chunpan* 春盤 (recipe #34, 1, 37a), or "Spring Plate," is traditionally a plate of fresh greens presented as an honor to some elderly or otherwise distinguished personage. This *chunpan*, Y *tʂʰynphɔn*, is a noodle soup and the term must represent a foreign word, in this case *chöppün* or *chöp bün[i]*, "noodle soup." On *mün* (here assimilated to the p of *chöp*) see Appendix II. Our colleague Olav Hekala (personal communication to PDB) notes that a *chunpan* can be a noodle soup in Korea. This may be a Mongol–era borrowing.

[72] The Chinese transcription (1, 44a), *qisige* 乞思哥, Y *kʰisẓkɔ*, is clearly Turkic *chiziq* and the *xi* 細 preceding *qisige* simply means "fine" and is not part of the transcription. Compare *bai* 白 *nabat*, "white" *nabat* (See Lao, 1969: 407). On *chiziq* see G. Doerfer, 1963–75: III, 2–3. In this recipe the finely sliced radish seems to substitute for the more traditional flour.

[73] The Chinese, in recipe #24 (1, 34a) is *zhijiabian shi* 指甲匾食, Y *tʂʅkjapjɛn ʂi*, "*zhijiabian*" or "finger–nail–tablet" food. This makes no sense and seems to be a transcription. The second element may be *kebap* or *kebabi* and the first can represent a *jish*, a form more like the modern Uighur *zix* than the expected *sis* or *shish*. This may be one of the earliest references to *shish–kebab*. In view of the lack of other references to early *shish–kebab* in the sources of the time this identification must be considered extremely tentative.

[74] The Chinese *jüemian* 撧麵 Y *tsɥɛmjɛn*, in recipe #17 (1, 31a), literally "*jüe*" noodles, makes no sense and must be a transcription.

[75] See the discussion of this word in Buell, 1999. In our view the *mantou* 饅頭, probably Y *mənthəw*, of the *YSZY* and of other contemporary sources has nothing to do whatever, other than sharing a name, with the unfilled steamed bun called *mantou* 饅頭 (or 蠻頭, *etc.*) still eaten, particularly in north China, where it has considerable antiquity, going back at least to Han times if not before. See, for example, the tradi-

Näwälä (Pr.) "meat, food"
Päräk (Tu.) "dumpling filled with fat and meat, e.g. *börek*"[76]
**Qazi* (Tu.) here: "a sheep intestine stuffed with spices" rather than the expected horse stomach
**quruq qima* (Tu.) chopped, parched meat[77]
**Shilön* (Tu. from Mongolian) "soup"[78]
**Shoyla Toyym* (Tu), "Porridge Abundance"
salma (Tu.) "small thin soup noodles"[79]

---

tions summarized in Murohashi Tetsuji, *Dai kanwa jiten*大漢和辭典, 13 volumes, Taibei 台北: Beiyi chupanshe 北一出版社, 1987: 12: 424a–b. The *YSZY*'s *mantou* is a Central Asia food, the later Uighur *manta* and Kazakh *manty etc*., probably derived from the *mamata* (if this is the correct reading; other possibilities are *yamata*, *tamata*) of Mahmud of Kashgar's dictionary. See Mahmud al–Kashgari, *Divanü lûgat–it–Türk tercümesi*, vols. 1–3 (Ankara, 1985), 445. *Mamata* is defined by Mahmud as "dough smeared on fat chicken or meat so that the fat will not run out when the meat is roasted." See Perry in Appendix II. This is interestingly exactly what is called for in one of Ni Zan's *mantou* recipes (*YLTYSZDJ*, pp 6–7). We also find something similar in the *YSZY*'s eggplant skin wrapped *mantou* (recipe #83). If Uighur *manta etc*. does derive from Mahmud's *mamata* (*mamata*>*mamta*>*manta*) then what was originally a dough–wrapped fat piece of meat has become a dough–skin–wrapped steamed bun with meat filling. This fact, and the similarly sounding name, is probably why Hu and his contemporaries choose to transcribe the name of this new bread food with the same characters used for the south Chinese *mantou* although the recent *mantou* has clearly been influenced by the type of *mantou*/*manta* found in Medieval and early modern sources such as the *YSZY*, complicating matters. Today too the *mantou* is little more than a variant of the ubiquitous *jiaozi* 餃子. On the popularity of the *manta*/*manty* throughout the Turkic world see Doerfer, 1963–75: IV, 23–4.

[76] On this word see Appendix II and Doerfer, 1963–75: II, 321. Note that the Chinese form, *pielie* 撇列, Y *pʰjɛljɛ*, clearly indicates an initial "p." The word may ultimately be from the Chuvash who gave the word to the Slavs, among whom it appears as *pirog*.

[77] The Chinese, in recipe #38 (1, 38a) for the meat portion of these "noodles" is *jiaorouqima* 焦肉乞馬, Y *tsjɛwriwkʰima* or *tsjɛwrykʰima*, a straightforward transcription of Uighur *quruq qima*. Note that the first two characters translate meaning as well as transliterate.

[78] In one recipe (*YSZY* 1, 48b), this word, apparently a Turkic form of Mongolian *šülen*, is written *shiluo* 時蘿, Y *ʂʅlɔ*, which, when the top character has the leaf radical, *i.e.*, 蒔蘿, is also used to write Persian *zhira*, "cumin," although in that case the borrowing is an old one and the modern *shihlo* should more properly be read *zila*. In any case, no cumin is called for and this *shihlo*, although the linguistic match is not perfect, is most likely Turkic *shilön*, and the recipe does call for the *piräk* to be cooked in water. See Lao, 1969: 411–2. Compare the similar recipe in the *JJBYSL* (14, 32a–b).

[79] On the transcription of this word see above. The *JJBYSL* gives the following recipe for *Shuihua* Noodles:

**Samsa* (Tu. from Pr.), *samusa*[80]
Sharba[t] (Ar.) "syrup"
**sürmä* (Tu. from Ar. sharba[t]?) "liquor," in the *YSZY*: "brandy"[81]
**tngri* (Tu.) here: a variety of Qaraqojha Wine[82]
Tutum Ash (Tu.) "noodles'[83]
[Tangut] *Um Ash* (Tu.) lamb–filled soup noodles made of flour[84]

> Use the best quality flour. During the spring, the summer and the autumn use freshly drawn water. Add oil and salt. First mix together uniformly. When the flour becomes dough–like, gradually add water. Press together into balls. Use the hands to [press] open. Make into [flat] lumps. Then sprinkle with oil and water. Combine by kneading one or two hundred times. After doing this three or four times, the dough will be very soft, like a cake. With the dough placed on a table, use an *aopeng* 拗捧 and roll out more than a hundred times. If one does not have an *aopeng* knead a hundred times with the hands. When the dough is ready, it can then be divided to make noodle fingernails. Put into recently cooled water. Soak for a couple of hours or so, waiting until the noodles are ready. Then put into the pot. [The noodles] will be ample and fine. Make them as one pleases. During the winter months soak the noodles in warm water. (18, 21b)

Compare the following a recipe for stuffed *salma* from the *Kitab al–Tibakhah* (Perry, 1985):

> *Salma*: Dough is taken and twisted and cut in small pieces and struck like a coin with a finger, and it is cooked in water until done. Then yogurt is put with it and meat is fried with onion for it and mint and garlic are put with it.

The *aopeng* called may be a Chinese variant of the characteristic Turkic rolling pin, called *oklava* in Turkey and *oqtaw* in Modern Kazakh. On the Turkish form see Algar, 1991: 174.

[80] The Chinese transcription in recipe #10 is *suanzi* 筭子, "abacus counter," Y *sɔntsz̨*, in this case conferring both the idea of a round pasta, and the foreign sound *samsa,* Turkic form of the more common Persian *sambusa*, in early times, *sambusak*.

[81] The transcription for this word, *suerma* 速兒麻, *Y surr̨ma*, makes it unmistakably Uighur *sürmä*. Doerfer (Doerfer, 1963-1975: III, 249-250) has *sorma*. The *suma* given by Muhmud of Kashgar, who may have misheard or mistranscribed his informant, may be a variant of **sürmä*. See Appendix II.

[82] The Chinese is *tiandi* 田地, Y *tʰjɛnti*. Since the wine is Uighur, this word should also be Uighur. We offer *tngri* as a plausible suggestion.

[83] On this food see Appendix II and Doerfer, 1963–75: II, 457–9. The characteristic of this the *tutmach* noodle, according to Perry, is that it is a sturdy, rolled out noodle.

[84] The form *uma[ch] ash*, from Chinese *wumashi* 兀麻食 (1, 28a), Y *umaşi*, with a softening of the "ch" sound of the ending, instead of the expected *umach*, corresponds to modern Turkistanian usage. See G. Doerfer, 1963–75: II, 123–4. This is the *ov-*

Umach (Tu.) "a hand–twisted noodle"[85]
****Yubqa*** (Tu.) "pot cooked bread stuffed with meat and onions"[86]

C. Miscellaneous Terms

Qaraqojha (Tu.) place name
**qashiq* (Tu.), "spoon"[87]
sashuq (Tu.) "small coin"

Two things are immediately striking about these words. One is the degree to which Turkic terminology, particularly for names of dishes, dominates with 36 out of 49 words. The second is the degree to which the *YSZY*'s Turko–Islamic vocabulary is expressive of a quite different cultural experience than does the text's Mongol terminology. List A, for example, includes cosmopolitan spices more or less universal in the Islamic World. The comparable listing of Mongolian words is mostly comprised of relatively obscure plants and animals more or less unique to the Mongol experience. In addition, List B is strongly indicative of an Islamic, in this case Turkic, emphasis on already processed or refined foodstuffs. It includes, for example, no less than 12 prepared bread foods, *i.e.*, breads, noodles, 3 words for foods utilizing prepared bread foods (**Chöppün*, **Shoyla Toyym,* **Ishkänä*), two words for refined liquors, and one for a refined sugar product, *Sharba[t]*.

Islamic World materia dietetica et medica

The following are Islamic world spices, raw and processed foods, and medicines in the *YSZY*. Many appear there for the first time in a Chinese source while others already had long histories of use in China prior to the *YSZY*, in some cases reaching back to Han times at least.

mach, "small soup noodles, pea–shaped dumplings," or, locally, "a vegetable porridge," of Appendix II.

85 The *maqi* 馬乞, Y *mak^{h}i*, of the text is apparently an alternative form, from some other Turkic language, for *wumashi* 兀麻食, i.e., *um ash*. This may be an indication that Hu used different Turkic sources for his recipes.

86 The full title of the recipe in (*YSZY*, 1, 48a) is "butter skin" *yanzi* 掩子, i.e., Y *jɛmtsʐ̩*. With a devoicing of the first vowel, *yanzi* could easily represent *yubqa* or some related word. The title makes it clear that a buttered, thin dough sheet is meant, not unlike modern phyllo, used today in making *yubqa* in Turkey. See Appendix II and Doerfer, 1963–75: IV, 211–12.

87 On this word see Doerfer, 1963–75: III, 390–1. The transcription is a relatively straight forward one (*achi* 阿赤, Y *ɔtʂ^{h}i*).

Such *materia dietetica et medica* were thus not new to Chinese dietary and food traditions. In this case, what is new in the *YSZY* are not the spices, foods and medicines themselves, but the uses to which older borrowings are now put in flavor and ingredient combinations that are unmistakably Western and Middle Eastern:

A. Spices:

Asafoetida (Pr. *kasni*)
Asafoetida root (Pr. *anguzhad*)
Attar of Roses
Basil
Black Pepper ("Iranian Pepper")
Camphor (Ar. *ka'fur*)
Cardamom
Cubebs
Cumin (Pr. *zhira*)
Fennel
Fenugreek Seeds
Long Pepper
Poppy Seeds ("Little Black Seeds")
Purple Perilla Leaves
Safflower
Saffron (*za'faran*)
Swiss Chard Seeds
Turmeric

B. Raw Foods:

Almonds (*badam*),
Aromatic Non–glutinous Rice
Bottle Gourds
Bulb Onions
Carrots ("Iranian Radishes")
Chickpeas ("Muslim beans")
Chigen 赤根 ("Red Root," true Spinach)
Durum or Hard Wheat (Ar. *qamh*)
Grapes
Hazelnuts
"Iranian Sesame Seeds"
Leek Juice

Leeks
Mulberry Fruits
"Muslim Green[s]" (Mint, Cress?)
Oil Rape
Oil Rape Sprouts
Pistachios (*pistä*)
Pomegranates
Purslane
Rape (*shajhimur*, *shaljam*)
Shallots ("Muslim Onions")
Sugar Beets
Swiss Chard
Walnuts
White Millet
White Sugar Beets

C. Processed or Fermented Foods:

Arajhi (Ar. *'araq*) Brandy
Bouillon ("clear broth")
Cane Sugar
Ghee
Glauber's Salts Solution
Grape Wine
Malt–Sugar
Mastajhi, mastic
Mäskä (Butter) Oil
"Muslim Lesser Oil" (Unrefined Sesame Oil?)[88]
Qatiq ("Dried Sour Milk")
**Sürmä* (Brandy)
White Lead ("Iranian Powder") Solution
White *Nabat* (Fine Cane Sugar)
Yogurt

Unlike many of the *YSZY*'s Near Eastern–influenced recipes, there is little about this which is particularly Turkic. The *YSZY*'s spices,

[88] "Muslim Lesser Oil" is not further identified in the text but, judging from the usage, must be a vegetable oil. The most likely possibility is unrefined sesame oil, the favored Muslim cooking oil in areas where olive oil was unavailable or too expensive (such as China). No "Muslim Greater Oil" is mentioned in the text but the *JJBYSL* (13, 18b) does mention a "Muslim Oil," almost certainly ghee.

foods and medicines from the Islamic World reflect more a common Middle Eastern (Irano–Arabic) than specifically Turkic cultural context. But in view of the predominance of Turkic cultural elements elsewhere within the Islamic culture of the *YSZY*, the Turkic forms of some Arabic and Iranian words, there can be no doubt whatever that the above *materia dietetica et medica* none the less largely occurs in the *YSZY* through Turkic intermediation.[89]

Turko–Middle Eastern Recipes

Turko–Middle Eastern influences find expression in two major categories of *YSZY* recipes in particular, the one comprised of a large number of mostly Turkic bread, noodle and grain foods, the other of various sweets jams, jellies, sweet nut butters, *sharba[t]*s, syrups *etc.*, representing traditions generalized throughout the Islamic world, but particularly widespread among the Turkic peoples. The latter are well known today for their "sweet tooth." The presence of so many recipes calling for large amounts of more or less refined crystal sugar is one of the most striking West Asian features of the entire *YSZY*.

In addition to these direct Turko–Middle Eastern influences, most other *YSZY* recipes, even including some medicinal ones at the end of *juan* 2, are either cooked with Islamic world *materia dietetica et medica* or prepared in what is clearly an Middle Eastern rather than a Chinese manner. These include the highly acculturated 27 *šülen* recipes whose Islamic content has already been noticed above. There may also be considerable influence of Arabic medicine in the *YSZY* as well, although it has perhaps been mediated through a highly similar Chinese medicine in most cases.

Bread, Noodle and Grain Foods

The category of breads and bread foods is a large and relatively uniform one in the *YSZY*, comprising no less than 16 recipes (7.3% of all recipes). A range of largely Turkic recipes is presented including both steamed and baked breads. The steamed bread recipes include 3 recipes (#81–2, #84) for Turkic **manta* (plus one imitation **manta* using eggplant skin as the covering, #83), 2 for what the text calls *paozi*

---

[89] The same observation can be made for the "Muslim (Huihui) recipes" occurring in the *JJBYSL* (13, 17a–19b). Of the 12 recipes given, no less than 5 have Turkic names while two others ("West of the River Lungs" and the *halwa*) are basically Turkic recipes. For a complete translation see Buell, 1999.

包子 (#89–90; the *YSZY*'s *baozi* are all **manta*), and one recipe (#93) for what is a yeasted loaf bread (**chuqmin*), although steamed in a special pot, and not baked. Baked bread recipes include 3 (#85–7) for baked Turkic *börek* (*piräk*), one made with thin sheets of dough ancestral to phyllo (to make a **yubqa*), 1 for a boiled *börek* (#88), and two (#91–2) for spiced buns (clearly to be baked, compare the *Khubz al–Abazir* on page 77). In addition to these bread recipes *per se*, there are also four *YSZY* recipes eaten over, wrapped up in or specifically with bread: recipes #8 and #28, to be eaten with long rolled bread (a textual note says this is like the yeasted steamed loaf bread **chuqmin*), recipe #33, literally a "companion (**ishkänä*)" to Iranian Bread (*Nan*), and recipe #63, a **chuqmin* (rolled bread) stuffing.

The *YSZY*'s grain and noodle dishes and noodles constitute another prominent tradition mostly from the Turkic Middle East. Grain foods and noodles had, of course, long histories in China by the time the *YSZY* was written. There were many that were completely indigenous. Others, above all those associated with the fine milling of wheat owe their origin to a much earlier era of dissemination of foods and technology from the Middle East and were, for all practical purposes, Chinese by the fourteenth century. Be that as it may, most *YSZY* noodles, noodle and grain dishes are clearly not part of the well–established Chinese grain and noodle food traditions of the era and are quite distinct: in terminology, since in many of the recipes the noodles are called by their Turkic names; often in technology, *e.g.*, in the possible use of durum, called in the *YSZY* by its Arabic name **qamh*, to make true pasta; and recipe context. The number of recipes calling for fried stuffed noodles, for example, is conspicuous.

Altogether 27 recipes in the *YSZY* (12.3%) are either noodle food recipes, or call for noodles. Conspicuously, 23 of these recipes are found among the exotic recipes of *juan* 1 (24.2%), meaning that *YSZY* noodle dishes and noodles are overwhelmingly clustered among those recipes most demonstrably non–Chinese in origin, although not always in detail. Of noodles called for in these 23 recipes, 15 are stuffed noodles, with 9 of the stuffed noodles fried. The following *YSZY* noodles are of definite or probable West or Central Asian origins. The list includes all those noodles with non–Chinese names, all stuffed noodles, all noodles made more or less exclusively with white flour, as opposed to the bean paste noodles typical of the Chinese practice of the day, the barley noodles, made from what is not a common Chinese flour, the hanging noodles, noodles apparently rack–dried much like early pasta in the West, and the "Euryale Blood Noodles." The latter probably reflect Mongolian taste even if made with a typically Chinese ingredient. Compare the use of Euryale flour to make **chöp* and, in one case, the text's "square" noodles, if they are that. They may also be foreign:[90]

> "Barley **Samsa* Noodles" (3 parts barley flour, 1 part bean paste) (#10)
> "Chicken–claw Vermicelli" (white flour) (#25)

---

[90] The Uighur *suyqaš* (<*suyuq–aš*) of the present day is characteristically a small square–shaped noodle and this noodle may be what the *YSZY* means with its mysterious *qizi* 䭲子, probably Y k^h*itsz̧*, of uncertain reading but probably to be read *qi* as done here, although *jizi* is also possible, yielding a strong phonological resemblance to the Uighur although the term, at least, is old in China and the phonological resemblance may be purely coincidental. In form at least, the first element recalls the Chinese character for go counter, i.e., *ji* 碁 (or 棋), and this points up the square shape of this noodle, a fact clearly indicated in the *JJBYSL*. Five kinds of *qizi* are called for in the text, "rice-heart" *qizi* in recipe 10, Euryale flour "swallow's tongue *qizi*, in recipe 15, "nail-headed" *qizi* in recipe 24, "water dragon" or "cash eye" *qizi*, in recipe 42, and flour *qizi*, in recipes 164 and 168. Of them, the *JJBYSL* (11, 23a–b) gives the following recipe for "Rice heart" *qizi*:

> Add cool water to the best flour. Add salt, combine and form into lumps. After having worked the dough, careful that it does not become too thin, cut into delicate squares [go counters]. After pressing through a fine bamboo sieve again use a knife and cut. After having pressed through a fine bamboo sieve and cut a thousand or a hundred times, re–cut any coarse noodles into fine. If there is excess flour, again press through a sieve etc. Cook in soup. When done, remove noodles with soup and put into a cup of cool water. Stir around. Fish noodles out and set out to dry. [To cook] use sesame oil. Add [as filling]: chunks of meat, pieces of sweet melon pickle, pieces of Sauce Melon, pieces of cucumber, basil, *etc.*

A recipe for Sauce Melon, in this case made from sweet melon, is given elsewhere in the *JJBYSL* (12, 66a–b):

> Take 10 immature sweet melons and skewer with bamboo spits. Apply 4 *liang* of salt. Put inside the melons. Squeeze out the liquid and let the melons dry. Apply evenly with 10 *liang* of "sauce." Dry in the sun on a hot day. Turn over the melons several times and dry again until completely dry. Put into a new porcelain container. Close container. Use salt and use "sauce," employing them to the best advantage in terms of the size and quantity of the melons.

This and other pickle recipes of the text are not particularly Chinese and the ultimate inspiration is probably Middle Eastern. We are grateful to Julia Fearing for discussing modern Uighur *suyqaš* with us.

**Chöp* (2 parts glutinous rice flour, one part bean paste) (#12)
"Euryale Flour Blood Noodles" (2 parts euryale flour, 1 part bean paste) (#16)
"Euryale Flour **Chöp*" (2 parts euryale flour, 1 part bean paste) (#18)
"Fine **Salma*" (#41)
Fine vermicelli (white flour) (#26–7, 34)
"Hanging Noodles" (pasta?) (#37)
"River Pigs" (white flour) (#13)
"Tangut *Um Ash*" (#5)
Tutum Ash (#40)
Umach (#43)[91]

Sweets

Although it was probably Indians who first refined sugar cane sap into sugar, it was the Arabs who developed sugar more or less into its modern forms and broadly disseminated the use of refined sugar and sugar products in foods and in medicine. This fact finds its full reflection in the *YSZY* with its many Islamic traditions, including Arab sweets in many forms.[92]

---

[91] For a discussion of many of these noodles see now Françoise Sabban, "Ravioli cristallins et tagliatelle rouges: les pâtes chinoises entre xiie et xive siècle," *Medievales* 16–7 (1989): 29–50.

[92] Refined sugar was already common in China by 1330 where it may have been known, in the south at least, for as long as a thousand years. It was, for example, already well known to Ji Han (Li, 1979: 55ff). In the Near East too sugar had been known since classical times where a great expansion of the sugar industry took place in early Islamic times (Watson 1981, 1983). In China, Wang Shao's 王紹 1153 *Tangshuang pu* 糖霜譜, "Treatise on Crystallized Sugar," among other sources, reflects a sophisticated knowledge of producing raw sugar from cane and then whiter sugar from the raw. For Ming, the *Tiangong kaiwu* 天工開物 describes an extremely sophisticated sugar technology, not much inferior in terms of products to modern industry. See *Sung Ying-hsing* 宋應星, *Tian-kung Kai-wu*, trans. by E–tu Zen Sun and Shiou–chuan Sun (University Park, 1966). Most of this probably already existed by late Yuan. The best white was close to ours today, but took a great deal more time and effort to produce than modern white sugar. It was expensive, a food for the emperor. China's sugar center was, and long remained, in the Canton Delta, where small holders produced much of it. Sugar is easier to produce on plantations than on small farms, because of the huge mills needed. It usually accompanies the most socially unequal and regressive of socioeconomic systems. See George Beckford, *Persistent Poverty* (Oxford, 1972) and Mintz, 1985. In the Delta, the maze of waterways eliminated the need for plantations. Cane could be boated to mills, or, in a more uniquely Chinese

Juan 2 is the repository for this kind of recipe, with a total of 21, 9.6% of all recipes. The recipes include 10 for various sweet jams and jellies,[93] *julab* and *rubb*,[94] for sauces, one of which may be a badly described *khabis*, fruit extracts, one is called a *sharba[t]* and syrups made with refined or crude granulated sugar,[95] or with crystallized honey. There are also 5 recipes for spiked, here freeze–distilled to concentrate alcohol,[96] and unspiked berry and fruit punches. One calls

---

approach, mills mounted on barges were actually moved from farm to farm. See now in detail the full monograph by Sucheta Mazumdar, *Sugar and Society in China: Peasants, Technology, and the World Markets*. (Cambridge, MA, 1998). Meanwhile, in India and Persia, the same technology developed. Indeed, China's early sugar technology was derived from theirs. Sugar became highly important in medicine in those areas, because of its soothing qualities and its value as a vehicle for other medicines, as well as because of alleged medical virtues and the fact that it and its products tend to be pleasing and cheering. Syrups, sharbats, confits, jams, preserves, and other confectionery became preferred ways to administer all kinds of medicinal substances, perhaps especially naturally sweet fruits. This technology is notably well reflected in the *YSZY*, a point that is particularly interesting since little else that is directly West Asian is found in the medical sections. In China, sugar was also medicinal, but in a different way: brown sugar was heating, "ice" (rock) sugar and raw sugar cane were cooling. All sugar was believed valuable in compounds to harmonize ingredients. On sweets in the Islamic world see Martin Levey, translator, *The Medical Formulary or Aqrabadhin of Al-Kindi* (Madison, 1966).

[93] Such fruit jams and jellies were completely foreign to Chinese tradition and not a feature of Chinese life except as minor medicinal preparations.

[94] According to Mintz (1985: 97–8): "to prepare [a *rubb*]..., fruits and flower petals were immersed in hot water to which sugar was added, and the whole preparation was boiled down until it was concentrated." This was distinct from a *julab*, which was prepared in a similar fashion but was less thick (Mintz, 1985: 98), and a *shurba*, a very viscid juice that would now break when two fingers were thrust into it, removed and then extended (Mintz, 1985: 97). For other categories see also Mintz, 1985: 98.

[95] *Sharbat* are also well represented (under that name) in the *JJBYSL* (11, 15b–17b).

[96] Recipes of this sort are a marker of an age when distillation was new and far from widespread, and is hard to pin down as to exact origin. Clearly this method would have been of special usefulness to the Mongols, given Mongolian climatic conditions, and would have readily adapted itself to distillation of fruit "beers" that must have been made on the steppe. This is because most natural fruits and berries begin fermentation on their own if left to sit and the results of alternately freezing and thawing, or semi–thawing, such "beers" must have been only too readily apparent to the Mongols. Turkic experience may have applied here as well since Uighurs and other Turkic groups would not only have been among the first to acquire ideas of distillation coming from the West; note, for example, that one word in the *YSZY*, for a brandy, *sürmä*, is apparently Uighur, but also, quite likely, made "beers" from fruits and berries and probably observed the same changes occasioned by alternately freez-

for ginseng, but is prepared in a completely Islamic way. One recipe is for a medicinal fruit candy, and 3 are for sweet medicinal cakes. Two call for Turkic *qatiq*, a dried sour milk, one for ingredients with Mongolian names (*tabilqa, cicigina*). None the less, all three are prepared in a Middle Eastern way using sugar as a major bonding agent. The *YSZY*'s medicinal foods, listed later in *juan* 2, also include two sugar–based recipes.

Other Recipes from the Islamic World

YSZY breads and bread foods, probably most noodle and grain foods, and virtually all *YSZY* sweets are from the Turko–Islamic world. We might add to the list the two special vegetable oil (#128–9) recipes in *juan* 2 along with the grape wine and two distilled liquors (Tu. *Arajhi* and **Sürma*) in *juan* 3. There are also many isolated examples of Turko–Islamic world recipes in the *YSZY*, including some not at all obvious such as recipe #59, Fish Cakes. It is strongly reminiscent of the Bagdhadi methods for cooking fish of the era.[97] Still other examples will be pointed out and discussed below.

Islamic World Influences on Other Material

Judging from examples and recipe categories discussed above, a third, perhaps more, of all *YSZY* recipes are direct transfers from the Turko–Islamic world. They are little modified by contact with the Chinese side of Mongol China, and the Chinese conceptual world of the *YSZY*. In addition to such direct Turko–Islamic world influence on the *YSZY* there is indirect influence as well. Two areas are of particular concern here: 1) a subtle and not so subtle Middle Eastern assimilation of most non–Islamic world foods in the *YSZY*; and 2) evidence for the presence of concepts of Islamic medicine and dietary theory as well as foodways in the *YSZY*. The latter is particularly difficult to document since Chinese and Arabic medicine had come to be very similar by the fourteenth century. Both had, by and large, for example, grown up on the same humoral base, both owed a great deal to Indian Ayurvedic traditions, and each continued to be in contact with the other. It is this

---

ing and thawing. On freeze distillation see the discussion in Joseph Needham, Ho Ping–yü and Lu Gwei–djen, *Science and Civilisation in China,* vol. 5: *Chemistry and Chemical Technology,* part IV: *Spagyrical Discovery and Invention: Apparatus, Theories and Gifts* (Cambridge, 1980), 151ff.

[97] Compare Heine, 1988: 82–6.

common base, and continuing contact between two fairly similar systems, which makes identification of Arabic elements in a Chinese medical text so difficult. In addition, Medieval Arabic medicine is only now beginning to be well studied.[98] Most texts still remain unpublished including quite a number directly relating to the cultural exchanges of the Mongol age. The tentativeness of any suggestions we make here is thus to be stressed. None the less, certain clear borrowings are evident and will be pointed out in more detail below, this including the material on the wet nurse in *juan* 1 (21b-22b). There is nothing like it in the Chinese tradition although very similar material is found in Ibn Sīnā, the probable origin of the section in question.[99]

Assimilation of Other People's Recipes

Perhaps the best examples of *YSZY* recipes reworked with the Turko–Islamic World palate in mind are the 27 *šülen*. These dishes are in essence Mongolian boiled, cauldron food, but the spicing (cinnamon, fenugreek seeds, *mastajhi*, saffron, turmeric, *kasni*, black pepper) is mostly Middle Eastern. The same is true for most of the additives, especially chickpeas used as a thickener, probably the aromatic non–glutinous rice, and certainly the *šaqimur/sajhimur* beets, carrots, bottle gourds, cheese, the "Tangut *Um Ash*," and probably the bouillon and sheep's liver sauce as well. The dishes themselves have been converted from relatively primitive Mongolian foods into the classic "dry soups" and "pilafs" of the classical Arabic food category *nashif*. Recipes for two foods of this category from a Medieval Arabic cookbook are quoted above. Compare the highly similar *YSZY* recipes for "Chinese Quince Soup" (#6) and for "*Šaqimur* Soup" (#4). Compare also usage of a Turkic word for small coin, to indicate how vegetables are to be cut up, with similar usage above, where the recipe (*Dinariya*) is named after the Arabic equivalent of such coin shapes.

In addition to the 27 *šülen*, there are other *YSZY* recipes showing strong West Asian influence. They include #7, for "Deer Head Soup," #51, "Broiled Sheep's Loins," and #30, "Bear Soup." In these recipes, typical Middle Eastern spices or condiments (*kasni*, turmeric, pepper, saffron, attar of roses) have either been used to bring out the flavor of

[98] See now Peter E. Pormann and Emilie Savage-Smith, *Medieval Islamic Medicine* (Washington, D.C, 2007) and on pharmacy Leigh Chipman, *The World of Pharmacy and Pharmacists in Mamlūk Cairo* (Leiden and Boston), 2010.

[99] Compare the material summarized directly from Ibn Sīnā in Hassan Kamal, *Encyclopaedia of Islamic Medicine* (Cairo, 1975), 138ff.

meat and other ingredients (the traditional role of *kasni* or asafoetida, although turmeric works perfectly well too), or to change a food's appearance. This is the purpose of the saffron in recipes #51 and #30. Turmeric can also color as well as change flavor. In addition, recipe #51 calls for quenching, a cooking technique extremely popular in Medieval Arabic cooking as studied by Heine.[100] The attar of roses called for in the same recipe is also a pure and typical Islamic cooking refinement. All three recipes, although spiced and cooked in a Muslim manner, none the less appear to be Mongolian in taste if not in essence. Certainly the Mongolian background to the boiled deer's head or the bear meat soup is unmistakable.

Influences of Arabic Medicine

Arabic medicine, like Chinese, was heavily based on herbal products, including, as in the Chinese tradition, animal and mineral as well as plant pharmaceutics. Among items notable in the *YSZY*, onions and eggs were conspicuous as aphrodisiacs.[101] Here we do not speak of the general stimulants, tonics, and nutrients of the body or the genital system that Chinese medicine employs, and that are miscalled "aphrodisiacs" in the pop Western literature. We have to deal with out–and–out aphrodisiacs. Such items were always popular with emperors, who were under some pressure to satisfy their large harems. Many foods and spices were considered aphrodisiacs in Medieval Islamic medicine as well.

Onions were also used for several other reasons in Medieval Arab medicine,[102] but not for any reasons discussed in the *YSZY*. Among other *YSZY* plants used medicinally in West Asia we may mention fennel, jujube, mallow, garlic, carrot, walnut, mint, fenugreek, asafoetida, chickpeas, cinnamon, black and long peppers, saffron, ginger, quince, sesame, sugar, ghee, liquorice, basil, barley, honey, turmeric, coriander, cumin, rose, and probably to a very minor extent some other items. Chickpeas, for example, were used for sores and eruptions, and, improbably, as an abortifacient; saffron, as in recipe #50, was cheering; ginger as a carminative, stomachic, skin stimulant, for all of which it is obviously effective; quince for coughs, a use also tradition-

[100] Heine, 1988: 66.

[101] Shaykh Nefzawi, *The Perfumed Garden*, trans. from the Arabic by Richard Burton, ed. Alan Hull Walston (Berkeley and New York, 1964).

[102] Levey, 1966: 230–1.

al in China. Mutton and other meats were, of course, used to nourish and for general purposes.

Most *YSZY* medical foods in *YSZY* are Chinese, not Near Eastern, and conversely the vast majority of major Near Eastern Medieval drugs are absent from the *YSZY*. The *YSZY*'s medical discourse is also in Chinese, and when foods and drugs also used in Near Eastern medicine occur in the *YSZY*, with some notable exceptions, it is almost always with those indications recognized by Chinese medicine. These are in some cases identical to the Near Eastern ones, mainly in cases where no one could possibly miss the medical effect, as with the carminative effects of ginger and apiaceous fruits.

But despite the overlay of Chinese medical tradition and terminology, Arabic medicine is reflected in the *YSZY*. It finds expression: 1) in specific *materia dietetica et medica* whose assigned properties in Arabic medicine have been implicitly transferred into the *YSZY*. One example is fennel, a common Arabic medicine stomachic, used in recipe #105, and #107.[103] Both are powders, typical of Medieval Arabic usage. Other examples are the heart–meat, saffron, and attar of roses[104] in recipes #50–51. It also finds expression: 2) in types of medicinals, dose forms in particular, above all those employing a sugar base, *e.g.*, the syrup recipes in *juan* 2 *etc.*;[105] 3) through specific medicinal recipes more or less representing intact transfers from medieval Arabic tradition into the *YSZY*, *e.g.*, recipe #105, also possibly #111 with its unique use of Western cardamom; and 4) possibly through certain generalized principles of lifestyle, hygiene and even food avoidances, although here it is very difficult to distinguish what is Chinese from what is not although some material, *e.g.*, the dictums on the wet nurse, do appear Muslim.

One primary source of influences of this type for the Chinese dietary manual may have been works of the popular Arabic tradition represented in the West by the various extant versions of the *Tacuinum Sanitatis*. In its present form, it is strikingly similar to *juan* 3 of

---

[103] Some of the other medicinals of this recipe, including the *Melia azederach*, appear very Chinese but were very important in Arabic medicine too, as was liquorice, in powdered form as here. The medicinal properties of orange peel were also known to Arabic doctors, although the form of the medicinal here is unquestionably Chinese.

[104] On this combination see Levey, 1966: 230–1. Sabban (1986b) long ago pointed out the Arab origins of these recipes.

[105] See Mintz, 1985: 96ff, for similar Arabic medicine contributions to the Medieval West.

the *YSZY*, although the latter is far more extensive and is largely based upon Chinese, rather than Middle Eastern, experience with herbs and foods. The *Tacuinum Sanitatis* is a straight adaptation of an eleventh century dietary/hygiene work by Ibn Butlan, the *Kitab Taqwim as–sihha*, part of a whole tradition of similar Arabic treatises.[106] Such works may have been known to Muslim doctors and dietitians working at the Mongol court in China and thus been used by Hu Sihui as sources.[107]

The Chinese Framework

Chinese influence in the *YSZY* is primarily presentation and theoretical content, *i.e.*, the culture of the work as a whole. It also finds expression in many Chinese "erratic blocks" of text, *e.g.*, biographies of the "Three Sages," "Doses and Foods of the Beneficent Immortals," the nucleus of the medicinal recipes, in the Chinese *materia dietetica* of *juan* 3, and in a pervading Chinese culinary influence that is in most respects even more significant than the Islamic.[108]

The most noticeable overall Chinese feature of the *YSZY* is that it was written with a largely Sinicized audience in mind. Its contents, as a consequence, reflect particular interests of this audience, and appeal to Chinese cultural values. The *YSZY* assumes Chinese attitudes towards foods and medicines, not sharply distinct categories to the Chinese. The *YSZY* also lists and gives pride of place to an impressive array of more or less purely Chinese *materia dietetica et medica*, particularly those enjoying considerable prestige in the Chinese cultural experience. Thus there is extensive discussion in *juan* 3 of rice and millet (1a–2b), and later a section on pork (14b–15a). Rice, millet and

[106] See Luisa Cogliate Arano, *The Medieval Health Handbook: Tacuinum Sanitatis* (New York, 1976). See also Ullmann, 1978: 99.

[107] The examples discussed above indicative of possible direct influence of Arabic humoral medicine upon the *YSZY* are only those which stand out. There may be many other not so obvious examples. The research of a specialist, one who can make detailed comparison of *YSZY* recipes with those contained in Arab sources, is needed. But what little we already know suggests that this will be a fruitful line of inquiry.

[108] It is interesting that so much of the Near Eastern material in sources inherited by the YSZY as "erratic blocks" appears to be quite old suggesting there may have been Near Eastern medical manuals floating around as major chunks of material, even whole texts. The YSZY is also rich in Daoist material, including fragments from the works of Ge Hong. See now Robert Ford Campany, *To Live as Long as Heaven and Earth: A Translation and Study of Ge Hong's Tradition of Divine Transcendents* (Berkeley, 2002).

pork are also mentioned frequently elsewhere in the *YSZY*, in "erratic" text blocks that are culturally Chinese and restate Chinese dietary values.

But appearances deceive. Rice, millet and pork, so prominent in *juan* 3 listings and in other culturally Chinese "erratic" blocks of text, are rarely called for in recipes. Rice is called for most often, but the recipes involved are nearly all Muslim, *e.g.*, "dry soups" of *juan* 1. The rice itself is probably a Middle Eastern variety.[109] Millet is used in only five recipes, one clearly Turko–Mongolian (recipe #45 "*Qima* Congee"), the others medicinal (recipes #103–104, and 212–213). Pork, *the* Chinese meat, is called for in only three recipes (recipe #66, "Galangal Sauce Hog's Head," and medicinal recipes #165, "Pig Kidney Congee," and #217, "Wild Pig Meat Broth," in *juan* 2). None is particularly Chinese.[110]

Thus, judging from these examples, "Chinese" listings in *juan* 3, and Chinese *materia dietetica* emphasized in "erratic" blocks elsewhere in the text, do not mesh well with contents of the recipes. Likewise, *juan* 3, the most Chinese segment of the entire text, fails to list many of the most important foreign ingredients (compare Tables B

[109] Rice was a common food called for by both the Chinese and West Asian culinary traditions of the time. In a Chinese–language dietary one would logically expect Chinese rices. But in fact virtually all *YSZY* recipes calling for rice specify a fragrant or aromatic rice. This is presumably something similar to the basmati rice of Punjab. Most Chinese do not like such markedly flavorful rices, finding them too much for daily fare. They are more characteristic of India, where aromatic rice was preferred in Moghul court pilafs, of the Arab and Persian world (*e.g.*, *domsiyah*), also of Uzbekistan (*dewzira*), places where rice is enough of a special dish to make a special flavor desirable. But some Chinese do like fragrant rice, *e.g.*, the old long–grain varieties of Thailand and Hong Kong, which are not as strong–tasting as basmati. This preference might have been more common in the rice–poor north of the era in so that the rice–usage here can represent both West Asian and Chinese traditions. In any case, the aromatic rice of the *YSZY* was probably not unappealing to the Chinese palate.

[110] The reason usually advanced for the virtual absence of pork in the *YSZY* is that Hu Sihui was a Muslim. He quite likely was, but his work includes recipes for other animals, *e.g.*, wolves, donkeys, horses, equally abominations to the orthodox. A more likely reason for the absence of pork recipes in the *YSZY* is the simple fact that there were no pig herds in Mongolia and it was not an animal with which the Mongols had had a great deal of experience. Recent Mongols also reject pork because the pig is considered a dirty animal consuming excrement and other filth but we do not know how far into the past this belief, rooted in recent Mongol conflicts with Chinese, extends. See Uradyn Erden Bulag, "Nationalism and Identity in Mongolia" (Ph.D. dissertation, Cambridge University, 1993). In any case, the absence of pork from *YSZY* recipes does show how different its food culture is from that of South China.

and C in Appendix I) and lists in all only about two–thirds of all *YSZY materia dietetica et medica*. This is another indication of a great disparity between the Chinese side of the *YSZY* and other cultural traditions represented in it, even an isolation of Chinese from non–Chinese traditions. This fact makes the visible "Chinese" culture of the text at times seem thin and superficial.

But there is one major exception to this pattern which changes the picture completely. Someone, presumably Hu himself, has gone to great trouble to ground the *YSZY* in the latest medical theories of the time, specifically in the correspondence medicine of the Song–Jin–Yuan school of Liu Wansu 劉完素 (1110–1200), Zhang Congzheng 張從正 (1156–1228), Chen Yan 陳言 (fl. 1161–1174), Li Gao 李高 (1180–1251) and Zhu Zhenheng 朱震亨 (1281–1358), a contemporary of Hu.[111] In its mature form this medicine, by no means the only medical tradition active in China at the time, or even the only Chinese medicine represented in the *YSZY*, combines the medical world view of the various texts of the *Yellow Emperor's Inner Canon* (*Huangdi neijing* 黃帝內經)[112] with Neoconfucianism. It also sought to apply

---

[111] See the discussion of these thinkers in Paul U. Unschuld, *Medicine in China: A History of Ideas* (Berkeley, 1985), 172ff. See also Rall, 1970. We are indebted to Paul Unschuld (unpublished letter of 16 July, 1990 to PDB) for pointing out to us the importance of Song–Jin–Yuan Correspondence Medicine in *YSZY*. On Yuan medicine and its public aspects in particular see now Shinno Reiko, "Medical Schools and the Temples of the Three Progenitors in Yuan China: A Case of Cross-Cultural Interactions," *Harvard Journal of Asiatic Studies* 7 (2007): 89-133.

[112] There are three distinct texts today known collectively as the *Yellow Emperor's Inner Canon*: the *Huangdi neijing lingshu* 黃帝內經靈樞, "Numinous Pivot of the Yellow Emperor's Inner Canon," possibly fifth century AD in its present form, the *Huangdi neijing suwen* 黃帝內經素問, "Everyday Questions of the Yellow Emperor's Inner Canon," the definitive version of which appeared in AD 762 although it was not printed to produce the currently transmitted text until Northern Song times, and the *Huangdi neijing taisu* 黃帝內經太素, "General Synopsis of the Yellow Emperor's Inner Canon," seventh century AD, as it currently exists. Although supposedly reproducing knowledge obtained directly from the greatest of all Chinese culture heroes, the Yellow Emperor (traditional dates 2697–2598 BC), and clearly incorporating much earlier material, some even going back to Han times or earlier, as is evident from a comparison with other early medical texts, the existing versions of the canon not only do not reproduce the sagely words of the Yellow Emperor, but are best taken as representing Southern and Northern Dynasties thought, codified in Tang times. A complete translation of the transmitted text of the *Huangdi neijing suwen* by a team led by Paul Unschuld will appear shortly (University of California Press).

premises primarily developed with acupuncture in mind in the *Yellow Emperor's Inner Canon* to herbal medicine.[113]

Through this grounding, even if thin in places and awkward in others, *e.g.*, "Roast Wolf Soup," recipe #32 in *juan* 1, where Hu Sihui freely admits that he has forced a Mongolian food into Chinese categories, the highly heterogeneous materials making up the dietary have gained consistency, and have been assimilated, if superficially, to the Chinese cultural experience. Thereby the foreign has been made acceptable to a broad Chinese audience, and even part of the Chinese tradition. Many animal drugs, most of apparent Mongolian origin, so popular in later Chinese medicine, for example, are first mentioned and first assigned medical properties in the *YSZY*. Hu Sihui's clear success in this area is the primary reason for the popularity of the text since the fourteenth century, and the high esteem that it is held in by Chinese dietitians even today. The Chinese medicine of the *YSZY* thus bears our closest scrutiny as its most important and enduring, if not always most obviously visible, Chinese element. For that reason we begin our discussion with it, followed by a consideration of Chinese culinary influences.

Song–Jin–Yuan Correspondence Medicine in the YSZY

Origins of Correspondence Medicine

As Paul Unschuld has shown persuasively,[114] Chinese medicine is not a single tradition but rather a variety of traditions which have sometimes interacted, and sometimes existed separately, even in isolation from one another, never forming a homogenous and unified whole.

---

[113] Although below we interpret the Song-Jin-Yuan school solely in Chinese terms, and most of its background is Chinese, or, if foreign, long absorbed foreign ideas, e.g., humoral traditions coming in at an early date, the resemblance of the ideas of some of the later exponents in particular to those coming from recent Arabic medicine appears unmistakable. This may in part be because of the participation by assimilated foreigners in the "Chinese" medicine of the period. One was Sa Qianzhai 薩謙齋 or *Satmish," to call him by his Uighur name (Sademishi 薩德彌實). Despite an active official career, *Satmish found the time to publish in 1326 a large collection of medical recipes, the *Rui zhu tang jingyan fang* 瑞竹堂經驗方, which survives and was later used by Li Shizhen, who cites the book 48 times, in compiling the *Bencao gangmu*. On the topic of possible foreign influence on the Song-Jin-Yuan school see new suggestions offered in Shinno, 2007. We thank Igor de Rachewiltz for his help in reconstructing Sa's Uighur name (emails to PDB of 26 and 27 September, 2009).

[114] See in particular Unschuld, 1985.

Practitioners have also been highly idiosyncratic to the extent that there are almost as many Chinese medicines as there are individual practitioners of it.[115]

Among the most ancient traditions of Chinese medicine are various forms of manipulation of the spirit world to ensure the health of the individual and of the community. In Shang times it was believed that illness by and large arose due to disharmony between the living and the spirits of the dead. When illness occurred, divination ascertained which ancestor was responsible and that ancestor was offered a bribe in the form of a sacrifice to restore health. Also producing illness were certain forces in nature including "evil wind (*feng* 風)," but these the Shang people likewise viewed as spiritual forces and sought to propitiate.[116]

Also very old in Chinese medicine is the belief that certain individuals are specially empowered to deal with the menaces of the spiritual world, for example the power of generalized forces such as evil wind, or, in later Chinese usage, demons.[117] In early texts these individuals are generally called *wu* 巫 (or *xi* 覡 when female), a term usually translated "shaman." Although the shaman performs many other functions including various ritual practices intended to ward off "demons"[118] and prevent illness in the first place, the primary focus in shamanic healing is on those illnesses believed caused by the stolen or errant soul of the person who is ill. To discover its location and recover it in a spiritual journey in which the shaman's own soul is placed in jeopardy, the shaman must go into a trance with the help of a powerful tutelary spirit which is the source of the shaman's power. If the effort

---

[115] We are indebted to Christopher Muench for this insight, growing out of our research on the Ah–Fong legacy in Idaho. See Christopher Muench, "One Hundred Years of Medicine: the Ah–Fong Physicians of Idaho," in *Chinese Medicine on the Golden Mountain, An Interpretive Guide*, ed. H. G. Schwarz (Bellingham, 1984), 51–80, and also Paul D. Buell and Christopher Muench, "Chinese Medical Recipes from Frontier Seattle," *Annals of the Chinese Historical Society of the Pacific Northwest*, II (1984): 100–43.

[116] Unschuld, 1985: 17–28.

[117] For an excellent introduction to the uncanny side of Chinese medicine as it still exists see in particular N. H. van Straten, *Concepts of Health Disease and Vitality in Traditional Chinese Society*, Münchener ostasiatische Studien 34 (Wiesbaden, 1983).

[118] On what Unschuld calls "demonic medicine" see Unschuld, 1985: 29ff.

is successful, the patient recovers; if not, the patient dies, perhaps taking the shaman with him.[119]

Of more recent origin are two other important traditions of Chinese medicine, herbal medicine and acupuncture. Although their invention is assigned to two of China's ancient sage kings, neither was systematized until late Zhou and Han times at the very earliest. Herbal medicine is the older of the two, since use of herbs in treating illness dates back to Shang times at least,[120] but herbal medicine as it is now practiced owes much to the experiments and theorizing of proto–Daoist alchemists of the last centuries BC. They sought to utilize drugs, special foods and herbs to purify the body and free the spirit for immortality.[121] The *YSZY* devotes considerable space to their exploits and details various prescriptions for achieving immortality. In its most ancient form, acupuncture appears to have been associated with efforts to expel demons with moxa–loaded stones and special metal implements, not unrelated to the ritual dagger of the shaman. These were applied directly to the body at special points, not always the same as today's acupuncture points, to attack the demons, drive them out of the body and thus cure.[122] In large part magical, acupuncture also grew out of the knowledge that stimulation of certain points of the body had a beneficial, therapeutic impact. In this regard acupuncture is closely related to moxacautery, another old Chinese healing tradition.[123] It is also related to therapeutic bleeding, a very old tradition

---

119 On shamanism in early China see A. Waley, *The Nine Songs: A Study of Shamanism in Ancient China* (London, 1955). See now also Gilles Boileau, "Wu and Shaman," *Bulletin of the School of Oriental and African Studies*, 65, 2 (2002), 350-378. On shamanism in general see also Mircea Eliade, *Shamanism: Archaic Techniques of Ecstasy*, Bollingen Series LXXVI, trans. from the French by Willard R. Trask (Princeton, 1964).

120 See Unschuld, 1985: 22.

121 On this tradition see, as an introduction, Joseph Needham and Lu Gwei–djen, *Science and Civilization in China,* vol. 5: *Chemistry and Chemical Technology,* part II: *Spagyrical Discovery and Invention: Magisteries of Gold and Immortality* (Cambridge, 1974). See also Campany, 2002. For a history of Chinese herbal literature see Unschuld, 1986. See also the discussion in Unschuld, 1985: 101ff. On the earliest Chinese medicine see now also Donald Harper, *Early Chinese Medical Literature, The Mawangdui Medical Manuscripts* (London, 1998).

122 On the earliest history of Chinese acupuncture see Yamada Keiji, *Shinhatsugen Chūgoku kagakushi shiryō no kenkyū* (Kyōto, 1985), 3–122.

123 On the relationship between the two in Han times see Yamada Keiji, *op. cit.*, 225–62. See also Yamada Keiji, *The Origins of Acupuncture, Moxibustion, and Decoction* (Kyoto, 1998).

found throughout Eurasia which is little distinct from acupuncture *per se* in China in the earliest sources, for example in the *Huangdi neijing suwen.*[124]

During Han times new political and philosophical currents and new technology radically altered the character and ideology of traditional Chinese medicine. China was unified under a single dynasty and a new national ideology, a combination of many philosophical streams present in late Zhou times, principally those later identified as Confucianist, Legalist, and Daoist.[125] Chinese medicine too was reinterpreted, where possible, to conform to the new ideology came to stress imperial authority, a rational political structure, and the domination of reason over superstition.[126] At the same time important new ideas reached China from the West. They probably included the idea of five elements, although the Chinese elements are different than the Indian, Humoral Medicine, and most likely the tradition of classifying foods and medicines as hot or cold. The Chinese also received, or developed, the technology necessary to make fine steel needles, beginning the development which has led to the acupuncture needles of today although it has taken many centuries for acupuncture needles as we know them today to completely replace the far cruder ones that were long in general use.

One result of all these changes was the emergence of an entirely new, syncretic medical theory, Correspondence Medicine. Perhaps first developed with moxacautery and acupuncture (and bloodletting) in mind, by the time of the *YSZY* it had been applied to herbal treatment as well. The system is founded in a theory of the universe based on the mutual interplay of forces, or more accurately of dynamic aspects, between the cosmos of the universe and the microcosmos formed by the human body. This view of mutual influences may have found its earliest expression in the universal belief in sympathetic

---

[124] See, as an introduction, discussion in Paul U. Unschuld, *Huang Di Nei Jing Su Wen, Nature, Knowledge, Imagery in an Ancient Chinese Medical Text.* Berkeley, Los Angeles and London, 2003), 268ff and *passim.*

[125] As an introduction to the Chinese philosophy of the time see A. C. Graham, *Disputers of the Tao*: *Philosophical Argument in Ancient China* (La Salle, 1989), 313ff, T. Roger Ames, *The Art of Rulership*: *A Study in Ancient Chinese Political Thought* (Honolulu, 1983), and the latest views in R. P. Peerenboom, *Law and Morality in Ancient China: The Silk Manuscripts of Huang–Lao* (Albany, 1993).

[126] For a detailed statement of this theory and its implications see now Paul U. Unschuld, *What is Medicine? Western and Eastern Approaches to Healing*, translated by Karen Reimers, Berkeley, Los Angeles, London, 2009.

magic, a style of thought certainly present in China, throughout its long history.

In the *YSZY,* as in most other works of its kind, the main surviving sympathy is one of bodily organs. Eating animal lungs benefits human lungs. Eating legs helps legs. Eating penis helps the male strength or male vitality. Some validation of these beliefs was provided by the obvious benefits of eating blood in cases of anemia, eating bones in cases that we would describe as low calcium nutrition, and the like. Deer antlers are a marginal case. Their popularity owes something to their phallic shape and rapid growth, also to their hormone and mineral content, although this was articulated in different terms by the Medieval Chinese, who did not conceptualize harmones and mineral nutrients as such.[127]

More basic, indeed the fundamental postulate in all subsequent Chinese medicine was the presence of *qi*. *Qi* may have first emerged with the meaning of vapour rising from hot food (at a sacrificial meal), but soon came to mean far more. By Han times at least *qi* had become the finest material in everything, permeating all things and explaining the very physics of the Chinese universe. As time passed it was visualized as flowing in channels throughout the cosmos and the human microcosm. As it circulated, it could be blocked, unblocked, augmented, diminished, redirected and so on; its flow could be manipulated.[128]

Another basis for mutual permeation in the Chinese system was ancient *yin–yang* cosmology. Equated to human conditions through contrast of female (predominantly *yin*) to male (predominantly *yang*), and the alternation of chills and fever, *yin–yang* proved a basis for early medical speculation. Naturally, it was soon assimilated to the idea of *qi*, and *yin qi* 陰氣 and *yang qi* 陽氣 were born.

By the early Han Dynasty, *yin–yang* and *qi* had been merged with the theory of the so–called five transitional phases (*wuxing* 五行), also called "elements" and symbolically designated as metal, wood, water, fire, and earth. Originally designed as an independent mode of categorizing all visible and conceivable phenomena, and of explaining

[127] Nontheless, a lot of medieval Chinese theory about body fluids or *qi* is so close to hormonal medicine that one has to conclude that the Chinese clearly inferred something close to the truth.

[128] The definitive study of *qi* is Manfred Kubny. *Qi, Lebenskraftkonzepte in China, Definition, Theorien und Grundlagen* (Heidelberg, 1995). The question of the circulation of *qi* and its connection with the circulation of blood continues to be debated.

changes in their rise, fall, and appearance, the five phases were now identified with specific proportions of *yin* and *yang*. Water, at one extreme, was the most *yin* and least *yang*, fire, at the other, the most *yang* and least *yin*. The other phases occupied intermediate positions. Earth, for example, was predominantly *yin* since it contains a substantial amount of water. Earth is also often identified as "center," and as neither *yin* nor *yang*. Metal, refined through fire, was the opposite, and wood an even mixture of *yin* and *yang*. Primarily through the agency of *qi*, the five phases are subject to universal change. As part of this change metal, for example, was believed to become another element, water. Water becomes wood, wood fire, fire earth and earth metal. There were also cross–sectional interactions recognized. Metal was said to become dominant over wood, water over fire, wood over earth, fire over metal, and earth over water.

Five transitional phases also give birth to other sets of five with some relevance in Chinese medicine and dietetics. They include: five directions (center included), equated with five flavors, five smells, five grains, five fruits, five "depots" (*wu zang* 五臟) and five "palaces" (*wu fu* 五府), sets of organs, and so forth. In Correspondence Medicine the Chinese organs, originally anatomical entities known from observation, were extended to cover whole fields of physiological activity and even psychological action. Thus the heart (*xin* 心) was not only a small organ in the chest. The term also referred to physiological processes thought to be associated with the heart, including much emotional and willed thought. Functions of mind were also assigned to other major organ systems and were not limited to the brain.

A final input came from the Western World. No later than the Wei Dynasty, perhaps earlier, the system of hot, cold, wet, and dry influences, already well known in the ancient Greek, Near Eastern and Indian worlds, appeared in China. Possibly, Buddhist medical missionaries introduced it.[129] This system fits naturally into the native concepts of heating and cooling associated with the *yin-yang*. According to this theory, environmental influences, particularly in foods, affect the body's balance. Fever can be produced by eating too much heating food, as well as rashes, flushing, sores and other burn–like effects. Cooling foods may produce pallor, chills, and weakness. Hot conditions can be cured by eating the safer cooling foods, and *vice*

---

[129] On this see E. N. Anderson, "Why is humoral medicine so popular?," *Social Science and Medicine* 25 (1987): 4: 331–7.

versa. Although the question of what was imported from the West and what invented locally remains to be resolved, the virtual identity and convergence of hot/cold systems found throughout Asia implies mutual influence.

By the time that all of these traditions had been combined into one, a whole new system of traditional Chinese medicine had emerged. Originally set forth in the various texts of the *Yellow Emperor's Inner Canon*, it was based upon "correspondences" within the microcosmos of the human body, and within the macrocosmos constituted by man and the rest of the universe. The new medical theory attempted to unify fundamentals of sympathetic magic with hot–cold Humoral Medicine, Chinese views of the basic structures of the body and of metabolism, the theory of *qi*, *yin–yang*, the five transitional phases, Confucian ideology, and a great deal of Chinese folk belief.

The Correspondence System Structures

In the classic Correspondence Medicine as it emerged from Song on[130] each physiological focus of man's body is primarily *yin* or *yang* and associated with one of the five transitional phases. Included are six pairs of complementary organs. There are six *yin* viscera (*liu-zang* 六臟), largely involved with control and volition: the heart (*xin*); the lungs (*fei* 肺); the spleen (*pi* 脾); the liver (*gan* 肝); the kidneys (*shen* 腎); and the heart enclosing network (*xinbao* 心包); and six *yang* organs (*liufu* 六腑), whose main function is to receive and process food and remove wastes from the body: the gall bladder (*dan* 膽); the sto-

[130] Although the roots of Correspondence Medicine extend back to Han times or before, as the Chinese set about explaining their universe in a rational and scientific manner, as opposed to formerly prevalent magical and religious views, correspondence theory only became the dominant paradigm, not just one view among many, from late Tang on. Its increased importance paralleled the rise of Neoconfucianism which made many of the same assumptions about the physical world and spoke much the same language as Correspondence Medicine. In many ways Song thinkers reinvented Chinese medicine, their reinvention assuming particular importance because it was under the Song that most medical texts were first codified and printed. Thus, even though the texts of the *Yellow Emperor's Inner Canon* predated the Song rethinking of Chinese medicine by many centuries, we still see them by and large, for example, through the eyes of their Northern Song editors since it is the editions of these texts produced by Song that have come down to us, except for a very few fragments. The same is true for most other major Chinese medical texts. See now Asaf Goldschmidt, *The Evolution of Chinese Medicine: Northern Song Dynasty, 960-1127* (London, 2008).

mach (*wei* 胃); the small intestine (*xiaochang* 小腸); the large intestine (*dachang* 大腸); the bladder (*pangguang* 膀胱); and the so–called triple burner (*sanjiao* 三焦). This last Chinese organ, without anatomical equivalent in Western medicine, may have been conceptualized for the same reason that the ancient Greeks and Romans believed in the existence of a very real fire or source of heat somewhere in the body. The body's changing temperature required an explanation, and the Chinese solution was the "triple burner." This notion, lacking an anatomically verifiable counterpart in the body, has been a topic of discussion throughout Chinese medical history. For example, some authors came to consider the triple burner as three groups of organs, with the upper burner (*shangjiao* 上焦) controlling the *yang* functions of lungs, respiration and digestion, the middle burner (*zhongjiao* 中焦), controlling the overall distribution of nutrients, and the lower burner (*xiajiao* 下焦), controlling accumulation and elimination of waste products.[131]

The 12 Chinese organs are groups interactively and associated with the five transitional phases as follows:

Metal«——————»Lungs/Large Intestine
Wood«——————»Liver/Gall Bladder
Water«——————»Kidneys/Bladder and Triple Burner
Fire«——————»Heart/Small Intestine
Earth«——————»Spleen/Stomach

In addition to their influences upon each other each organ also governs certain parts of the body. The kidneys, for example, govern bone and the ears, which are thus *yin* and associated with water.

Also part of Correspondence Medicine physiology are *qi* and "blood" (*xue* 血), but there is enormous disagreement in the sources concerning their nature. In recent Theory, *qi* has been seen as the body's primary *yang* force, and "blood," not always identical with anatomical blood, as a reservoir of *yin*. There is no evidence that such

131 The upper burner is also often said to refers to organs above the diaphragm, including the heart and liver, the middle burner to organs between the diaphragm and the navel, and the lower burner to lower organs, e.g., intestines, bladder, kidneys, and even the liver, but the Chinese are always listing those organs together with the three burners, and entirely separately from them. They are thus quite possibly to be understood as stand-ins for the metabolism in general. The Chinese knew perfectly well that the metabolism generated heat and the idea of these organs likely derived from the insight.

a distinction was made when the *YSZY* was written. Some sources also distinguish various kinds of *qi*, e.g., *qi* in general, and *jingqi* 精氣, the body's "vital air." There is also considerable disagreement in the sources regarding the vessels (*luomai* 絡脈) through which *qi* and "blood" are supposed to move. Other bodily systems recognized by Correspondence Medicine as separate entities are the brain, the five sense organs (nose, eyes, mouth, tongue, and ears), the bodily apertures *qiao* 竅), including the openings of the above sense organs, also the genitals, the skin, flesh, muscles, tendons, ligaments, hairs, sweat pores, and other *foci*. They are frequently referred to in the *YSZY*.

The Correspondence System Illness, Diagnosis and Treatment

In the Correspondence Medicine many illnesses are interpreted as states of disharmony or disharmonies within the body. Disharmony is normally caused either by an unbalanced intrusion, into the body, of environmental factors, such as wind, cold, heat, *etc*., or by excessive drainage of one's inherent resources through excessive emotions. The former situation leads to "repletion," while the latter ends in "depletion," of factors that should be present, in the organism, in balanced proportions. In addition, traumatic events, including burns, bites, parasitic infestation, and other direct, visible impacts on the body, were also perceived as causes of illness.

Since, in correspondence medicine, the body, like the universe itself, reflects *yin–yang* dualism and the Theory of Five Phases, certain bodily systems were considered particularly sensitive to a given cause of illness. Although there is considerable disagreement in the sources about the precise nature of the influences involved, some recent practitioners of Correspondence Medicine have believed that each of the seven emotions (*qiqing* 七情), *i.e.*, happiness, anger, anxiety, contemplation, grief, fear, or fright affects one organ in particular. For example, too much happiness harms the heart, too much anxiety the lungs and too much fear the kidneys. Specific types of climatic influences are also believed to affect just one organ. But any illness was none the less still generalized in the body due to the interconnection of bodily systems.

Teeth and the stomach are, for example, believed in acupuncture theory to be connected by the same *qi* vessel. Therefore any cause of illness affecting the one necessarily affects the other. The stomach also affects the spleen, and systems associated with the spleen, since both the stomach and the spleen are associated with the phase "earth." Some systems distinguish even more complex relationships.

To diagnose such generalized patterns of illness Correspondence Medicine has employed many diagnostic tools. Among recent practitioners they most often include:

1) Observation (*wangzhen* 望診): appraisal of the physical appearance of a patient, especially facial features, his essential quality of life (*shen* 神, "spirit"), careful observation of bearing and posture, and close examination of various parts of the body, especially those thought associated with specific organs;

2) Smelling and listening (*wenzhen* 聞診): detection of the general odor of the body and of its parts; perception of minor body sounds;

3) Inquiry of the patient, his associates and relatives (*wenzhen* 問診): questioning about any feelings of chill or fever, sweating, headache or other pain, patterns of defecation and urination, appetite, any congestion in the chest, or condition of heating, the presence of thirst, and the patient's perception of his own body smell.

Pulse taking (*qiezhen* 切診), although today considered one of the "four diagnostic methods" (*Si zhenfa* 四診法), has never been general in Chinese medicine. Some physicians have done it, some have not. There is also considerable disagreement in the sources about precisely how pulse indications are to be interpreted.

The final diagnosis weighed various signs (*hou* 候), physical manifestations of disease (*xing* 形) and what Paul Unschuld[132] calls pathoconditions (*zheng* 症), which may or may not be identical to the disease being diagnosed. Exactly how they were interpreted and how the diagnosis was expressed varied considerably from school to school. In the *YSZY* the terminology of disease and thus of diagnosis seems largely traditional. In some theoretical systems elaborate efforts are made to create a terminology specifically adapted to the system in question. Chinese diagnoses are often easily equivalent to Western categories, but just as often are not.

In Correspondence Medicine many kinds of treatment are possible. One, acupuncture, by Hu Sihui's time involved insertion of needles,

[132] Unpublished letter of 16 July, 1990 to PDB.

almost always in groups, at several recognized points along major and minor vessels to stimulate or retard various organs and systems. Related to it was moxibustion, burning of an artemisia extract on or near the skin largely at the same points used in acupuncture. By Hu's time herbal[133] and dietary medicine had also become possible methods of treatment in terms of Correspondence Medicine, thanks to the integrative efforts of the Jin–Song–Yuan School, the work of Wang Haogu 王好古 and his very popular *Tangye bencao* 湯液本草 in particular.[134]

Herbal and Dietary Traditions and Their Role in Correspondence Medicine

The origins of Chinese herbal medicine in China's age–old experience with herbs and in the experiments of proto–Daoist physiological alchemy have already been alluded to above. When these Proto–Daoist traditions were systematized[135] and assimilated to five phase and hot–cold, wet–dry theory, the Chinese system of medicine and food classification currently in use developed.

In this system, well–developed in the *YSZY*, each medicine or food is assigned to one of five categories:

Re 熱, "heating,"
Wen 溫, "warming,"
Ping 平, "neutral,"
Liang 涼, "cooling,"

---

[133] In actuality "herbal" is somewhat of a misnomer since not only plants but also minerals and parts of animals are used. Of 1,892 *materia medica* listed as the basis of main entries in the *BCGM*, 1,173 or 62.0% are of herbal origin, 444 or 23.5% are of zoological origin and 275 or 14.5% are of mineralogical origin. Most medicinals in common use in Chinese herbal medicine today are in fact of herbal origin, reflecting a long-term shift away from animal, insect and mineral substances, in some cases with herbal treatments carefully structured to replace minerals in particular. Only a few animal drugs are still being used today because many animals have become rare or endangered species and materials from them all but unavailable. The *materia medica et dietetica* of the *YSZY*, in view of the nature of this text as a dietary, includes very few minerals, and but does include a high proportion of foods of animal origin, many of them quite exotic, a reflection of the Mongolian traditions so strong in the text.

[134] On this text see as an introduction Ulrike Unschuld, "Traditional Chinese Pharmacology: An Analysis of its Development in the Thirteenth Ceutury," *Isis* 68 (1977): 224-248.

[135] For a history of the Chinese herbal literature which played such an important part in this systemization see Unschuld, 1986.

Han 寒, "chilling,"

and to one (sometimes two together) of five flavor groups:

Xin 辛, "acrid,"
Gan 甘, "sweet,"
Suan 酸, "sour,"
Ku 苦, "bitter,"
Xian 鹹, "salty."

Herbal and dietary texts such as the *YSZY* also usually indicate whether or not a medicine or food has a strongly medicinal effect or is even toxic (both are *youdu* 有毒, "has poison") and any other negative or positive effects on the body.

During Jin, Song, and Yuan times this classification system and other perceived properties of herbs and foods[136] were carefully coordinated with the disease categories of Correspondence Medicine. Efforts were made to create a theoretical system allowing generalized use of specific herbs with specific properties to treat specific disease categories or to respond to specific physiological problems.[137] Most often groups of herbs or foods were used, to balance one another or fine tune a specific remedy. Although the use of combinations of balancing herbs may have grown out of Chinese practical experience, once herbal medicine was integrated with Correspondence Medicine during the thirteenth and fourteenth centuries such combinations by and large became *de rigueur*, as they are in much of the *YSZY*.

The following entries for rice (3, 1a), and the meat of the *tarbaqan*, *Marmota bobak*[138] (3, 19b), are typical of the system. That the latter is

---

[136] For example, one very old way of classifying drugs involved assignment to one of the following four categories:

1. *Jun* 君, "lord" drugs, major ingredients to treat major dysfunctions;
2. *Chen* 臣, "minister" drugs, to accelerate the effects of major ingredients;
3. *Zuo* 佐, "assistant" drugs, to assist further the major ingredients and prevent side effects;
4. *Shi* 使, "envoy drugs," to "induce or carry through the mission of the principle" [drugs].

See the discussion in Frank Liu and Liu Yan Mau, *Chinese Medical Terminology* (Hong Kong, 1980), 161.

[137] See the discussion in Unschuld, 1985: 179ff.

[138] *Tarbaqa[n]*: the large Mongolian marmot was an important meat and fur source in former times. Like the Central Asian ground squirrels (it is itself only a large ground squirrel) it is a major vector for plague, since the flea *Xenopsylla cheopis*,

a Mongolian rather than a Chinese food makes little difference, except that Hu, the first to describe the medicinal properties of *tarbaqan* meat, has not assigned it a hot/cold category. Later herbals call the meat neutral and the fat, mentioned by Hu, warming:[139]

> Paddy rice is sweetish–bitter in flavor, neutral and lacks poisons. It is good for warming the middle burner. It makes one very heated and constipated. Too much should not be eaten. This is the same as *nuomi* 糯米. (Sumen 蘇門 [paddy rice] is best. It is often used to make liquor.)
>
> *Tarbaqa*[*n*] (One name is Tubo 土撥 Rodent)[140] [Meat] is sweetish in flavor and lacks poison. It is good for "pheasant sores."[141] If eaten boiled, it benefits a person. The *Tarbaqa[n]* lives beyond the mountains, in the grasses and swamps. The northern people [= The Mongols] dig them out and capture them to eat. Although they are fat, they make no oil when boiled. The broth lacks flavor. If too much is eaten it is difficult to accomplish transformation. It excites the *qi* slightly.

---

which actually carries the plague from animal to animal or animal to human, is at home on this marmot. In the early twentieth century, major plague outbreaks were traced to marmot trappers who were often newcomers and did not know that one should avoid sick animals. This insight is based on the pioneer work of Wu Lien-teh. See Carol Benedict, *Bubonic Plague in Nineteenth Century China* (Stanford, 1996).

[139] See the entries on *tarbaqan* ("Snow Pig") meat, oil, and bones in the *Zhongzao da zidian*, vols. 1–3 (Hong Kong, 1979) (*ZYDZD*), II, 2088–9.

[140] If this name is not simply a variant of *tarbaq*[*an*] it could mean "Tibetan" Rodent. The problem is that *M. bobak* does not live in Tibet. However, the similar *M. himalayana* does, and this may be our "Tibetan" marmot.

[141] The identity of this disease complex is uncertain. According to Li (Hu Sihui, 1988: 294), it is characterized by oozing sores, not unlike the buboes of plague. It may be an earlier, less virulent form of the plague, to which the Mongols may have been largely immune in any case according to Ell. See Stephen R. Ell, "Immunity as a factor in the epidemiology of Medieval plague," *Reviews of Infectious Diseases* 6: 6 (November–December, 1984): 866–79. See also Colin McEvedy, "Plague and leprosy in the Middle Ages: a paradoxical cross–immunity," *International Journal of Leprosy and other Micobacterial Diseases* 55: 2 (June, 1987): 345–50. Perhaps the association of the *tarbaqa*[*n*] with black plague was known and the beast attributed magical, or real, powers to cure the sores produced by black plague, the "pheasant sores" of our text. For a full recent survey of the Black Death see Ole Bennedictow, *The Black Death, 1346-1353, the Complete History*, Woodbridge, Suffolk: The Boydell Press, 2004. See also Colin McEvedy, "The Bubonic Plague," *Scientific American* 258 (February, 1986): 2: 118–23.

When treating with diet or medicine, a traditional Chinese doctor was supposed to weigh known properties of foods and herbs and choose those best suited to counteract dysfunction and restore balance in the body. This, at least, is the practice today, and seems to have been so in Hu's time as well. If the body was overheated, cooling foods would be indicated, and vice versa, with particular cooling foods preferred to particular conditions. Certain flavors were thought to promoting smooth functioning of certain organs. Other flavors had the opposite effect. (Compare pages 25b–26a of *juan* 2 of the *YSZY.*)

The Residue of Demons and Folklore

The *YSZY*, as a Chinese document, falls squarely within the bounds of the extensive Chinese herbal literature (*bencao*) as described by Unschuld.[142] It has been unquestionably accepted as part of this tradition by later Chinese medical commentators, who have made the *YSZY* a major source for the early modern expansion of the range of Chinese *materia dietetica* and *medica.* See, for example, the table of Mongolian *materia dietetica* and *medica* above. The two entries quoted above, on paddy rice and the *tarbaqa[n],* also make clear the subordination of *YSZY* medicine and *materia dietetica* to Correspondence Medicine. This fusion of Correspondence Medicine, herbalism and diet therapy was fairly new at the time, a product of medical theory developments over the previous couple of centuries.

Hu inherited this grand system and accordingly placed his herbal squarely within the theoretical context of the flow of *qi*, the supplementing and strengthening of bodily organs,[143] and correspondences of flavors and of qualities. He lived with the logical extensions of what had once been a system grounded in empirical observation. By his time, the logic had taken over, and empirical observation was

142 See Unschuld, 1986.

143 The concept of *bu* 補, "supplementing, strengthening," is the easiest Chinese category to understand in modern Western medical terms. Almost all easily digestible foods high in protein, vitamins and/or minerals are considered to have the desired effect of *bu* by the Chinese. Almost no other foods are, except for those made part of the system by extension, *e.g.*, non–nourishing parts of otherwise nourishing animals. Sympathetic magic and folk belief also exert their influence. Brains, for example, supplement brains, and the like. Other specific claims are based on the system of correspondences. The supplementation theory is also found widely outside of China. In the Indian subcontinent, too, easily digestible protein foods are called "strengthening" and are fed to parturient women (Najma Rizvi, personal communication to ENA). The same general belief system prevails in Southeast Asia as well.

forced into its straitjacket. Chinese herbal literature, including the *YSZY*, did not fit the mold very well. Even when assimilated to Correspondence Medicine, it continued to develop and to incorporate, often haphazardly and piecemeal, the new knowledge that was constantly accumulating.

By Jin and Yuan times the sheer weight of new information appeared overwhelming. New knowledge was accumulating far more rapidly than it could be absorbed. One reason was the continued expansion of China's geographical horizons due to overseas trade and improved overland connections with Inner Asia and the Islamic World. Also extremely important was the coming of printing and an explosion in the publication of medical literature of every sort. More knowledge was more readily available to a larger audience. There were also ideological factors, principally the establishment of Neoconfucianism as the official state philosophy for all of China by Yuan times. The need for the synthesis of new empirical fact and for reformulation of medical theory to explain discrepancies between pragmatically observed reality and theory had become pressing and unavoidable.

But in spite of Hu's good intentions, and the theoretical efforts of Liu and other original medical thinkers of the time, what most impresses us in the *YSZY* is the degree to which Hu's medical ideas are not formulated in terms of Correspondence Medicine, or any other system. Hu was no slave to tradition. He drew upon folk belief and folk experience as well as Correspondence Theory in presenting his medical ideas.

For example, Hu scores all major foods by heating/cooling category, and according to their effects on *qi*. He also discusses the effects many of them have on particular organs and anatomical parts, their role in humoral therapy. But, like other pragmatists of the Chinese herbal tradition, Hu also specifies which cannot be eaten together, which cure particular diseases or cause particular conditions, and which have magical effects. He often does so without relating such properties to Correspondence Medicine or any other system. In general, this reflects a very old system of avoiding certain foods at certain seasons—Sun Simiao's *Qianjin beiji fang* 千金備急方, "Emergency Recipes Worth Thousands in Gold," of 652 utilizes this system continually.[144] Thus, although Correspondence Medicine is pervasive in the *YSZY*, it is not the only belief system present. Nor is Correspondence Medicine assimilation of medical information imparted by the *YSZY* very thorough.

One example of the knowledge incorporated into the *YSZY* and systematized is the section on "Animal Transformations" (2, 51a–52a). This is a list of uncanny or unnatural apparitions, evidently considered inedible because of their anomalous appearance. Most are perfectly harmless by any other standard, *e.g.*, a crab with only one claw. But some indicated dangers have clear empirical roots.

"A liver that is colored green–black" is one that any sensible person would avoid, for obvious reasons. Dried meat that has not dried fully, or moves when placed in water, or stays warm at night (from putrefying), would be carefully avoided by the modern biophysician as well as by the Medieval believer in the dangers of the uncanny.

In the same tradition but more complicated is the list of dangerous properties of foods (2, 44a–45b). Many are based upon purely empirical observations: "if fresh ingredients are colored [*i.e.*, discolored] and stink, they cannot be eaten." "If the various meats smell and are

---

144 Sun Simiao or Sun Zhenren, is also attributed a *Sun zhenren shiji* 孫真人食忌 "Sun Zhenren's Dietary Prohibitions," which now survives only in fragments. The material, which focuses on food and everyday objects treating illness with passing discussion of food prohibitions, is quoted more than a score of times by Li Shizhen in his BCGM. In addition to this work, *juan* 30 of Sun's *Qianjin beiji fang* circulated separately as the *Qianjin shizhi* 千金食治, "Treatments with Victuals, Worth a Thousand in Gold." This material was available to Hu Sihui who imitates or directly adapts its contents at several places in the *YSZY*. Other important texts on dietary medicine available to him may have included the *Shiliao bencao* 食療本草, "Materia Medica of Curative Victuals," originally written during the Tang by Meng Xian 孟詵 (621-713) as the *Buyang fang* 補養方, "Recipes for Supplementation and Nourishment," but later revised by Zhang Ding 張鼎, also of the Tang, to produce the *Shiliao bencao*, certainly the fragments of it were widely quoted and available, the *Shi xing bencao* 食性本草, "Dietetic Materia Medica," written during the Five Dynasties period by Chen Shi liang 陳士良, if the work still survived, and the Southern Song *Shizhi tong shuo* 食治通說, "General Discussion of Using Foods to Cure." On the early dietary literature see Ute Engelhardt, "Dietetics in Tang China and the First Extant Works of Materia Dietetica," in Elisabeth Hsu, ed., *Innovation in Chinese Medicine* (Cambridge, 2001), 173-191.

spoiled, they cannot be eaten." (2, 44a). But there are also avoidances based on systems of mutual influence: "One should not eat pepper in the tenth month. It wounds a person's heart" (2, 45b).

The section also reproduces old Chinese beliefs, such as the idea that a horse's liver is poisonous. We suspect horses sometimes ate poisonous herbs whose toxins accumulated in the liver. There are also folk beliefs of uncertain origin, such as "the various brains cannot be eaten." Modern Chinese and Mongols certainly do eat brains and there are even recipes for brains in the *YSZY*. Is this an Islamic prohibition? It may be caused by the association of the brain with the marrow system and blood, unclean in Islam. The list, much of which is repeated in the list of anomalies, is divided between excellent sanitary advice, logical if incorrect beliefs, and the perfectly inexplicable. These last are the types of beliefs that accumulate in every culture, despite much evidence against them.

Even harder to explain in the *YSZY* and elsewhere is the enormous and ongoing popularity of prohibitions of particular food combinations. This is still widespread Chinese folk culture, in spite of such brave experiments as Libin Cheng's sampling of many feared combinations.[145] In Yuan it seems to have become an obsession. Hu Sihui's several pages of prohibitions are outdone by Jia Ming's 賈銘 *Yinshi xuzhi* 飲食須知, "What One Ought to Know about Eating and Drinking," written down in early Ming but from Yuan–era data. Yet there appears to be absolutely no empirical, theoretical, logical or other justification, for any of this material. Nor is there much agreement among authors as to what combinations are bad. Perhaps it was simply the favored way of explaining any stomach upset or illness.

Unschuld explains Hu's theories as "largely based on concepts of magic correspondence."[146] While generally true, it is the particular type of magic that concerns us. Moreover, the many purely practical tips indicate that empirical experience was not ignored. We cannot see any logic in the prohibited combinations, and hesitate to explain them by magical correspondence. The few explained in text are explained strictly in terms of diseases they cause, and the same is true today among folk believers in prohibited combinations. A few, like persimmon and crab, have carried through from Hu's day to our own.

---

[145] Cheng Libin, "Are the so–called Poisonous Food–Combinations Really Poisonous?" *Contributions from the Biological Laboratory the Science Society of China, Zoological Series* II, 9 (1936): 307–16.

[146] Unschuld, 1986: 216.

In short, we see several things mixed in Hu's medical lore:

1) Medieval and Early Modern Chinese Correspondence Medicine;

2) Common sense and empirical observation: There is more reliance upon common sense and empirical observation than a modern reader may realize. Herbal remedies with weak but verifiable effects have been replaced in our time by more powerful and effective drugs, leading many to forget how valuable the old remedies were. Nutritional advice, too, was more important in pre–industrial days than now. Not only poverty, but also the unbalanced diet of the rich, led to widespread malnutrition;

3) Chinese folk belief imperfectly assimilated to Correspondence Theory;

4) Supernatural medicine, including attention to fox spirits and the like;

5) Folklore of the type the Christian Church calls "superstitions," in this case, miscellaneous beliefs that probably represent some crystallization of misinterpreted experience. The prohibited or avoided food combinations often go back to such mistaken logic;

6) Known Mongol interest in purity and tabus;

7) Near Eastern medicine, appearing in several minor points, such as the cheering effects of saffron and the heavy medical use of jams and sugar preserves.

Hu was a good dietitian, working with what he had, but it is no wonder that he was sometimes led into contradictions. Quotes from Chinese classics and probably from Mongol lore did not always accord with his experience. Neither he nor his editors attempted to bring them into agreement.

In any case, there is a great deal of assimilated and unassimilated new knowledge in the *YSZY*. Some of it was correct, and has withstood the test of time. Some was based on truth, but has been over–generalized or mistakenly generalized. Some was simply wrong: the result of natural errors in an age before microscopes, control–case studies, double–blind tests, and antiseptic fields transformed medical research. There are also examples where a series of correct observations have been too easily explained, *post hoc*, through the Correspondence

Theory, in culturally–logical but untested ways. In all of this Hu was typical of a greater tradition of Chinese herbal medicine, one reason why the *YSZY* has been so well accepted by later Chinese tradition, in spite of the foreignness of much represented there.

Chinese Culinary Traditions and the YSZY

Chinese culinary influence upon the *YSZY* is substantial and pervasive. It is not easily isolated and defined since Chinese and non–Chinese influences are blended smoothly into a whole. There is the added problem of defining just what was "Chinese" when the *YSZY* was written. Sabban sees a Chinese structure to *YSZY* recipes, methods, spicing and culinary refinements in general, on a "Mongol" base of mutton, game and wheat products.[147] If we include Turks as "Mongols," there is clearly some truth to this, but Sabban's judgment somewhat oversimplifies a complex culinary tradition. Hu Sihui wrote his recipes down in Chinese and had to use, as a matter of necessity, Chinese cooking terminology, although it is very awkward in places. It is also true, as Sabban has noted, that *YSZY* recipes, even recipes completely Near Eastern or Central Asian in essence, have been adapted with the needs of an imperial cooking staff which must have been largely Chinese using locally available foodstuffs in mind. None the less, to see everything as a Chinese "refinement" of foods to suit the Mongolian taste is a mistake.

Additionally, comparatively few *YSZY* recipes represent relatively un–varnished Chinese culinary tradition, in contrast to Ni Zan's cookbook, for example, where the majority of recipes are purely Chinese. Most are found among the medicinal foods of *juan* 2. A few are also found in *juan* 1 but often exhibit West Asian refinements in spicing or cooking technique. One example is the otherwise typically Chinese Recipe #31, "Carp Soup," employing both black and long pepper. The marination called for is more typical of the Baghdadi cooking of the era than of Chinese. Yet recipes in some ways accommodated or adapted to Chinese culinary traditions are, as Sabban suggests, quite common. Many clearly non–Chinese recipes call for Chinese seasonings. One example is the "sauce" of recipe # 30 in *juan* 1, "Bear Soup." "Sauce" normally means sauce made by fermenting soy beans, or soy beans and wheat, *etc*. Flower pepper and processed Mandarin

[147] Sabban, 1986b: 167ff.

orange peel, to give only a few examples, are other frequent Chinese culinary additions to otherwise foreign dishes.

Other common flavorings in the *YSZY* may also represent Chinese influence. Some 49 out of 95 recipes in *juan* 1 and all the more detailed recipes in the *juan* 2 call for Chinese bunching onions. Bunching onions often replace Western globe onions in the *YSZY*'s Near Eastern recipes. This is certainly a Chinese touch but the Mongol taste for onions must be borne in mind as well. Also Chinese touches may be the widespread use of tsaoko cardamoms (34 occurrences among the "exotic recipes," 18 more in *juan* 2), although this spice certainly has a south and Southeast Asian context as well as Chinese, and ginger (35 occurrences). Tsaoko cardamom is a signature spice of the *YSZY* as a whole, flavoring 52 or 23.7% of the recipes, one of the dietary's most pervasive culinary influences. Ginger is employed widely in the world but the usage in the *YSZY* is generally Chinese, although the ginger is employed in an unusual pickled form, preserved in distilled liquor,[148] in nine of the recipes. Among the book's most thoroughly Chinese touches are its bean starch noodles, although often used in a most un–Chinese way,[149] glutinous rice powder, Chinese cabbages, Chinese radish, Chinese yams, lotus rhizome, and probably its Chinese chives, although not all are exclusive to China.[150] Also Chinese are turtle, Yangtse River porpoise, and most of the southern herbs, medicines, and teas in *juan* 2.[151] Conspicuously there are no

---

148 A recipe is given in the *JJBYSL*, 12, 63a:

> Take tender ginger before the spring rains. The quantity does not matter. Remove the shoots and sprouts. Scour and wash. Use distilled liquor and pickling salts. Apply evenly. Put into a porcelain jar. Put a lump of sugar on top. Stop the opening with bamboo leaves. Seal with clay.

149 The technology and terminology of the *YSZY*'s bean flour noodles are frequently Near Eastern or Central Asian and in some cases, at least, bean flour is probably a substitution for semolina. Cook testing has shown, for example, that the *JJBYSL*'s recipe (13, 18b) for a proto–baklava works best if semolina is re–substituted for the bean flour called for in the recipe.

150 The Chinese radish was used outside China and Chinese chives were, of course, well known to the Mongols as a gathered and probably medicinal food and were among those wild plants gathered by Hö'elün in feeding her orphans.

151 Despite the clear Central Asian interests of Hu or his colleagues in the list of teas given, it is highly significant that examples of all the major Chinese teas of the time are also given, this including brick teas, the preferred form of tea for long boiling and flavoring, as done by the Turks and Mongols, under the Tang, powdered teas, which had become popular in earlier Song times, and the late Song leaf (and bud)

recipes for really non–Chinese game like swans and marmots, although these are discussed in the catalogue section of the *YSZY*. Deer and bears were familiar to Chinese gourmets, and even wolves were at least known. They did appear in later herbals.

In Appendix I, Table A lists all foods, medicinals, and ingredients called for anywhere in the text of the *YSZY*. By way of contrast, Tables B and C list ingredients called for in the three major *YSZY* recipe groups and how often they are mentioned. Table B lists ingredients and how often they are used for the 95 recipes for "exotic delicacies" listed in *juan* 1. Table C lists ingredients and how often they are used for the "soups and decoctions" and the medical recipes in *juan* 2. Tables B and C show that there are considerable differences in culinary or medicinal usage between the recipes in the various parts of the text. The recipes and ingredients from *juan* 2 are far more Chinese than those in *juan* 1.

Sabban, who makes a listing of the various spices called for in *YSZY* recipes,[152] is profoundly impressed by their range and variety and points up the connection of *YSZY* foods with the "haute cuisine" of the Medieval European courts of the era.[153] Since the Mongol court was probably consciously assimilating itself to the great courts not only of the European world but of the Middle East and points beyond, this is understandable. Much of the spicing is Chinese and this is a major source of Chinese influence throughout the text. Some is not and this may include the undefined spices and spice mixtures called for in several recipes. Judging from two surviving listings found in the *JJBYSL*,[154] the spice mixtures of the time were combinations of West and East.

---

teas, which have continued to be the favored form of tea today. Only missing are the oxidized and pressed leaf teas known as fermented teas today (there are actual fermented teas as well). These had simply not emerged yet. The result, in the *YSZY*, is a minor masterpiece in its description of the range of teas available at the time to the court and others. The range discussed suggests, even if it does not spell out, a definite connoisseurship.

[152] Sabban, 1983, 1986b.

[153] Unpublished letter of 7 June, 1993 to PDB.

[154] *JJBYSL*, 14, 40a–b:

> Great Spice Combination for a Large (or Imperial) Kitchen (made by powdering the following and forming it into pellets with **chuqmin* dissolved in water):
> [Processed] Stinking Elm (*Ulmus macrocarpa*) pulp
> lesser galangal (*Alpinia officinarum*)

In any case, despite the many Chinese seasonings and ingredients called for in the *YSZY*, the range of dishes there is a great deal less Chinese. The commonest dish in the *YSZY* is a thick soup or stew (*šülen*). Sabban compares these soups to the favorite potage of Medieval Europe[155] which like the soups of the *YSZY* were frequently masterpieces of the culinary art, carefully spiced and made with choice and carefully selected ingredients.[156]

Usually this type of dish is based on mutton, sometimes on chicken, often on some other animal of alleged special medical value. It is almost always started by boiling the meat or bones with (large) cardamoms. Many recipes involve chickpeas, called "Muslim beans" in the book. That term also applies to broad beans, but they are not implied here. In the *YSZY* the chickpeas are skinned and mashed into a hummus and added during the initial stage of cooking. Sometimes additional chickpeas are added to the final soup.

In many recipes the soup was boiled dry, as in pilaf or in the Mexican *sopa seca*, a derivative of pilaf. Many of the others involve so much thickening, *e.g.*, with rice, flour, bean flour, barley grain, *etc.*, that they cook solid. This is common Near Eastern practice. The "Bar-

---

long pepper (*Piper longum*)
greater galangal (*Alpinia galanga*)
grains–of–paradise (*Amomum villosum* and *A. xanthioides*)
Sichuan pepper (*Zanthoxylum simulans* and *Z. bungeanum*)
dried ginger
roasted cinnamon
zhira (*shihluo* 蒔羅, Persian "cumin")
fennel
Mandarin orange peel (peel of *Citrus reticulata*)
apricot kernel (*Prunus armeniaca*)

Quick Spice Combination for Flavoring (made by finely pounding the following and forming into small "pills" with water):
makdunis (*maqin*, Y *mak*^{h}*in*, L *ma:kñin*) 馬芹, "Muslim celery," *i.e.*, Iranian parsley)
black pepper
fennel
dried ginger
cinnamon
Sichuan pepper

On possible Middle Eastern influences see also Buell, 1999.

155 Sabban, 1986b: 181 f.

156 See O. Redon, F. Sabban, S. Serventi, *La gastronomie au Moyen Age, 150 recettes de France et d'Italie* (Paris, 1991), 333.

ley Soup" (recipe #2) is in fact almost exactly like a common dish of Iraq and neighboring areas. Kitchen experience confirms the implications of instructions such as "cook until dry" or "eat with long bread." The stews were probably picked up in or placed on buns, as is the near–universal rule for such dishes in West and Central Asia and, derivatively, China. Such dishes as the "*Mastajhi* Soup" and the Bal–po [Nepal] Soup cook into thick stews, if one uses a reasonable quantity of water. Much water evaporates in the long process of cooking the tough muscles of nomadic sheep. The rest is absorbed by large volumes of dry beans and starches.

On the other hand, many of the "soups" are straightforward broths or congees, both of which are characteristically watery. This is especially true of the strictly medicinal recipes. Of course, all the decoctions and teas are liquid. So this cookbook implies a watery diet. This is, of course, because the Mongols lived in desert and semidesert environment and had active outdoor lives. They needed the liquid. As we have already noted the Mongol honorific word for "food," *šülen*, also means "soup." The Mongols may have picked up, or long shared the Chinese awareness that unboiled plain water carries diseases.[157] At this time, tea was still an uncommon luxury in north China, let alone Mongolia where it first became generally popular in late Ming times at earliest. The liquid in the diet came almost entirely from broths and soups. Also, this is a medical book. Chinese medicines are usually taken as soups or teas.

Sabban notes that the Chinese diet of today is less soupy.[158] Some comments may be made: first, even the non–medical cuisine of the far northwest, especially perhaps of the Ningxia Hui, is still very soupy. Second, the cuisine of Fujian province is at least as much so. Fukienese think nothing of serving three or four soup dishes at a banquet, and even the dessert is apt to be a sweet soup. So, Chinese traditions may have reinforced Mongolian, and even Middle Eastern, since the Turks and Arabs of the era liked their soups too. Many of the soups of modern European haute cuisine have Middle Eastern prototypes.

[157] Of course sources of fresh water in Mongolia were, in the fourteenth century at least, considerably less polluted than equivalent sources in China, due not only to the smaller population and smaller resulting pressures on such waters, but also to Mongol religious prohibitions intended to prevent any offense to the "lords of the land and waters," above all through pollution or misuse of any natural environmental resources, including all sources of fresh water. On this see Roux, 1984: 132ff.

[158] Sabban: 1986b: 182–3.

The cooking methods of the *YSZY* also reflect a variety of sources. Some are Turkic, some Mongolian, and some Chinese. The refinements are certainly Central and West Asian in large part. The base was by and large shared with northwest China, except for the more exotic game items. One very notable non–Chinese touch is the use of fat-tailed sheep fat as the main cooking oil. This is rendered from the mass of fat and connective tissue forming the enormous enlargement of the buttocks and tail in certain Central and West Asian sheep varieties. It is exceedingly popular in Central Asia today, but has never caught on with the Chinese. Another conspicuously un–Chinese trait in the *YSZY* is the lack of pork.

But despite this the cooking techniques of the *YSZY* appear heavily assimilated to the then Chinese practices of North China, although in many ways these were not unlike those associated with the Baghdadi cooking of the era. Thus *YSZY* recipes call for fine slicing, typical of Chinese cuisine today, but use a Turkic word for "small coin" to describe the end product. Compare the same function of "dirhem" in Arabic cooking manuals. The careful timing of many recipes, with different ingredients added at different times, is also best explainable as due to a Chinese cooking milieu, although the practice was certainly known in the Arabic West. There are no stir–fry recipes in the *YSZY*, but the elaborate baking so characteristic of the Baghdadi cooking of the time is largely absent as well, although there are buns and baked breads, and some casserole–like dishes. Hu Sihui may perhaps have had to limit his approach due to the known Mongol preference for boiled foods. Still, even when foods are boiled there are many Chinese touches. In spite, for example, of a heavily Turkic terminology for *YSZY* grain foods, many of the noodles appear typically Chinese. Others, despite exotic Turkic names, *e.g.*, *chöp*, have been assimilated to Chinese tradition to the extent that bean paste is the primary ingredient of these *fen*. But in any case noodle technology had by then been established in China for more than a thousand years. Only durum pasta was new, and the names and complicated rolling techniques of many Turkic noodle variations. So, with Sabban, one gets the sense of a Mongol, but also Turkic, cuisine influenced by and fusing with Chinese food. The Mongols adopted Chinese food partly because it was good for them, like modern Americans seeking a low–cholesterol dinner.

Hu Sihui and his collaborators made a concerted effort to improve nutritionally what the Mongols wanted to eat. Despite this, the *YSZY* imperial diet was not a healthy one. Mutton and the other meats used so extensively are high in fat and cholesterol. There is little fiber, in spite of use of whole grain flours to make most of the breads and other grain foods, and almost no vegetables or fresh sources of vitamins A and C other than the occasional sheep's milk and sheep's milk products (and Kumiss). On the whole, it is a heavy diet: greasy meat, stodgy grains, and beans. The spices greatly helped digestion, in modern medical terms as well as in the *YSZY* belief system. The cooks did the best they could with what they had, and produced excellent dishes, but we find that a steady diet of *YSZY* food is highly conducive to dyspepsia and general ill health. After a diligent phase of kitchen–testing, one craves greens, fresh fruit, and whole grains. Two days on the latter diet are necessary to restore proper functioning. No wonder the Mongol courtiers needed so many dietary remedies.

In modern times, many of the foods of the *YSZY* are still used, whether in the Near East or in China and Central Asia, for tonic, strength–building, and digestion–easing purposes. They are mostly used by well–to–do and often older persons who have subsisted on a poor diet that runs to the opposite extreme: too much grain and vegetables, too few good sources of iron, calcium and easily digested protein. This was not the problem of the Mongol court. It seems possible that the medical thrust of the *YSZY* dietary is misguided, from this perspective. The meat/tsaoko/galangal/ginger stews were ideal for Chinese living on coarse grains and coarse vegetables; they were not well chosen for people living on meat, yogurt, cheese, and white flour. In so far as the Mongol court's pre–eminent problem was, as we suspect, alcohol, these recipes would have had a good effect. B vitamins are abundantly represented, especially in the many organ meats. Mineral nutrition would have been good. It is also worth noting that the high protein and mineral levels would have kept the immune system well prepared to resist disease.

In summary, this is an unbalanced diet, but not without redeeming virtues. The Mongols were probably somewhat acculturated to life in Beijing, with its unmilled grain and fibrous cabbages. It is perhaps against such a background that we should consider *YSZY* cuisine. Many of the specific ingredients have, in general, the virtues represented for them. Meat is strengthening, blood builds blood because of its protein and heme iron, foxglove stimulates, mallow and bottle gourd are diuretic and "cooling," *i.e.*, beneficial for deficiency of vitamins A and C. The more complex "made dishes" are well–

balanced and relatively digestible. Many of the dishes in the first section merely "augment the middle burner and increase *qi*," which appears to be a Chinese way of saying that they are nutritious. Many others have no indicated value at all. Most of the rest operate by sympathetic magic. Heart, for example, nourishes heart in a process of association that we currently do not credit.

In the "soups and decoctions" in *Juan* 2, most of the Near Eastern or Indian recipes do not have an indicated medical value. The Chinese ones include several that produce saliva and quench thirst, *i.e.*, they are basically just drinks for dehydrated nomads. A large number of them, however, have medical values that accord with those in the classic herbals.

The final *YSZY* recipe group is more strictly medical. These recipes are arranged by the conditions they treat, beginning with deficiency and ending with bleeding and piles. The largest group treats deficiency, insufficiency, weakness, and lack of strength, often in particular organs. These are treated by a combination of highly nutritious foods with stimulant and carminative spices and drugs, which are very effective for this purpose. Then follow several hydrating and diuretic foods of varying effectiveness; both in the third and first groups we see mallow correctly employed as a gentle diuretic. Some recipes are strictly magical in emphasis, *e.g.*, with references to the supernatural shape–changing fox. Some are hard to evaluate because of the ambiguity of Yuan medical terms. We have only an imperfect idea of what was really meant by the terms now translated as "diabetes" and "apoplexy" in the texts of the era. One suspects strongly that much of this ambiguity would be resolved, to the credit of the Yuan doctors, if we could understand fully their interpretations of illness. A food that is worthless for curing what is *now* translated as "apoplexy" may have worked perfectly well for the condition specified by *zhongfeng* 中風 in Yuan.

The dangers of over–translating can be shown from Anderson's field work in South China. There, many foods were eaten for purposes of "cooling" the body. This, in the medical texts, implied curing fever and various "hot" diseases. It turned out that the villagers and fishermen were actually using fresh vegetables to treat low–level deficiencies of vitamins A and C, which, to them, were the focal hot conditions. Needless to say, the treatment worked perfectly. A similar knowledge of the relationship of disease categories and actual behavior is needed for the Yuan. Unfortunately we may be several centuries too late. Further study of surviving documents may provide further clues.

The Social Context of YSZY Foodways

In our analysis above we have focused on the foods, foodways and medical traditions of the *YSZY* as cultural artifacts in and of themselves. In addition, they also had a direct social function as an assemblage, one which can easily be categorized in terms of social science theory. Functionalist and structural–functionalist explanations of foodways show that food marks social categories and events, communicates social states and conditions, and defines roles and situations. In particular, much attention has been paid to food as a marker of status.[159] Status marking is consciously and specifically intended in the *YSZY*. The Yuan court was creating a cuisine that would be splendid, refined, exclusive, and yet identifiably Mongol. Rare spices, exotic ingredients and recipes were grafted onto a local stock. Cuisine of court banquets from several parts of the world is intended for show. The Yuan court no doubt wished to be the most splendid of all. They did not forget ethnicity, taking care to have Mongol and other marker foods.

It seems likely, though we have no direct evidence, that the wide variety of ethnic foods had another function too, to please or accommodate guests coming from all parts of the Old World. The cookbook implies, by giving health values for all the major dishes that the court was itself the major consumer of foods described. But perhaps a visiting ambassador from, say, Northern India would have been served with appropriate dishes from his homeland as a mark of courtesy.

Surprisingly, there are no indications of foods served at particular festivals, nor of any intended sequencing of dishes in a meal. However, medical directions do include many rules about the season, time of day, state of mental or physical health of the individual, and other matters of occasion and context. Thus, *YSZY* food is connected with time and setting, as in other societies.[160] Food functions not only to maintain health and strength. It also serves to mark many, if not all, social divisions and situations. Claude Levi–Strauss,[161] Mary Doug-

---

[159] See in particular Pierre Bourdieu, 1979 and Jack Goody, *Cooking, Cuisine and Class* (Cambridge, 1982).

[160] See Goody, 1982.

[161] See, for example, Claude Levi–Strauss, *La Pensée sauvage* (Paris, 1962).

las,[162] and others have discussed at length the structuring of foodways in society. We have been unable to analyze all aspects of the structure of Hu's cuisine, primarily because of lack of evidence about how the cuisine was actually served and consumed. Further research may allow more to be said in this regard. We confine ourselves here to analysis of the form and content of recipes.

There is clear distinction between food and drink, meat and non–meat, between primarily exotic dishes with incidental medical values and primarily medical dishes with incidental good eating qualities, between fancy and simple dishes. The classic Chinese contrast between grain staples and "made–dish topping" is conspicuously absent. Most of the dishes involve starch staple and meat cooked together. Many such dishes survive to this day in Northwest China. They are eaten there as one–dish meals, or as hearty dishes to eat with bread, rather than as toppings for boiled grain.

On the other hand, several of the classic contrasts of traditional Chinese cuisine are conspicuously absent in the *YSZY*. The balance of stir–fried and steamed dishes is gone. Almost everything in the *YSZY* is boiled, following Mongol cosmological health practices, since boiling was believed to bring out the essence of food. Balances of heating and cooling humoral essences are maintained, but balances of literal temperature are not. There is no indication of the complex interplay of hot and cool dishes that one finds in many Chinese feasts. Balance of dry and soupy dishes may be implied in the *YSZY*, since many dishes of both kinds occur, but nothing is stated explicitly. One cannot pursue such *argumenta ex nihil* far, because the *YSZY* is clearly not a guide to presentation and meal planning, only to the actual cooking and health values of dishes.

The *YSZY* is notable in the wide range of foods listed. In addition to the recipes, a long account of various food ingredients is given. No insects are mentioned, but few other categories of edible beings are excluded. If the Yuan rulers were as eclectic as this book suggests, they had as few food tabus as any known people. But we do not know whether any individual actually ate all the foods mentioned. We also do not know, in most cases, what was liked, what was disliked, and what was abhorred[163] by particular people or groups.

---

162 See Mary Douglas, *Natural Symbols* (London, 1970) and her *Implicit Meanings* (London, 1975).

163 See Angela Logue, *The Psychology of Eating and Drinking* (San Francisco, 1986). See also E. N. Anderson, *Everyone Eats* (New York, 2005).

On the medical prescriptions, we are on surer ground. Here the operations of classic processes of human inference[164] are at work. Empirical observations are over–generalized. Much is based on assumptions. Much is deduced from principles of cosmology widely shared in China. The anthropologist's old favorites, sympathetic and contagious magic, are much in evidence. We have discussed this in reference to particular medical beliefs. This is not to denigrate the nutritional science of the *YSZY*, which is based to a great extent on shrewd, rigorous and empirically verifiable observations. High–protein foods do build strength; high–vitamin foods do cure many diseases, those now recognize as avitaminoses; and putrid foods do cause sickness. Unusual or unnatural looking items are indeed best avoided, as Hu recommends.

Much more analysis of Song and Yuan medicine is needed before we can discuss these questions in detail, but our impression is that most of the *YSZY*'s medical lore is based on a tradition that made logical, but often false, extensions and extrapolations from valid basic principles. But much also comes from an earlier stratum of folklore, for example, the fox with its mysterious powers and associations with mental disease, immortals wandering on air, and other strange beings.

As we have seen, most *YSZY* food and lore is loosely integrated within the Chinese Correspondence System. This system is one of the best known examples of a logical and cosmological framework erected to integrate a mass of empirical observations and low–level inferences. It has served China well for two thousand years as a structure for organizing information and as a way to help learn, remember and code medical data. Hu classified foods in terms of effects on *qi* and placement within Correspondence and *yin/yang* theory. By so doing he had a ready–made way to organize foods and his thoughts about them. Without such a framework, he probably could not have put together such an orderly, comprehensive, and coherent book.

But the real question is how Hu Sihui and his court patrons decided what finally became canonical, in so far as the *YSZY* is a canon. The officers of the Mongol–Turkic–Chinese court and its cooks had to negotiate the creation of a particular court cuisine. Their methods and purposes are, to a point, clear. They took a basically Mongolian diet, determined ultimately by the realities of steppe existence, but at the Yuan court also by tradition and a probably romanticized view of the

[164] See Richard Nisbett and Lee Ross, *Human Inference* (Englewood Cliffs, 1980).

great Mongol heritage, and made it into an appropriate cuisine for a sophisticated world empire. This they did by grafting onto it the finest delicacies of the whole Asian continent: the spices, exotic combinations, herbs and medicines, the varied techniques of many cultures. They laid it forth to show their sophistication and their control; it was part of their display, part of a discourse on power. Through food as through ritual, ceremony, clothing, language uses, and other cultural forms they made visible not only their mastery of much of the world, but also their intention to be true world rulers, not mere locals who could not adapt their culture to a new role. Finally, they assimilated medical traditions, mostly Chinese, to their own ways, to make the diet as healthy and protective of long life as possible. Within loose constraints of tradition and perceived medical efficacy, they designed a diet worthy of the power and refinement of a great empire.

The implications of this for the theory of food history are many. Local ecology rarely provides more than very loose guidelines for people deciding what to eat, especially if those people are rich and powerful enough to draw on a large area. Cultural tradition and psychological considerations restrict the field more, but are only some of the influences affecting decision–making. Health beliefs constrain the field considerably more tightly, and determine many of the foods eaten or avoided. These beliefs may be accurate, empirical observations; logical although often incorrect extensions of those observations; or purely mistaken beliefs, derived from magical reasoning or from simple misinterpretation of the world. They are none the less powerful, and they often persist for millennia without empirical check.

The Chinese and Mongols and Turks of the time observed the clear and dramatic effects of certain foods on certain conditions, such as that of fresh vegetables rich in vitamin C on scurvy. There is constant empirical testing and consequent alteration of behavior in the food systems of Chinese folk communities, as we have had much opportunity to observe. By contrast, inaccurate beliefs persist only when powerful logic drives them, that is, when they follow so naturally from broader principles that plausibility makes them almost irresistible, or when they involve foods and practices rare enough or ambiguous enough to withstand the cold truths of daily experience. Within the framework of ecological, medical and cultural factors individuals make their own daily choices. They weigh personal taste, social setting, expense, and many other immanent factors in terms of the immediate social reality in which they live and act. No cultural history or ethnography can afford to ignore this.

III. Conclusion

A few genuinely exotic recipes are marked off but the rest of the foods are, by implications, more or less part of a Turko–Mongol–Chinese fusion. Some elements of this fusion even pre–dated Mongol conquest due to centuries of Altaic presence and influence in the Chinese north. The result of it all was a distinctive cuisine not obviously close to anything today.

By contrast with other Asian cooking traditions, almost everything in the *YSZY* is boiled. Surprisingly little is roasted or grilled, to the point where *shao* 燒, "roast," simply means "cook" in most recipes. The very characteristic Chinese method of stir–frying is virtually unknown in the *YSZY*. Also, garlic, a signature spice in much of China today, is strikingly rare. It is called for only twice in the *YSZY*, both in Turkic dishes where the garlic is a minor ingredient of a cream/mint/garlic sauce. The recipe is, incidentally, very good, and of Middle Eastern affinity. There is another mention of large garlic among the medical foods, but this may be the much milder–flavored elephant garlic. Sabban points out that other Chinese cookbooks of the time also seem to downplay garlic.[165] Buddhist influence may be responsible. Buddhists traditionally held that such rank foods offended deities and Buddhas.

Otherwise *YSZY* cuisine is very close to the perhaps assimilated cuisine of Ningxia, Gansu 甘肅 and Shanxi 陜西 today. The high use of mutton, great focus on soups, especially noodle soups, a well–developed dumpling technology, the importance of Chinese onions, simple spicing, love of a variety of animal foods, lack of much use of rice and fish, and relative downplaying of soybean foods all link these provinces with the *YSZY* rather than with the modern food of east and south China. The vinegar that is called for in 39 *YSZY* recipes is probably another touch linking the cuisine of the *YSZY* with China's Northwest. The vinegar used in modern "Hui" cooking is often a wine vinegar instead of the traditional Chinese rice, or rice–wheat vinegar. The *YSZY*'s vinegar is probably also wine– rather than rice–based.

---

165 Sabban, 1986b: 180.

Differences between *YSZY* and modern Northwest cuisine include a fondness in that area for stir–frying, and rather more use of garlic, pork, and soy products, but Ningxia Muslim cooking in particular is still very close to the *YSZY*. It lacks, of course, pork. There is also little demonstrable Western influence in the Northwest today, no mastic, asafoetida or *sharbat*. Disruption of Central Asian trade routes since the Yuan is no doubt the primary reason.

Mongol influence shows itself primarily in the discussion of game in the species section of the book, although soups as the main dietary emphasis strongly represent Mongol traditions as well. Some of the Mongol gathered foods called for by *YSZY* recipes may also reflect Mongol medicinal tradition. Among the recipes, one may mention the recipes for wolf; for horse tripes; and for sheep parts such as dried thorax; to say nothing of the whole earth–baked sheep in willow leaves. Game is much in evidence in the systematic section of the book, but recipes are restricted to rather standard ones for wolf, bear, deer, and in the medicinal section the medicinal use of fox, badger, otter, pheasant, and wild boar.

Turkic influence is plain not only in terminology, several "Mongolian" words are given in a Turkic form, and in many specifically Turkic *YSZY* foods, principally bread foods. It is also found in the many west Asian traditions for which Turks were the principal intermediators. There are notable differences from the Central Asia (Turkic or Afghani) foodways of today. The most striking and obvious is the comparative lack of the real Central Asian staples of the present: bread; shishkebab, with one possible recipe; and yogurt. There are bread recipes, and more bread is implied in directions like "eat with buns." Something like *shaobing* 燒餅 is obviously meant, although in one case reference is clearly to a pocket or pita bread, but we have no recipes or discussion. Yogurt too is down to a very lowly place. It is not mentioned at all in the recipes although its use is clearly intended with *Tutum Ash*. In part this is due to the fact that the *YSZY*'s Chinese terminology confuses liquid butter, cream, and yogurt all called *suyou* 酥油. The various noodle and dumpling dishes are very much like those of modern Turkic Central Asia, but not much like Afghanistan equivalents. Finally, pilaf, now so important in these areas, is strongly implied but is not found in unequivocal form in the *YSZY*, although many of the rice dishes are close to it and obviously related.

In making these comparisons we must bear in mind differences between the well–known Turkic foodways of the present, and the less well documented traditions of the past. For one example, shishkebab recipes are rare in Middle Eastern cookbooks contemporary with the *YSZY* and seem to be a relatively recent innovation.[166] Also, most of the Turkic peoples of Central Asia were still relatively close to their steppe traditions in the fourteenth century. The bread and bread–food traditions of the present may have only begun to take root among them.

Farther afield are Arabo–Persian words like "mastic," "arak" (in a Turkic form, "*arajhi*"), and "*sharba[t]*," and characteristic spices of the area, notably asafoetidas with Persian names. But no recipe is exactly like an Arab or Persian one although some are very close. We find a "Barley Soup," almost identical to an Iraqi dish. The poppy seed rolls also would not seem out of place in west Asia or east Europe. The recipes for grilled sheep parts marinated with saffron and rose attar are unmistakably Arab.

A stronger influence is North India. A couple of recipes in *Juan* 1 are explicitly identified as being from there. One of them ("*Se-aBru* soup," #49) seems hard to pin down to any specific area, in spite of its Tibetan name and Tibetan mediation. The other ("Bal–po soup") is called Nepalese (#3). It is not much like today's Nepalese food, which shows recent Indian and Tibetan influences, but it is very much like the food of Kashmir. A modern Kashmiri dish called *qalia,* based on mutton, Chinese radish, thickener, and an analogous spice mix, is strikingly similar. It is even topped with fresh coriander leaves. Two key differences between the *YSZY*'s "Bal–po Soup" and *qalia* tell us much about the *YSZY*. In *qalia*, the meat is first fried and the thickener is yogurt. Another Kashmiri touch is the use of both ground dried ginger and fresh ginger in several *YSZY* recipes, often along with asafoetida. This exact spice mix is very common in Kashmir and, to our knowledge, nowhere else.[167] Evidently, it was more widespread in 1330, but still a northwest Indian influence is obvious and unmistakable in the *YSZY* and was most likely transmitted through many Tibetan monks at court, some known to have been actively involved in imperial dietary medicine,[168] among others. Such spices as ground ginger, long pepper, turmeric, and pomegranate are associated with India in the *YSZY* and seem to measure the influence.

---

[166] See Heine, 1988: 65ff on the preparation of meat in the medieval Arabic cookbook tradition.

[167] See Krishna Prasad Dar, *Kashmiri Cooking* (New Delhi, 1977).

[168] See Buell, forthcoming.

Last, some recipes seem like nothing on earth today. This is especially true of the long, complicated and detailed recipe for "*Qurim* bonnets" (#90). It would seem the creation of some genius in the kitchen of the Yuan court, possibly Hu himself. It mixes Chinese and west Asian ingredients with gay abandon, but is based on a thoroughly Mongolian mix of sheep parts. It is, like the *YSZY* itself, a reflection of a long lost era of unique cultural interaction and of fusion, by Mongol rulers with pretensions of universality.

Part B

* * *

TEXT AND TRANSLATION

TRANSLATOR'S NOTE

I. TRANSLATION

The translation of the *YSZY* which follows is full and complete in all particulars. It retains the organization of the original and like it is divided into a section for prefaces and three main divisions, each comprised of one *juan* of the original. Each part, including the three prefaces, is preceded by a reproduction of its full text except where indicated as printed in the *sibu congkang xubian* facsimile of the 1456 edition. A complete translation follows with full annotation and apparatus. Bold numbers and capital letters in brackets refer to the pages of the original text; numbers preceding recipes are recipe numbers, referred to in the introduction. *Juan* 1 includes a complete table of contents for the entire text.

Every effort has been made to make the translation consistent. Wherever possible a single English term has been used throughout to translate a single Chinese term. When this has not been possible, and the deviation is significant, the fact is so indicated in the notes. In every case translations of Chinese terms appearing in the text reflect the particular usage of the *YSCY*. This may be at variance with usage elsewhere. This is often true for cooking terms.[1]

Botanical, zoological and mineral terminology has also been standardized. For Latin names we have generally followed the *ZYDZD*, but have corrected frequently to accord with recent taxonomic revisions. Popular names, by and large, are from Hu Shiu-ying, *An Enumeration of Chinese Material Medica*. Hong Kong: The Chinese University Press, 1980. Hu Shiu-ying reproduces relatively well-known nineteenth century Chinese customs terminology. For popular names not in Hu we have used a variety of sources including: the largely outdated, but still useful works of B. E. Read; Pierre Pfeffer's superb *Asia: A Natural History* (London: Hamish Hamilton, 1968); Algirdas Knystautas, *The Natural History of the USSR* (London: Century,

[1] For an excellent survey of traditional Chinese cooking terminology see F. Sabban, "Le système des cuissons dans la tradition culinaire chinoise," *Annales, economies, sociétés, civilisations* 2 (Mars-Avril) 1983: 341-68.

1987); and Rodolphe Meyer de Schauensee, *The Birds of China* (Washington, DC: Smithsonian Institution Press, 1984). For most Western food plants our authority has been, unless otherwise indicated, G. B. Masefield, M. Wallis, S. G. Harrison, and B. E. Nicholson. *The Oxford Book of Food Plants* (Oxford: Oxford University Press, 1969).

It should be stressed that traditional Chinese botanical, zoological and mineral terminology is less precise than Western and is rather different in intent. It relies in large part upon a classification system based (in part) on magical correspondences and in other medicinal and dietary properties of substances as seen by the Chinese (see Chapter 2), rather than upon any Linnaean or Darwinian perception of the proper place of things in a biological order, a Chinese "great chain of being."[2] Chinese folk classification of plants and animals does recognize biologically related families (*e.g.*, *gua* 瓜 = cucurbits), based upon their physical similarities and past Chinese pragmatic experience. But in their fullest development, traditional Chinese classification systems can also produce groupings and terminology quite different from anything Western.

The Chinese, for example, sometimes employ a single name for unrelated species due to similar appearances and identically perceived medicinal and dietary properties, *e.g.*, the *YSZY*'s *caoguo*, probably covering a variety of species of large cardamom. Two substances can also have the same name when one has replaced the other as a food or medicine, even in cases where one was originally an animal product, the substitution a plant. This strange practice is understandable in part because traditional Chinese pharmacists rarely saw the substances they used in their unprocessed, natural forms, something particularly true for generally extremely rare animal products.[3] Conversely, sever-

[2] For an introduction to the terminological problems of the *YSCY* see Paul D. Buell, "The *Yin-shan cheng-yao*, a Sino-Uighur Dietary: Synopsis, Problems, Prospects," In Paul U. Unschuld, ed., *Approaches to Traditional Chinese Medical Literature* (Dordrecht, 1989), 109-127.

[3] The long-term tendency in Chinese medicine has been for plant materials to replace medicinals from animal and mineral sources, in part due to the rarity of some animal materials on account of the extinction or near extinction of many species in China and immediately neighboring areas, also because of the highly poisonous qualities of minerals once widely used in physiological alchemy. Regulations of the United States and other Western countries where traditional Chinese medicine is widely practiced outside China have also played a role in promoting this development as well since they prohibit trafficking in products from species facing extinction and strongly discourage, if they do not outright prohibit, use of extremely toxic substances as me-

al different terms can apply to parts of one and the same plant, *e.g.*, the different terms for the herb and root of the Chinese garlic chive in the *YSZY*.

All of this makes the translation of traditional Chinese biological terminology particularly difficult. For the *YSZY* there is the added problem that the terminology is often employed in a manner somewhat divergent from other, more standard sources. Part of the problem is that the dietary was written at a time when the codification and amalgamation of Chinese terminology had just begun, and represents its own Northern tradition. Another obstacle is that Hu Sihui has been creative in his usage and that in many cases the *YSZY*'s Chinese botanical and zoological terminology is no more than an approximation of usage in West and Central Asia. This fact is made abundantly clear by the illustrations, which often depict a plant or animal different from what one should expect from the Chinese terminology alone.

In addition to these questions of Chinese terminology and usage, there is the added difficulty of a *YSZY* biological environment which has been little studied and is certainly not well understood. This is true for modern East and Central Asian biology as well, with study and classification perhaps a century behind the standard set for well-settled parts of Europe and the United States. In this connection, the authors are aware of the considerable disagreements among botanists and zoologists regarding the taxonomy of some plants and animals mentioned by the *YSZY*, and in other sources used in this study. Where relevant we note these disagreements but make no attempt to settle them. We leave this task to specialists and in most cases simply follow our authorities.

Also fraught with problems is *YSZY* medical terminology. Like Chinese botanical, zoological and mineral terminology, traditional Chinese medical terminology is not readily equivalent to that used in the West. The world views of Chinese and Western medicine are, for example, utterly different, as are their respective terminological intents. Much of *YSZY* usage is formulated in terms of the generalized categories of Chinese folk medicine, *e.g.*, "head pain," "lower back pain." It is translated in equivalent general terms, as literally as possible. In a few cases a more complex terminology expressive of the full diagnostic categories of traditional Chinese medicine is used. Frequently *YSZY* terminology refers to symptoms, diseases, and syndromes still recognized by traditional Chinese physicians. For many,

---

dicines or in foods. We are grateful to Christopher Muench (personal communication to PDB) for this information.

standard English translations exist and can be found in the many Western language dictionaries of traditional Chinese medical usage.[4] But in other cases *YSZY* formulations are unique to the text, or are of uncertain application. We know far too little about the disease environment of Hu Sihui's time to allow us to give exact translations. To guard against any possible over-interpretation of the text, we have always translated as literally as possible when there is any uncertainty. This is particularly necessary in view of the added problem of exactly what Hu intended to communicate with his Chinese categories, and the strong possibility that he has used categories of Chinese medicine to translate West Asian or even Mongolian ideas.

Here the problem of inexact medical terminology impinges upon the equally great problem of inexact cultural focus. We have noted in the introductory chapters the great differences of content, for example, between a largely Chinese *juan* 3 and the recipes. There are similar differences of cultural content among the three major groups of recipes themselves, and even between "erratic blocks" of seemingly Chinese materials. Some material in these blocks represents elite traditions, some popular, and some traditions unique and specific to Mongol China, with its many non-Chinese cultural influences. These facts necessarily make the *YSZY* extraordinarily complex and a culturally inconsistent work.

This has meant that the question of what culture or mix of cultures a particular part of the text represents had to be foremost in our minds as we made our translation. Little or nothing in the *YSZY* can be taken at face value. For example, not only do many *YSZY* recipes represent more or less pure Central and West Asian cooking traditions, very roughly translated into Chinese categories, but some recipes may even be translations from a Turkic language. In such cases the adaptation of terminology to Chinese culinary experience may be superficial and highly inaccurate, and more of a hindrance than a help to proper un-

---

[4] For a useful listing of Western language and other reference works on traditional Chinese medicine see Paul U. Unschuld, *Chinese Life Sciences, Introductory Readings in Classical Chinese Medicine* (Taos, NM, 2005), 341-79. For convenience, we have relied on Ou Ming 歐明, *et al.*, *Chinese-English Glossary of Common Terms in Traditional Chinese Medicine* (Hong Kong, 1982), for English translations of well-known symptoms, diseases and syndromes, with a few modifications made to suit the fourteenth century. We freely acknowledge the limitations of this approach but feel that a full study of the disease and pathological environment of the *YSZY*, the context of the other Chinese medicines of the era, is simply beyond the scope of this introductory study.

derstanding. There are similar problems even with those portions of the text more or less purely Chinese.

For example, there is throughout the Chinese culture of the *YSZY* a great tension between elite traditions and folk belief. This finds expression in particular in the sometimes strange formulations of the *YSZY* avoidances. Some of the influences may not even be Chinese, especially if we assume that traditions represented are those of culturally diverse North China. Thus, even Chinese "erratic blocks" of text cannot be taken at face value.

Therefore, *YSZY* is by no means an easy text to translate. Parts, the recipes in particular, appear deceptively easy but can be in practice quite misleading. Language in them tends to be highly technical and is often expressed in terms unique to the Mongol era or the *YSZY* itself. Recipe texts are usually highly abbreviated and some are mutilated.[5] In some cases, detailed comparison with similar recipes found in other texts such as the *JJBYSL* as necessary before any real sense could be made out of some recipe texts. In such cases missing text and explanations have been supplied in brackets. Brackets are used throughout the translation to indicate any materials added by the translators and not found in the original. As with other *YSZY* texts, over-translation has been carefully avoided. Recipes too are translated as literally as possible.[6]

As an example of the type of problems encountered in translating the recipes the reader may profitably compare the following two recipes for "West of the River Lungs." The first is from the *JJBYSL* (13, 19a-b). The second is taken from *juan* 1 (42b) of the *YSZY*. Note that Hu has reversed the first two characters of the title, instead of the *JJBYSL*'s Xihe 西河, a term usually referring to the Uighurs in Yuan-era texts, he writes instead hexi 河西, a term usually to be understood as "Tangut":

1. "West of the River Lungs"

> Connect heart, sheep lungs, one set. Clean in water. Use 4 *liang* 兩 of bean paste and broth. Work into meat. Use 4 *liang* of flour and scallion juice. Work into meat. Honey, 3 *liang*, half a *jin* 近

[5] This may be due in part to damaged Yuan printing blocks used in making the Ming edition.

[6] We are extremely grateful to Paul Unschuld and Donald Harper for help in translating some of the more difficult recipes. We would also express our thanks to participants in the 1986 Munich conference on traditional Chinese medical terminology for critiquing some of our early translation efforts.

of butter, pine nuts, walnuts; remove the skin and clean, pound with a 10 *liang* weight. Filter finely and remove dregs. Stir together and combine. Pour onto the lung. When covered completely, put into cooking pot. Cook until done. Put on the table on a Tatar plate.[7] First baste and marinate lung. Put the excess broth into sesame paste. Cook until done. Make into entrees.

2. "Tangut Lungs"

Ingredients: Sheep's lung (one), leeks (six *jin*. Take the juice), flour (two *jin*. Make into paste), ghee (half a *jin*), black pepper (two *liang*), juice of sprouting ginger (two *he* 合).

Use salt. Flavor evenly. Submerge the lungs in water and cook. When done baste with the juice and eat.

Leaving aside slight differences in ingredients, the two recipes are clearly recipes for more or less the same dish but the *YSCY* version is so abbreviated as to be largely incomprehensible.

The original recipes thus assumed a great deal about their reader. The reader must not only know how to cook, but how to cook with the specific culinary traditions of the Mongol court in mind. Since the *YSZY*, with all its imperfections, is itself our best source for understanding these traditions, with little documented elsewhere, we can often only guess at what has been left out. When philological means fail, where internal comparisons are impossible or unfruitful, or where no parallel Medieval or Modern traditions exist, our only alternative has been cook-testing, to see which of several possibilities yields the best results.

In conclusion, although the translation which follows is well-based, and as reliable as we have been able to make it, a great deal remains conjecture, with much further research needed. We accept this limitation of our work in view of the infancy of the field of cross-cultural food and medicine studies, and the uniqueness of our document. It is also true that (like others who go first) we will necessarily make errors in what is the first translation of its kind from a Chinese source. We thus offer our work as a challenge to those who come after. Just as we have drawn heavily upon pioneer work by Laufer, Schafer, Sabban and others, and corrected them in some cases, we invite a new generation of scholars to refine our view, to make improvements, and to go on from here.

---

[7] This Tatar, or Dadan 大單, plate is presumably the large serving plate called *tabaq* in the *YSZY* (1, 47a).

II. Weights and Measures

In the translation below we have made no attempt to translate Chinese weights and measures. The following equivalents must be borne in mind when interpreting the recipes: a *qian* 錢 is today 3.12 g or .011 oz and is one-tenth of a *liang* 兩. Sixteen *liang* make a *jin* 斤 (about 500 g). A *sheng* 升 is today 516.19 ml, and is comprised of 10 *he* 合. Ten *sheng* make a *dou* 斗. Units of length relevant to the translation are the *cun* 寸, which is 33.3 mm and comprised of ten *fen* 分, and the *chi* 尺, ten *cun*, or about one third of a meter. In the thirteenth and fourteenth centuries, if Matsui is correct, and we believe that he is, about a standard Mongol-era base of weights and measures,[8] a *qian* was slightly larger, 4 g, and a *jin* was thus 640 g, while a *sheng* was 84.66 ml and a *he* one-tenth of that. These figures are quite different than those found in most standard reference sources (e.g., see the table in Farquhar, 1990: 443-44), which will now require revision. Possibly standards also existed for units of length and land measure too, but these are not discussed by Matsui.

III. Cooking with the *YSZY*

The *YSZY* is emphatically a medical work. True, many of the recipes do not have specific medical claims made for them, but all would have been seen as warming or beneficial in some way. In this regard, it is important to recall that nutrition has always held pride of place in Chinese medical practice. Foods are the preferred form of therapy and no sharp distinction is made between them and medicine. Thus in the second two groups of recipes primarily gustatorial recipes are freely mixed with purely medical items. This seems an unlikely combination to the American reader at least, but was a perfectly straightforward one for the Chinese or Mongol. Culturally-grounded readers would not see any mixing, merely a running account of things that are taken by mouth and influence health.

None the less, the reader should not lose track of the cookbook value of the work. It is certainly not just a medical formulary. The recipes include many that are highly sophisticated and give us every reason to respect both the skill and the eclecticism of the Yuan court chefs. As we have seen, they could take such an exotic matter as a

[8] Matsui 2004.

Kashmiri recipe (recipe #3) and develop a form of it adapted to their own cooking rules, boiling instead of frying, or cutting the rank mutton taste with tsaokos or other large cardamoms. Kitchen testing reveals that they did a brilliant job. The dish is very Kashmiri in taste, yet more subtle. The spicing is absolutely superb.

In following the *YSCY* recipes the modern cook does well to observe what instructions there are. This is a typical Chinese cookbook; it specifies only what a good cook would not know. Much is left to the discretion of the chef: the specific spice mixes in several recipes, the amount of water for boiling, the time of cooking, *etc*. However, important matters are given very carefully. The modern cook is advised to follow, to the letter, directions on the ordering of events, on ingredients and specific quantities; and other culinary matters. Otherwise, use your own discretion.

Hu Sihui follows standard Chinese practice in giving quantities where absolutely necessary, but otherwise leaving amounts (once again) to the discretion of the cook. This makes it somewhat difficult for anyone not experienced in Asian food. We suggest that the novice cook follow these guidelines:

1. Look for similar recipes in Chinese and Near Eastern cookbooks. Kenneth Lo's Chinese cookbooks have many Northern and Northwestern recipes; for Near Eastern, see especially Claudia Roden, 2000. Use the amounts indicated. Naturally, characteristically Chinese ingredients like soy sauce and fresh ginger should be used in Chinese amounts, while Near Eastern ingredients should be used in accord with the Near Eastern cookbooks. Kashmir preserves an ancient Central Asian style sometimes virtually identical with *YSZY* recipes, and if you can find a Kashmiri cookbook, use it as your guide on things like asafoetida and ground ginger.

2. The recipes work best if spiced with a fairly light hand by Asian standards. This still makes many of them, particularly the Indian and Arabic-style ones, very spicy by Euro-American standards, but they are definitely subtle, like the classic Near Eastern and North Chinese traditions they resemble, not like the spicier cuisines of southern Asia.

3. Cooking temperatures, unless otherwise indicated, should be moderate. Baking, for instance, should be at about 190 C.

Chinese stir-frying with its fiery heat is notably absent here. Meat should be fairly evenly cooked to "medium" doneness. Boiling should be gentle. Hu preached moderation, and his recipes work best if we take him as seriously as he evidently intended.

4. Most of the recipes produce hearty soups or fluffy dishes in which starches absorb the broth, producing the soft texture that Mexicans call "dry soup" (*sopa seca*).

5. As is often true in the Middle East, but rarely in China, these recipes are good when lukewarm and often better after sitting a while. Some even call for a waiting period during preparation, to give time for spices to flavor the main ingredients. This process goes on after cooking finishes.

6. Parts of the sheep that are unavailable, or undesirable to the modern cook can be replaced, up to a point, by available cuts. Sheep tail and rump fat can be dispensed with entirely, since modern lamb is fatty. This does alter the consistency and flavor of the dishes quite appreciably, but those of us who have had the authentic Central Asian items usually prefer the taste of the unauthentic version. Sheep tail fat is pretty strong stuff. Sheep feet can be left out or replaced by calves' feet. Wolf and bear can be replaced by lamb and pork respectively. Unavailable spices and minor ingredients will simply have to be left out, but you can always add a pinch of something as improvisation suggests. Alas, recipes involving such items as dried sheep's thorax must remain untried, unless you know an exceptionally cooperative sheep-rancher.

7. In improvising, to whatever degree, be guided by Hu's commitment to moderation, simple elegance, and delicate sophistication. Avoid strong seasonings, get the best ingredients, cook them so that their best flavor is brought out, and spice so as to highlight but not mask that flavor. Whatever may be said of Hu's specific medical beliefs, no one could fault his overall strategy of judicious cooking (simple without being dull), gently seasoned, thoroughly done but not overcooked. It does indeed maximize health benefits as well as flavor.

Note also the following on some specific ingredients: lesser galangal, often required in these recipes, is similar to ginger in appearance but not in taste. It is usually sold in the Western world under the Indonesian names *laos* or *lengkuas*. Most oriental markets carry small bottles of powdered *laos*, usually the "Conimex" brand, and some have the frozen whole root. Either is acceptable. It is a southern plant and the court in Beijing may well have used the powder.

Regular cardamoms can be substituted for tsaokos, but, if this is done, the cook must use perhaps twenty or more, for the tsaokos are much larger and more strongly flavored. Try to find the tsaokos or some other closely equivalent large cardamom. They result in a far better product. They are found in most Asian markets under the name "large" or "black cardamoms," if not called "tsaoko."

Lamb: the recipes make it clear that the Mongols had small sheep. A regular leg of lamb is amply large enough, if not too large. A big one overwhelms the other ingredients in these recipes. In boiling the lamb for the many two-stage dishes, leave it underdone in the first boiling; otherwise the second final stage will cook all the flavor out of it. Those who cannot stand lamb may substitute beef or chicken in any of these dishes. Obviously, this creates a new dish, but in Persian cooking such things are often done, and elsewhere in the Near East it is not unknown. The Chinese, too, vary their recipes; and indeed several of the *YSZY* recipes are virtually identical except for the main meat.

With all recipes involving mashed chickpeas, extreme care must be taken to avoid burning. These recipes must be stirred constantly or cooked over very low heat.

Remember to put in such items as greens, saffron, and other delicate-flavored quick-cooking items at the very end of the cooking process. Hu carefully lists these ingredients last, when he uses them, making it obvious that this was what he intended.

Some trouble may be involved in all this, but the results are worth the effort in nearly every case. Most recipes in the *YSZY* are simple and excellent. They are sophisticated. Their simplicity is that of a classic cuisine, not of a naive one. Doubters need only try the recipe for lamb marinated in saffron and rosewater, or the stuffed eggplant.

PREFACES

* * *

CHINESE TEXT

忽思慧
飲膳正要卷一

四部叢刊續編子部: Title, (Imperial Preface) 1B, 2A-2B; (Main Preface) 1A-2A, 3A- 4B; (Author's Preface) 5A-6A

中國古代版畫叢刊: (Imperial Preface) 1A

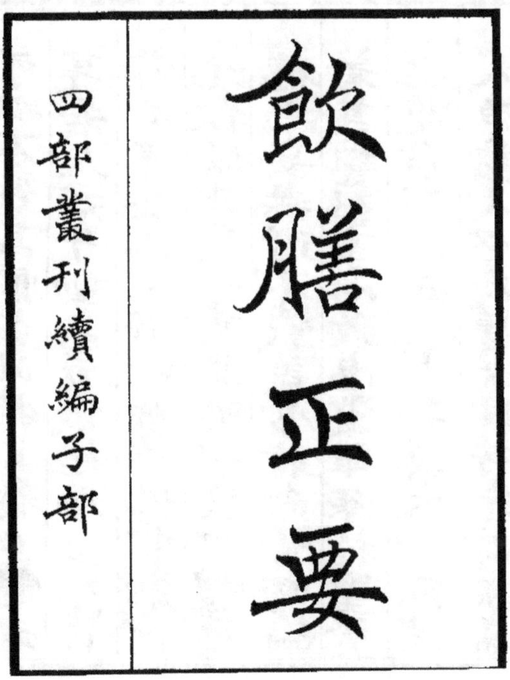
飲膳正要

四部叢刊續編子部

Title

1A
Imperial Preface

御製飲膳正要序

朕惟人物皆稟天地之氣以生者也
然物又天地之所以養乎人者苟用
之失其所以養則至於戕害者有矣
如布帛菽粟雞豚之類日用所不能
無其為養甚大也然過則失中不及
則未至其為戕害一也其為養甚大
者尚然而況不為養而為害之物焉

1B

可以不致其慎哉此特其養口體者
耳若夫君子動息威儀起居出入皆
當有其養焉又所以養德也嘗觀前
元飲膳正要一書其所以養口體養
德之要無所不載蓋當時尚醫所論
著其執藝事以致忠愛雖深於聖賢
之道者不外是也夫善莫大於取諸
人取諸人以為善大舜所先肆朕嘉

2A

是書而用之。以資攝養之助。且鋟諸
梓以廣惠利於人。亦庶幾乎好生之
仁。雖然生稟於天。非人之所能為。若
或戕之與立巖墻之下者同。有不由
於人乎。故此非但攝養之助。而抑順
受其正之大助也。

2B

景泰七年四月初一日

1A
Yu Ji's
Preface

臣聞古之君子善脩其身者動息節宣以養生飲
食衣服以養體威儀行義以養德是故周公之制
禮也天子之起居衣服飲食各有其官皆統於冢
宰蓋慎之至也
今上皇帝天縱聖明文思深遠御延閣閱圖書旦暮
有恒則尊養德性以酬酢萬幾得內聖外王之道
焉於是趙國公臣常普蘭奚以所領膳醫臣忽思
慧所撰飲膳正要以進其言曰昔
世祖皇帝食飲必稽於本草動靜必準乎法度是以
身躋上壽貽子孫無疆之福焉是書也當時尚醫

1B

之論著者云噫進書者可謂能執其藝事以致其
忠愛者矣是書進上
中宮覽焉念
祖宗衛生之戒知臣下陳義之勤思有以助
聖上之誠身而推其仁民之至意命中政院使臣拜
住刻梓而廣傳之茲舉也蓋欲推一人之安而使
天下之人舉安推一人之壽而使天下之人皆壽
恩澤之厚豈有加於此者哉書之既成大都留守
臣金界奴傳
勅命臣集序其端云臣集再拜稽首而言曰臣聞易

2A

之傳有之大哉乾元萬物資始至哉坤元萬物資
生天地之大德不過生生而已耳今
聖皇正統於上乾道也
聖后順承於中坤道也乾坤道備於斯爲盛斯民斯
物之生於斯時也何其幸歟顧颺言之使天下後
世有以知夫高明博厚之可見如此於戲休哉
天曆三年五月朔日謹序
奎章閣侍書學士翰林直學士中奉大夫
知制誥同脩國史臣虞集譔

3A Official Preface

伏覩
國朝奄有四海遐邇罔不賓貢珍味奇品咸萃內
府或風土有所未宜或燥濕不能相濟儻司庖厨
者不能察其性味而槩於進
獻則食之恐不免於致疾欽惟
世祖皇帝聖明按周禮天官有師醫食醫疾醫瘍醫
分職而治行依典故設掌飲膳太醫四人於本草
內選無毒無相反可久食補益藥味與飲食相宜
調和五味及每日所造珍品
御膳必須精製所職何人所用何物

3B

進酒之時必用沉香木沙金水晶等盞斟酌適中
執事務合稱職每日所用標注於曆以驗後效至
於湯煎瓊玉黃精天門冬蒼术等膏牛髓枸杞等
煎諸珍異饌咸得其宜以此
世祖皇帝聖壽延永無疾恭惟
皇帝陛下自登
寶位國事繁重萬機之暇遵依
祖宗定制如補養調護之術飲食百味之宜進加日
新則
聖躬萬安矣臣思慧自延祐年間選充飲膳之職于

4A

茲有年久叨
天祿退思無以補報敢不竭盡忠誠以答
洪恩之萬一是以日有餘閑與趙國公臣普蘭奚
將累朝親侍
進用奇珍異饌湯膏煎造及諸家本草名醫方術
幷日所必用穀肉菓菜取其性味補益者集成一
書名曰飲膳正要分為三卷本草有未收者今即
採摭附寫伏望
陛下恕其狂妄察其愚忠以
燕閒之際鑑

4B

先聖之保攝順當時之氣俟棄虛取實期以獲安則
聖壽躋於無疆而四海咸蒙其
德澤矣謹獻所述飲膳正要一集以
聞伏乞
聖覽下情不勝戰慄激切屏營之至
天曆三年三月三日飲膳太醫臣忽思慧進上
中奉大夫太醫院使臣耿允謙校正
奎章閣都主管事資政大夫大都留守內宰隆禧總管提調織染雜造人匠都總管府事臣張金界奴校正
資德大夫中政院使儲政院使臣拜住校正
集賢大學士銀青榮祿大夫趙國公臣常普蘭奚編集

5A Author's Preface

天之所生地之所養天地合氣人以稟天地氣生並
而為三才三才者天地人人而有生所重乎者心也
心為一身之主宰萬事之根本故身安則心能應萬
變主宰萬事非保養何以能安其身保養之法莫若
守中守中則無過與不及之病調順四時節慎飲食
起居不妄使以五味調和五藏五藏和平則血氣資
榮精神健爽心志安定諸邪自不能入寒暑不能襲
人乃怡安夫上古聖人治未病不治已病故重食輕
貨蓋有所取也故云食不厭精膾不厭細魚餒肉敗
者色惡者臭惡者失飪不時者皆不可食然雖食飲

5B

非聖人口腹之欲哉蓋以養氣養體不以有傷也若
食氣相惡則傷精若食味不調則損形形受五味以
成體是以聖人先用食禁以存性後制藥以防命蓋
以藥性有大毒有大毒者治病十去其六常毒治病
十去其七小毒治病十去其八無毒治病十去其九
然後穀肉菓菜十養一儘之無使過之以傷其正雖
飲食百味要其精粹審其有補益助養之宜新陳之
異溫凉寒熱之性五味偏走之病若滋味偏嗜新陳
不擇製造失度俱皆致疾可者行之不可者忌之如
姙婦不慎行乳母不忌口則子受患若貪爽口而忘

6A

避忌則疾病潛生而中不悟百年之身而忘於一時
之味其可惜哉孫思邈曰謂其醫者先曉病源知其
所犯先以食療不瘥然後命藥十去其九故善養生
者謹先行之攝生之法豈不爲有裕矣

PREFACES

* * *

TRANSLATION

YINSHAN ZHENGYAO

[Prefaces]

[Introduction to the [Ming] Imperial Edition of the *Yinshan Zhengyao*]

[**1A**] WE believe that people and things all rely upon the *qi* of Heaven and Earth in order to live. But things are also the means by which heaven and earth nourish people. If in using things, we lose that by which they nourish, then WE suspect that we will put ourselves into a position whereby we will attain serious harm. In the case of things such as linen and silk, pulses and grains, chickens and pigs: we use them daily and cannot be without them. Their value as nourishment is extremely great. But if they are in excess, the mean is low; while if they are insufficient [their function] is not attained. This is the same as their being seriously harmful. If things which are especially nourishing are like this, how much more so things which are not nourishing and are harmful. How [**1B**] can we not be circumspect in such matters? And these are merely what one nurtures the mouth and the body with, nothing more. As for the gentleman's motion and rest, gravity and deportment, rising and retiring, going and coming: all must have their nurture. They must also have what is needed to nourish intrinsic virtue [*de*]. WE have examined the entire book *Yinshan zhengyao* of the former Yuan dynasty. With regard to the essentials for nourishing mouth and body, and for nourishing intrinsic virtue, everything is there. The work was written by a leading doctor of the day. His taking up literary activity to convey his loyalty and love, although deep in the way of sages and worthies, was nothing more than this. Now of goodness, nothing is greater than accepting things from another man. Thinking that accepting things from another man was good, it was first done by Great Shun. I praise [**2A**] this book and use it. I rely on it as an aid for hygiene and nourishment. Moreover, I have engraved it on catalpa wood [printing blocks], so that it might propagate its benefits and advantages to human beings. This also is close to the benevolence of loving life. Although life relies on heaven, yet it is not something that men are able to do anything about. If someone injures it, it is exactly the same as standing below a towering wall. It is something out of human control. Thus this book is not just an aid for hygiene and nourishing. It is also a great aid for training to receive the correct [way of living].

[**2B**] Seventh year of Qingtai [1456], 4th month, first decade, first day.

[Yu Ji's Preface:]

[1A] (minister)[1] [I] have heard that the gentlemen of olden days were good at cultivating their persons. In activity or repose they were restrained or loose in order to nourish life. Drink, food, and clothing were used to nourish the body. With gravity and deportment they practiced duty thereby cultivating intrinsic virtue. For this reason, when the Duke of Zhou regulated ritual, the emperor's rising and resting, robes and ritual clothing, drinking and eating, each had its official. They were all controlled by the minister of state. This was extreme circumspection!

As to The PRESENT EMPEROR, Heaven has allowed him sagely brilliance, HIS literate contemplation is deep and profound. In HIS management of the court and council chamber, HE examines documents and books morning and evening, on a regular basis. Thus HE honors and nourishes the qualities of [HIS] intrinsic virtue in order to respond to the myriad of subtle manifestations. He is able thereby to achieve the way of sagelyness within and kingliness without. Thus the Dynastic Duke of Zhao (minister) Chang Buralgi brought the book *Yinshan zhengyao*, written by (minister) Hu Sihui, a dietary physician under his control, to present it. His words were: "Formerly whenever

THE EMPEROR SHIZU [Qubilai] would eat or drink, he had to investigate [the properties of his food] in the herbal manuals. Whenever HE would be active or quiet, he had to balance [his activity or repose] according to restrictions. For this reason HIS health improved and he attained a great age. HE thereby stored up inexhaustible good fortune for his descendants." Now this book [**1B**] is considered to be the exposition of a leading doctor of the time. I dare say that, indeed, with regard to the one presenting the book, it can be said [to be a matter of the author's] ability to use his taking up literary activity to convey his loyalty and love. When this book had been presented

HER MAJESTY Examined it. SHE thought about the admonitions of

[1] The word "minister," always printed in half-size, is used in this preface to designate all subordinates of the emperor. The text also begins a new line when Yuan emperors are mentioned, and indents other text. We follow the former but not the latter convention.

THE IMPERIAL ANCESTORS to guard life. She understood the diligence of the subordinate in setting forth duty. She thought that it had things that would aid

HIS SAGELY HIGHNESS in perfecting his person, and would promote his supreme intention of being humane to the people. She ordered the (minister) Baiju, officer of the Bureau for the Establishment of the Empress, to engrave catalpa wood and disseminate it widely. Now this undertaking intends to promote the security of the ONE MAN and thereby to cause all the people of the empire to be secure. It promotes the longevity of the ONE MAN thereby to achieve the longevity of all the people of the empire. In terms of substantial imperial bounty, assuredly there can be no improvement over this! When the book was ready, the Governor of Daidu, (minister) Jin Jienu, disseminated the work.

[THE EMPEROR] ordered (minister) [me, Yu] Ji to write a preface at its head. (minister) [I Yu] Ji repeatedly bow, knock the head and say: (minister) "[I] have heard that [**2A**] it is there in the commentary to the *Changes*. Great is Heavenly Principle. The myriad things avail of it to come into being. Exceeding is the Earthly Principle. The myriad things avail of it to live. Of the great intrinsic virtues of heaven and earth, none exceeds giving life to the living. And at the present

THE SAGELY EMPEROR maintains an orthodox succession above. This is the Heavenly Principle.

THE SAGELY EMPRESS accords and receives his influence in the center. This is the Earthly Principle. The presence of the Heavenly and Earthly Principle in this is a source of flourishing. That these people and these things should be born at this time, what a wonderful thing! [I] Would soar up to tell it, to provide a way for later generations of the empire to know that it is possible to receive great intelligence and extreme bounty like this. Oh how glorious indeed!"

Respectfully prefaced, Tianli, third year [1330], fifth month, new moon

Written by (minister) Yu Ji, Attendant Literary Scholar of the Hall of Literature, Primary Literary Scholar of the Hanlin, Middle Level Grandee, the Scholar-in-charge-of-edicts-and-patents-and-at-the-same-time-compiler-of-dynastic-history.

[Hu Sihui's Preface:]

[**3A**] [I] Dare to Observe that the present dynasty grandly holds the four seas. There is none, near or far, who does not come to court and offer tribute. Rare dainties and exotic things are all collect in the imperial treasury. But, perhaps, wind and land [*i.e.*, the local environment] have something unsuitable about them. Perhaps dry and wet [*i.e.*, moisture levels] are unable to complement one another. If those in charge of the kitchen are unable to investigate the natures and flavors of these [foods], and simply present all of them to the emperor to eat, and if he eats them, I fear that he will not avoid becoming sick. Now [I] dare to think that

EMPEROR SHIZU had sagely brilliance. HE Saw that the Tianguan chapter of the *Zhouli* has separate offices for a chief physician, dietary physician, a doctor of internal medicine, and a doctor for ulcerous afflictions; and governing according to old canons, HE therefore appointed four persons as chief physicians in charge of diet. They were to choose from the herbals supplementing and beneficial medicinal foods which are not poisonous, which do not conflict with each other, and which can be eaten over the long term; along with drink and food spices which can be blended together to mutual benefit, and the rare things to be made on each day. The imperial cuisine had to be compounded very carefully. Each person had his area of expertise. Each thing had its proper use.

[**3B**] When liquor was presented, cups of garuwood, *shajin* [stone],[2] rock crystal, and the like had to be used. In their considerations, they accorded with the mean. In taking charge of official actions, they acted in accordance with functions. Each day they would make calendar entries of what was used, as proof for future imitation. As for soups, various rare delicacies such as concentrates of red jade, Solomon's seal, Chinese asparagus, tsangshu and the like, decoctions of ox marrow, Chinese matrimony vine [fruits] and the like, all attained their benefit. For this reason

EMPEROR SHIH-TSU enjoyed sagely longevity without sickness from beginning to end. I respectfully consider that from the time of

YOUR MAJESTY THE EMPEROR'S mounting of the precious position, dynastic affairs have been complicated and difficult. In YOUR

---

[2] According to the dictionaries, this is an unidentified green stone with large golden, star-shaped flakes.

leisure from the myriad activities, you have honored and accorded with regulations set by

YOUR IMPERIAL ANCESTORS; such things as methods for supplementing and nourishing, and protecting oneself, the benefits of the hundred flavors in drinking and eating. I dare say that, with each passing day, THE SAGELY BODY has a myriad of securities [more]. Since (minister) [I, Hu] Sihui, was chosen to fill the office of dietary physician during the Yanyou period [1314-1320], [**4A**] a number of years have passed. [I] have long enjoyed the favor of Heaven. I have regretted that I had nothing with which to repay THE EMPEROR'S kindness. I dare not utterly exhaust my loyalty and sincerity to reply to a myriad and one liberal benefits. For this reason I have daily used my excess leisure and, together with (minister) Chang Bulargi, the dynastic duke of Zhao, have taken the exotic delicacies presented for the imperial use in personal service to various courts, made into soups, dry concentrates, decoctions; and recipes of famous doctors from herbals written by various persons; along with the grains, meats, fruits, and vegetables of daily use, noting their properties and flavors; and the ones strengthening and augmenting, and compiled them together into a book. It is called *Yinshan zhengyao* and is divided into three *juan*. Where the herbals have omissions, we have now collected [the relevant material] and written it out as a supplement. We humbly anticipate

YOUR MAJESTY'S anger at our madness, and his consideration of our stupid loyalty. Here in the capital city, we follow the example [**4B**] set by

FORMER SAGE [EMPERORS] in preserving health. We accord with the *qi* of the time and hope to gather fruit from barren waste. We expect, I dare say, that with the achievement of security, the

[EMPEROR'S] SAGELY LONGEVITY will be increased to the unlimited, and that the entire empire will enjoy the benefits of the favor of his intrinsic virtue. We respectfully present the completed *Yinshan zhengyao*, which we have written, that it might be brought to the EMPEROR'S attention. We humbly beg that

THE SAGELY [EMPEROR] will deign to consider the feelings of subordinates. We come awestruck, roused to make an effort in spite of our agitation.[3]

---

[3] Compare the translation of this preface in Unschuld, 1986: 215-6.

Tianli third year, third month, third day

Presented to the Emperor by the Chief Dietary Physician (minister) Hu Sihui.

Edited by the Middle Level Grandee, Officer of the Chief Medical Office (minister) Geng Jiuqian.

Edited by the Hall of Literature Chief Officer-in-charge, the Grandee-who-brings-affairs-to-the-attention-of-the-Emperor and Who-is-relied-upon-to-govern, The Governor of Daidu, Imperial Steward, Chief Administration Officer of the Beneficent Omen Administrative Office[4] for Controlling Craftsmen of Textiles, Dye Stuffs, and Various Commodities Chang Jinchienu.

Edited by the Grandee-who-is-relied-upon-for-intrinsic-virtue, Officer of the Bureau for the Establishment of the Empress, Officer of the Bureau for the Establishment of the Heir Apparent (minister) Baiju.

Compiled by The Chief Literary Scholar, Grandee of the Silver-green-glorious emolument, Dynastic Duke of Zhao (minister) Chang Buralgi.

[Hu Sihui's Introduction:]

[**5A**] Whatever is given life by Heaven and nourished by Earth represents the combined *qi* of Heaven and Earth. Man relies upon the *qi* of Heaven and Earth to live. Together they are the Three Powers. The Three Powers are Heaven, Earth, and Man. But Man has that which weighs in life, the heart. The heart is the lord and master of the entire body. It is the foundation of the myriad things. Therefore if the body is secure, the heart can then respond to the myriad changes. It controls the myriad things. If it is not protected and nourished, how can it make the body secure? Among methods for protecting and nourishing, none is better than keeping to the mean. If one keeps to the mean, then there will be no excess and illness which does not respond to treatment. If one accommodates oneself to the four seasons and is restrained and careful in drink and food; if one is not foolish in rising and resting; if one causes the five flavors to accord with the five viscera and the five viscera are in balance, the blood and *qi* will rely on this to flourish. If the essence and spirit are strong and energetic; if the heart and will are secure and established; the various pathological in-

[4] This office was part of the establishment of the empress but separate from the Bureau for the Establishment of the Empress.

fluences will not be able to enter on their own, and cold and heat will be unable to invade. A person will then be healthful and secure. Now as for the sages of high antiquity, they treated those not yet ill, they did not [have to] treat those already ill. Thus they placed emphasis on food, and de-emphasized things. They therefore had their own way of living. Therefore it is said: in food one should not disdain delicate food. In minced meat [or fish] one should not disdain fine food. In the case of putrid fish or rotten meat, [food] which has a bad color, or a bad odor, or which is badly cooked or unseasonal, none of it can be eaten. However, food and drink [**5B**] is definitely not a matter of what a sage's mouth or stomach wants. It is a matter of nourishing *qi* and nourishing the body, and not being harmful. If the *qi*s of foods mutually damage one another, the essence is then harmed. If the flavors of foods are not in accord, the form is then damaged. The form takes up the five spices to form the body. For this reason sages first of all used food prohibitions to preserve their natures. Secondly, they created medicines to protect their lives. But medicines because of their nature have great poison. If a highly poisonous medicine is used to treat illnesses, it eliminates six out of ten. If a normally poisonous [medicine] is used to treat illnesses, it eliminates seven of ten. If a little poisonous [medicine] is used to treat illnesses, it eliminates eight of ten. If a non-poisonous [medicine] is used to treat illnesses, it eliminates nine of ten. Then, as for grain, meat, fruit and vegetables, they are nourishing for all [illnesses] and get rid of them completely. One should not allow them to be in excess and thereby harm one's proper state of health. Although one drinks and eats a hundred flavors, one requires the essence. One should investigate whether or not they benefit in strengthening and augmenting, in aiding and nourishing, the peculiarities of the foods fresh and stale; their warming, chilling, cooling and heating properties; and illnesses from overindulgence in the five flavors. If one consumes thick flavors excessively; if one does not select for freshness and staleness; if preparations are out of proportion, then all of these things together will result in illness. If something is possible, proceed. If something is impossible, avoid it. If a pregnant woman is not cautious in her behavior, if a wet nurse does not practice food avoidances, the child will then suffer harm. If one is avaricious for whatever tastes good, and forgets [**6A**] avoidances, illness will then arise secretly and one will be completely unaware. The body of a hundred years is forgotten with the flavor of a single moment. This is extremely pitiful! Sun Simiao said: "As for what is called medicine, it is first of all to understand the origins of illness, knowing what it is that has violated the body. One should treat illness first with diet. If [patient] does not recover, only then should medicine be ordered." It eliminates nine out of ten. Therefore, those good at nurturing life must cautiously practice [dietary medicine] in advance. This is a method for hygiene. I dare say that this cannot but enrich![5]

[5] Compare the translation of this introduction in Unschuld, 1986: 213-14.

JUAN 1 (MAIN TEXT)

* * *

CHINESE TEXT

忽思慧
飲膳正要 卷一 (Continued)

四部叢刊續編子部: 7A-15A, 16A-34B, 36B-38B, 39B-50A

中國古代版畫叢刊: 15B, 35A, 39A

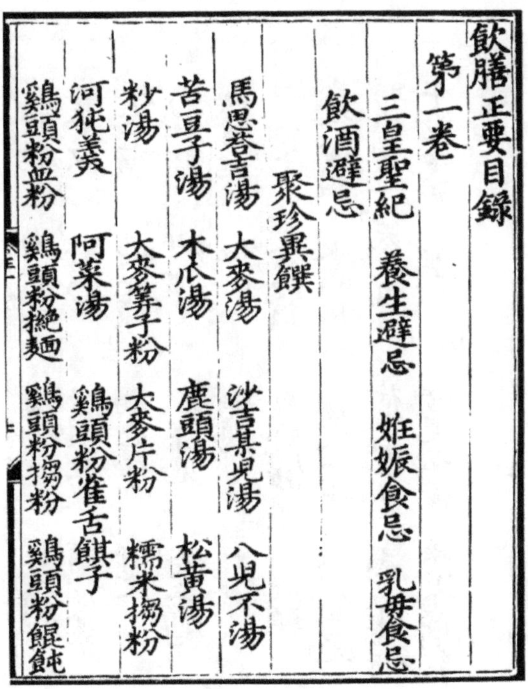

飲膳正要目錄

第一卷

7A
Table of Contents

7B

雜羹 葷素羹 珎珠粉 黄湯
三下鍋 葵菜羹 瓠子湯 團魚湯
盞蒸 臺苗羹 熊湯 鯉魚湯
炒狼湯 圍像 春盤麵 皂羹麵
山藥麵 掛麵 經帶麵 羊皮麵
禿禿麻食 細水滑 水龍餶子 馬乞
搠羅脫因 乞馬粥 湯粥 粱米淡粥
河西米湯粥 撒速湯 炙羊心 炙羊腰
攢雞 炒鵪鶉 盤兎 河西肺
薑黄腱子 鼓兒簽子 帶花羊頭 魚彈兒

8A

芙蓉雞 肉餅兒 塩腸 腦瓦刺
薑黄魚 攢鴈 豬頭薑豉 蒲黄瓜虀
攢羊頭 攢牛蹄 細乞思哥 肝生
馬肚盤 煠腜兒 熬蹄兒 熬羊胸子
魚膾 紅絲 燒鴈 雞鵝 鴨子 水扎同
柳蒸羊 倉饅頭 鹿妳肪饅頭 茄饅頭
剪花饅頭 水晶角兒 酥皮奄子 撇列角兒
時蘿角兒 天花包子 荷蓮兜子 黑子兒燒餅
牛妳子燒餅 䭔餅 頹兒必湯 米哈訥關列孫
第二卷

8B

諸般湯煎

桂漿　桂沉漿　荔枝膏　梅子丸
五味子湯　人參湯　仙术湯　杏霜湯
山藥湯　四和湯　薑棗湯　茴香湯
破氣湯　白梅湯　木瓜湯　橘皮醒酲湯
渴忒餅兒　官桂渴忒餅兒　答必納餅兒　橙香餅兒
牛髓膏子　木瓜煎　香圓煎　株子煎
紫蘇煎　金橘煎　櫻桃煎　桃煎
石榴漿　小石榴煎　五味舍兒別　赤赤哈納
松子油　杏子油　酥油　醍醐油

9A

馬思哥油　枸杞茶　玉磨茶　金字茶
范殿帥茶　紫笋雀舌茶　女須兒　西番茶
川茶　藤茶　夸茶　燕尾茶
孩兒茶　温桑茶　清茶　炒茶
蘭膏　酥簽　建湯　香茶

諸水

玉泉水　井華水　鄒店水

神仙服餌

瓊玉膏　地仙煎　金髓煎　天門冬膏
服地黃　服蒼术　服茯苓　服遠志

9B

五加皮酒　服桂　服松子　松節酒
服槐實　服枸杞　服蓮花　服栗子
服黃精　神枕法　服菖蒲　服胡麻
服五味　服藕實　服蓮子 蓮蕊　服何首烏
四時所宜　五味偏走
食療諸病
生地黃雞　羊蜜膏　羊藏羹　羊骨粥
羊脊骨粥　白羊腎羹　豬腎粥　枸杞羊腎粥
鹿腎羹　羊肉羹　鹿蹄湯　鹿角酒
黑牛髓煎　狐肉湯　烏雞湯　醍醐酒

10A

山藥飥　山藥粥　酸棗粥　生地黃粥
椒麵羹　蓽撥粥　良薑粥　吳茱萸粥
牛肉脯　蓮子粥　雞頭粥　雞頭粉羹
桃仁粥　生地黃粥　鯽魚羹　炒黃麵
乳餅麵　炙黃雞　牛奶子煎蓽撥　獾肉羹
黃雌雞　青鴨羹　蘿蔔粥　野雞羹
鵓鴿羹　雞子黃　葵菜羹　鯉魚湯
馬齒菜粥　小麥粥　驢頭羹　驢肉湯
狐肉羹　熊肉羹　烏雞酒　羊肚羹
葛粉羹　荊芥粥　麻子粥　惡實菜

10B

烏驢皮羹 羊頭膾 野猪臛 獺肝羹
鯽魚羹
食物利害 食物相反 食物中毒
禽獸變異
第三卷
米穀品
稻米 粳米 粟米 粱米 白粱 黃粱
黍米 丹黍 稷米 河西米 菉豆 白豆
大豆 赤小豆 回回豆子 青小豆 豌豆 匾豆
小麥 大麥 蕎麥 芝麻 胡麻 餳

11A

蜜 麵 醋 醬 豉 鹽
酒 虎骨酒 枸杞酒 地黃酒 松節酒 茯苓酒 松根酒 羊羔酒 五加皮酒 腽肭臍酒 小黃米酒 葡萄酒 阿剌吉酒
速兒麻酒
獸品
牛 羊 黃羊 羖䍽 馬 野馬
象 駝 野駝 熊 驢 麋
鹿 獐 犬 猪 野猪 獺
虎 豹 麅 麂 麝 狐
犀牛 狼 兔 狸 塔剌不花 黃鼠 猴
禽品

11B

天鵝 鵞 鴈 鴜鷀 水札 丹鷄
野雞 雞角 鴨 野鴨 鸂鶒 鴛鴦 鵓鴿 鳩
鴒 寒鴉 鵪鶉 雀 蒿雀

魚品

鯉魚 鯽魚 魴魚 白魚 黃魚 青魚 鮎魚
沙魚 鮮魚 河豘 鮑魚 石首 阿八兒忽魚 乞里麻魚
鼈 蟹 蝦 螺 蚌 蛤蜊 鱸魚 蜎

菓品

桃 梨 柿 木瓜 梅 李
柰 石榴 林檎 杏 柑 橘

12A

橙 栗 棗 櫻桃 葡萄 胡桃
松子 蓮子 鷄頭 芰實 荔枝 龍眼
銀杏 橄欖 楊梅 榛子 榧子 沙糖
甜瓜 西瓜 酸棗 海紅 香圓 株子
平坡 八擔仁 必思荅

菜品

葵菜 蔓菁 芫荽 芥 葱 蒜
韭 冬瓜 黃瓜 蘿蔔 胡蘿蔔 天淨菜
瓠 菜瓜 葫蘆 蘑菰 菌子 木耳
竹筍 蒲筍 藕 山藥 芋 萵苣

12B

白菜 蓬蒿 茄子 莧 芸薹 波稜
莙薘 香菜 蓼子 馬齒 天花 回回葱
甘露 榆仁 沙吉木兒 出莙薘兒
山丹根 海菜 蕨 薇 苦買 水芹

料物

胡椒 小椒 良薑 茴香 甘草 芫荽子
乾薑 生薑 蒔蘿 陳皮 草果 桂
薑黃 蓽撥 縮砂 蓽澄茄 五味子 苦豆
紅麯 黑子兒 馬思荅吉 咱夫蘭 哈昔泥
穩展（阿魏根） 臙脂 梔子 蒲黃 回回青

13A
Three Sages

太昊伏羲氏

風姓之源皇熊氏之後生有聖德繼天而王爲萬世帝王之先位在東方以木德王爲蒼精之君都陳時神龍出於滎河則而畫之爲八卦造書契以代結繩之政立五常定五行正君臣明父子別夫婦之義制嫁娶之理造屋舍結網罟以佃漁服牛乘馬引重致遠取犧牲供祭祀故曰伏羲氏治天下一百一十年

炎帝神農氏

姜姓之源烈山氏之後生有聖德以火承木位在南方以火德王爲赤精之君時人民茹草飲水採樹木

13B

之實而食蠃蛖之肉多生疾病乃求可食之物嘗百
草種五穀以養人民日中為市作陶冶為斧斤造耒
耜教民耕稼故曰神農都曲阜治天下一百二十年

黃帝軒轅氏

姬姓之源有熊國君少典之子生而神靈長而聰明
成而登天以土德王為黃精之君故曰黃帝都涿鹿
受河圖見日月星辰之象始有星官之書命大撓探
五行之情占斗罡所建始作甲子命容成作曆命隸
首作筭數命伶倫造律呂命岐伯定醫方為衣冠以
表貴賤治干戈作舟車分州野治天下一百年

14A

飲膳正要卷第一

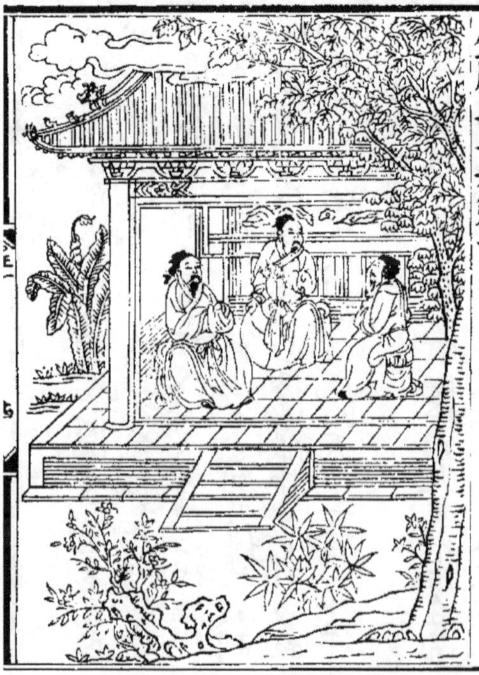

14B Nurturing Life

養生避忌

夫上古之人其知道者法於陰陽和於術數食飲有節起居有常不妄作勞故能而壽今時之人不然也起居無常飲食不知忌避亦不慎節多嗜慾厚滋味不能守中不知持滿故半百衰者多矣夫安樂之道在乎保養保養之道莫若守中守中則無過與不及之病春秋冬夏四時陰陽生病起於過與蓋不適其性而強故養生者既無過耗之弊又能保守真元何患乎外邪所中也故善服藥者不若善保養不善保養不若善服藥世有不善保養又不能善服藥倉卒

15A

病生而歸咎於神天乎善攝生者薄滋味省思慮節嗜慾戒喜怒惜元氣簡言語輕得失破憂阻除妄想遠好惡收視聽勤內固不勞神不勞形神形既安病患何由而致也故善養性者先饑而食食勿令飽先渴而飲飲勿令過食欲數而少不欲頓而多蓋飽中饑饑中飽飽則傷肺饑則傷氣若食飽不得便卧即生百病

凡熱食有汗勿當風發痙病頭痛目澀多睡

夜不可多食　卧不可有邪風

凡食訖溫水漱口令人無齒疾口臭

15B

汗出時不可扇生偏枯　勿向西北大小便
勿忍大小便令人成膝勞冷痺痛
勿向星辰日月神堂廟宇大小便
夜行勿歌唱大叫　一日之忌暮勿飽食
一月之忌晦勿大醉　一歲之忌暮勿遠行
終身之忌勿燃燈房事　服藥千朝不若獨眠一宿
如本命日及父母本命日不食本命所屬肉
凡人坐必要端坐使正其心
凡人立必要正立使直其身
立不可久立傷骨　坐不可久坐傷血

16A

行不可久行傷筋　卧不可久卧傷氣
視不可久視傷神　食飽勿洗頭生風疾
如患目赤病切忌房事不然令人生內障
沐浴勿當風腠理百竅皆開切忌邪風易入
不可登高履險奔走車馬氣亂神驚魂魄飛散
大風大雨大寒大熱不可出入妄為
口勿吹燈火損氣　凡日光射勿凝視損人目
勿望遠極目觀損眼力　坐卧勿當風濕地
夜勿燃燈睡魂魄不守　晝勿睡損元氣
食勿言寢勿語恐傷氣　凡遇神堂廟宇勿得輒入

16B

凡遇風雨雷電必須閉門端坐焚香恐有諸神過
怒不可暴怒生氣疾惡瘡
遠唾不如近唾近唾不如不唾
虎豹皮不可近肉鋪損人目
避色如避箭避風如避讎莫喫空心茶少食申後粥
古人有云入廣者朝不可虛暮不可實然不獨廣凡
早皆忌空腹
古人云爛煮麵軟煮肉少飲酒獨自宿
古人平日起居而攝養今人待老而保生蓋無益
凡夜卧兩手摩令熱揉眼永無眼疾

17A

凡夜卧兩手摩令熱摩面不生瘡䵟
一呵十搓一搓十摩久而行之皺少顏多
凡清旦以熱水洗目平日無眼疾
凡清旦刷牙不如夜刷牙齒疾不生
凡清旦鹽刷牙平日無齒疾
凡夜卧被髮梳百通平日頭風少
凡夜卧濯足而卧四肢無冷疾
盛熱來不可冷水洗面生目疾
凡枯木大樹下久陰濕地不可久坐恐陰氣觸人
立秋日不可澡浴令人皮膚麄燥因生白屑

17B

常默元氣不傷　少思慧燭內光
不怒百神安暢　不惱心地清涼
樂不可極慾不可縱

18A
Avoid-
ances

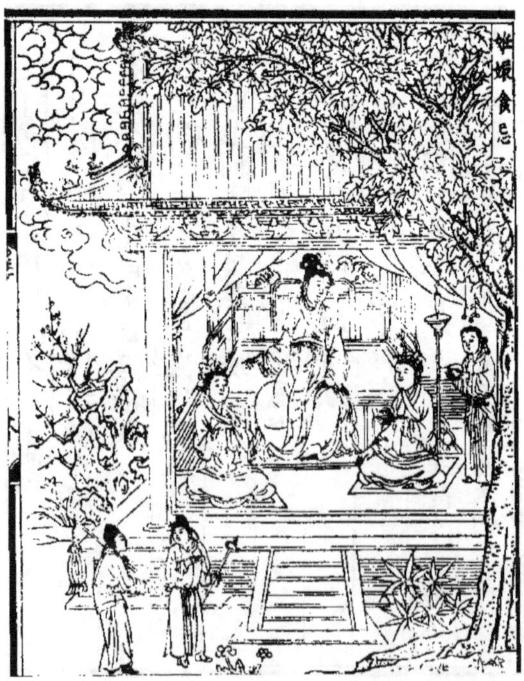

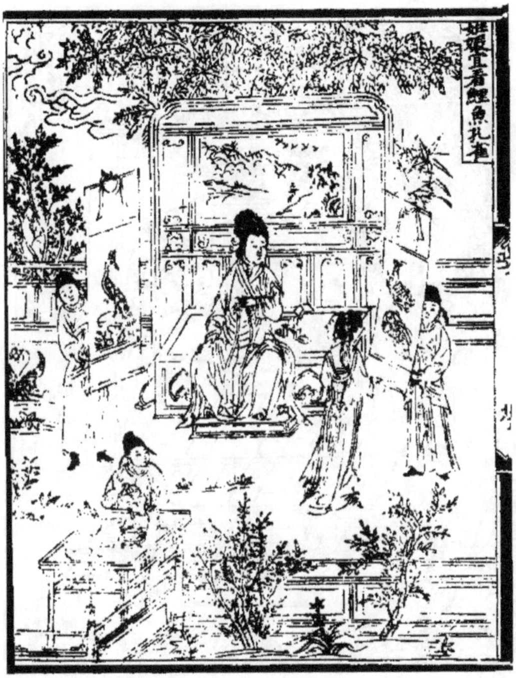

18B
Carp
and
Cranes

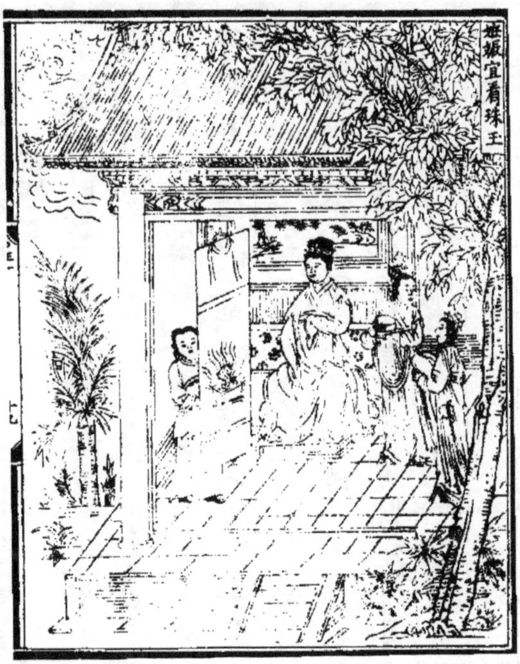

19A
Pearls
and
Jade

19B Geese And Dogs

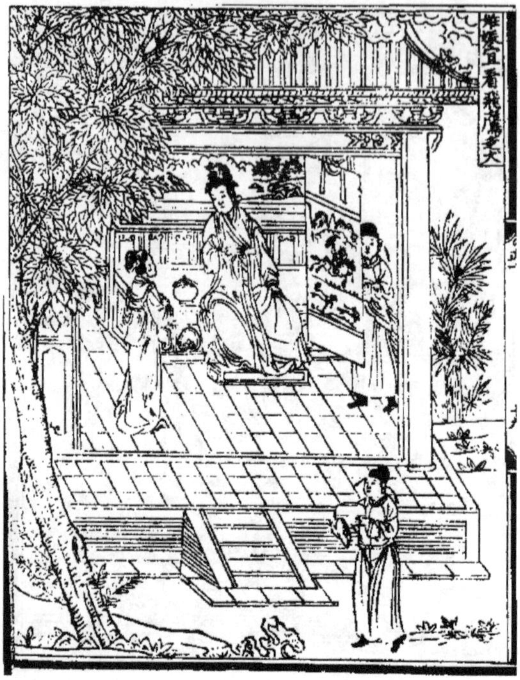

20A Avoidances for Pregnant Women

姙娠食忌

上古聖人有胎教之法古者婦人姙子寢不側坐不
邊立不蹕不食邪味割不正不食席不正不坐目不
視邪色耳不聽淫聲夜則令瞽誦詩道正事如此則
生子形容端正才過人矣故太任生文王聰明聖哲
聞一而知百皆胎教之能也聖人多感生姙娠故忌
見喪孝破體殘疾貧窮之人宜見賢良喜慶美麗之
事欲子多智觀看鯉魚孔雀欲子美麗觀看珎珠美
玉欲子雄壯觀看飛鷹走犬如此善惡猶感況飲食
不知避忌乎

20B

妊娠所忌

食兎肉令子無聲缺唇　食山羊肉令子多疾

食鷄子乾魚令子多瘡　食桑椹鴨子令子倒生

食雀肉飲酒令子心淫情亂不顧羞恥

食鷄肉糯米令子生寸白虫

食雀肉豆醬令子面生䵟黯

食鼈肉令子項短　食驢肉令子延月

食冰漿絕產　食騾肉令子難產

21A
Wet
Nurses

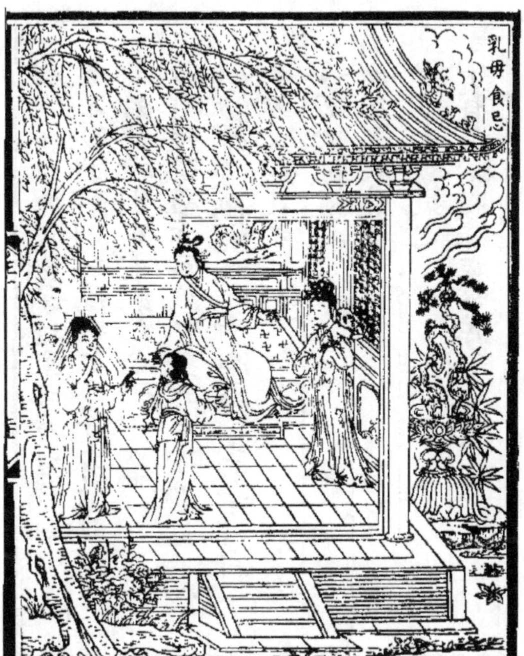

21B

乳母食忌

凡生子擇於諸母必求其年壯無疾病慈善性質寬裕溫良詳雅寡言者使為乳母子在於母資乳以養亦大人之飲食也善惡相習況乳食不遂母性若子有病無病亦在乳母之慎口如飲食不知避忌倘不慎行貪爽口而忘身適性致疾使子受患是母令子生病矣

乳母雜忌

夏勿熱暑乳則子偏陽而多嘔逆

冬勿寒冷乳則子偏陰而多咳痢

22A

母不欲多怒怒則氣逆乳之令子顛狂

母不欲醉醉則發陽乳之令子身熱腹滿

母若吐時則中虛乳之令子虛羸

母有積熱蓋赤黃為熱乳之令子變黃不食

新房事勞傷乳之令子瘦瘁交脛不能行

母勿太飽乳之

母勿太飢乳之

母勿太寒乳之

母勿太熱乳之

子有瀉痢腹痛夜啼疾

22B

乳母忌食寒凉發病之物
子有積熱驚風瘡瘍
乳母忌食濕熱動風之物
子有疥癬瘡疾
乳母忌食魚蝦鷄馬肉發瘡之物
子有癖疳瘦疾
乳母忌食生茄黃瓜等物

23A

凡初生兒時
以未啼之前用黃連浸汁調朱砂少許微抹口內
去胎熱邪氣令瘡疹稀少
凡初生兒時
用荊芥黃連煎水入野牙猪膽汁少許洗兒在後
雖生斑疹惡瘡終當稀少
凡小兒未生瘡疹時
用臘月兎頭并毛骨同水煎湯洗兒除熱去毒能
令斑疹諸瘡不生雖有亦稀少
凡小兒未生斑疹時

23B

以黑子母驢乳令飲之及長不生瘡疹諸毒如生
者亦稀少仍治小兒心熱風癇

24A
Liquor

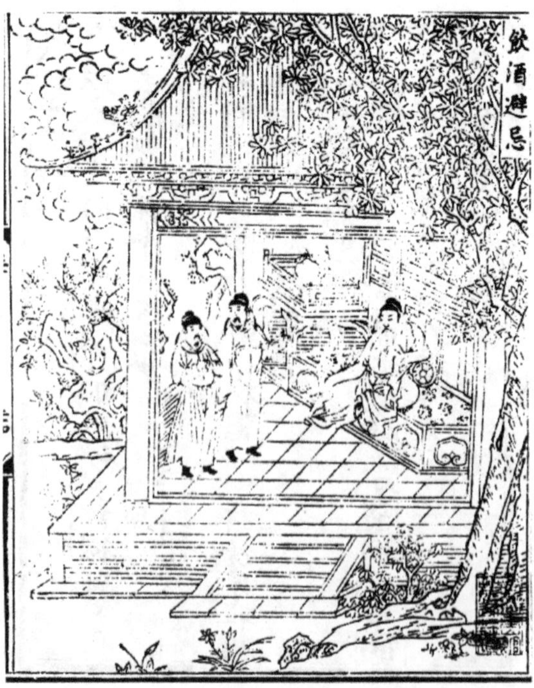

24B

飲酒避忌

酒味苦甘辛大熱有毒主行藥勢殺百邪去惡氣通
血脉厚腸胃潤肌膚消憂愁少飲尤佳多飲傷神損
壽易人本性其毒甚也醉飲過度喪生之源
飲酒不欲使多知其過多速吐之為佳不爾成痰疾
醉勿酩酊大醉即終身百病不除
酒不可久飲恐腐爛腸胃漬髓蒸筋
醉不可當風卧生風疾　醉不可向陽卧令人發狂
醉不可令人扇生偏枯　醉不可露卧生冷痺
醉而出汗當風為漏風　醉不可卧黍穰生癩疾

25A

醉不可強食嗔怒生癰疽
醉不可走馬及跳躑傷筋骨
醉不可接房事小者面生䵟欬嗽大者傷臟澼痔疾
醉不可冷水洗面生瘡　醉醒不可再投損後又損
醉不可高呼大怒令人生氣疾
晦勿大醉忌月空　醉不可飲酪水成噎病
醉不可便卧面生瘡癤內生積聚
大醉勿燃燈叫恐鬼魂飛揚不守
醉不可飲冷漿水失聲成尸噎
飲酒酒漿照不見人影勿飲

25B

醉不可忍小便成癃閉膝勞冷痺

空心飲酒醉必嘔吐　醉不可忍大便生腸澼痔

酒忌諸甜物　酒醉不可食猪肉生風

醉不可強舉力傷筋損力

飲酒時大不可食猪羊腦大損人煉真之士尤宜忌

酒醉不可當風乘凉露脚多生脚氣

醉不可卧濕地傷筋骨生冷痺痛

醉不可澡浴多生眼目之疾

如患眼疾人切忌醉酒食蒜

26A
Delicacies

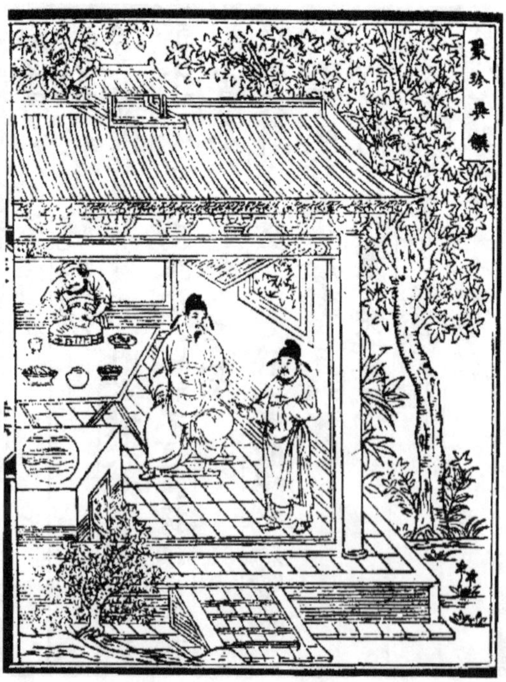

26B

聚珍異饌

馬思荅吉湯

補益温中順氣

羊肉一脚子卸成事件　草果五箇　官桂二錢

回回豆子半升擣碎去皮

右件一同熬成湯濾淨下熟回回豆子二合香
粳米一升馬思荅吉一錢塩少許調和勻下
事件肉芫荽葉

大麥湯

温中下氣壯脾胃止煩渴破冷氣去腹脹

27A

羊肉一脚子卸成事件草果五箇

大麥仁二升滚水淘洗淨微煑熟

右件熬成湯濾淨下大麥仁熬熟塩少許調和令勻
下事件肉

八兒不湯係西天茶飯名

補中下氣寛胷膈

羊肉一脚子卸成事件草果五箇

回回豆子半升擣碎去皮蘿蔔二箇

右件一同熬成湯濾淨湯內下羊肉切如色數大熟
蘿蔔切如色數大咱夫蘭一錢薑黃二錢胡椒二錢

27B

哈昔泥半錢芫荽葉鹽少許調和勻對香粳米乾飯
食之入醋少許
沙乞某兒湯
補中下氣和脾胃
羊肉一脚子卸成事件 草果五箇
回回豆子半升搗碎去皮 沙乞某兒五箇係蔓菁
右件一同熬成湯濾淨下熟回回豆子二合香粳米
一升熟沙乞某兒切如色數大下事件肉鹽少許調
和令勻
苦豆湯

28A

補下元理腰膝溫中順氣
羊肉一脚子卸成事件 草果五箇 苦豆一兩係葫蘆巴
右件一同熬成湯濾淨下河西兀麻食或米心餜子
哈昔泥半錢鹽少許調和
木瓜湯
補中順氣治腰膝疼痛脚氣不仁
羊肉一脚子卸成事件 草果五箇
回回豆子半升搗碎去皮
右件一同熬成湯濾淨下香粳米一升熟回回豆子
二合肉彈兒木瓜二斤取汁沙糖四兩鹽少許調和

28B

或下事件肉

鹿頭湯

補益止煩渴治脚膝疼痛

鹿頭蹄一付退洗淨卸作塊

右件用哈昔泥豆子大研如泥與鹿頭蹄肉同拌勻用回回小油四兩同炒入滾水熬令軟下胡椒三錢哈昔泥二錢蓽撥一錢牛妳子一盞生薑汁一合塩少許調和一法用鹿尾取汁入薑末塩同調和

松黄湯

補中益氣壯筋骨

29A

羊肉一脚子卸成事件 草果五箇

回回豆子半升搗碎去皮

右件同熬成湯濾淨熟羊胷子一箇切作色數大松黄汁二合生薑汁半合一同下炒葱塩醋芫荽葉調和勻對經捲兒食之

粆湯

補中益氣建脾胃

羊肉一脚子卸成事件 草果五箇 回回豆子半升去皮

右件同熬成湯濾淨熟乾羊胷子一箇切片粆三升白菜或蕁麻菜一同下鍋塩調和勻

29B

大麥筭子粉

補中益氣建脾胃

羊肉一脚子卸成事件 草果五箇 回回豆子半升去皮

右件同熬成湯濾淨大麥粉三斤豆粉一斤同作粉

羊肉炒細乞馬生薑汁二合芫荽葉塩醋調和

大麥片粉

補中益氣建脾胃

羊肉一脚子卸成事件 草果五箇 良薑二錢

右件同熬成湯濾淨下羊肝醬取清汁胡椒五錢熟

羊肉切作甲葉糟薑二兩瓜虀一兩切如甲葉塩醋

30A

調和或渾汁亦可

糯米粉搊粉

補中益氣

羊肉一脚子卸成事件 草果五箇 良薑二錢

右件同熬成湯濾淨用羊肝醬熬取清汁下胡椒五

錢糯米粉二斤與豆粉一斤同作搊粉羊肉切細乞

馬入塩醋調和渾汁亦可

河㹠羹

補中益氣

羊肉一脚子卸成事件 草果五箇

30B

右件同熬成湯濾淨用羊肉切細乞馬陳皮五錢去
白葱二兩細切料物二錢鹽醬拌餡兒皮用白麪三
斤作河豘小油煠熟下湯內入鹽調和或清汁亦可

阿菜湯

補中益氣

羊肉一脚子卸成事件 草果五箇 良薑二錢

右件同熬成湯濾淨下羊肝醬同取清汁入胡椒五
錢另羊肉切片羊尾子一箇羊舌一箇羊腰子一付
各切甲葉蘑菰二兩白菜一同下清汁鹽醋調和

鷄頭粉雀舌餌子

31A

補中益精氣

羊肉一脚子卸成事件 草果五箇

回回豆子半升擣碎去皮

右件同熬成湯濾淨用鷄頭粉二斤豆粉一斤同和
切作餌子羊肉切細乞馬生薑汁一合炒葱調和

鷄頭粉血粉

補中益精氣

羊肉一脚子卸成事件 草果五箇

回回豆子半升擣碎去皮

右件同熬成湯濾淨用鷄頭粉二斤豆粉一斤羊血

31B

和作撥粉羊肉切細乞馬炒葱醋一同調和
鷄頭粉撧麵
補中益精氣
羊肉一脚子卸成事件 草果五箇
回回豆子半升擣碎去皮
右件同熬成湯濾淨用鷄頭粉二斤豆粉一斤白麵
一斤同作麵羊肉切片兒乞馬入炒葱醋一同調和
鷄頭粉撥粉
補中益精氣
羊肉一脚子卸成事件 草果五箇 良薑二錢

32A

右件同熬成湯濾淨用羊肝醬同取清汁入胡椒一
兩次用鷄頭粉二斤豆粉一斤同作撥粉羊肉切細
乞馬下塩醋調和
鷄頭粉餛飩
補中益氣
羊肉一脚子卸成事件 草果五箇
回回豆子半升擣碎去皮
右件同熬成湯濾淨用羊肉切作餡下陳皮一錢去
白生薑一錢細切五味和勻次用鷄頭粉二斤豆粉
一斤作枕頭餛飩湯內下香粳米一升熟回回豆子

32B

二合生薑汁二合木瓜汁一合同炒葱塩勻調和

雜羹

補中益氣

羊肉一脚子卸事件 草果五箇

回回豆子半升擣碎去皮

右件同熬成湯濾淨羊頭洗淨二箇羊肚肺各二具羊白血雙腸兒一付並煑熟切次用豆粉三斤作粉蘑菰半斤杏泥半斤胡椒一兩入青菜芫荽炒葱塩醋調和

葷素羹

33A

補中益氣

羊肉一脚子卸成事件 草果五箇

回回豆子半升擣碎去皮

右件同熬成湯濾淨豆粉三斤作片粉精羊肉切條道乞馬山藥一斤糟薑二塊瓜虀一塊乳餅一箇胡蘿蔔十箇蘑菰半斤生薑四兩各切鷄子十箇打煎餅切用麻泥一斤杏泥半斤同炒葱塩醋調和

珍珠粉

補中益氣

羊肉一脚子卸成事件 草果五箇

33B

回回豆子 半升擣碎去皮

右件同熬成湯濾淨羊肉切乞馬心肝肚肺各一具

生薑二兩糟薑四兩瓜虀一兩胡蘿蔔十箇山藥一

斤乳餅一箇鷄子十箇作煎餅各切次用麻泥一斤

同炒葱鹽醋調和

黄湯

補中益氣

羊肉一脚子卸成事件 草果五箇

回回豆子 半升擣碎去皮

右件同熬成湯濾淨下熟回回豆子二合香粳米一

34A

升胡蘿蔔五箇切用羊後脚肉丸肉彈兒肋枝一箇

切寸金薑黄三錢薑末五錢咱夫蘭一錢芫荽葉同

鹽醋調和

三下鍋

補中益氣

羊肉一脚子卸成事件 草果五箇 良薑二錢

右件同熬成湯濾淨用羊後脚肉丸肉彈兒丁頭餌

子羊肉指甲匾食胡椒一兩同鹽醋調和

葵菜羹

順氣治癃閉不通性寒不可多食今與諸物同製

34B

造其性稍温
羊肉一脚子卸成事件　草果五箇　良薑二錢
右件同熬成湯熟羊肚肺各一具切蘑菰半斤切胡
椒五錢白麵一斤拌鷄爪麵下葵菜炒葱塩醋調和

瓠子湯
性寒主消渴利水道
羊肉一脚子卸成事件　草果五箇
右件同熬成湯濾淨用瓠子六箇去穰皮切掠熟羊
肉切片生薑汁半合白麵二兩作麵絲同炒葱塩醋調
和

35A

團魚湯
主傷中益氣補不足
羊肉一脚子卸成事件　草果五箇
右件熬成湯濾淨團魚五六箇煮熟去皮骨切作塊
用麵二兩作麵絲生薑汁一合胡椒一兩同炒葱塩
醋調和

盞蒸
補中益氣
攢羊背皮或羊肉三脚子卸成事件　草果五箇
良薑二錢　陳皮二錢去白　小椒二錢

35B

右件用杏泥一斤松黃二合生薑汁二合同炒葱塩五味調匀入盞内蒸令軟熟對經捲兒食之

臺苗羹

補中益氣

羊肉一脚子卸成事件 草果五箇 良薑二錢

右件熬成湯灑淨用羊肝下醬取清汁豆粉五斤作粉乳餅一箇山藥一斤胡蘿蔔十箇羊尾子一箇羊肉等各切細入臺子菜韮菜胡椒一兩塩醋調和

熊湯

治風痺不仁脚氣

36A

熊肉二脚子煑熟切塊 草果三箇

右件用胡椒三錢哈昔泥一錢薑黃二錢縮砂二錢咱夫蘭一錢葱塩醬一同調和

鯉魚湯

治黃疸止渴安胎有宿瘕者不可食之

大新鯉魚十頭去鱗肚洗淨 小椒末五錢

右件用芫荽末五錢葱二兩切酒少許塩一同淹拌清汁内下魚次下胡椒末五錢生薑末三錢蓽撥末三錢塩醋調和

炒狼湯

36B

古本草不載狼肉今云性熱治虛弱然食之未聞
有毒今製造用料物以助其味暖五藏溫中
狼肉一脚子卸成事件 草果三箇 胡椒五錢
哈昔泥一錢 蓽撥二錢 縮砂二錢 薑黃二錢
咱夫蘭一錢
右件熬成湯用葱醬鹽醋一同調和
圖像
補益五藏
羊肉一脚子煮熟細切 羊尾子二箇熟切細
藕二枝 蒲筍二斤 黃瓜五箇 生薑半斤

37A

乳餅二箇 糟薑四兩 瓜虀半斤 鷄子一十箇煎作餅
蘑菰一斤 蔓菁菜 韭菜各切條道
右件用好肉湯調麻泥二斤薑末半斤同炒葱鹽醋
調和對胡餅食之
春盤麵
補中益氣
白麵六斤切細麵 羊肉二脚子煮熟切條道乞馬
羊肚肺各一箇煮熟切 鷄子五箇煎作餅裁旛
生薑四兩切 韭黃半斤 蘑菰四兩 臺子菜
蓼牙 胭脂

37B

右件用清汁下胡椒一兩塩醋調和

皂羹麵

補中益氣

白麵六斤切細麵羊胷子二箇退洗淨煮熟切如色數塊

右件用紅麵三錢淹拌熬令軟同入清汁內下胡椒

一兩塩醋調和

山藥麵

補虛羸益元氣

白麵六斤鷄子十箇取白生薑汁二合豆粉四兩

右件用山藥三斤煑熟研泥同和麵羊肉二脚子切

38A

丁頭乞馬用好肉湯下炒葱塩調和

掛麵

補中益氣

羊肉一脚子切細乞馬掛麵六斤蘑菰半斤洗淨切

鷄子五箇煎作餅糟薑一兩切瓜虀一兩切

右件用清汁下胡椒一兩塩醋調和

經帶麵

補中益氣

羊肉一脚子炒焦肉乞馬蘑菰半斤洗淨切

右件用清汁下胡椒一兩塩醋調和

38B

羊皮麵

補中益氣

羊皮二箇挦洗淨煮軟 羊舌二箇熟

羊腰子四箇熟各切如甲葉 蘑菰一斤洗淨 糟薑四兩各切如甲葉

右件用好肉釅湯或清汁下胡椒一兩塩醋調和

禿禿麻食係手撇麵

補中益氣

白麵六斤作禿禿麻食 羊肉一脚子炒焦肉乞馬

右件用好肉湯下炒葱調和勻下蒜酪香菜末

細水滑絹邊水滑一同

39A

補中益氣

白麵六斤作水滑 羊肉二脚子炒焦肉乞馬

鷄兒一箇熟切絲 蘑菰半斤洗淨切

右件用清汁下胡椒一兩塩醋調和

水龍䭔子

補中益氣

羊肉二脚子熟切作乞馬 白麵六斤切作錢眼䭔子

鷄子十箇 山藥一斤 糟薑四兩 胡蘿蔔五箇

瓜虀二兩各切細 三色彈兒內一色肉彈兒外二色粉鷄子彈兒

右件用清汁下胡椒二兩塩醋調和

39B

馬乞係手搓麵或糯米粉鷄頭粉亦可

補中益氣

白麵六斤作馬乞 羊肉二脚子熟切乞馬

右件用好肉湯炒葱醋塩一同調和

搠羅脱因係畏兀兒茶飯

補中益氣

白麵六斤和按作錢様 羊肉二脚子熟切 羊舌二箇熟切

山藥一斤 蘑菰半斤 胡蘿蔔五箇 糟薑四兩切

右件用好釃肉湯同下炒葱醋調和

40A

乞馬粥

補脾胃益氣力

羊肉一脚子卸成事件熬成湯濾淨 粱米二升淘洗淨

右件用精肉切碎乞馬先將米下湯內次下乞馬米葱塩熬成粥或下圓米或折米或渴米皆可

湯粥

補脾胃益腎氣

羊肉一脚子卸成事件

右件熬成湯濾淨次下粱米二升作粥熟下米葱塩或下圓米渴米折米皆可

40B

粱米淡粥

補中益氣

粱米 二升

右先將水滚過澄清濾淨次將米淘洗三五遍熬成粥或下圓米渴米折米皆可

河西米湯粥

補中益氣

羊肉 一脚子卸成事件 河西米 二升

右熬成湯濾淨下河西米淘洗淨次下細乞馬米葱塩同熬成粥或不用乞馬亦可

41A

撒速湯 係西天茶飯名

治元藏虛冷腹内冷痛腰脊酸疼

羊肉 兩脚子頭蹄一付 草果 四箇 官桂 三兩 生薑 半斤

哈昔泥 如回回豆子兩箇大

右件用水一鐵絡熬成湯於石頭鍋内盛頓下石榴子一斤胡椒二兩塩少許炮石榴子用小油一杓哈昔泥如豌豆一塊炒鵝黄色微黒湯末子油去淨澄清用甲香甘松哈昔泥酥油焼煙薫瓶封貯任意

炙羊心

治心氣驚悸鬱結不樂

41B

羊心一箇帶系桶 咱夫蘭三錢
右件用玫瑰水一盞浸取汁入塩少許簽子簽羊心
於火上炙将咱夫蘭汁徐徐塗之汁盡爲度食之安
寧心氣令人多喜

炙羊腰
治卒患腰眼疼痛者
羊腰一對 咱夫蘭一錢
右件用玫瑰水一杓浸取汁入塩少許簽子簽腰子
火上炙将咱夫蘭汁徐徐塗之汁盡爲度食之甚有
効驗

42A

攢鷄兒
肥鷄兒十箇撏洗淨熟切攢 生薑汁一合 葱二兩切
薑末半斤 小椒末四兩 麪二兩作麪絲
右件用煑鷄兒湯炒葱醋入薑汁調和

炒鵪鶉
鵪鶉二十箇打成事件 蘿蔔二箇切 薑末四兩
羊尾子一箇各切如色數 麪二兩作麪絲
右件用煮鵪鶉湯炒葱醋調和

盤兔
兎兒二箇切作事件 蘿蔔二箇切

42B

羊尾子一箇切片 細料物二錢
右件用炒葱醋調和下麵絲二兩調和
河西肺
羊肺一箇 韮六斤取汁 麵二斤打糊 酥油半斤
胡椒二兩 生薑汁二合
右件用塩調和匀灌肺煑熟用汁澆食之
薑黄腱子
羊腱子一箇熟 羊肋枝二箇截作長塊 豆粉一斤
白麵一斤 咱夫蘭二錢 梔子五錢
右件用塩料物調和搽腱子下小油煠

43A

鼓兒簽子
羊肉五斤切細 羊尾子一箇切細 鷄子十五箇 生薑二錢
葱二兩切 陳皮二錢去白 料物三錢
右件調和匀入羊白腸内煑熟切作鼓樣用豆粉一斤白麵一斤咱夫蘭一錢梔子三錢取汁同拌鼓兒簽子入小油煠
帶花羊頭
羊頭三箇熟切 羊腰子四箇 羊肚肺各一具煑熟切攢胭脂染
生薑四兩 糟薑二兩各切 鷄子五箇作花樣 蘿蔔三箇作花樣
右件用好肉湯炒葱塩醋調和

43B

魚彈兒

大鯉魚十箇去皮骨頭尾 羊尾子二箇同剁為泥 生薑一兩切細

葱二兩切細 陳皮末三錢 胡椒末一兩 哈昔泥二錢

右件下鹽入魚肉內拌勻丸如彈兒用小油煠

芙蓉鷄

鷄兒十箇熟攢 羊肚肺各一具熟切 生薑四兩切

胡蘿蔔十箇切 鷄子二十箇煎作餅刻花樣 赤根芫荽打糝

胭脂 梔子染 杏泥一斤

右件用好肉湯炒葱醋調和

肉餅兒

44A

精羊肉十斤去脂膜筋搥為泥 哈昔泥三錢 胡椒二兩

蓽撥一兩 芫荽末一兩

右件用鹽調和勻捻餅入小油煠

鹽腸

羊苦腸水洗淨

右件用鹽拌勻風乾入小油煠

腦瓦剌

熟羊胷子二箇切薄片 鷄子二十箇熟

右件用諸般生菜一同捲餅

薑黃魚

44B

鯉魚十箇去皮鱗 白麵二斤 豆粉一斤 芫荽末二兩
右件用塩料物淹拌過搽魚入小油煠熟用生薑二
兩切絲芫荽葉胭脂涂蘿蔔絲炒葱調和

攢鴈

鴈五箇煮熟切攢 薑末半斤
右用好肉湯炒葱塩調和

猪頭薑豉

猪頭二箇洗淨切成塊 陳皮二錢去白 良薑二錢 小椒二錢
官桂二錢 草果五箇 小油一斤 蜜半斤
右件一同熬成次下芥末炒葱醋塩調和

45A

蒲黃瓜虀

淨羊肉十斤煮熟切如瓜虀 小椒一兩 蒲黃半斤
右件用細料物一兩塩同拌勻

攢羊頭

羊頭五箇煮熟攢 薑末四兩 胡椒一兩
右件用好肉湯炒葱塩醋調和

攢牛蹄馬蹄熊掌一同

牛蹄一付煮熟攢 薑末二兩
右件用好肉湯同炒葱塩調和

細乞思哥

45B

羊肉一脚子煮熟切細 蘿蔔二箇熟切細 羊尾子一箇熟切
哈夫兒二錢
右件用好肉湯同炒葱調和
肝生
羊肝一箇水浸切細絲 生薑四兩切細絲 蘿蔔二箇切細絲
香菜蓼子各二兩切細絲
右件用塩醋芥末調和
馬肚盤
馬肚腸一付煮熟切 芥末半斤
右件将白血灌腸刻花様澀脾和脂剁心子攅成炒

46A

葱塩醋芥末調和
煠膁兒係細項
膁兒二箇卸成各一節 哈昔泥一錢 葱一兩切細
右件用塩一同淹拌少時入小油煠熟次用咱夫蘭
二錢水浸汁下料物芫荽末同糁拌
熬蹄兒
羊蹄五付退洗淨煮軟切成塊 薑末一兩 料物五錢
右件下麵絲炒葱醋塩調和
熬羊胷子
羊胷子二箇退毛洗淨煮軟切作色數塊 薑末二兩 料物五錢

46B

右件用好肉湯下麵絲炒葱塩醋調和

魚膾

新鯉魚五箇去皮骨頭尾 生薑二兩 蘿蔔二箇 葱一兩

香菜蓼子各切如絲胭脂打糝

右件下芥末炒葱塩醋調和

紅絲

羊血同白麵依法煮熟 生薑四兩 蘿蔔一箇

香菜蓼子各一兩切細絲

右件用塩醋芥末調和

燒鴈燒鷄鵝燒鴨子等一同

47A

鴈一箇去毛腸肚淨 羊肚一箇退洗淨包鴈 葱二兩 芫荽末一兩

右件用塩同調入鴈腹內燒之

燒水扎

水扎十箇擇洗淨 芫荽末一兩 葱十莖 料物五錢

右件用塩同拌勻燒或以肥麵包水扎就籠內蒸熟亦可或以酥油水和麵包水扎入爐鏊內爐熟亦可

柳蒸羊

羊一口帶毛

右件於地上作爐三尺深周回以石燒令通赤用鐵芭盛羊上用柳子蓋覆土封以熟為度

47B

倉饅頭

羊肉羊脂葱生薑陳皮各切細

右件入料物塩醬拌和為餡

鹿妳肪饅頭或做倉饅頭或做皮薄饅頭皆可

鹿妳肪羊尾子各切如指甲片生薑陳皮各切細

右件入料物塩拌和為餡

茄子饅頭

羊肉羊脂羊尾子葱陳皮各切細嫩茄子去穰

右件同肉作餡却入茄子內蒸下蒜酪香菜末食之

剪花饅頭

48A

羊肉羊脂羊尾子葱陳皮各切細

右件依法入料物塩醬拌餡包饅頭用剪子剪諸般花樣蒸用胭脂染花

水晶角兒

羊肉羊脂羊尾子葱陳皮生薑各切細

右件入細料物塩醬拌匀用豆粉作皮包之

酥皮奄子

羊肉羊脂羊尾子葱陳皮生薑各切細或下瓜哈孫係山丹根

右件入料物塩醬拌匀用小油米粉與麵同和作皮

撇列角兒

48B

羊肉羊脂羊尾子新韭各切細
右件入料物塩醬拌匀白麵作皮鏊上炮熟次用酥
油蜜或以葫蘆瓠子作餡亦可
時蘿角兒
羊肉羊脂羊尾子葱陳皮生薑各切細
右件入料物塩醬拌匀用白麵蜜與小油拌入鍋內
滾水攪熟作皮
天花包子或作蟹黃亦可 藤花包子一同
羊肉羊脂羊尾子葱陳皮生薑各切細
天花滾水燙熟洗淨切細

49A

右件入料物塩醬拌餡白麵作薄皮蒸
荷蓮兜子
羊肉三脚子切 羊尾子二箇切 雞頭仁八兩
松黃八兩 八檐仁四兩 蘑菰八兩 杏泥一斤
胡桃仁八兩 必思荅仁四兩 胭脂一兩
梔子四錢 小油二斤 生薑八兩 豆粉四斤
山藥三斤 雞子三十箇 羊肚肺各二付 苦腸一付
葱四兩 醋半餅 芫荽葉
右件用塩醬五味調和匀豆粉作皮入盞內蒸用松
黃汁澆食

49B

黑子兒燒餅

白麵五斤 牛妳子二升 酥油一斤 黑子兒一兩微炒

右件用鹽減少許同和麵作燒餅

牛妳子燒餅

白麵五斤 牛妳子二升 酥油一斤 茴香一兩微炒

右件用鹽減少許同和麵作燒餅

飪餅 經捲兒一同

白麵十斤 小油一斤 小椒一兩炒去汗 茴香一兩炒

右件隔宿用酵子鹽減溫水一同和麵次日入麵接
肥再和成麵每斤作二箇入籠內蒸

50A

頗兒必湯 即羊辟膝骨

生男女虛勞寒中羸瘦陰氣不足利血脉益經氣

頗兒必三四十箇水洗淨

右件用水一鐵絡同熬四分中熬取一分澄濾淨去
油去滓再凝定如欲食任意多少

米哈訥關列孫

治五勞七傷藏氣虛冷常服補中益氣

羊後脚一箇去筋膜切碎

右件用淨鍋內乾爁熟令蓋封閉不透氣後用淨布
絞紐取汁

JUAN 1 (MAIN TEXT)

* * *

TRANSLATION

YINSHAN ZHENGYAO

[*JUAN* ONE]

[**7A**] *Yinshan zhengyao* Table of Contents

Meat and Vegetable Broth
Pearl Noodles
Yellow Soup
Three in the Cooking Pot
Mallow Leaf [*Malva* sp] Broth
Long Bottle Gourd [*Lagenaria siceraria* var *clavata*] Soup
Turtle Soup
Cup Steamed
Oil Rape Shoots Broth
Bear Soup
Carp Soup
Roast Wolf Soup
**Ishkäne*
**Chöppün* Noodles
Black Broth Noodles
Chinese Yam Noodles
Hanging Noodles
**Jingtei* Noodles
Sheep's Skin Noodles
Tutum Ash
Fine **Salma*
Water Dragon *Qizi*
**[U]mach*
**Shoyla Toyym*
Qima Congee
Soup Congee
Millet Insipid Congee
**Qamh* [*Triticum durum*] Soup
**Se-aBru* Soup
Broiled Sheep's Heart
Broiled Sheep's Loins
Deboned Chicken Morsels
Roasted Quail
Rabbit Plate
"Tangut" Lungs
Turmeric[–colored] Tendons
Drum **Qazi*
Sheep Heads Dressed in Flowers
Fish Cakes
[**8A**] Cotton Rose[–Petal] Chicken
Meat Cakes

Salt Stomach
Näwälä
Turmeric[–colored] Fish
Deboned Wild Goose Morsels
Galangal Sauce Hog's Head
Cat–tail "Sweet Melon Pickles"
Deboned Sheep's Head Morsels
Deboned Ox Hoof Morsels
Fine **Chizig*
Liver and Sprouting [Ginger]
Horse Stomach Plate
Scalded **Jasa'a*
Boiled Sheep's Hooves
Boiled Sheep's Breast
Fine Fish Hash
Red Strips
Roast Wild Goose
Roast Eurasian Curlew
Willow–steamed Lamb
Quick **Manta*
Deer Milk Fat **Manta*
Eggplant **Manta*
Cut Flowers **Manta*
Quartz Horns
Butter Skin **Yubqa*
Päräk Horns
**Shilön* Horns
Pleurotus ostreatus [Mushroom] *Baozi*
**Qurim* Bonnets
Poppy Seed Buns
Cow's Milk Buns
**Chuqmin*
Borbi[n] Soup
Miqan–u kö[n]lesün

Juan 2:

[**8B**] Various Hot Beverages and Concentrates:

Cassia Syrup
Cassia–Garuwood Syrup
Lichee Paste

Oriental Flowering Apricot [*Prunus mume*] Pellet
Red Currant Puree
Ginseng Puree
Immortal's Tsangshu Puree
Apricot Frost Puree
Chinese Yam Puree
Puree of Four
Ginger–Jujube Puree
Fennel Puree
Decoction for Stagnant *Qi*
Oriental Flowering Apricot Puree
Chinese Quince Puree
Detoxifying Dried Orange Peel Puree
Qatiq Cakes
Cinnamon *Qatiq* Cakes
Tabilqa Cakes
Fragrant Orange Spice Cakes
Cow Marrow Paste
Chinese Quince Concentrate
Citron Concentrate
Hazelnut Concentrate
Purple Perilla Concentrate
Kumquat Concentrate
Cherry Concentrate
Peach Concentrate
Pomegranate Syrup
Rose Hips Concentrate
Red Currant *Sharba*[*t*]
Cicigina
Pine Seed Oil
Apricot Seed Oil
Liquid Butter
Ghee
Mäskä Oil
Chinese Matrimony Vine Fruit Tea
Jade Mortar Tea
Golden Characters Tea
[**9A**] Fan Tianshuai Tea
Purple Shoots Sparrow Tongue Tea
Nuxuer Tea
Tibetan Tea

Sichuan Tea
Rattan Tea
Kua Tea
Swallow Tail Tea
Children's Tea
Warm Mulberry Tea
Clear Tea
Roasted Tea
Orchid Paste
**Süttiken*
Fortified Broth
Aromatic Tea

Various Waters:

Spring Water
Well Splendor Water
Zhou Shop Water

Doses and Foods of the Beneficent Immortals:

Red Jade Paste
Earth Immortal Decoction
Golden Marrow Decoction
Chinese Asparagus Paste
Taking Chinese Foxglove
Taking Tsangshu
Taking China Root
Taking Chinese Senega
[**9B**] Wuchiapi Liquor
Taking Cassia
Taking Pine Nuts
Pine Knot Liquor
Taking Pagoda Tree Fruits
Taking Chinese Matrimony Vine [Leaves]
Taking Lotus Flowers
Taking Chestnuts
Taking Solomon's Seal
The Method for the Spirit Pillow
Taking Sweetflag
Taking Sesame Seeds
Taking Schisandra

Juan 3:

Grain Foods:

Paddy Rice
Non–Glutinous Rice
Foxtail Millet
Millet
Green Millet
White Millet
Yellow Millet
Panicled Millet
Red Panicled Millet
Ji Panicled Millet
**Qamh*
Mung Beans
White Beans
Soybeans
Adzuki Beans
Chickpeas
Green Small Beans
Garden Peas
Hyacinth Beans
Wheat
Barley
Buckwheat
Sesame Seeds
"Iranian" Sesame Seeds
Malt–Sugar
Honey
Yeast
Vinegar
Sauce
Salted Bean Relish
Salt

[**11A**] Liquor:

Tiger Bone Liquor
Wolfthornberry Liquor
Chinese Foxglove Liquor
Pine Knot Liquor
China Root Liquor

Pine Root Liquor
Lamb Liquor
Acanthopanax Bark Liquor
Olnul "Navel" Liquor
Small Coarse Grain Liquor
Grape Wine
Arajhi Liquor
**Sürmä* Liquor

Animal Foods:

Ox
Sheep
Gazelle
The Blue Sheep
Horse
Wild Horse
Elephant
Camel
Wild Camel
Bear
Donkey
Sika Deer
Red Deer
River Deer
Dog
Pig
Wild Boar
Otter
Tiger
Leopard
Pere David's Deer
Musk Deer
Muntjac Deer
Fox
Rhinoceros
Wolf
Hare

Wildcat[1]
Tarbuqa[n]
Weasel
Monkey

Poultry:

[**11B**] Swan
Oriental Swangoose
Wild Goose
Crane
Eurasian Curlew
Chicken
Pheasant
Eared Fowl
Duck
Wild Duck
Tufted Duck[2]
The Mandarin Duck
Pigeon
Dove
Great Bustard
Collared Crow
Common Quail
Sparrow
Bunting

Fish:

Carp
Golden Carp
Chinese Bream
"White Fish"
"Yellow Fish"
"Green Fish"
Sheatfish
Sawfish

---

[1] In the body of the text the entry on the wildcat occurs after the *tarbuqan* and before the weasel, not as here. The text also has an entry on the badger preceding the wildcat; the badger is omitted here.

[2] In the text the entry on the Mandarin duck occurs before the entry on the tufted duck.

Mud Eel
Baoyu
Puffer
Sciaenid Fish
Abarqu Fish
Qilam Fish
Softshelled Turtle
Crab
Shrimp
Sea Snail
Trough Shells
Wei
Fresh Water Mussels
The Prickly Sculpin

Fruits:

Peach
Chinese Pear
Persimmon
Chinese Quince
Flowering Apricot
Japanese Plum
Prinsepia
Pomegranate
Crab Apple
Apricot
Mandarin Orange
Tangerine
Sweet Orange
Chestnut
Jujube
Cherry
Grapes
Walnut
[**12A**] Pine Nut
Lotus Seed
Euryale ferox Fruit
Trapa bispinosa Fruit
Lichee
Longan
Ginkgo Nut

Chinese Olive
Chinese Myrica Fruit
Hazelnut
Torreya Nut
Cane Sugar
Sweet Melon
Watermelon
Sour Jujube
Flowering Apricot Red
Citron
Acorns
Pingpo
Badam Nut
Pistä

Vegetables:

Mallow
Swiss Chard
Chinese Parsley
Mustard Greens
Chinese Onions
Garlic
Chinese Chives
Winter Melon
Cucumbers
Chinese Radish
Carrot
Tianjing Vegetable
Long Bottle Gourd
Oriental Pickling Melon
Pear–Shaped Bottle Gourd
**Möög* Mushroom
Junzi [Fungi]
Tree Ears
Bamboo Shoots
Cattail Shoots
Sacred Lotus Rhizome
Chinese Yam
Taro
Lettuce
[**12B**] Bokchoy

Penghao [*Chrysanthemum* spp]
Chinese Eggplant
Amaranth Greens
Oil Rape
Spinach
White Sugar Beet
Basil
Smartweed
Purslane
Pleurotus ostreatus [Mushroom]
Shallot
Chinese Artichoke
Elm Seeds
Shajhimur
Chugundur
Lily Root
Seaweed
Bracken
Vetch
Sonchus spp greens
Water–celery

Spices:

Black Pepper
Chinese Flower Pepper
Lesser Galangal
Fennel
Liquorice[3]
Coriander
Dried Ginger
Sprouting Ginger
Zhira
Mandarin Orange Peel
Tsaoko Cardamom
Cassia
Turmeric
Pippali
Grain–of–paradise

---

[3] Liquorice, coriander seeds, dried ginger, and sprouting ginger are out of place here.

Cubebs
Schisandra Fruits
Fenugreek Seeds
Red Yeast
Poppy Seeds
Mastajhi
Za'faran
Kasni
Anjudan (same as *Angwa*)
Safflower
Zhizi
Cattail [Pollen]
"Muslim" Green

[13A] Vast Heaven Fuxi

He was first of the surname Feng and was the descendant of Huangxiong. He had sagely virtue at birth. He succeeded to Heaven and became ruler. He was the first of the emperors and kings of ten thousand generations. His position was in the east and he ruled by virtue of wood. He was the lord of the Green Essence. He made his capital at Chenshi. The beneficent spirit dragon appeared at Yonghe. When this happened, Fuxi marked down its [design] to make the eight diagrams. He created writing and incisings on bamboo and wood to replace the method of knotted cords. He established the five cardinal relationships, and determined the five transitional phases. He defined lord and minister, clarified father and son, separated the duties of man and wife, and ordered marriage. He invented housing. He plaited together nets and snares to hunt and fish. He hitched up oxen and rode on horses to move heavy goods and attain distances. He selected sacrificial victims to supply rites and sacrifices. Therefore it is said that Fuxi ruled the empire well for one hundred ten years.

The Brilliant Emperor Shennong

He was the first of the surname Chiang and was the descendent of Lieshan. He had sagely virtue at birth. He received wood with fire. His position was in the south and he ruled by virtue of fire. He was lord of the Red Essence. People of his time ate herbs and drank water, and collected the fruits of trees. [**13B**] They also ate the meat of the *luomang* ["naked *mang*"[4]] and many developed illnesses. Shennong thereupon sought things they could eat. He sampled the hundred herbs and planted the five grains to support the people. Markets were held during the day. Shennong invented potting and the casting of metal. He made axes and fashioned digging tools and taught the people to till and sow grain. Therefore it is said: Shennong made his capital in Qufu and ruled the empire well for 120 years.

The Yellow Emperor Xianyuan

He was the first of the surname Qi. He was the son of Shaotianzi, the lord of Xiong Guo. He was born beneficent and numinous, grew up to great intelligence and when mature attained to Heaven. He ruled by virtue of earth. He was the lord of the Yellow Essence. Therefore it is said: the Yellow Emperor made his capital at Zhuolu and received the

---

[4] The *luomang* was apparently a variety of mole cricket.

"River Map." After he had observed the configurations of sun, moon, stars, and planets there were first books on astrology. He ordered Great Yao to probe the natures of the five transitional phases. He inquired by oracle about that which the Dipper establishes. He originated the cycle of 60 and ordered Yong Cheng to create the calendar. He ordered Li Shou to create mathematics. He ordered Ling Lun to make the 12 standard pitch pipes. He ordered Qi Bo to set medical recipes. He made clothing to express differences of social position. He put the weapons of war into order. He made boats and chariots and divided cultivated area from wasteland. He ruled the empire well for 100 years.

[14A] [Uncaptioned illustration]

[14B] Nurturing Life and Avoiding Things to Be Shunned[5]

Those of the very ancients who knew the Way had methods based in *yinyang*, and kept in harmony with magical calculations. They practiced moderation in their drinking and eating, and there was a regimen to their activity and repose. They were not disorderly in their actions. Therefore they could attain to a great age. People of today are not like that at all. There is no regimen in their activity and repose. They do not know how to avoid things which should be shunned in their drinking and eating, and also are not careful about moderation. They are much addicted to lust. They like strongly–flavored food; cannot keep the mean; and do not know how to be satiated. Therefore most, I think, will be decrepit at fifty. The way of peace and joy resides in nourishing. For the Way of nourishing, nothing is better than keeping the mean. Where there is keeping to the mean, then there will be no excess and illnesses which do not respond to treatment. Spring, autumn, winter, and summer are the *yinyang* of the four seasons. Falling ill is due to excess, that is, not according with the character of the seasons, and overdoing it. Thus those who would nurture life are without the defect of excess and waste. They can also preserve their true natures. How can they be harmed through being targeted by external miasmas? Thus being good at nourishing is better than taking medicines. But it is better to take medicines if one is not good at nourishing. If there are those in the world who are not good at nourishing, and are also not good at taking medicines, they will suddenly **[15A]** fall ill. And will they not assign the blame to beneficent Heaven? Those who

[5] The material below is drawn from the *Huangdi neijing suwen*.

are good at protecting their lives; prefer lightly–flavored food; spare their minds; moderate their desires; limit their emotions; are frugal of their primordial *qi*, laconic in their speech, even–tempered about gain and loss. They make a clean breast of anxiety; eliminate wild fantasy; keep away from likes and dislikes; accumulate personal experience. They insist on inner steadfastness. They do not weary the spirit and do not weary the form. If spirit and form are at peace, where can illness come from? Thus those who are good at nurturing their natures, are hungry before eating. When they eat they do not eat to satiation. They are thirsty before drinking, and do not drink to excess. In eating there should be frequent meals of small intake. There should not be a few set meals with eating to excess, lest one experience hunger amidst satiation or satiation amidst hunger. If one eats to satiation it wounds the lungs. If one is hungry it wounds the *qi*. If one eats to satiation one will not sleep well. The hundred illnesses then arise.

Whenever hot food is served there will be sweating. One should stay out of the wind. It will produce convulsions, headache, eye astringency,[6] and excessive drowsiness.

One should not eat much at night.

When sleeping one should not be [exposed to] evil wind.[7]

Whenever you finish eating, rinse the mouth with warm water. This will cause a person to be without tooth disease and bad breath.

[**15B**] One should not fan the body when sweating. It will produce a hemiplegia.

One must not defecate or urinate towards the northwest.[8]

---

[6] Ou, 1982 defines this as "dryness and uneasy feeling of the eye" (53).

[7] Wind here refers to environmental influences causing disease and is not literally wind.

[8] This is probably a Mongolian rather than a Chinese prohibition. Although the preferred Mongolian direction is southeast, and not northwest, special consideration was shown this direction as well. See Gongor: 1970–78: II, 94–5. The Mongolian yurt (*ger*) also normally faced southeast and urination or defecating towards the northwest may have meant disrespect for its sacred world. Note, for example, the strong traditional prohibition against urination inside a dwelling mentioned by John of Plano Carpini. (Beazley, 1967: 48). Mongols living at the Yuan court may also have been fearful of offending the land and water spirits of Mongolia, if they urinated or defecated in the direction (from Daidu) of the old Mongolian homeland. On Altaic views of the spiritual potency of earth and water see Jean–Paul Roux, 1984: 132ff. Our colleague Henry Schwarz notes that this prohibition may have a practical aspect too due to the prevailing direction of the wind in Mongolia.

One must not hold back a bowel movement or urine. It will cause a person to develop knee impairment caused by overstrain, and chill numbness pain.[9]

One must not defecate or urinate towards stars or planets, the sun or the moon, temples for spirits or ancestral halls.

If traveling by night, one must not sing or call out loudly.

A daily avoidance: one should not eat to satiation in the evening.

A monthly avoidance: one must not become greatly tipsy on the last day of the month.

An annual avoidance: one must not go on a long trip in the evening.

A lifetime avoidance: one must not have sexual intercourse in a brightly lit room.

It is better to sleep alone for a single night than take drugs for a thousand mornings.

On one's own birthday, or on the birthdays of one's parents, do not eat the meat of animals associated with these days.[10]

Whenever a person is sitting, he must certainly sit still and formally. It will rectify the heart.

Whenever a person is standing, he must certainly stand up straight. This will straighten the body.

If one should stand, one should not stand for long periods. Standing wounds the bones.

If one sits, one should not sit for long periods. Sitting wounds the blood.

[**16A**] If one walks, one should not walk for long periods. Walking harms the sinews.

If one lies down, one should not lie down for long periods. Lying down wounds the *qi*.

---

[9] According to the Ou, 1982 (111) a cold pain is a "painful region with cold feeling." Here there is also a feeling of numbness.

[10] Reference is to birthdays dated according to the Chinese cycle of 60, combinations of the 10 celestial stems and 12 earthly branches. Each of the latter is associated with an animal, and it is the meat of these animals which must be avoided. If one is born on a *jiachen* 甲辰 day, for example, one would avoid eating the meat of the dragon.

If one looks at something, one should not look for long periods. It harms the spirit.

If one has eaten to satiation, one must not wash the head. [It will cause a person] to contract “wind diseases.”

If one is afflicted with “red eye disease [conjunctivitis],” one should practice complete sexual abstinence. If not, it will cause a person to develop an internal screen [an internal oculopathy].

If one bathes, one must stay out of the wind. The hundred apertures of the pores will all be open. One must absolutely avoid the easy entry of evil wind.

One should not ascend to a high place with insecure footing, ride fast in a chariot or on a horse. The *qi* will be thrown into disarray, and the spirit will be frightened. The souls will fly away and be lost.

If there is a great wind, great rain, great cold or great heat, one cannot go and come in an unseemly manner.

The mouth must not blow on the flame of a lamp. It will harm the *qi*.

Whenever the daylight is dazzling, one must not stare fixedly. It harms the eyes.

One must not stare off into the distance as far as the eye can see. It harms the power of the eye.

In sitting or lying down one must not be exposed to the wind, or in a damp place.

One must not sleep at night in bright light. The souls will not protect [the body].

One must not doze during the daytime. It harms the primordial *qi*.

One must not talk when eating, and one must go to bed without conversation. One should fear wounding the *qi*.

Whenever one encounters a temple or shrine, one must not abruptly enter.

[**16B**] Whenever one encounters wind and rain, thunder and lightning, it is obligatory to shut the gate, sit up straight, and light incense. One should fear the various spirits passing by.

If one is angry, one must not become violently angry. Anger produces *qi* illnesses and malignant boils.

It is better to spit short distances than long distances. It is better not to spit at all than spitting short distances.

Skins of tiger and leopard should not be put close to a meat rack. It harms the eye.

Avoiding lust is like avoiding an arrow. Avoiding dissipation is like avoiding an enemy. No one should drink tea on an empty stomach. Eat little congee after the *shen* hour [3:00–5:00 PM].

There was an ancient person who said: "He who has entered the wilderness, cannot have an empty stomach in the morning, and cannot be full in the evening." Not only those who have entered the wilderness, all of us should avoid an empty stomach whenever it is early.

There was an ancient person who said: "Cook noodles until soft. Cook meat until tender. Drink little liquor. Sleep alone."

The ancients practiced hygiene and nourished [themselves] in their ordinary daily activity and repose. People of the present wait until old age to protect life. This effort is without benefit.

Whenever one lies down at night, if one rubs the two hands together to make them warm, and massages the eyes, one will continue to be without ocular disease.

[17A] Whenever one lies down at night, if one rubs the two hands together to make them warm, and rubs the face, then *chuanggan*[11] will not develop.

In one expelling of the breath one should rub the hands together ten times. During each rubbing of the hands, there should be ten manipulations. If one continues this for a long time, wrinkles will be few and one's color extremely good.

Every morning, bathe the eyes with hot water. One will normally be without eye disease.

Brushing the teeth at night is better than brushing the teeth in the morning. Tooth disease will not arise.

If one brushes the teeth with salt every morning, one will normally be without tooth disease.[12]

---

[11] *Chuanggan* is a skin disease characterized by dark discolorations.

[12] The "tooth disease" in question must be periodontal since salt solutions do improve the health of gums, although having no effect upon tooth decay directly.

If the hair is combed one hundred times whenever one goes to bed, one will normally have very little "head wind [recurrent headache]."

Whenever ones goes to bed at night, if one goes to bed after washing the feet, the four extremities will be without chill–type diseases.

When the extremely hot weather arrives, one should not wash the face with cold water. It produces eye disease.[13]

One should not sit for a long time in any place there is withered wood, which is below a large tree and which has long been shaded and damp. It is to be feared that the *yinqi* [of the place] will touch a person.

One should not bathe during the days at the beginning of autumn. It causes one's skin to rough and dry. *Boxie* [apparently seborrheic dermatitis] is produced as a result.

[**17B**] If one is as a rule silent, the primordial *qi* will not be wounded.

If one has few cares, quick–witted understanding will shine.

Do not be angry. The hundred spirits [*i.e.*, one's own intellectual capacities] will be peaceful and pleasant.

Do not be vexed. The place of the heart will be pure and cool.

Joy should not be excessive. Desire should not be given free reign.

[18A] [Illustration Caption] Food Avoidances During Pregnancy

[18B] [Illustration Caption] During Pregnancy it is Beneficial to see Carp and Peacocks.

[19A] [Illustration Caption] During Pregnancy it is Beneficial to see Pearls and Jade.

[19B] [Illustration Caption] During Pregnancy it is Beneficial to see a Flying Wild Goose and a Running Dog.

[Instructing Children in the Womb]

[**20A**] Sages of high antiquity had a method for instructing children in the womb. Women of ancient times did not sleep on their sides when pregnant with a child; did not sit on the side; and did not stand to the side. They did not eat evil flavors. If meat was not cut straight they did

[13] Technically *mu* 目 refers to the eyeball, *yan* 眼 to the eye in general, including tissues around the eye. Hu Sihui may or may not have used *mu* and *yan* in these restrictive senses.

not eat it. If a mat was not straight, they did not sit on it. Their eyes did not see depraved colors [*i.e.*, lustful sights]; their ears did not hear lewd sounds. And at night they had blind musicians intone the *Poetry*, and discuss orthodox things. As a result of their doing this, I dare say that they gave birth to children whose appearance was correct and whose talents were superior. Thus Tairen gave birth to Wenwang. He was intelligent and had sagely wisdom. He could hear one thing and know a hundred. These were all abilities learned in the womb. Sages are born very much influenced [by what happens before birth]. Pregnant women therefore avoid funerals and mourning, ravaged bodies, and persons crippled by disease or exhausted by poverty. It is suitable for them to see worthy and good things, joyful and happy things, pleasant and beautiful things. If one wants a child with great knowledge, one should view carp and peacocks. If one wants a child who will be pleasant and beautiful, one should view precious pearls and beautiful jade. If one wants a child who will be brave and strong, one should view flying wild geese and racing dogs. If even good or bad things like this influence [children in the womb], how much more will this be the case if one does not know avoidances in drinking and eating?

[20B] Things to Avoid during Pregnancy

If the mother has eaten hare meat, it will cause the child to be mute and have a hare–lip.

If the mother has eaten goat meat, it will cause the child to be ill frequently.

If the mother has eaten eggs and dried fish, it will cause the child to have many sores.

If the mother has eaten mulberry fruits and duck eggs, it will cause the child to be a breech birth.

If the mother has eaten sparrow meat and has drunk liquor, it will cause the child to have lust in his heart, and to be dissolute without any sense of shame.

If the mother has eaten chicken and glutinous rice, it will cause the child to produce tapeworms.

If the mother has eaten sparrow meat and bean sauce, it will cause the child to develop an extremely dark discoloring of the face.

If the mother has eaten turtle meat, it will cause the child to have a short neck.

If the mother has eaten donkey meat, it will cause the child to be late.

If the mother has eaten any thick frozen fluids, it will cause a miscarriage.

If the mother eats mule meat, it will make for a difficult birth.[14]

[21A] [Illustration Caption] Avoidances for a Wet Nurse:

[21B] Avoidances for a Wet Nurse[15]

Food Avoidances for a Wet Nurse

Whenever one has produced children, one should choose among various mothers. One must seek for one who is strong and without illness; who is compassionate and well–meaning; whose character is liberal and generous; who is warm and good, careful and polished; and who is of few words, and make her wet nurse. The child needs the milk of the wet nurse for nourishment. This is also food that can be drunk by grown–ups. Good and evil are from their respective practice; how can milk food not be in accord with the nature of the wet nurse? Whether or not a child has, or has not an illness, depends upon the caution in diet of the wet nurse. If she does not know avoidances in her drinking and eating; if she is not cautious in her actions; if she is covetous of whatever immediate thing tastes good; if she forgets the body and does not control her nature, it will result in illness and cause the child to contract it as well. This is a matter of the wet nurse causing the child to contact disease, I think.

Various Avoidances for a Wet Nurse

A wet nurse must not nurse during the heat of summer. [If this is the case] the child will be inclined towards *yang*, and will vomit a great deal.

---

14 Compare the translation of this section in Unschuld, 1986: 216–17.

15 To the best of our knowledge, this is the first section of its kind in a Chinese medical source. By contrast, similar material is well known in Greek and Arabic medicine and Arabic medicine is almost certainly the source here. On the Arabic material, see Porman and Savage-Smith, 2007: 107 and A. Gl'adi, *Children of Islam: Concepts of Childhood in Medieval Muslim Society* (Basingstoke, 1992). See also the summary of such material from Ibn Sīnā in Hassan Kamal, *Encyclopaedia of Islamic Medicine* (Cairo, 1975), 138-141.

A wet nurse must not nurse during the cold of winter. [If this is the case] the child will be inclined towards *yin*, and will cough and have diarrhea a lot.

[**22A**] A wet nurse should not wish to be very angry. When she is angry the *qi* is contrary. If she nurses, the child will become wild.

A wet nurse should not wish to be tipsy. When one is tipsy the *yang* is issued forth. If she nurses, the child's body will become hot and the bowels full.

If a wet nurse should ever spit, then the center will [suffer from] deficiency. If she nurses, this will cause the child to suffer from deficiency emaciation.

If a wet nurse has retained heat, and if there are red [or] yellow [skin] fever symptoms, and she nurses, the child will become jaundiced and will not eat.

If the wet nurse is exhausted and wounded from recent intercourse, and she nurses, the child will be thin and sickly. Its shins will cross, and the child unable to walk.

A wet nurse must not nurse a child after eating to over–satiation.

A wet nurse must not nurse a child when she is extremely hungry.

A wet nurse should not nurse a child when the weather is extremely cold.

A wet nurse should not nurse a child when the weather is extremely hot.

If a child has leaking [heat] diarrhea, abdominal pain or morbid nocturnal crying illness [**22B**] the wet nurse should avoid eating foods that make cold or cool and give rise to illness.

If the child has retained heat, infantile convulsions, or sores and ulcers, the wet nurse should avoid eating foods that make damp and hot and move wind.

If the child has an illness with scabies or ringworm sores, the wet nurse should avoid eating fish, shrimp, chicken, and horse meat foods which give rise to sores.

If the child has severe constipation, infantile malnutrition[16] or emaciation disease, the wet nurse should avoid eating fresh eggplant, cucumber *etc*.

[23A] When a Woman Has Just Given Birth:

Before the child has cried, take the juice of soaked golden thread [rhizome of *Coptis chinensis*], mix evenly with a little cinnabar, and smear a little inside the child's mouth. It gets rid of womb heat and evil *qi*, and will make sores and pustules extremely few.

When a Woman Has Just Given Birth:

Take chingchieh [*herba* or flower of *Schizonepeta tenuifolia*] and golden thread [rhizome] boiled in water. Add a little gall bladder juice from a male wild boar and wash the child. Afterwards, although he will develop malignant boils of macule, they will be very uncommon until the end of the child's life.

When a Child Has Not Contracted Sores and Eruptions:

Take the head of a hare of the twelfth lunar month, along with the fur and bones, and decoct together in the same water. Wash the child. It removes heat and gets rid of poison, and can prevent the various sores of macule from developing. Although they may develop, it will happen very rarely.

Whenever a Child Has Not Contracted Macule:

[**23B**] Have the child drink the milk of a small black mother donkey. When it grows up, the child will not develop the various poisons of sores and eruptions. If they do appear, they will be very few in number. This will likewise cure a small child's heart of heat and wind convulsions.[17]

[24A] [Illustration Caption] Things to Avoid and Shun When Drinking Liquor

[24B] Things to Avoid and Shun When Drinking Liquor:

The flavor of liquor is bitter, sweet–acrid. It is greatly heating and has

---

[16] The Chinese term *gan* can indicate any number of different conditions of infantile malnutrition, including rickets, the apparent usage here, and parasitic infestation.

[17] This syndrome is apparently the same as *jingfeng* 驚風, "infantile convulsions."

poison. It is good for putting into effect the powers of medicines. It destroys the hundred evil factors, removes evil *qi*, puts through blood and pulse, fills bowels and stomach, moistens muscle, eliminates care and melancholy. It is best to drink little. If one drinks much, it wounds the spirit and shortens life. It changes a person's basic nature. Its poison is extreme. If one drinks and gets tipsy excessively, this is the origin of destruction of life.

If one drinks liquor, it is undesirable to allow oneself to over drink. If one realizes that one has drunk too much, it is best to spit it out quickly. If not, it results in phlegm disease.

If one becomes tipsy, one should not become helplessly, excessively intoxicated. If so, to the end of one's life, one will not be able to eliminate the hundred illnesses.

One cannot drink liquor for an extended period of time. One should be afraid of corrupting bowels and stomach, of soaking the marrow, and steaming the sinew.

If one is tipsy one should not sleep facing the wind. It can produce wind diseases.

If one is tipsy one cannot sleep facing the sun. It will cause a person to go mad.

If one is tipsy one cannot have a person fan one. It will produce a hemiplegia.

If one is tipsy one cannot sleep exposed. It will produce chill numbness.

If one sweats while exposed to the wind when tipsy, it gives rise to leaking wind.[18]

If one is tipsy one cannot sleep [on] millet stalks. It produces leprosy.

[**25A**] If one is tipsy one cannot eat voraciously, or become rebuking or angry. It produces boils.

If one is tipsy one cannot ride on a horse. When the horse jumps it wounds sinew and bone.

If one is tipsy one cannot engage in sexual intercourse. If it is a minor intercourse, it produces black facial discolorings [and] coughing. If it

[18] The syndrome is characterized by excessive sweating, especially after eating, chills and thirst.

is a major intercourse, it wounds the viscera, and [produces] bloody stool and perianal abscesses.

If one is tipsy one cannot wash the face with chilled water. It produces sores.

If one is tipsy and sobering up, one cannot get drink again. This is damage on top of damage.

If one is tipsy one cannot call loudly, or be extremely angry. It causes one to produce *qi*.

One must not become extremely tipsy on the last day of the moon. One should avoid the emptiness of the moon.

If one is tipsy one cannot drink fermented milks. They create throat stoppage illness [dysphagia].

If one is tipsy one should not lie down casually. The face will produce furuncles. Internally, abdominal mass will be produced.

When one is greatly tipsy one must not shout with lamps lit. It is to be feared that the souls will fly away, and will not guard the body.

If one is tipsy one cannot drink thick frozen fluids. One loses the voice. It forms cadaverous throat stoppage.

If one drinks liquor, and the liquor is thick so that one's reflection does not appear in it, do not drink it.

[**25B**] If one is tipsy one cannot retain urine. It will result in dysuria, knee joint impairment caused by overstrain, and chill numbness.

If one drinks liquor on an empty stomach, one will vomit when tipsy.

If one is tipsy one cannot retain excrement. It will produce dysentery peri–anal abscesses.

Various sweet things are liquor avoidances.

If one is tipsy with liquor, one cannot eat pork. It produces "wind."

If one is tipsy, one cannot strongly exert oneself. It wounds sinew and damages strength.

When one is drinking liquor, one can absolutely not eat pig or sheep brain. It greatly damages a person. For a gentlemen practicing physiological alchemy, the avoidance is all the greater.

If one is tipsy with liquor, one cannot expose the feet to be cooled by the wind. It often produces [evil] foot *qi*.

One cannot sleep in a damp place when tipsy. It wounds sinew and bone. It produces chill numbness pain.

If one is tipsy one cannot bathe. It often produces eye disease.

In the case of a person who has contracted eye disease, getting tipsy from liquor and eating garlic is a strong avoidance.

[26A] [Illustration Caption] Strange Delicacies of Combined Flavors

[26B] Strange Delicacies of Combined Flavors

[1.] *Mastajhi* [Mastic] Soup[19]

It supplements and increases, warms the center, and accords *qi*.

Mutton (leg; bone and cut up), tsaoko cardamoms (five), cinnamon (2 *qian*), chickpeas ["Muslim beans"] (one–half *sheng*; pulverize and remove the skins).

Boil ingredients together to make a soup. Strain broth.[20] [Cut up meat and put aside.] Add 2 *he* of cooked chickpeas, 1 *sheng* of aromatic non–glutinous rice,[21] 1 *qian* of *mastajhi*. Evenly adjust flavors with a little salt. Add [the] cut–up meat and [garnish with] coriander leaves.

---

[19] The recipes immediately following, and some occurring later, are acculturated variations of the Mongol cauldron–cooked mutton soup (*šülen*), analyzed in Chapter 2. In this case the external influence is Near Eastern, specifically Irano–Mesopotamian, where chickpeas are still employed in cooking in much the same way, and have been for a thousand years or more. See J. Najor, 1981: 156–57. Dishes of the same type are found throughout the Near East (see Roden, 1970: 253–55), and in Iberia thanks to the Moors. Its most far–flung representative surely is a stew of mutton, chickpeas, and rice, cooked down together, and described by Cleofas Jaramillo, a lady of old Hispanic New Mexico, in 1942. See Cleofas M. Jaramillo, *The Genuine New Mexico Tasty Recipes* (Santa Fe, 1981). The mastic and cinnamon, as opposed to cassia, called for here are a thoroughly west Asian touch, as is the removal of chickpea skins prior to mashing (Heine, 1988: 69), but the tsaokos represent adaptation of the recipe to locally available spices. In Near Eastern cooking, chickpeas are added to dishes to even out flavors, absorb them, and provide otherwise lacking consistency, the case here. Note that the addition of a quantity of chickpeas to a dish during the last stages of cooking was typical of early Arabic cuisine as represented in Medieval cookbooks. See Heine, 1988: 69.

[20] On this practice in Medieval Arabic cooking see Heine, 1988: 64.

[21] On the use of rice in Medieval Near Eastern cooking see Heine, 1988: 39–40.

[2.] Barley[22] Soup

[22] This dish is a variant of the *Harisa* common today in the Near East and surrounding areas where it is usually made with wheat but is otherwise identical to the present dish. According to Charles Perry (unpublished letter of 2 January, 1994, to PDB), "the traditional essence of *Harisa* is that after the porridge is cooked, the meat is taken out and the porridge is beaten smooth (*tuhras*) with a wooden bat. The meat is then used as a garnish on the smooth porridge." This is quite similar to what is called for here although there is no reference to beating. This dish is a rather heavy, stodgy item.

Barley, *damai* 大麥, "large wheat/barley," *mou* 牟:

Barley is uniquely tolerant of cold, heat, drought, salt, altitude, and short growing seasons. It is the ideal crop for desert and mountain regions, the Himalayas and Karakorams, for example, where it is grown at over 15,000 feet, higher than any other grain. Many varieties exist adapted to specific local conditions. Some mature in only two to three months, others require as little as four inches of rainfall. Barley produces crops in land white with salt and alkali, where few other plants will grow. It is not especially high–yielding or versatile, and is not grown where any other grain will flourish. In early modern China barley yielded a lowly 1200 kg/ha (Perkins, 1969: 287), now over 1500 (Ben. Stavis, *Making Green Revolution*, 1974: 67). In China barley is the major crop of interior border regions, especially Tibet and parts of Xinjiang. There it is usually grown in the winter, rotated with rice in southern mountains, with various summer crops in the north, and with buckwheat in the Tibet–Mongolian mountain arc and in Manchuria. At the highest altitudes and latitudes it becomes a summer crop. Himalayan cultivators specialize in six–row barleys whereas barleys elsewhere are usually two–rowed, and many of their barleys are unusual (hooded, naked, irregular...), suggesting that area which has been a center of barley diversity for millennia. The naked barley, with very reduced chaff, is convenient for threshing. It is thus preferred in many barley–staple areas of Tibet.

Barley originated in the east Mediterranean area, where it was one of the earliest domesticates. It occurs with sheep, goats, and wheat in sites ten to twelve thousand years old. Barley appeared in China about the same time as wheat, as their shared named implies. They are not distinguished in early texts.

In China barley was normally used as flour, sometimes mixed with ground legumes. It was made into porridge, flat cakes, and, noodles. It was sometimes mixed with marrow and similar foods. The product could also be sweetened. Chinese do not brew with barley, but the Tibetans and other Central Asian peoples do. Pearl barley is common in China, known by a name once used for Job's–tears, which it has largely replaced as food, and as a medicinal. It is used in soups and for cooking with rice to "extend" supplies. In Tibet, barley that is not malted and brewed into Tibetan beer (*chang*) is parched and finely ground as *tsamba*. This is the Tibetan staple food and is usually consumed mixed with tea and cured butter in a paste. Since the *tsamba* is first parched (*i.e.*, dry–roasted in the open) before grinding, it is fully cooked, and makes a nourishing instant ration. A bag of it and a pot of boiling tea make the Tibetan's meal. It had spread to the Mongols by the mid–thirteenth century and is now extremely popular in Mongolia as well, although largely an imported food.

Folk medicine in modern south China holds that barley strengthens the body and helps it fight off disease. Pearl barley is thus a standard component of strengthening

It warms the center and brings down *qi*. It strengthens spleen and stomach, controls polydipsia, and destroys chill *qi*. It gets rid of abdominal distension.

[**27A**] Mutton (leg; bone and cut up), tsaoko cardamoms (five), hulled barley (two *sheng*; scour wash in boiling water; parboil the grains.)

Boil ingredients to make a soup. Strain [broth. Cut up meat and put aside]. Add [the] hulled barley and boil until cooked. Evenly adjust flavors with a little salt. Add [the] cut–up meat.

[3.] Bal–po Soup (This is the name of a Western Indian food)[23]

It supplements the center, and brings down *qi*. It extends the diaphragm.

Mutton (leg; bone and cut up), tsaoko cardamoms (five), chickpeas (half a *sheng*; pulverize and remove the skins), Chinese radish.

Boil ingredients together to make a soup. Strain [broth. Cut up meat and Chinese radish and put aside]. Add to the soup [the] mutton cut up into *sashuq* [coin]–sized pieces, [the] cooked Chinese radish cut up into *sashuq*–sized pieces, 1 *qian* of *za'faran* [saffron], 2 *qian* of Turmeric, 2 *qian* of Black ["Iranian"] Pepper [**27B**], half a *qian* of *kasni*, [asafoetida], coriander leaves. Evenly

---

and tonic soups and stews. As in the *YSZY*, it is considered heating. Perhaps the *YSZY* is referring to its strength–giving properties when it calls barley the best of grains *juan* 3, 4a). The text may also be referring to the popularity of barley among the Mongolian, Turkic, and even Tibetan courtiers, whose foodways are the main focus of the *YSZY*. The influence is not from the Near East since, according to Charles Perry (unpublished letter of January 2, 1994, to PDB), "Barley has always been considered a plebeian grain in the Arabic and Persian world...and Medieval as well as modern cookbooks rarely bother to give any recipes involving it."

Today, barley sprout tea is used as a diuretic.

Sources: John Lossing Buck, *Land Utilization in China* (Chicago, 1937); Harlan, 1975; Ho, 1975; Leonard and Martin, 1963; Perkins, 1969.

[23] Tibetan Bal–po is normally Nepal, but in the fourteenth century also neighboring Kashmir as well. This recipe is typical of the area. A close variant is still made in Kashmir. It differs primarily in using chilies, unknown in the Asia of 1330, and yogurt, rarely called for as such in the *YSZY*. Similar dishes are widespread in the Near East and northwest India. Kitchen–testing confirms the Kashmir–type flavor. This is an excellent dish.

adjust flavors with a little salt. Eat over cooked aromatic non–glutinous rice. Add a little Vinegar.

[4.] *Šaqimur* [Rape Turnip] Soup[24]

It supplements the center, and brings down *qi*. It harmonizes spleen and stomach.

Mutton (leg; bone and cut up), tsaoko cardamoms (five), chickpeas (half a *sheng*, pulverize and remove the skins), *šaqimur* (five); like *Manqing* [silver beet or Swiss chard]).

Boil ingredients together and make a soup. Strain [broth. Cut up meat and *šaqimur* and put aside]. Add 2 *he* of cooked chickpeas, 1 *sheng* of aromatic non–glutinous rice, [the] cooked *šaqimur* beet cut up into *sashuq*–sized pieces. Add [the] cut–up meat. Evenly adjust flavors with a little salt.

[5.]Fenugreek Seed[25] Soup

[**28A**] It supplements lower primordial energy [*yuanqi* 元氣], orders loin and knee, warms the center, and accords *qi*.

Mutton (leg; bone and cut up), tsaoko cardamoms (five), fenugreek seeds (1 *liang*; a kind of *hulba[t]* [*i.e.*, Fenugreek Seeds]).

Boil ingredients together and make a soup. Strain [broth]. Add Tangut *Um Ash*, or "Rice Heart *Qizi*," half a *qian* of *kasni*. Adjust flavors with a little salt.

[6.] Chinese Quince Soup[26]

It supplements the center, and accords *qi*. It cures pain of loin and knee, and [evil] foot *qi* insensitivity.

Mutton (leg; bone and cut up), tsaoko cardamoms (five), chick-

---

[24] This dish is a variant of recipe #1. It is delicately flavored, excellent though bland. The rape– or Chinese turnip is probably a local substitution for the regular turnip, much used in the similar dishes of the Irano–Mesopotamian area.

[25] Fenugreek has been a common Near Eastern food since before agriculture was born, and asafoetida is a virtually certain marker of Iranian influence. Here again we are dealing with a typical Irano–Mesopotamian dish.

[26] Another Irano–Mesopotamian item. Whole quinces can be substituted for the quince juice. Even then, this is a rather stodgy dish. Stew of mutton and quince is common in Iran and neighboring areas. Chinese quince is a different species from the Near Eastern, but probably the recipe implies that any quince will do.

peas (half a *sheng*; pulverize and remove the skins).

Boil ingredients together into a soup. Strain [broth. Cut up meat and put aside]. Add 1 *sheng* of aromatic non–glutinous rice, 2 *he* of cooked chickpeas, "meat pellets", two *jin* of Chinese quince (take the juice), 4 *liang* of granulated sugar. Adjust flavors with a little salt. [**28B**] [The] cut–up meat can perhaps be added.

[7.] Deer Head Soup[27]

It supplements and increases, controls polydipsia, and cures ache of foot and knee.

Deer's head [and] hooves (one set; remove hair and clean; bone and divide into pieces).

For the ingredients, take a large chunk of *kasni*, grind up into a mush and apply evenly to deer head, [and] hoof meat. Fry both the [marinated] head and hoof meat in 4 *liang* of vegetable oil ["Muslim lesser oil"]. Quench roasted head and hoof meat in boiling water,[28] boil until soft. Add 3 *qian* of black pepper, 2 *qian* of *kasni*, 1 *qian* of long pepper [*Piper longum*], 1 cup of cow's milk, 1 *he* of juice of sprouting ginger. Adjust flavors with a little salt.

[Variation:] In one method, use deer's tail to obtain broth. Add ground ginger. Adjust flavors with salt.

[8.] Pine Pollen [Juice] Soup[29]

---

[27] The spicing adds an Iranian touch to what is almost certainly a Mongol recipe. Note the unusual use of cow's milk.

[28] On this practice in the Arab World see Heine, 1988: 66.

[29] "Pine pollen juice", along with other pine products, was believed by the Chinese interested in sympathetic magic to promote longevity since the pine lives for centuries. Its use here, together with sprouting ginger, may be a marker of Chinese influence on this basically Irano–Mesopotamian dish. More likely, given the known Mongolian love of pine nuts, the "pine pollen" here is little more than crushed pine nuts, in which case this dish is one more example of dishes cooked with the Mongolian palate in mind.

Here we encounter for the first time a common instruction: add onions, salt, vinegar, and, sometimes, coriander leaves at the end. Ethnographic analogy from both the Near East and north China shows that this is to be done after cooking, either by the eater or the cook. Modern restaurants in northwest China have at each table a vinegar cruet and a salt shaker. Usually the vinegar is a white grain product, Chinese rice vinegar or something similar. Dark, rich, thick vinegar such as that of Shanxi or Zhejiang is possible, and makes an interesting substitute. Experimenters should try both with different dishes. Note that the directions do NOT specify soy sauce, pepper, or (of

It supplements the center, and increases *qi*. It strengthens sinew and bone.

[**29A**] Mutton (leg; bone and cut up), tsaoko cardamoms (five), chickpeas (half a *sheng*; pulverize and remove the skins).

Boil ingredients together into a soup. Strain [broth]. Fry together: one cooked sheep's thorax (cut up into *sashuq*–sized pieces), 2 *he* of pine pollen juice, half a *he* of juice of sprouting ginger. [Add to soup and] evenly adjust flavors with onions, salt, vinegar and [garnish with] coriander leaves. Eat with Long Rolled Bread.

[9.] Russian Olive [Fruit] Soup[30]

It supplements the center, and increases *qi*. It strengthens spleen and stomach.

Mutton (leg; bone and cut up), tsaoko cardamoms (five), chickpeas (half a *sheng*; remove the skins).

Boil ingredients together into a soup. Strain [broth]. Add together to the pot: a cooked dried sheep's thorax (sliced up), 3 *sheng* of Russian olive fruits, Chinese cabbage or nettle leaf. Evenly adjust flavors with salt.

---

course) chilies, all things that one finds on the modern table along with the vinegar and salt.

[30] The *sha* of the original is a term for coarse sugar. However, even the Mongols, with their great love of sugar, would find 3 *sheng*, 153.3 cubic inches (!) a little hard going. We have thus taken the *sha* here as a miswriting of *sha* 沙, *i.e.*, as an abbreviation for *shaguo* 沙果 (also *shazao* 沙棗) the fruits of the oleaster or Russian olive. Both Russian olive and nettles, while not used much or at all elsewhere in Asia, are known Mongolian gathered foods (see our discussion in the introduction), and their appearance in the recipe, along with such an uncommon, by Chinese standards, food as sheep thorax, strongly suggests that this is a traditional Mongolian one, but it has been modified by court cooks, *e.g.*, the tsaoko cardamom and chickpeas, and includes Chinese cabbage as an alternative to suit Chinese taste. The recipe is basically a Mongol variant on the mutton–chickpea base. *Eleagnus* berries are small and sour, and cranberries make a good substitute. Nettle leaves are available almost anywhere in the United States and may be gathered, with care and heavy gloves. Use only the tender youngest leaves. However, spinach is a perfectly good substitute with similar flavor and nutritional value.

[10.] [29B] Barley **Samsa* Noodles[31]

They supplement the center, and increase *qi*. They strengthen spleen and stomach.

Mutton (leg; bone and cut up), tsaoko cardamoms (five), chick-peas (half a *sheng*; remove the skins).

Boil ingredients together into a soup. Strain [broth. Set aside meat]. Make [**samsa*] noodles from a combination of 3 *jin* of barley flour, 1 *chin* of bean paste. [Fill with] mutton and fry. Adjust flavors with a fine *qima*, 2 *he* of juice of sprouting ginger, coriander leaves, salt, and vinegar.

[11.] Barley Strip–Noodles[32]

They supplement the center, increase *qi,* and strengthen spleen and stomach.

Mutton (leg; bone and cut up), tsaoko Cardamoms (five), lesser galangal [*Alpinia officinarum*].

Boil ingredients together into a soup. Strain [broth. Set meat aside.] Add sheep's liver sauce ([decoct and] take the bouillon), and 5 *qian* of black pepper. Cut [the] cooked mutton into [small, thin pieces like] armor scales, cut up 2 *liang* of pickled ginger and [add along with] 1 *liang* of sweet melon [*Cucumis melo*] pickles cut–up like "armor scales."

[**30A**] Adjust flavors with salt and vinegar. A thick broth can also be used.

[12.] Glutinous Rice Flour **Chöp*[33]

They supplement the center, and increase *qi*.

Mutton (leg; bone and cut up), tsaoko cardamoms (five), lesser galangal (two *qian*).

---

[31] *Samsa*, from Persian *sambusa*, also occur in the *CCPYSL*, but under the latter, Persian form of their name (see 13,17b, 14, 34a). The ginger and bean paste introduce a Chinese flavor to this dish.

[32] A Central Asian food with Near Eastern and Chinese spicing. Note that there are no actual barley or noodles, the sliced mutton and pickles providing the whitish, noodle–like appearance.

[33] In spite of their Uighur name, the glutinous rice noodles are a thoroughly Chinese touch.

Boil ingredients together into a soup. Strain [broth. Set aside meat]. Use sheep's liver sauce (decoct and take the bouillon). Add 5 *qian* of black pepper. Combine two *jin* of glutinous rice flour, and one *jin* of bean paste and make the **chöp*. Cut up [the] mutton into a fine *qima* and add [as stuffing]. [Put into soup and] adjust flavors with salt and vinegar. A thick broth can also be used.

[13.] River Pig Broth[34]

It supplements the center, and increases *qi*.

Mutton (leg; bone and cut up), tsaoko cardamoms (five).

[**30B**] Boil ingredients together into a soup. Strain [broth. Set meat aside]. Take [the] mutton (cut up finely into *qima*), five *qian* of mandarin orange peel (remove the white),[35] 2 *liang* of White Onions (cut up finely), two *qian* of spices, salt, and [sheep's liver] sauce, and make the stuffing. Use 3 *jin* of white flour to make the skins. Make the "River Pigs." Cook by frying in vegetable oil ["lesser oil"] and when done put into the soup. Adjust flavors with salt. Bouillon can perhaps also be used.

[14.] **Achchiq* ["Bitter"] Soup

It supplements the center, and increases *qi*.

Mutton (leg; bone and cut up), tsaoko cardamoms (five), lesser galangal (two *qian*).

Boil ingredients together into a soup. Strain [broth. Set meat aside]. Add sheep's liver sauce. Decoct bouillon from broth and sauce. Add 5 *qian* of black pepper. In addition, cut up [the] mutton into strips. Cut up into "armor scales" one sheep's tail, one sheep's tongue, one set of sheep kidneys and add together with two *liang* of **möög* [mushrooms], and Chinese cabbage. Adjust flavors with broth, salt and vinegar.

---

[34] One of the more Chinese–influenced of these basically Turkic noodle foods. The mandarin peel/onion/mixed spice/soybean sauce mix is, of course, thoroughly Chinese. The dumplings are fried like modern *guotie* 鍋貼 before being added to soup. They are supposed to look like "river pigs," *i.e.*, fresh water porpoises, swimming in the soup.

[35] The "white" is the white interior skin of the *chenpi*.

[15.] Euryale Flour Swallow's Tongue *Qizi*[36]

[**31A**] They supplement the center, and increase vital energy.

Mutton (leg; bone and cut up), tsaoko cardamoms (five), chickpeas (half a *sheng*; pulverize and remove the skins).

Boil ingredients together into a soup. Strain [broth. Set meat aside]. Use two *jin* of euryale flour, 1 *jin* of bean paste, work together and cut into *qizi*. Use [the] mutton cut up into a fine *qima* [and] one *he* of juice of sprouting ginger [as stuffing. Stuff *qizi*] and fry. [Add to soup and] adjust flavors with onions.

[16.] Euryale Flour Blood Noodles[37]

They supplement the center, and increase the vital air.

Mutton (leg; bone and cut up), tsaoko cardamoms (five), chickpeas (half a *sheng*; pulverize, remove the skins).

Boil ingredients together into a soup. Strain [broth. Set meat aside]. Use two *jin* of euryale flour, one *jin* of bean paste, and sheep's blood [**31B**] and combine to make **chöp*. [Use] mutton cut into a fine *qima* [as stuffing. Stuff **chöp* and] Fry. [Add to soup and] adjust flavors of everything together with onions and vinegar.

[17.] Euryale Flour **Jüzmä*

They supplement the center, and increase the vital air.

Mutton (leg; bone and cut up), tsaoko cardamoms (five), chickpeas (half a *sheng*; pulverize and remove the skins).

Boil ingredients together into a soup. Strain [broth. Set meat aside]. Use two *jin* of euryale flour, one *jin* of bean paste, one *jin* of white [wheat] flour to make the noodles. Cut [the] mutton into strip *qima*, stuff noodles and fry. [Add to soup and] adjust flavors of everything together with onions and vinegar.

---

[36] Euryale is a Chinese water lily relative whose fruit is starchy and is thus ground for flour. Euryale seeds are strictly a Chinese food, and are exceedingly important in Chinese medicine. Quite possibly they are a high quality substitute for the starch of some Mongol gathered seed. The Western cook will probably have to substitute ordinary noodles here and in similar recipes.

[37] Recipes # 16–18 are variations on a Turkish or Irano–Mesopotamian dish with some Chinese touches; the euryale at least and probably the bean powder.

[18.] Euryale Flour **Chöp*

They supplement the center, and increase the vital air.

Mutton (leg; bone and cut up), tsaoko cardamoms (five), lesser galangal (two *qian*).

[**32A**] Boil ingredients together into a soup. Strain [broth. Set meat aside]. Use sheep's liver sauce. Take the bouillon of the combined soup and sauce. Add one *liang* of black pepper. Then use two *jin* of euryale flour, one *jin* bean paste and make into **chöp*, [stuff with the] mutton cut up into a fine *qima* and add. Adjust flavors with salt and vinegar.

[19.] Euryale Flour *Hundun*[38]

They supplement the center, and increase *qi*.

Mutton (leg, bone and cut up), tsaoko cardamoms (five), chick-peas (half a *sheng*; pulverize and remove the skins).

Boil ingredients together into a soup. Strain [broth. Set meat aside]. Cut [the] mutton into stuffing. Add 1 *qian* of salted mandarin orange peel (remove the white), 1 *qian* of sprouting ginger (cut up finely). Spice evenly with the "five spices." Then use two *jin* of the euryale flour, and one *jin* of bean paste, make into "Fluffy–pillow *Hundun*," and put into the soup. Fry together a *sheng* of aromatic non–glutinous rice, two *he* of cooked chickpeas, [**32B**] two *he* of juice of sprouting ginger, one *he* of quince juice. [Add to soup and] evenly adjust flavors with onions and salt.

[20.] Sundry Broth[39]

It supplements the center, and increases *qi*.

Mutton (leg, bone[40] and cut up), tsaoko cardamoms (five), chick-peas (half a *sheng*; pulverized. Remove the skins).

---

[38] This is the same general dish as # 16–18 but with the added Chinese touch of ginger and its juice.

[39] This is the first of many dishes in which the broth is thickened by apricot kernel paste. This is unquestionably a local adaptation of the Near Eastern habit of mixing crushed nuts, specifically almonds, into such stews. Kitchen–testing with almonds makes this clear, if one knows the Near Eastern analogs. However, Hu has been careful to scale down his amounts to a relatively low level, because the flavor of Chinese apricot kernel paste is stronger and more bitter than that of almond paste.

[40] Part of this formula has been omitted in the text.

Boil ingredients together into a soup. Strain [broth]. Cook together: two sheep's heads (clean), two sets each of sheep stomachs and lungs, one set of white blood, paired sheep intestines.[41] When done cut up [and add to soup]. Then use three *jin* of bean flour to make noodles, Stuff with half a *jin* of **möög* [mushrooms], half a *jin* of apricot kernel[42] paste, one *liang* of black pepper. Fry [with] mint[43] and coriander leaves. Adjust flavors with onions, salt, and vinegar

[21.] Meat and Vegetable Broth[44]

[41] Reference is apparently to the fatty deposits often found on sheep intestines. See, however, the explanation given by Li in Hu Sihui, 1988: 47.

[42] Apricot: the apricot, a very important food tree in China, is either a Chinese native or an ancient introduction from Central Asia. It is primarily a tree of montane west Asia, but its range may have extended as far as north China, where it was cultivated so early that transmission across Central Asia seems unlikely. The apricot is closely related to the *mei* 梅, differing mainly in having larger fruits, less showy flowers, and slightly different growth habits. It is currently important in Xinjiang, which exports dried apricots of high quality. The fruit is of minor medical import, but the seed kernels are widely used in Chinese medicine, for cough, sore throat, *etc*. The kernels must first be ground and cooked or dried to get rid of the cyanide–generating glycoside compounds that makes the fresh kernels dangerously poisonous. The powder is typically mixed with hot water or hot milk and drunk. It makes an extremely soothing and refreshing drink when one has a sore, irritated or dusty throat, and the heat and volatile oils do well by the nasal passages. Children especially are often treated for sore throats with this drink. Various compound medicines also use the kernels. The oil of the kernels is sometimes expressed and variously used. The kernels are often called "almonds" or "Chinese almonds," and the powder is "almond powder" on labels in English. The true almond is very rare in China, and is known as a kind of apricot [*bayanren* 八檐仁 "*badam* apricot," from *badam*, the Persian word for the almond], so the mistake is natural. The whole dried kernels are often sold, but the powder is commoner, at least in modern times.

[43] *Qingcai*, "green vegetable," is usually bokchoy, *Brassica chinensis*, called *bocai* 白菜 (*i.e.*, bokchoy) in the *YSZY* (3, 49a). The usage here makes that unlikely since the *qingcai* of the recipe is a cilantro-like garnish. We suspect that the *qingcai* of the text is identical to the Huihui *qing* listed at the very end of *juan* 3 (59a) and is mint.

[44] This is the first of a number of dishes that combine Near Eastern, Mongol, Turkic, and Chinese ingredients in a particularly creative and original way. These we find the most interesting and significant recipes in the *YSZY*. They clearly represent the apex of court cuisine. Among identifiable groups of recipes, they are the most complex and subtle.

In this one, on the usual Irano–Mesopotamian and Turkic base, we have such Chinese ingredients as Chinese yams, sprouting ginger and apricot kernel paste (for almond paste). The custom of frying eggs into a sheet (Chinese *jindan* 燼蛋) and cutting it into strips to add to soup is thoroughly Chinese, but Irano–Mesopotamian cooking does use eggs in such dishes. Sometimes the eggs are hard–boiled and cut up for

[**33A**] It supplements the center, and increases *qi*.

Mutton (leg; bone and cut up), tsaoko cardamoms (five), chick-peas (half a *sheng*; pulverized. Remove the skins).

Boil ingredients together into a soup. Strain [broth. Set meat aside]. [Use] three *jin* of bean flour to make "strip–noodles." Cut select mutton into long *qima*. Cut up: one *jin* of Chinese yams[45], two lumps of pickled ginger, one sweet melon pickle, one cheese,[46] ten carrots ["Iranian radishes"], half a *sheng* of **möög* [mushrooms], and four *liang* of sprouting ginger, ten eggs fried into an omelet and sliced. Use one *jin* of sesame seed paste and half a *jin* of apricot kernel paste and fry [everything together]. [Add to soup and] adjust flavors with onions, salt, and vinegar.

[22.] Pearl Noodles[47]

They supplement the center, and increase *qi*.

Mutton (leg; bone and cut up), tsaoko cardamoms (five), [**33B**] chickpeas (half a *sheng*; pulverized. Remove the skins).

Boil ingredients together into a soup. Strain [broth. Set aside meat]. Cut mutton into *qima*. Cut up each of the following: one sheep's heart, one sheep's liver, a set of sheep's lungs, two *liang* of sprouting ginger, four *liang* of pickled ginger, one *liang* of sweet melon pickles, ten carrots, one *jin* of Chinese yams, one cheese, ten eggs fried into an omelet. Then fry everything together using one *jin* of sesame paste. [Add everything to soup and] adjust flavors with onions, salt, and vinegar.

---

topping; sometimes they are stirred into the broth to cook there, an idea that may come from China. Chinese *jindan* are made like an omelet, but are not folded over, thus forming a thin sheet, and are allowed to cook hard, not "wet." Vegetable oil is used, but never butter. The combination of sesame and apricot kernel/almond paste makes an exquisite taste and texture. The pickles almost certainly represent Middle Eastern influence, as elsewhere in the *YSZY*.

45 Chinese yam: true Chinese yams, genus *Dioscorea*, cannot be found in the United States or in most of China today, but closely related Japanese yams, *imo*, are available. One type, *naga imo,* is a delicacy–crisp with a sticky sap, and edible raw or cooked. Not all *imo* are *Dioscorea.* The term now cover other root crops.

46 This cheese was probably like the Baghlan of Afghanistan, a white cheddar type. It could be cut into cubes or grated and put into the soup. Chances are also good that it was a white fresh cheese like the Mexican *queso blanco* or *queso ranchero*, and then would be crumbled into the soup, towards the end, as Mexicans do.

47 A dish similar to the preceding one, essentially a variant of it.

[23.] Yellow Soup[48]

It supplements the center, and increases *qi*.

Mutton (leg; bone and cut up), tsaoko cardamoms (five), chick-peas (half a *sheng*; pulverized. Remove the skins).

Boil ingredients together into a soup. Strain [broth]. Add two *he* of cooked chickpeas, one *sheng* of aromatic non–glutinous rice [**34A**], and five carrots (cut up). Use “meat pellets” [made from] the “meat pill” of the rear hoof of a sheep, one [sheep’s] rib (cut up into small, square pieces), three *qian* of turmeric, five *qian* of ground ginger, one *qian* of *za’faran*, and coriander leaves. Adjust flavors with salt and vinegar.

[24.] Three in the Cooking Pot

It supplements the center, and increases *qi*.

Mutton (leg; bone and cut up), tsaoko cardamoms (five), lesser galangal (two *qian*).

Boil ingredients together into a soup. Strain [broth]. Use “meat pellets” [made from] the “meat pill” of the rear hoof of a sheep, “nail–headed *Qizi*,” “mutton **jis–kebabi* food” and one *liang* black pepper. Adjust flavors with salt and vinegar.

---

[48] This dish uses rice instead of noodles as the starch thickener, and like most dishes in this section specifies aromatic non–glutinous rice, *i.e.*, Basmati type as opposed to the much less markedly–flavored rice of China. Near Eastern and northwest Indian cooking, in which rice was then a luxury, usually call for a rice with a good flavor. The Chinese, for whom rice is common fare, prefer it not to taste too strongly. Even the best flavor becomes tiresome eventually. The odd combination of turmeric, ground ginger, and saffron makes this dish striking and memorable. We are not aware of such a combination anywhere else, though it clearly echoes spice mixes of Iran and northwest India, and probably more directly, of the Uighur cuisine. It is a variant or local representative of a class of yellow rice dishes that extends from Mesopotamia to Indonesia. Everywhere, they are colored with saffron, turmeric, or both, and are dishes of hospitality and festivity. The carrots called for here carry the color deeper, and the result is visually stunning. The ritual importance of yellow rice in Java has received a classic description in Clifford Geertz’ *The Religion of Java* (Glencoe, 1960). The liquid is totally absorbed by the rice. In this recipe, meatballs of two types are used. We have no recipes for them, and in kitchen–testing simply used small grilled patties of ground lamb. The original was probably fancier, but this proved excellent.

[25.] Mallow Leaf Broth[49]

It [Mallow Leaf] accords *qi*. It treats retained urine that does not pass. Its nature is cold and one cannot eat a lot. In the present case we have cooked the mallow leaf with various things [**34B**] intended to make its nature slightly warming.

Mutton (leg; bone and cut up), tsaoko cardamoms (five), lesser galangal (two *qian*).

Boil ingredients together into a soup. [Use as stuffing] one set each of cooked sheep's stomach and lungs (cut up), half a *jin* of **möög* [mushrooms] (cut up). Combine five *qian* of black pepper and one jin of white flour to make "chicken–claw vermicelli." Add to soup. Fry mallow leaf [and add]. Adjust flavors with onions, salt, and vinegar.

[26.] Long Bottle Gourd [*Lagenaria siceraria var. depressa*] Soup[50]

It [the long bottle gourd] is cooling by nature. It is good for diabetes. It benefits the water paths.

Mutton (leg; bone and cut up), tsaoko cardamoms (five).

Boil ingredients together into a soup. Strain [broth. Set aside meat]. Use six long bottle gourds (remove the pericarps and skins, dice), [the] cooked mutton (cut into strips). Make fine vermicelli from half a *he* of juice of sprouting ginger and two *liang* of white flour. Fry everything together. [Add to soup and] adjust flavors with onions, salt, and vinegar.

[27.] [35A] Turtle Soup[51]

---

[49] Mallow leaves are a diuretic, as the recipe specifies. They also are rich in vitamin A and C while being low–calorie and "cooling" and sour to the mouth, all traits that make them cooling in Chinese medicine. Here they seem an afterthought, unless the idea is to use an enormous amount of them in the recipe. The lack of specification of quantity implies that one adds as many leaves as one wills. Hu specifies exact quantities when a dish requires it.

[50] Adding long bottle gourds to soup for their cooling values is still standard in China.

[51] This is a Chinese dish, Mongolized. Turtles are not used in Near Eastern cooking since they are forbidden in Islam. They were not a major part of the Mongolian fauna. Turtle soup, very similar for this except for the mutton, is still a part of Chinese health cuisine.

It is good for a wounded center, and increases *qi*. It supplements [in cases of] insufficiency.

Mutton (leg; bone and cut up), tsaoko cardamoms (five).

Boil ingredients together into a soup. Strain [broth]. Cook five or six turtles. When done, remove the skin and bones, and cut into lumps [and add to soup]. Use two *liang* of flour to make fine vermicelli. Roast together with one *he* of juice of sprouting ginger, one *liang* of black pepper. [Add to soup and] adjust flavors with onions, salt, and vinegar.

[28.] Cup Steamed[52]

It supplements the center, and increases *qi*.

Sheep's back skin from which the hair has been removed, or mutton (three legs; bone and cut up), tsaoko cardamoms (five), lesser galangal (two *qian*), prepared mandarin orange peel (two *qian*; remove the white), Chinese flower pepper ["lesser pepper;" *Zanthoxylum* sp][53] (two *qian*).

[35B] [Take] ingredients and fry[54] together with one *jin* of almond paste, two *he* of pine pollen [juice], and two *he* of juice of sprouting ginger. Adjust flavors evenly with onions, salt and spices [five spices]. Put into a liquor cup and steam until tender. When cooked eat with long rolled bread.

---

52 This dish, still a mainstay of Hunan cooking, is made there with pork, not mutton, and somewhat different flavoring. The product is a small individual–size meatloaf filling the cup.

53 Chinese flower pepper: This native spice occurs in many species. It is now called brown, flower or *Sichuan* pepper to distinguish it from other spices, but the *YSZY* uses the Chinese adjective "small" to separate it from black pepper. *Zanthoxylum* is not related to either black or red pepper, but is a thorny plant known botanically as "prickly ash." Many species occur in East Asia and the southeastern United States. Many of the Asian ones are used as spices. They share a slight citrus flavor, a numbing quality, and a peppery spiciness. The part used is the small fruit. Fruits usually grow twinned on a short stalk, making them a miniature model of the male genitalia. As such, they are a standard literary trope or euphemism in old Chinese writings, from the *Book of Songs* onward. They are China's principal native true spice, *i.e.*, dry, hard, intensely aromatic plant part, as opposed to culinary herbs. Intensive use of brown pepper and herbs preadapted west China for acceptance of the chili pepper now so popular there. It is not, as sometimes alleged, due to Indian influence that *Sichuan* food is hot. Brown pepper is still used as a stimulant and warming drug. The various species have different properties, somewhat imperfectly distinguished.

54 There are major omissions in this recipe. We follow Li (Hu Sihui, 1988: 53–4).

[29.] Oil Rape Shoots Broth[55]

It supplements the center, and increases *qi*.

Mutton (leg; bone and cut up), tsaoko cardamoms (five), lesser galangal (two *qian*).

Boil ingredients together into a soup. Strain [broth]. Use sheep's liver, make into a sauce. [Decoct and] take the bouillon. Make noodles with five *jin* of bean paste [and add to soup]. Cut up finely and add: one cheese, one *jin* of Chinese yams, ten carrots, one sheep's tail, mutton. Adjust flavors with oil rape [sprouts], Chinese chives,[56] one *liang* of black pepper, salt, and, vinegar.

[30.] Bear Soup[57]

---

[55] This complex dish of uncertain origin is another example of creativity, but the primary influences are Irano–Mesopotamian and Mongol. Oil rape can be any of several species of *Brassica* used for seed oil. Species occur throughout Asia. Presumably, the court of Beijing would use whatever was locally available. In kitchen testing, we left out the liver sauce and sheep tail, and used regular noodles instead of bean flour noodles. Bean flour noodles tend to fall apart and dissolve into a soup. Possibly Hu assumed that one would use enough wheat flour to make a noodle; otherwise, these noodles must be made of pure washed starch of bean or pea, like many modern Chinese noodles, and not of the actual flour. This is an excellent, subtle, and highly nutritious recipe.

[56] Chinese chives are different species from Western chives. Chinese chives have a pronounced garlic flavor and are known as "garlic chives" in the vegetable marketing trade. As the scientific name suggests, they differ from Western chives by being distinctly tuberous. The leaves are used for garnish and as a vegetable to stir–fry with other vegetables. Often they are blanched, earth is hilled around them as the they grow, and the resulting "chive yellows" are very choice. The Chinese proverb says: "The chive that sticks its head up is the one that gets cut." This gives rise to the phrase "chive–cutting mentality" in China where the tendency to be afraid to do or say anything original or challenging is all too common. In antiquity Chinese *jiu* was pronounced *kiôg*, a word which may be compared to Mongolian *gogod* which is almost certainly related. Since *jiu* occurs in Tibetan as *giu* the borrowing is mostly likely from Sino–Tibetan to Mongolian, unless Mongolian, Chinese, and Tibetan have all borrowed the word from some other language partially ancestral to all.

[57] Bear is a Mongol dish but is here cooked according to a Near Eastern recipe. The only Chinese touch is the "sauce," probably soy sauce, traditionally added by the eater, at the last moment, as here. The use of the alternative "sheep's liver sauce," is, in any case, altogether different in the *YSZY*. We have tried this recipe with beef, which in our experience is much like bear meat. The result was excellent. Lamb or pork, also somewhat bear–like, could be used. The spices have the function of reducing the rank gaminess all too common in bear, as in sheep meat. This must have been a small bear, if the spices were to flavor two whole legs, although leg, as elsewhere, may simply be a standard measure of meat.

It treats migratory arthralgia insensitivity and [evil] foot *qi*.

[**36A**] Bear meat (two legs; cook. When done cut into chunks), tsaoko cardamoms (three)

[Boil] ingredients [together into a soup]. Use three *qian* of black pepper, one *qian* of *kasni*, two *qian* of turmeric, two *qian* of grain–of–paradise [seed of *Amomum villosum* or *A. xanthioides*], one *qian* of *za'faran*. Adjust flavors of everything together with onions, salt, and sauce.

[31.] Carp Soup[58]

It treats jaundice, stops thirst, and pacifies the womb. If a person is ill with chronic abdominal mass he should not eat it.

Large young carp (ten; remove the scales and intestines; clean), finely ground Chinese flower pepper (five *qian*).

Marinate ingredients with a combination of five *qian* of ground coriander, two *liang* of onions (cut up), a little liquor, salt. Put fish into bouillon. Then add five *qian* of finely ground black pepper, three *qian* of sprouting ginger, and three *qian* of ground long pepper. Adjust flavors with salt and vinegar.[59]

[32.] Roast Wolf Soup[60]

[**36B**] Ancient *bencao* do not include entries on wolf meat. At present we state that its nature is heating. It treats asthenia. I have never heard that it is poisonous for those eating it. In the case of the present recipe we use spices to help its flavor. It warms[61] the five internal organs, and warms the center.

---

58 A fairly standard Chinese recipe for a Chinese fish, this is one of the few thoroughly Chinese recipes in this section. The liquor rules out a Near Eastern origin and the combination of flavorings is classic Chinese.

59 Compare similar Medieval Arabic methods to cook fish discussed in Heine, 1988: 82ff.

60 This is just a typical lamb recipe, except for the main ingredient. One can imagine the Yuan court chefs staring in horror as some uncouth nomad *qan* threw down a freshly–slain wolf on their board and yelled: "Cook that!" since Islam forbids eating canines, and north Chinese had probably lost the dog–eating habit by this time. Not having a wolf, we in fact kitchen–tested this recipe with leg of lamb, and found it excellent.

61 Note that this "warm" translates a different character (*nuan* 暖) than the warm (*wen* 溫) in the next phrase. The medical difference escapes us.

Wolf meat (leg; bone and cut up), tsaoko cardamoms (three), black pepper (five *qian*), *kasni* (one *qian*), long pepper (two *qian*), grain–of–paradise (two *qian*), turmeric (two *qian*), *za'faran* (one *qian*).

Boil ingredients together into a soup. Adjust flavors of everything using onions, sauce, salt, and vinegar.

[33.] ****Ishkäne***[62]

It supplements and increases [for] the five internal organs.

Mutton (leg; cook. When done cut up finely), sheep's tail (two; [cook]. When done cut up finely). Cut into long strips: sacred lotus rhizome (two), cattail rhizome [*Typha* sp] (two *jin*), cucumbers (five), sprouting ginger (half a *jin*), [**37A**] cheeses (two), pickled ginger (four *liang*), sweet melon pickles (half a *jin*), eggs (ten. Fry into an omelet), **möög* [mushrooms] (one *jin*), Swiss chard, Chinese chives.

Use a "good meat soup" and blend together ingredients. Fry [*i.e.*, cook dry] with two *jin* of sesame paste, and half a *jin* of finely ground ginger. Adjust flavors with onions, salt and vinegar. Eat with "Iranian buns."

---

62 This topping for Iranian bread (or its Chinese derivative *shaobing*) is truly unique. We know of nothing like it anywhere else. It is also very different from anything else in the *YSZY*. A very Mongol flavor is implied, if it is not a straight borrowing from nomadic Turks. The "Iranian cakes" are Persian bread (*nan*), still a staple food in Ningxia and Xinjiang. In the Chinese Islamic Restaurant, a Ningxia Hui restaurant near Los Angeles, we have eaten similar stews with their incomparable *nan*–style bread. This particular stew, however, is one of the *YSZY*'s amazing, unique, and creative blendings of Mongol, Near Eastern, and Chinese elements (*cf.* recipes # 21–23, *etc.*). For the rhizomes, potatoes make a tolerable substitute. The combination of cheese, cucumber, and ginger *etc*., is unusual but superb, perhaps the best thing in the *YSZY*. Compare the following, much simpler dish, but still an addition to bread, with beef substituted for mutton, from Cromwell's England, entitled "A Turkish Dish of Meate:"

> Take an interlarded piece of beef, cut it into thin slices, and put into a pot that hath a close cover, or stewing pan; then put into it a quantity of whole pepper, two or three whole onions, and let this boil very well, then take out the onions, and dish it on sippets, the thicker it is the better.

See Madge Lorwin, *Dining with William Shakespeare* (New York, 1976), 28–9, quoting Robert May, *The Accomplisht Cook*, 1660.

[34.] **Chöppün* Noodles[63]

They supplement the center, and increase *qi*.

White flour (six *jin*; cut into fine vermicelli), mutton (two legs; cook. When done, cut into strip *qima* [and stuff vermicelli]), one set each of sheep intestines and lungs (Cook. When done cut up.), eggs (five; fry into an omelet. Cut into "streamers"), sprouting ginger (four *liang*), root and tuber of the Chinese chive[64] (half a *jin*), **möög* [mushrooms] (four *liang*), oil rape leaf, smartweed shoots, safflower.

[**37B**] Use bouillon for the ingredients. Add one *liang* of black pepper, Adjust flavors with salt and vinegar.

[35.] Black Broth Noodles[65]

They supplement the center, and increase *qi*.

White flour (cut fine vermicelli), sheep's thorax (two; pluck and clean; cook. When done cut into *sashuq*–sized chunks).

Use three *qian* of "red flour"[66] to marinate ingredients. Boil until tender. Put everything together into bouillon. Add one *liang* of black pepper, salt and vinegar. Flavor [evenly].

[36.] Chinese Yam Noodles

They supplement [for] deficiency emaciation. They increase primordial energy.

White flour (six *jin*), eggs (ten; take the white), juice of sprouting ginger (two *he*), bean paste (four *liang*).

Use three *jin* of Chinese yams. Cook. When done grind up into a paste and combined with ingredients to make noodles. Cut up two legs of mutton into [**38A**] "nail–headed *qima*" [as stuffing]. Use a "good meat broth," add [noodles] and fry. Adjust flavors with onions and salt.

---

63 The Uighur name clarifies the origin of this dish, another unique and surprising one.

64 Compare, however, Li in Hu Sihui, 1988: 59.

65 Recipes 35–39 are five ordinary Central Asian noodle dishes.

66 If this is not a Middle Eastern *kaimakh*, the *hongmian* of the text is probably an error for *hongqü* 紅曲, red wine dregs, a common additive in Chinese cooking.

[37.] Hanging Noodles[67]

They supplement the center, and increase *qi*.

Mutton (leg; cut up into a fine *qima*), hanging noodles (six *jin*), **möög* [mushrooms] (half a *jin*; wash; cut up.), eggs (five; fry), pickled ginger (one *liang*; cut up), sweet melon pickles (one *liang*; cut up).

Use bouillon for ingredients. Add one *liang* of black pepper. Adjust flavors with salt and vinegar.

[38.] **Jingtei* Noodles[68]

They supplement the center, and increase *qi*.

Mutton (leg; roast the meat. [Make] **quruq* [dried] *qima*),[69] **möög* [mushrooms] (half a *chin*; wash and cut up).

Use bouillon for ingredients. Add one *liang* of black pepper. Adjust flavors with salt and vinegar.

[39.] [38B] Sheep's Skin Noodles

They supplement the center, and increase *qi*.

Sheep's skins (two; remove the hair; clean; cook until tender), sheep's tongues (two; cook.), sheep's loins (four; cook. Cut up each [*i.e.*, previous ingredients] like "armor scales"), **möög* [mushrooms] (one *jin*; cleaned), pickled ginger (four *liang*. Cut up each like "armor scales").

Use a good rich meat soup, or bouillon for the ingredients. Add one *liang* of black pepper. Adjust flavors with salt.

[40.] *Tutum Ash* (This is a kind of kneaded noodle)[70]

---

[67] Note that in the west, in the *Tacuinum sanitatis*, "hanging noodles" are pasta.

[68] Note that this dish, and the one following, have ingredients looking like noodles, but do not actually contain noodles.

[69] More properly this is *quruq et*.

[70] This is the *Tutmajh* of the later Middle Eastern cookbooks, still a standard dish. See, for example, Arto der Haroutunian, *Middle Eastern Cookery* (London, 1982), 80; Roden, 1970: 135. *Tutmajh* is one of the earliest (pre–Ottoman) Turkic borrowings by a broader Middle Eastern food culture. In the Near East it is flavored with mint, probably the "fragrant herb" here, and not basil. A different word specifically meaning "mint" is used for mint in the medicinal recipes of the following sections.

They supplement the center, and increase *qi*.

White flour (six *jin*. Make into *tutum ash*), mutton (leg. Roast the meat. [Make into] **quruq qima* [and stuff *tutum ash*]).

Use a Good Meat Soup for ingredients. Add the noodles and roast [cook dry]. Adjust flavors evenly with onions. Add garlic, cream [or yogurt],[71] finely ground mint (or basil).

[41.] Fine **Salma* (same as "Thin Silk Border" **Salma*)[72]

[**39A**] They supplement the center, and increase *qi*.

White flour (six *jin*; make **salma*), mutton (two legs; roast the meat. [Make into] **quruq qima* [and stuff **salma*]), chicken (one; cook and cut up finely), **möög* [mushrooms] (half a *jin*; wash; cut up).

Use bouillon for ingredients. Add one *liang* of black pepper. Adjust flavors with salt and vinegar.

[42.] Water Dragon *Qizi*

They supplement the center, and increase *qi*.

Mutton (two legs; cook; cut up into *qima*), white flour (six *jin*. [Make dough and] cut into "cash eye *qizi*"[73]), [stuff *qizi* with *qima*], eggs (ten), Chinese yams (one *jin*), pickled ginger (four *liang*), carrots (five), sweet melon pickles (two *liang*. Cut up each finely), "Three Color Meat Patties." (The inside color is of a meat patty. The outer two colors are noodle and chicken patties.)

Use bouillon for ingredients. Add two *liang* of black pepper. Adjust flavors with salt and vinegar.

[43.] [39B] *[U]mach* (a kind of hand twisted noodle. It can be glutinous rice flour or euryale flour.)

It supplements the center, and increases *qi*.

White flour (six *jin*; make *[u]mach*), mutton (two legs; cook. Cut

---

[71] As Doerfer's authorities (Doerfer, 1963–1975: II: 458) make clear, *Tut[u]ma[ch] Ash* was traditionally eaten with yogurt.

[72] Recipes 41–44 are further noodle items of a sort that would not be out of place in Ningxia or Xinjiang today.

[73] Note the Chinese term for a small coin here in place of the usual Turkic *sashuq*.

into *qima* [and stuff *[u]mach*]).

Use a good meat soup for ingredients and roast [cook dry]. Adjust flavors of everything together with onions, vinegar, and salt.

[44.] **Shoyla Toyym* (Name of an Uighur Food)

It supplements the center, and increases *qi*.

White flour (six *jin*; knead; make into coin shapes), mutton (two legs; cook; cut up), sheep's tongues (two; cook; cut up), Chinese yams (one *chin*), **möög* [mushrooms] (half a *jin*), carrots (five), pickled ginger (four *liang*; cut up).

Use a good rich meat soup, add all ingredients and roast [cook dry]. Adjust flavors with onions and vinegar.

[45.] [40A] *Qima* Congee[74]

It supplements spleen and stomach, and increases the power of *qi*.

Mutton (leg; bone and cut up. Boil into a soup. Strain [broth. Set meat aside]), millet grains (two *sheng*; scour and wash. [Add to soup]).

[Prepare] ingredients, use select mutton. Cut up into a chunk *qima*. First take [millet] grains and add to the soup. Then add the *qima*, rice, onions, and salt. Boil to make the congee. One can perhaps add polished rice, *zhemi* [uniform washed grains of fine millet], or dried rice. All are possible.

[46.] Soup Congee

It supplements spleen and stomach, and increases kidney *qi*.

Mutton (leg; bone and cut up).

Boil ingredient into a soup. Strain. Then add two *sheng* of millet grains to make a congee. When the congee is cooked, add rice, onions and salt. One can perhaps add polished rice, *zhemi* or dried rice. All are possible.

---

[74] Recipes 45–48 are several ordinary congees, in spite of the exotic name of the first, and the relatively exotic ingredient of the last.

[47.] [40B] Millet Insipid Congee

It supplements the center, and increases *qi*.

Millet grains (two *sheng*).

[For the ingredient] first boil water, settling out impurities and straining. Then scour clean the millet, three to five times. Boil to make a congee. One can perhaps add polished rice, *zhemi* or dried rice. All are possible.

[48.] **Qamh [Triticum durum]* Soup[75]

It supplements the center, and increases *qi*.

Mutton (leg; bone and cut up), **qamh* (two *sheng*).

Boil ingredients into a soup. Strain [broth. Cut up meat into *qima*.] Add the **qamh* (scoured clean). Then add fine *qima*, rice, onions and salt. Boil together into a congee. It is also possible not to use *qima*.

[49.] [41A] **Se-aBru* [Pomegranate] Soup (This is the name of a Western Indian Food)[76]

---

[75] Charles Perry notes, in an unpublished letter of 2 January, 1994, to PDB, that this "*qamh* soup resembles Medieval Arab dishes like *Tifshil* and *Tannuniyya*, porridges containing meat...[except that] they are cooked in a cooling bread oven overnight, rather than directly over a fire because it takes a long time to cook whole wheat." This recipe may thus be a version of a Middle Eastern one, but adapted to the Mongol taste and love of boiling.

[76] The name of this astonishing recipe is Tibetan since the pomegranate is Se-aBru, today pronounced sedu, with a relatively soft "d," in modern Tibetan. Here this word is represented by the modern Chinese and early Mandarin *sasu* 撒速, in Tang times **satsəwk*. The tree is also known in Tibetan as the *seu-shin* or, more properly, *Bal–po'i seu–shin*, "the *seu* Tree of Nepal" in Tibetan. The recipe itself, as Hu indicates, came from Kashmir or Nepal *via* Tibet. It is another example of a recipe transmitted rather than originated by Tibet. We have tried it with pomegranate juice, the standard Near Eastern concentrate, rather than the whole fruit. It cooks down to what is, essentially, potted meat. The idea is evidently to produce a product that will store, under its oil–and–ghee preserving coating, for a long time. The fumigation of the jar presumably has a sterilizing value. Made with pomegranate juice, and far less oil and ghee, this is a rich, subtle, strongly lamb–flavored food. The Indian ascription is interesting here; asafoetida and pomegranate give a much more Iranian than Indian flavor. There is no Indian spicing here. If this is an Indian dish it represents very strong Iranian influence. This is hardly surprising since at the time northwest Indian food was still Iran–influenced. To what extent the Tibetan transmission of this dish has colored it remains to be seen.

It treats deficiency chill of the primordial storehouse, chill pain of the abdomen, and aching pain along the spinal column.

Mutton (two legs, the head, and a set of hooves), tsaoko cardamoms (four), cinnamon (three *liang*), sprouting ginger (half a *jin*), *kasni* (big as two chickpeas)

Boil ingredients into a soup using one **telir* of water. Pour into a stone top cooking pot. Add a *jin* of pomegranate fruits, two *liang* of black pepper, and a little salt. The pomegranate fruits should be baked using one cup of vegetable oil and a lump of asafoetida the size of a garden pea. Roast [*i.e.*, cook dry ingredients] until a fine yellow in color, slightly black. Remove debris and oil in the soup. Strain clean. Use the smoke produced from roasting *jiaxiang* [*operculum* of *Turbo cornutus* and related spp], Chinese spikenard [*Nardostachys chinensis*], *kasni*, and butter to fumigate a jar.[77] Seal up and store [the *Se-aBru* Soup] as desired.

[50.] Broiled Sheep's Heart[78]

It treats heart energy agitation, and depressed melancholy.

[**41B**] Sheep's heart (one, including major veins), *za'faran* (three *qian*).

[For] ingredients use one shallow cup of attar of roses. Dissolve [the *za'faran*] and take the juice. Add a little salt. Spit the sheep's heart on a spit and broil over the fire. Baste regularly with the [attar–]*za'faran* juice. Continue until the basting juice is gone. If one eats this it pacifies heart *qi*. It makes a person very happy.[79]

[51.] Broiled Sheep's Loins

They treat lumbago due to strain and ocular ache.

Sheep's loins (one pair), *za'faran*.

[For] ingredients use one shallow cup of attar of roses. Dissolve [the *za'faran*] and take the juice. Add a little salt. Spit the sheep's loins on spits and broil over the fire. Baste regularly with the [at-

---

[77] Compare Lao's translation of this passage in Lao 1969: 411.

[78] This and the following are two forms of a purely Arabian recipe. Virtually identical dishes are still eaten in Saudi Arabia today. Such recipes contrast sharply with the Irano–Mesopotamian–based foods comprising most of the other Near Eastern recipes. Recipe #51 is particularly excellent.

[79] We have here a clear case of the influence of Arabic humoral medicine.

tar–]*za'faran* juice. Continue until the basting juice is gone. If eaten it will have great efficacy.

[52.] [42A] Deboned Chicken Morsels[80]

Fat chickens (ten; pluck; clean; cook and cut up. Debone as morsels), juice of sprouting ginger (one *he*), onions (two *liang*; cut up), finely ground ginger (half a *jin*), finely ground Chinese flower pepper (four *liang*), [wheat] flour (two *liang*; make into vermicelli).

[For] the ingredients take the broth used to boil the chickens and fry [cook dry]. Add onions and vinegar. Adjust flavors with juice of sprouting ginger.

[53.] Roasted Quail[81]

Quail (20; cut up into pieces), Chinese radishes (two; cut up), finely ground ginger (four *liang*), sheep's tail (one; cut into *sashuq*–sized pieces), flour (two *liang*; make vermicelli).

[For] ingredients take the broth used to cook the quail and fry [cook dry]. Adjust flavors with onions and vinegar.

[54.] Plate Rabbit

Ingredients: Rabbit (two; cut up into pieces.), Chinese radishes (two cut up), **[42B]** sheep's tail (one; cut into strips.), fine spices (two *qian*).

[For] ingredients use [sesame oil?] and fry.[82] Adjust flavors with onions and vinegar. Add two *liang* of vermicelli. Adjust flavors.

[55.] "Tangut" Lungs[83]

Sheep's lung (one), leeks (six *jin*; take the juice), flour (two *jin*; make into paste), butter (half a *jin*), black pepper (two *liang*), juice

[80] This is a standard Chinese chicken and noodles recipe and is still found in various forms.

[81] Recipes #53–55 are several local Central Asian recipes.

[82] This recipe is hopelessly garbled. Compare the "plate rabbit" in the *CCPYSL* (13, 11b).

[83] This recipe is characteristicly Uighur and still popular today. Compare the more complicated recipe for sheep's lung in Rinjing Dorje, *Food in Tibetan Life* (London, 1985), 87.

of sprouting ginger (two *he*).

[For] ingredients use salt and adjust flavors evenly. Submerge the lungs in water and cook. When done baste with the juice and eat.

[56.] Turmeric[–Colored] Tendon[84]

Sheep's tendon (one; cook.), sheep ribs (two; cut into long chunks), bean paste (one *jin*), white flour (one *jin*), *za'faran* (two *qian*), gardenia nuts [*Gardenia jasminoides*] (five *qian*).

[For] ingredients use salt and spices and adjust flavors. Dip tendon [and sheep rib chunks] in batter [*i.e.*, made from the bean paste, white flour, *za'faran* and gardenia nuts]. Put into vegetable oil and fry.

[57.] [43A] Drum **Qazi*[85]

Mutton (five *jin*; finely cut), sheep's tail (one; finely cut), eggs (15), sprouting ginger (two *qian*), onions (two *liang*; cut up), prepared mandarin orange peel (two *qian*; remove the white), spices (three *qian*).

Flavor ingredients evenly. Put into a sheep's white bowel and cook. When done cut up into drum shapes. Use one *jin* of bean paste, one *jin* of white flour, one *qian* of *za'faran*, three *qian* of gardenia nuts. Take the juice, and apply together to the drum **qazi*. Put into vegetable oil and fry.

[58.] Sheep's Heads Dressed in Flowers[86]

Sheep's heads (three. When cooked, cut up), sheep's loins (four), sheep's stomach and lungs (one set of each; cook. When done, cut

---

84 This is one of the few fried foods in the *YSZY*. It is also the nearest thing, indeed, the only thing even slightly similar, to the grilled and stir–fried meats now called "Mongolian barbecue" in China and in Chinese restaurants elsewhere. It is not much like anything currently served.

85 These spiced fresh lamb sausages, sliced and fried, are perhaps closest to the *mkanik* sausages of modern Lebanon and Syria but have Chinese and Central Asian ingredients and seem another creative Turko–Mongol adaptation. The title implies a "spit" but no "spit" is called for. In this case, unlike some previous recipes, the *qianzi* or early Mandarin *tsʰjɛmtsʐ̩*, Tang Chinese, *tsʰiamtsʐ̩*, is probably a transcription of Turkic *qazi* (Uighur *qezi*).

86 If there is one most distinctive recipe in the *YSZY*, this is it. It seems to express all that is most creative about Sino–Mongol–Turkic cuisine.

up. Debone as morsels. Dye with safflower), sprouting ginger (four *liang*), pickled ginger (two *liang*; cut up each), eggs (five; cut into flower shapes), Chinese radishes (three; cut into flower shapes).

[For] ingredients use a good meat soup and fry. Adjust flavors with onions, salt, and vinegar.

[59.] [43B] Fish Cakes[87]

Large carp (10; remove the skin, bones, head, and tail), sheep's tail (two; mince together into a paste), sprouting ginger (one *liang*; cut up finely), onions (two *liang*; cut up finely), finely ground prepared mandarin orange peel (three *qian*), finely ground black pepper (one *liang*), *kasni* (two *qian*).

[To the] ingredients [other than the carp] add salt. Add to the fish and work meat. Roll into cakes like crossbow bullets. Fry in vegetable oil.

[60.] Cotton Rose–[Petal] Chicken[88]

Chickens (10. When cooked, debone as morsels), sheep's stomach and lungs (each one set; cook; cut up), sprouting ginger (four *liang*; cut up), carrots (10; cut up), eggs (20; fry into omelets. Cut into flower shapes), spinach [true spinach, *Spinacia oleracea*][89]

---

[87] This is another creative recipe. Minced–fish cakes flavored with ginger onion, mandarin peel, and pepper are quite Chinese, but the asafoetida and the rest of the recipe, including the frying, seems more Irano–Mesopotamian. This and the bream recipes in the medical section may be compared with a modern recipe which involves frying a carp in vegetable oil, then stewing it with soy sauce, sugar, yellow rice "wine," and, just before serving, diced ginger, garlic, and vinegar. See People's Medical Publishing House, *The Chinese Way to a Long and Healthy Life* (New York, 1988), 295–6. This dish is said to relieve flatulence, indigestion and heart–burn, and alleviate poor health, coughing and asthma, symptoms not too far from those of the diseases treated by bream and carp soup in the medical section of the *YSZY*. Compare nearly identical Medieval Arab methods of cooking discussed in Heine, 1988: 82–86.

[88] The name of the recipe is apparently primarily due to the flower–shapes of the eggs and the flower–petal appearance assumed by other ingredients after cooking. Like several recipes involving vegetables, cut–up Chinese omelet, and thickening paste, this is a unique, distinctive, subtle, highly flavorful, and wonderfully textured dish, and one without obvious antecedents. The thickening with nut paste is Irano–Mesopotamian, but the rest of the recipe could have various origins.

[89] Spinach is called *bocu[cai]* 波蔟菜 in chapter three, not *qigen[cai]* as here. Perhaps Hu Sihui wishes to indicate here a specifically Western variety of spinach.

and coriander (a garnish), safflower [and] gardenia nuts (dyes), apricot kernel paste (one *jin*).

[For] ingredients use a good meat soup and roast. Adjust flavors with onions and vinegar.

[61.] Meat Cakes[90]

[**44A**] Select mutton (10 *jin*; remove the fat, membrane, and sinew. Mash into a paste), *kasni* (three *qian*), black pepper (two *liang*), long pepper (one *liang*), finely ground coriander (one *liang*).

[For] ingredients use salt. Adjust flavors evenly. Use the fingers to make "cakes." Put into vegetable oil and fry.

[62.] Salt Stomach[91]

Sheep's bitter bowel (Wash clean with water).

Apply salt to ingredient. When it has dried in the wind, put into vegetable oil and fry.

[63.] *Näwälä*[92]

Cooked sheep's thoraxes (two; cut into thin strips), eggs (20; cooked).

[For] ingredients use all kinds of fresh vegetables. Roll up together in bread.

[64.] Turmeric[–Colored] Fish[93]

[**44B**] Carp (10; remove the skin and scales), white flour (two *jin*), bean paste (one *jin*), finely ground coriander (two *liang*).

---

[90] These are *köfte*, Near Eastern meatballs. The spicing indicates an Irano–Mesopotamian relationship. *Köfte* of one sort or another, differing in spicing, exist throughout West and South Asia. This particular recipe produces a delicately spiced and excellent result. They can be grilled or pan–fried like hamburgers, rather than deep–fried in vegetable oil, if one prefers a lower–calorie dish. These are a straightforward kebab which would not attract special notice on a Lebanese meze tray today.

[91] This dish appears to be a Mongol specialty.

[92] This somewhat unclear recipe seems generic Inner Asian, with a Persian name added, perhaps merely for distinction.

[93] This recipe is, like most of the *YSZY* fish dishes, essentially a Chinese contribution.

[For the] ingredients, after making a marinate using salt and spices, marinate fish and fry in vegetable oil. When done, use two *liang* of sprouting ginger (cut into strips), coriander leaves, safflower dye, radish slices, and fry. Adjust flavors with onions.

[65.] Deboned Wild Goose Morsels[94]

Wild geese (five; cook. When done cut up. Debone as morsels), finely ground ginger (half a *jin*).

[For] ingredients use a good meat soup and roast. Adjust flavors with onions and salt.

[66.] Galangal Sauce Hog's Head[95]

Hog's head (two; wash; cut up into chunks), prepared mandarin orange peel (two *qian*; remove the white), lesser galangal (two *qian*), Chinese flower pepper (two *qian*), cinnamon (two *qian*), tsaoko cardamom (five), vegetable oil (one *jin*), honey (half a *jin*).

Boil ingredients together until done. Then add finely ground mustard and roast. Adjust flavors with onions, vinegar and salt.

[67.] [45A] Cattail "Sweet Melon Pickles"[96]

Cleaned mutton (10 *jin*; cook. When done cut up to look like sweet melon pickles), Chinese flower pepper (one *liang*), cattail [rhizome] (half a *jin*).

[For] ingredients use one *liang* of fine spices. Apply evenly with salt.

---

[94] A straightforward game recipe, with a Irano–Mesopotamian refinement. Tough wild geese would need the boiling.

[95] This dish is more Chinese than Near Eastern; Islam largely eliminated hogs from the roster in the latter direction. The mandarin peel, lesser galangal, honey–vinegar combination, and Sichuan pepper remove all doubt, although the honey–mustard combination gives this a flavor more reminiscent of modern American ham–cooking. The boiling into stew is a Mongol touch. In short, this is another highly creative dish, with the characteristic smooth, rich, understated, and subtle flavor that is the hallmark of Hu's, or the Yuan court's, cuisine. A lean, preferably rather bony cut of pork, such as shoulder or leg, can be substituted for hog's head. With a trimmed loin roast, the dish is one of the best in the book.

[96] Another combination recipe: Chinese spices on a Central Asian dish. Perhaps the *guaji* here is another transcription of *qazi*, in this case, of Uighur *qezi*.

[68.] Deboned Sheep's Head Morsels[97]

Sheep's head (five; cook. When done debone as morsels), finely ground ginger (four *liang*), black pepper (one *liang*).

[For] ingredients use a "good meat soup" and roast. Adjust flavors with onions, salt and vinegar.

[69.] Deboned Ox Hoof Morsels (Horse's Hoof, Bear's Paw are entirely the same)

Ox hooves (one set; cook. When done debone as morsels.), finely ground ginger (two *liang*).

[For] ingredients use a good meat soup and roast. Adjust flavors with onions and salt.

[70.] Fine **Chizig*

[**45B**] Mutton (leg; cook. When done cut up finely), Chinese radish (two; cook; cut up finely), sheep's tail (one; cook; cut up), *ka'fur* [Camphor] (two *qian*).

[For] ingredients use a good meat soup and roast. Adjust flavors with onions.

[71.] Liver and Sprouting [Ginger]

Sheep's liver (one; drench in water; cut into fine strips), sprouting ginger (four *liang*; cut into fine strips), Chinese radish (two *liang*; cut into fine strips), basil, smartweed (each two *liang*; cut up into fine strips).

[For] ingredients use salt. Adjust flavors with vinegar and finely ground mustard.

[72.] Horse Stomach Plate[98]

Horse stomach and intestines (one set; cook. When done cut up.), finely ground mustard (half a *jin*).

[For] ingredients, take the white blood irrigating bowel and cut in-

---

97 Recipes #68–75 are a group of minor local recipes.

98 This is a somewhat refined version of the dish called *qarta* by the Kazakhs.

to flower shapes. [Take] the astringent spleen,[99] combine with fat [*i.e.*, suet] and mince as filling. [**46A**] When made into morsels, fry. Adjust flavors with onions, salt, vinegar, and finely ground mustard.

[73.] Scalded **Jasa'a* (a delicacy)

**Jasa'a* (two; unload; make each into a knot), *kasni* (one *qian*), onions (one *liang*; cut up finely).

[For] ingredient use salt and work together with everything else. Fry quickly [scald] in vegetable oil. When done, then use two *qian* of *za'faran* dissolved in water. Add spices. Sprinkle with finely ground coriander.

[74.] Boiled Sheep's Hooves

Ingredients: Sheep's hooves (five hooves; remove the hair and wash; cook until tender; cut up into chunks), finely ground ginger (one *liang*), spices (five *qian*).

[To] ingredient add vermicelli and fry. Adjust flavors with onions, vinegar, and salt.

[75.] Boiled Sheep's Breast

Sheep's breasts (two; remove the hair and wash. Cook until tender. Cut up into *sashuq*–sized pieces), finely ground ginger (two *liang*), spices (five *qian*).

[**46B**] [For] ingredient use a good meat soup. Add flour vermicelli and fry. Adjust flavors with onions and vinegar.

[76.] Fine Fish Hash[100]

Young carp (five; remove the skins, bones, head, and tail), sprouting ginger (two *liang*), Chinese radishes (two), onions (one *liang*), basil and smartweed (cut each into fine strips; mix with saf-

---

[99] According to Li (Hu Sihui, 1988:87) this refers to various greases, fluids, and miscellaneous substances of horse intestines, other than the intestines themselves, and the suet.

[100] Another truly exceptional dish, with both West and East Asian components combined into a creation that bears no close resemblance to anything today. This unique dish defies analysis. It is presumably a Mongol or Turkic localism, elaborated by the court chefs.

flower).

[To] ingredients add finely ground mustard and fry. Adjust flavors with onions, salt and vinegar.

[77.] Red Strips[101]

Sheep's blood combined with white flour (Cook according to recipe), sprouting ginger (four *liang*), Chinese radish (one), basil and smartweed (each one *liang*; cut up into fine strips).

[For] ingredients use salt. Adjust flavors with vinegar and finely ground mustard.

[78.] Roast Wild Goose (Roast Cormorant and Roast Duck are the same)[102]

[**47A**] Wild goose (one; remove the feathers, bowels, and stomach and clean.), sheep's stomach [and attached skin] (one; remove the hair; clean and use to wrap up the wild goose), onions (two *liang*), finely ground coriander (one *liang*).

Use salt and flavor ingredients together [with the onions and ground coriander]. Put into the goose's stomach [put goose into sheep's stomach] and roast.

[79.] Roast Eurasian Curlew

Eurasian curlews (10; pluck; clean), finely ground coriander (one *liang*), onions (ten stalks), spices (five *qian*).

Apply [coriander, onions and spices] uniformly [to] ingredients and roast. One may dress the curlews in a thick flour and steam–roast until done in a cage; this is also possible. One may dress the curlews with liquid butter combined with flour, and brazier cook in a brazier; this is also possible.

---

[101] Blood makes a unique binder for noodles, but blood cooking technology is well developed in China, and Central Asia has it too where Islam has not forbidden such foods.

[102] More local game recipes. Note the similarity of the treatment of the goose in this recipe to Turkic sausage preparation methods, *e.g.*, *qazi*, although here the inspiration is probably Mongolian.

[80.] Willow–Steamed Lamb[103]

A sheep (one; with hair).

[For] ingredient construct a brazier on the ground three *qi* deep. Surround with stones. Heat the stones until red hot. Use a **tabaq* to hold the lamb. On top use willow [branches] to cover and seal with earth. Cook until done.

[81.] [47B] Quick **Manta*[104]

Mutton, mutton fat, onions, sprouting ginger, prepared mandarin orange peel (cut up each finely).

[To] ingredients add spices, salt and sauce, and combine into stuffing.

[82.] Deer Milk Fat[105] **Manta* (One can [also] perhaps make "Quick **Manta*," or perhaps "Thin–skin **Manta*," Both are possible.)

[Dried] deer milk fat, sheep's tail (cut up each into slices like finger nails), sprouting ginger, prepared mandarin orange peel. (Cut up each finely.)

[To] ingredients add spices, and salt, and combine to make stuffing.

[83.] Eggplant **Manta*[106]

[103] A perfectly straightforward pit barbecue, this recipe must go back to the oldest Siberian stratum in the cuisine. It is not significantly different from Native American pit cooking, from Cahuilla barbecue to Mayan *pib*; the Hawaiian *luau* and its many Pacific relatives are also essentially the same. There is probably an ancient relationship with the American forms, perhaps going back to the original crossing of the Bering Strait.

[104] Further recipes of the typical sort, this time for stuffed dumplings.

[105] This is not deer's milk but the fatty part ("milk fat") of a deer udder chopped up and dried as a delicacy. We are thankful to F. Sabban for pointing this out.

[106] Stuffed vegetables are a hallmark of Turkish and neighboring cuisines. The Uzbek magazine *Contact*, 4–6 (1993), for example, included on page 34 a recipe for a *pomidor–manti*, or stuffed tomato. This stuffed eggplant bears a close resemblance to certain contemporary Turkish stuffed eggplant dishes although the mandarin orange peel is a Chinese touch no doubt added by an irrepressible Yuan chef. The recipe demonstrates, once again, the creative union of two or more cuisines that characterizes much of the best recipes in the *YSZY*. It is worth recording that, at a large potluck party involving several *YSZY* recipes and modern dishes, this particular dish dis-

Mutton, sheep's fat, sheep's tail, onions, prepared mandarin orange peel (cut up each finely), "tender" eggplant (remove the pith).

[For] combine ingredients with meats into a stuffing. But [instead of making a dough covering] put it inside the eggplant [skin] and steam. Add garlic, cream [or yogurt *etc.*], finely ground mint [or basil]. Eat.

[84.] Cut Flowers **Manta*[107]

[**48A**] Mutton, sheep's fat, sheep's tail, onions, prepared mandarin orange peel. (Cut up each finely.)

[To] ingredients add, according to recipe, spices, salt and sauce. Make the stuffing. Form the **Manta*. Use scissors to cut out into various flower shapes. Steam. Use safflower to dye the flowers.

[85.] Quartz Horns

Mutton, sheep's fat, sheep's tail, onions, prepared mandarin orange peel, sprouting ginger. (Cut up each finely.)

[To] ingredients add fine spices, salt and sauce and mix [everything] together uniformly. Use bean paste to make skins. Make the horns.

[86.] Butter Skin **Yubqa*

Mutton, sheep's fat, sheep's tail, onions, prepared mandarin orange peel, sprouting ginger. (Cut up each finely. One can perhaps add *jha'uqasu[n]*. This is a kind of lily root.)

[To] ingredients add spices, salt, and sauce and mix [everything] together uniformly. Use vegetable oil, rice flour and [white wheat] flour, combine to make the skins.

[87.] *Päräk* Horns

[**48B**] Mutton, sheep's fat, sheep's tail, young leeks. (Cut up each finely).

---

appeared in record time. This excellent eggplant dish shares with the *Tutum Ash* recipe its mint–garlic–cream sauce, distinctive and excellent.

[107] Several further minor recipes for dumplings. "Horn" is standard modern Chinese for dumpling with pointed ends, like *börek*.

[To] ingredients add spices, salt, and sauce and mix [everything] together uniformly. Use white flour to make the skins. Bake on a flat iron. When done, then use liquid butter and honey. Perhaps one can use pear–shaped bottle gourd meat to make stuffing. This is also possible.

[88.] **Shilön* Horns

Mutton, sheep's fat, sheep's tail, onions, prepared mandarin orange peel, sprouting ginger. (Cut each up finely).

[To] ingredients add spices, salt and sauce and mix [everything] together uniformly. Take white flour, honey and vegetable oil and mix together. Put into boiling water in a cauldron. When cooked make skins.

[89.] *Pleurotus ostreatus* [Mushroom] *Baozi* (Some make them from crab spawn. This is also possible. Wisteria *Baozi* is entirely the same.)

Mutton, sheep's fat, sheep's tail, onions, prepared mandarin orange peel, sprouting ginger. (Cut up each finely), *Pleurotus ortreatus* [mushrooms] (Scald in boiling water. When cooked, clean and cut up finely.)

[**49A**] [To] ingredients add spices, salt, sauce and make stuffing. [Use] white flour to make a thin skin. Steam.

[90.] **Qurim* "Bonnets" [*i.e., boqtas*][108]

---

[108] This recipe combines a thoroughly and unmistakably Irano–Mesopotamian base, lamb with all kinds of nuts (the "pine pollen" surely means the nuts here), with Chinese ingredients such as sprouting ginger, bean paste, Chinese yams, and Chinese omelet, and those Turko–Mongol favorites, internal organs of sheep. The result is made into dumplings steamed in individual cups or steamers, perhaps like the "Lion Heads" of modern North China. The name recalls the great ritual feasts of the Mongolian past and the shapes of the *boqtaq* or high head dresses of Mongolian noble women. The nuts are used in such small quantities that they do not provide any significant taste to the whole. Probably, there was one of each kind of nut per dumpling, possibly on top as an ornament. In spite of its complexity this is a very bland and rather uninteresting dish. In cooking, potatoes can be used for Chinese yams, though potatoes provide too strong and marked a taste to be fully appropriate. Use regular wonton skins instead of bean flour. It is a mystery how bean flour is prepared such that it will hold up as a skin, for steaming, for a large meatball. One possibility is that the balls were

Mutton (three legs; cut up.), sheep's tail (two; cut up.), euryale seeds,[109] (eight *liang*) pine pollen (eight *liang*), *badam* [almonds] (four *liang*), **möög* [mushrooms] (eight *liang*), apricot kernel paste (one *chin*), walnuts (eight *liang*), *pistä* nuts [Pistachio nuts] (four *liang*), safflower (one *liang*), fruit of *Gardenia jasminoides* (four *qian*), vegetable oil (two *jin*), sprouting ginger (eight *liang*), bean paste (four *jin*), Chinese yams (three *jin*), eggs (30), sheep's stomach and lungs (two sets each), [and] [sheep's] bitter bowel (one), onions (four *liang*), vinegar (half a bottle), coriander leaves.

[For] ingredients [except pine pollen juice and the bean paste] use salt. Adjust flavors evenly with sauce and the five spices. Use bean paste to make skins. Steam in cups. Apply pine pollen juice and eat.

[91.] [49B] Poppy Seed Buns[110]

White flour (five jin), cow's milk (two *sheng*), liquid butter (one *jin*), poppy seeds (one *liang*. Slightly roasted).

[For] ingredients use salt and a little soda and combine with the flour. Make the buns.

[92.] Cow's Milk Buns

White flour (five *jin*), cow's milk (two *sheng*), liquid butter (one *jin*), fennel (one *liang*. Slightly roasted).

[For] ingredients use salt and a little soda and combine with the flour. Make the buns.

[93.] **Chuqmin* (same as "long bread")

White flour (ten *jin*), vegetable oil (one *jin*), Chinese flower pepper (one *liang*; roast and discard the juice), fennel (one *liang*; roast).

---

dipped in a thick bean–flour batter. It is possible that the reference is to washed bean starch made into flat sheets, like modern bean starch noodles.

109 This could also be the pulp of *Polygonatum* spp, traditionally gathered by the Mongols as a starch.

110 Needless to say, pastries of this sort are staples of Middle Eastern cooks even today. The use of cow's milk in this recipe is clear indication that "little black seeds" are poppy seeds, and not black cumin. Black cumin is used on breads, not in them. These buns are indistinguishable from ordinary poppy seed buns of today.

[Mix] ingredients and keep overnight. Use leaven, salt, soda and warm water. Combine this with flour [dough]. The next day add flour to thicken. Combine again into a dough. Divide each *jin* [of dough] into two loaves. Put into a *chong* and steam.

[94.] [50A] *Borbi*[*n*] Soup (this is the *piteng* bone [*i.e.*, knee joint] of a sheep.)

It is good for *xulao* diseases of men and women, cold–evil attack emaciation, insufficiency of *yin qi*. It benefits blood and pulse, and increases vital [healthy] energy.[111]

Borbi[*n*] (30 or 40; clean with water).

Boil ingredient in one **telir* of water. It will boil down to one–fourth. Strain clean, remove oil and the sediment and let coagulate again. If one wishes to eat, eat as much as desired.

[95.] *Miqan–u kö[n]lesün*[112]

It treats the five kinds of impairments and, the seven kinds of wounds, deficiency chill of organ *qi*. If taken regularly it supplements the center, and increases *qi*.

One sheep's rear leg (remove tendons and membrane; cut up and pulverize).

[For] ingredient use a clean cooking pot. Cook by dry scorching. Make sure the top is airtight and does not allow *qi* [*i.e.*, air] to pass. Afterwards use a clean cloth, knot up tightly and take the juice.

[111] Not to be confused with *jingqi* 精氣, "vital *qi*."

[112] An informant, Chung Chih–hui, notes that Taiwan Daoists use the same method in preparing dog meat today. We are grateful to Ms. Chung for pointing this fact out to us. It may indicate some alchemical connections for this type of cooking, although purely Mongolian roots are possible as well.

JUAN 2

* * *

CHINESE TEXT

忽思慧
飲膳正要卷二

四部叢刊續編子部: 1A-14A, 15A-18A, 19A-39B, 40B, 41B-51B

中國古代版畫叢刊: 14B, 18B, 40A, 41A

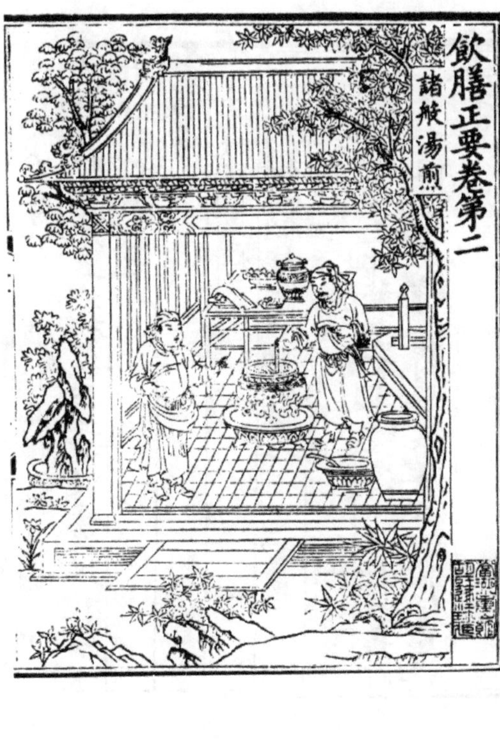

1A
Various
Soups

1B

諸般湯煎

桂漿

生津止渴益氣和中去濕逐飲

生薑三斤取汁 熟水二斗 赤茯苓三兩去皮為末 桂三兩去皮為末

麴末半斤 杏仁一百個湯洗去皮尖生研為泥 大麥蘖半兩為末

白沙蜜三斤煉淨

右用前藥蜜水拌和勻入淨磁礶內油紙封口數重泥固濟冰窖內放三日方熟綿濾冰浸暑月飲之

桂沉漿

去濕逐飲生津止渴順氣

2A

紫蘇葉一兩剉 沉香三錢剉 烏梅一兩取肉 沙糖六兩

右件四味用水五六椀熬至三椀濾去滓入桂漿一升合和作漿飲之

荔枝膏

生津止渴去煩

烏梅半斤取肉 桂一十兩去皮剉 沙糖二十六兩 麝香半錢研

生薑汁五兩 熟蜜一十四兩

右用水一斗五升熬至一半濾去滓下沙糖生薑汁再熬去柤澄定少時入麝香攪勻澄清如常任意服

梅子丸

2B

生津止渴解化酒毒去濕

烏梅一兩半取肉 白梅一兩半取肉 乾木瓜一兩半

紫蘇葉一兩半 甘草一兩炙 檀香二錢 麝香一錢研

右為末入麝香和勻沙糖為丸如彈大每服一丸噙化

五味子湯代葡萄酒飲

生津止渴暖精益氣

北五味一斤淨肉 紫蘇葉六兩 人參四兩去蘆剉 沙糖二斤

右件用水二斗熬至一斗濾去滓澄清任意服之

人參湯代酒飲

3A

順氣開胷膈止渴生津

新羅參四兩去蘆剉 橘皮一兩去白 紫蘇葉二兩

沙糖一斤

右件用水二斗熬至一斗去滓澄清任意飲之

仙朮湯

去一切不正之氣溫脾胃進飲食辟瘟疫除寒濕

蒼朮一斤米泔浸三日竹刀子切片焙乾為末 茴香二兩炒為末

甘草二兩炒為末 白麵一斤炒 乾棗二升焙乾為末 鹽四兩炒

右件一同和勻每日空心白湯點服

杏霜湯

3B

調順肺氣利胷膈治欬嗽
粟米五升炒為麵 杏仁二升去皮尖麸炒研 鹽三兩炒
右件拌匀每日空心白湯調一錢入酥少許尤佳
山藥湯
補虛益氣溫中潤肺
山藥一斤煮熟 粟米半升炒為麵 杏仁二斤炒令過熟去皮尖切如米
右件每日空心白湯調二錢入酥油少許山藥任意
四和湯
治腹內冷痛脾胃不和
白麵一斤炒 芝麻一斤炒 茴香二兩炒 鹽一兩炒

4A

右件並為末每日空心白湯點服
棗薑湯
和脾胃進飲食
生薑一斤切作片 棗三升去核炒 甘草二兩炒 鹽二兩炒
右件為末一處拌匀每日空心白湯點服
茴香湯
治元藏虛弱臍腹冷痛
茴香一斤炒 川楝子半斤 陳皮半斤去白 甘草四兩炒
鹽半斤炒
右件為細末相和匀每日空心白湯點服

4B

破氣湯
治元蔵虛弱腹痛胷膈閉悶
杏仁一斤去皮尖麸炒別研 茴香四兩炒 良薑一兩
蓽澄茄二兩 陳皮二兩去白 桂花半斤 薑黃一兩
木香一兩 丁香一兩 甘草半斤 塩半斤
右件為細末空心白湯點服
白梅湯
治中熱五心煩燥霍亂嘔吐乾渴津液不通
白梅肉一斤 白檀四兩 甘草四兩 塩半斤
右件為細末每服一錢入生薑汁少許白湯調下

5A

木瓜湯
治脚氣不仁膝勞冷痺疼痛
木瓜內箇蒸熟去皮研爛如泥 白沙蜜二斤煉淨
右件二味調和勻入淨磁器內盛之空心白湯點服
橘皮醒醒湯
治酒醉不解嘔噫吞酸
香橙皮一斤去白 陳橘皮一斤去白 檀香四兩 葛花半斤
菉荳花半斤 人參二兩去蘆 白荳蔻仁二兩
鹽六兩炒
右件為細末每日空心白湯點服

5B

渴忒餅兒

生津止渴治嗽

渴忒一兩二錢 新羅參一兩去蘆 菖蒲一錢各為細末

白納八三兩研係沙糖

右件將渴忒用葡萄酒化成膏和上項藥末令勻為

劑印作餅每用一餅徐徐噙化

官桂渴忒餅兒

生津止寒嗽

官桂二錢為末 渴忒一兩二錢 新羅參一兩二錢去蘆為末

白納八三兩研

6A

右件將渴忒用玫瑰水化成膏和藥末為劑用訶子

油印作餅子每用一餅徐徐噙化

荅必納餅兒

清頭目利咽膈生津止渴治嗽

荅必納二錢為末即草龍膽 新羅參一兩二錢去蘆為末 白納八五兩研

右件用赤赤哈納即北地酸角兒熬成膏和藥末為劑印作

餅兒每用一餅徐徐噙化

橙香餅兒

寬中順氣清利頭目

新橙皮一兩焙去白 沉香五錢 白檀五錢 縮砂五錢

6B

白荳蔻仁五錢 蓽澄茄三錢 南鵬砂三錢別研
龍腦二錢別研 麝香二錢別研
右件爲細末甘草膏和劑印餅每用一餅徐徐噙化
牛髓膏子
補精髓壯筋骨和血氣延年益壽
黄精膏五兩 地黄膏三兩 天門冬膏一兩
牛骨頭内取油二兩
右件将黄精膏地黄膏天門冬膏與牛骨油一同不
住手用銀匙攪令冷定和匀成膏每日空心温酒調
一匙頭

7A

木瓜煎
木瓜十箇去皮穰取汁熬水盡 白沙糖十斤煉淨
右件一同再熬成煎
香圓煎
香圓二十箇去皮取肉 白沙糖十斤煉淨
右件一同再熬成煎
株子煎
株子一百箇取淨肉 白沙糖五斤煉淨
右件同熬成煎
紫蘇煎

7B

紫蘇葉五斤 乾木瓜五斤 白沙糖十斤煉淨

右件一同熬成煎

金橘煎

金橘五十箇去子取皮 白沙糖三斤

右件一同熬成煎

櫻桃煎

櫻桃五十斤取汁 白沙糖二十五斤 同熬成煎

桃煎

大桃一百箇去皮切片取汁 白沙蜜二十斤煉淨

右件一同熬成煎

8A

石榴漿

石榴子十斤取汁 白沙糖十斤煉淨

右件一同熬成煎

小石榴煎

小石榴二斗蒸熟去子研為泥 白沙蜜十斤煉淨

右件一同熬成煎

五味子舍兒別

新北五味十斤去子水浸取汁 白沙糖八斤煉淨

右件一同熬成煎

赤赤哈納係酸刺

8B

赤赤哈納不以多少水浸取汁

右件用銀石器內熬成膏

松子油

松子不以多少去皮搗研為泥

右件水絞取汁熬成取浮清油綿濾淨再熬澄清

杏子油

杏子不以多少連皮搗碎

右件水煮熬取浮油綿濾淨再熬成油

酥油

牛乳中取浮凝熬而為酥

9A

醍醐油

取上等酥油約重千斤之上者煎熬過濾淨用大磁甕貯之冬月取甕中心不凍者謂之醍醐

馬思哥油

取淨牛妳子不住手用阿赤係打油木器也打取浮凝者為馬思哥油今亦云白酥油

枸杞茶

枸杞五斗水淘洗淨去浮麥焙乾用白布筒淨去蒂蕚黒色選揀紅熟者先用雀舌茶展溲碾子茶芽不用次碾枸杞為細末每日空心用

9B

匙頭入酥油攪匀温酒調下白湯亦可忌與酪同食

玉磨茶

上等紫筍五十斤篩筒淨　蘇門炒米五十斤

篩筒淨一同拌和匀入玉磨内磨之成茶

金字茶

係江南湖州造進末茶

范殿帥茶

係江浙慶元路造進茶芽味色絕勝諸茶

紫筍雀舌茶

選新嫩芽蒸過為紫筍有先春次春探春味皆

10A

不及紫筍雀舌

女須兒出直北地面味温甘　西番茶出本土味苦澀煎用酥油

川茶　藤茶　夸茶皆出四川　燕尾茶出江浙江西

孩兒茶出廣南　温桑茶出黑峪

凡諸茶味甘苦微寒無毒去痰熱止渴利小便

消食下氣清神少睡

清茶

先用水滚過濾淨下茶芽少時煎成

炒茶

用鐵鍋燒赤以馬思哥油牛妳子茶芽同炒成

10B

蘭膏 玉磨末茶三匙頭麵酥油同攪成膏沸湯點之

酥簽 金字末茶兩匙頭入酥油同攪沸湯點之

建湯 玉磨末茶一匙入碗內研勻百沸湯點之

香茶 白茶一袋 龍腦成片者三錢
百藥煎半錢 麝香二錢 同研細用香粳米
熬成粥和成劑印作餅

11A

泉水 甘平無毒治消渴反胃熱痢今西山有玉泉水甘
美味勝諸泉

井華水 甘平無毒主人九竅大驚出血以水噀面即住及
洗人目瞖投酒醋中令不損敗平旦汲者是也今
內府御用之水常於鄒店取之緣自至大初
武宗皇帝幸柳林飛放請
皇太后同往觀焉由是道經鄒店因渴思茶遂
命普蘭奚國公金界奴朶兒只煎造公親詣諸井

11B

選水惟一井水味頗清甘汲取煎茶以進
上稱其茶味特異
內府常進之茶味色兩絕乃
命國公於井所建觀音堂蓋亭井上以欄翼之刻
石紀其事自後
御用之水日必取焉所造湯茶比諸水殊勝隣左有
井皆不及也此水煎熬過澄瑩如一常較其分兩
與別水增重

12A
Doses of Immortals

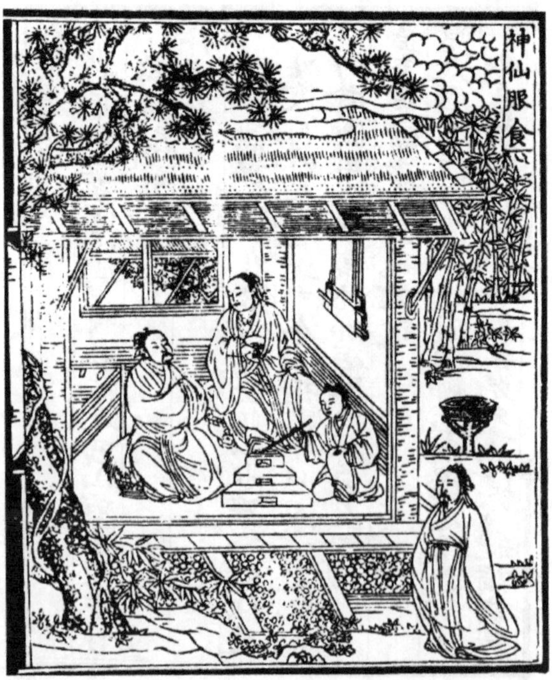

12B

神仙服食

鐵甕先生瓊玉膏

此膏填精補髓腸化為筋萬神具足五藏盈溢髓血滿髮白變黑返老還童行如奔馬日進數服終日不食亦不飢開通強志日誦萬言神識高邁夜無夢想人年二十七歲以前服此一料可壽三百六十歲四十五歲以前服者可壽二百四十歲六十三歲以前服者可壽一百二十歲六十四歲以上服者可壽百歲服之十劑絕其慾修陰功成地仙矣一料分五處可救五人癱疾分十處可救十

13A

人勞疾修合之時沐浴至心勿輕示人

新羅參二十四兩去蘆　生地黃一十六斤汁

白茯苓四十九兩去黑皮　白沙蜜一十斤煉淨

右件人參茯苓為細末蜜用生絹濾過地黃取自然汁搗時不用銅鐵器取汁盡去滓用藥一處拌和勻入銀石器或好磁器內封用淨紙二三十重封閉入湯內以桑柴火煑三晝夜取出用蠟紙數重包瓶口入井口去火毒一伏時取出再入舊湯內煑一日出水氣取出開封取三匙作三盞祭天地百神焚香設拜至誠端心每日空心酒調一匙頭

13B

地仙煎
治腰膝疼痛一切腹内冷病令人顏色悅澤骨髓
堅固行及奔馬
山藥一斤 杏仁一升湯泡去皮尖 生牛妳子二升
右件將杏仁研細入牛妳子山藥拌絞取汁用新磁
瓶密封湯煑一日每日空心酒調一匙頭
金髓煎
延年益壽塡精補髓久服髮白變黑返老還童
枸杞不以多少採紅熟者
右用無灰酒浸之冬六日夏三日於沙盆内研令爛

14A

細然後以布袋絞取汁與前浸酒一同慢火熬成膏
於淨磁器内封貯重湯煑之每服一匙頭入酥油少
許溫酒調下
天門冬膏
去積聚風痰癲疾三蟲伏尸除瘟疫輕身益氣令
人不飢延年不老
天門冬不以多少去皮去根鬚洗淨
右件擣碎布絞取汁澄清濾過用磁器沙鍋或銀器
慢火熬成膏每服一匙頭空心溫酒調下
道書八帝經

14B

欲不畏寒服天門冬茯苓為末服之每日頻服大
寒時汗出單衣
抱朴子云
杜紫微服天門冬御八十妾有子一百四十人日
行三百里
列仙子云
赤松子食天門冬齒落更生細髮復出
神仙傳
甘始者太原人服天門冬在人間三百年
修真秘旨

15A

神仙服天門冬一百日後怡泰和顏羸劣者強三
百日身輕三年身走如飛
抱朴子云
楚文子服地黃八年夜視有光手上車弩
抱朴子云
南陽文氏值亂逃於壺山飢困有人教之食术遂
不飢數年乃還鄉里顏色更少氣力轉勝
藥經云
必欲長生當服山精是蒼术也
抱朴子云

15B

任季子服茯苓一十八年玉女從之能隱彰不食
穀面生光
孫真人枕中記
茯苓久服百日百病除二百日夜晝二服後役使
鬼神四年後玉女來侍
抱朴子云
陵陽仲子服遠志二十年有子三十人開書所見
便記不忘
東華真人煑石經
舜常登蒼梧山曰厥金玉香草即五加也服之延

16A

年故云寧得一把五加不用金玉滿車寧得一斤
地榆安用明月寶珠昔魯定公母單服五加皮酒
以致長生如張子聲楊始建王叔才于世彥等皆
古人服五加皮酒而房室不絕皆壽三百歲有子
三二十人世世有服五加皮酒而獲年壽者甚衆
抱朴子云
趙他子服桂二十年足下毛生日行五百里力舉
千斤
列仙傳
偓佺食松子能飛行健走如奔馬

16B

神仙傳
松子不以多少研為膏空心温酒調下一匙頭日
三服則不飢渴久服日行五百里身輕體健
神仙傳
治百節疼痛久風虛脚痺痛松節釀酒服之神驗
神仙傳
槐實於牛膽中漬浸百日陰乾每日吞一枚十日
身輕二十日白髮再黑百日通神
食療云
枸杞葉能令人筋骨壯除風補益去虛勞益陽事

17A

春夏秋採葉冬採子可久食之
太清諸本草
七月七日採蓮花七分八月八日採蓮根八分九
月九日採蓮子九分陰乾食之令人不老
食療云
如腎氣虛弱取生栗子不以多少令風乾之每日
空心細嚼之三五箇徐徐嚥之
神仙服黃精成地仙
昔臨川有士人虐其婢婢乃逃入山中久之見野
草枝葉可愛即拔取食之甚美自是常食之久而

17B

不飢遂輕𢖍夜息大木下聞草動以為虎懼而上
木避之及曉下平地其身豁然淩空而去或自一
峯之頂若飛鳥焉數歲其家採薪見之告其主使
捕之不得一日遇絶壁下以網三面圍之俄而騰
上山頂其主異之或曰此婢安有仙風道骨不過
靈藥服食遂以酒饌五味香美置往来之路觀其
食否果来食之遂不能遠去擒之問以述其故所
指食之草即黄精也謹按黄精寛中益氣補五藏
調良肌肉充實骨體堅強筋骨延年不老顏色鮮
明髮白再黑齒落更生

18A
Spirit
Pillow

神枕法
漢武帝東巡泰山下見老翁鋤於道背上有白光
高數尺帝怪而問之有道術否老翁對曰臣昔年
八十五時衰老垂死頭白齒落有道士者教臣服
棗飲水絶穀并作神枕法中有三十二物内二十
四物善以當二十四氣其八物毒以應八風臣行
轉少黑髮更生墮齒復出日行三百里臣今年一
百八十矣不能棄世入山顧戀子孫復還食穀又
已二十餘年猶得神枕之力往不復老武帝視老
翁顏狀當如五十許人驗問其隣人皆云信然帝

18B

乃從授其方作枕而不能隨其絕穀飲水也
神枕方
用五月五日七月七日取山林柏以爲枕長一尺
二寸高四寸空中容一斗二升以柏心赤者爲蓋
厚二分蓋致之令密又使可開閉也又鑽蓋上爲
三行每行四十九孔凡一百四十七孔令容粟大
用下項藥
芎藭 當歸 白芷 辛夷
杜衡 白朮 藁本 木蘭
蜀椒 桂 乾薑 防風

19A

人參 桔梗 白薇 荊實
肉蓯蓉 飛廉 柏實 薏苡仁
款冬花 白衡 秦椒 蘪蕪
凡二十四物以應二十四氣
烏頭 附子 藜蘆 皁角
莽草 凡石 半夏 細辛
八物毒者以應八風
右三十二物各一兩皆㕮咀以毒藥上安之滿枕中
用囊以衣枕百日面有光澤一年體中諸疾一一皆
愈而身盡香四年白髮變黑齒落重生耳目聰明神

19B

方驗秘不傳非人也武帝以問東方朔荅云昔女廉
以此傳玉青玉青以傳廣成子廣成子以傳黃帝近
者穀城道士淳于公枕此藥枕百餘歲而頭髮不白
夫病之來皆從陽脉起今枕藥枕風邪不得侵人矣
又雖以布囊衣枕猶當復以幃囊重包之須欲卧時
乃脫去之耳詔賜老翁疋帛老翁不受曰臣之於君
猶子之於父也子知道以上之於父義不受賞又臣
非賣道者以陛下好善故進此耳帝止而更賜諸藥

神仙服食

菖蒲尋九節者窨乾百日為末日三服久服聰明

20A

耳目延年益壽

神仙服食

胡麻食之能除一切痼疾久服長生肥健人延年
不老

抱朴子

服五味十六年面色如玉入火不灼入水不濡

抱朴子云

韓聚服菖蒲十三年身上生毛日誦萬言冬袒不
寒須得石上生者一寸九節紫花尤善

食醫心鏡

20B

藕實味甘平無毒補中養氣清神除百病久服令
人止渴悅澤
日華子云
蓮子并石蓮去心久食令人心喜益氣止渴治腰
痛泄精瀉痢
日華子云
蓮花蘂久服鎮心益色駐顏輕身
日華子云
何首烏味甘無毒久服壯筋骨益精髓黑髭鬓令
人有子

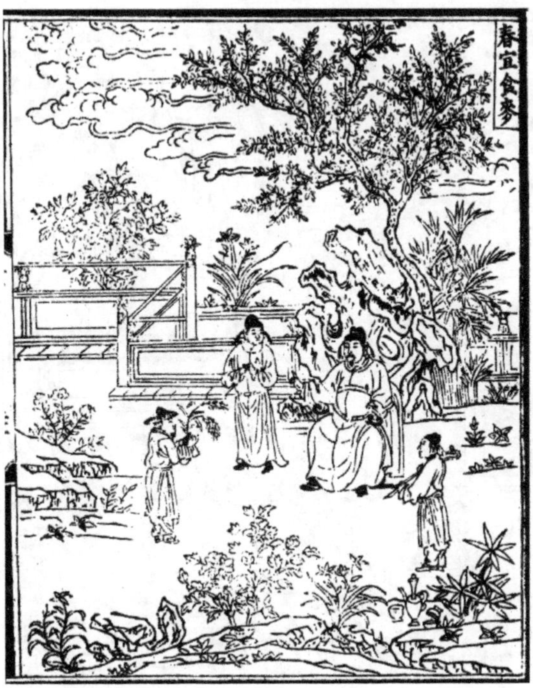

21A
Four
Seasons:
Spring

21B

四時所宜

春三月此謂發陳天地俱生萬物以榮夜卧早起廣步於庭被髮緩形以使志生生而勿殺予而勿奪賞而勿罰此春氣之應養生之道也逆之則傷肝夏為寒變奉長者少

春氣温宜食麥以凉之不可一於温也禁温飲食及熱衣服

22A
Summer

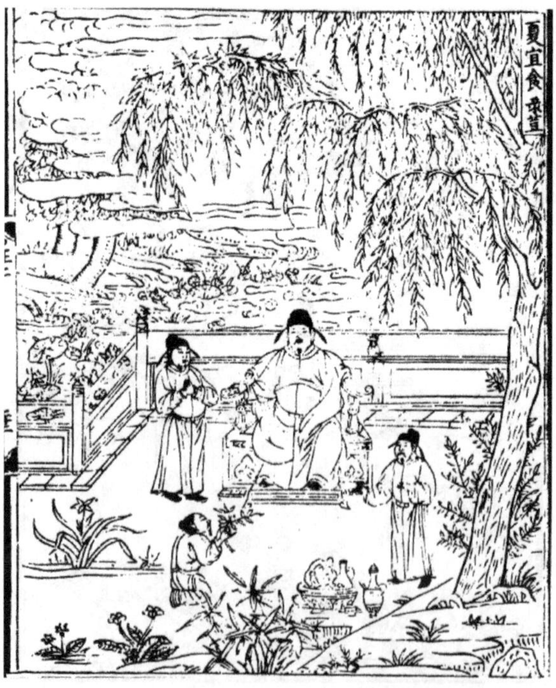

22B

夏三月此謂蕃秀天地氣交萬物華實夜卧早起無
厭於日使志無怒使華英成秀使氣得泄若所愛在
外此夏氣之應養長之道也逆之則傷心秋為痎瘧
奉收者少冬至重病
夏氣熱宜食菽以寒之不可一於熱也禁温飲食飽
食濕地濡衣服

23A
Autumn

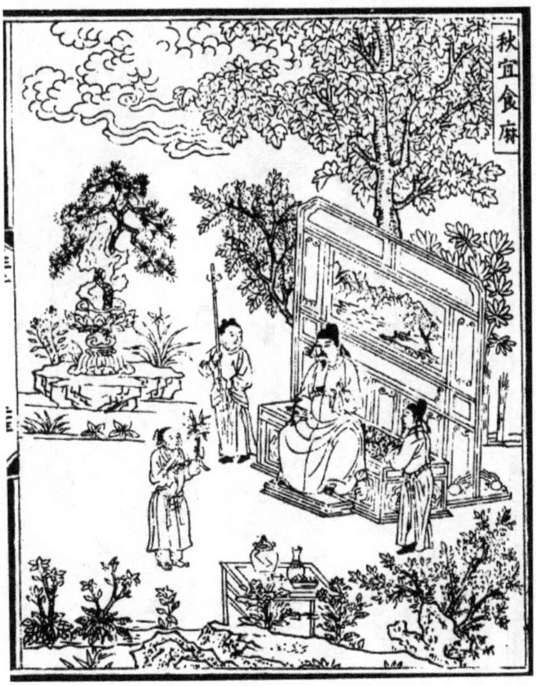

23B

秋三月此謂容平天氣以急地氣以明早卧早起與
雞俱興使志安寧以緩秋形收斂神氣使秋氣平無
外其志使肺氣清此秋氣之應養收之道也逆之則
傷肺冬為飧泄奉藏者少
秋氣燥宜食麻以潤其燥禁寒飲食寒衣服

24A
Winter

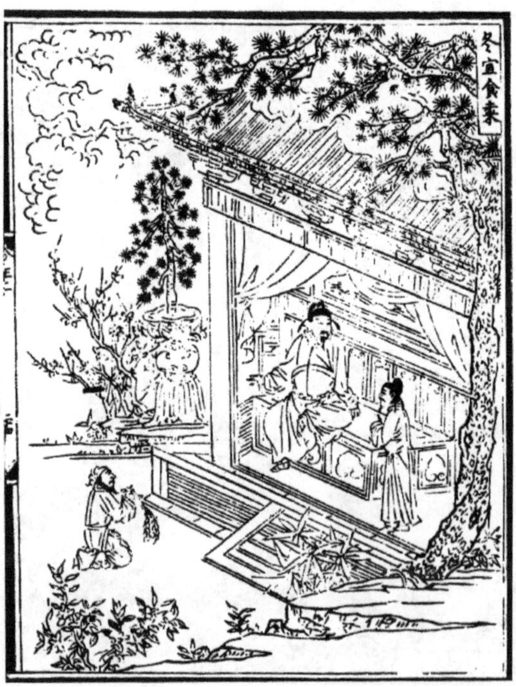

24B

冬三月此謂閉藏水氷地坼無擾乎陽早卧晚起必
待日光使志若伏若匿若有私意若已有得去寒就
温無泄皮膚使氣亟奪此冬氣之應養藏之道也逆
之則傷腎春為痿厥奉生者少
冬氣寒宜食黍以熱性治其寒禁熱飲食温炙衣服

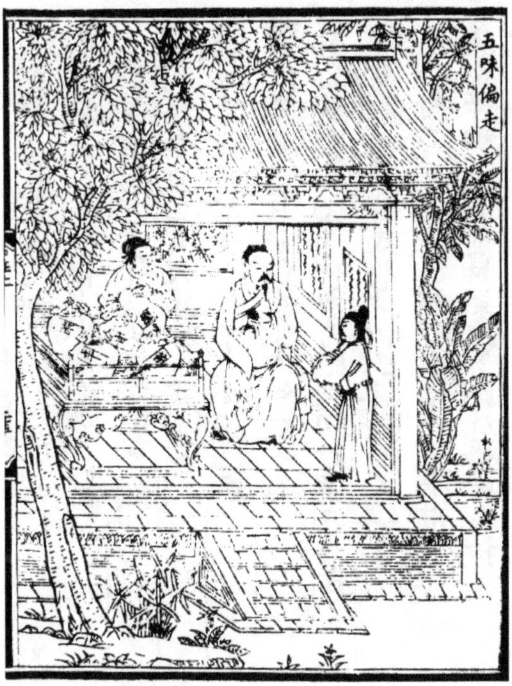

25A
Five
Flavors

25B

五味偏走

酸澀以收多食則膀胱不利爲癃閉
苦燥以堅多食則三焦閉塞爲嘔吐
辛味薰蒸多食則上走於肺榮衛不時而心洞
鹹味湧泄多食則外注於脉胃竭咽燥而病渴
甘味弱劣多食則胃柔緩而虫過故中滿而心悶
辛走氣氣病勿多食辛
鹹走血血病勿多食鹹
苦走骨骨病勿多食苦
甘走肉肉病勿多食甘

26A

酸走筋筋病勿多食酸
肝病禁食辛宜食粳米牛肉葵棗之類
心病禁食鹹宜食小荳犬肉李韭之類
脾病禁食酸宜食大荳豕肉栗藿之類
肺病禁食苦宜食小麥羊肉杏薤之類
腎病禁食甘宜食黄黍雞肉桃葱之類
多食酸肝氣以津脾氣乃絶則肉胝䐢而唇揭
多食鹹骨氣勞短肥氣折則脉凝泣而變色
多食甘心氣喘滿色黑腎氣不平則骨痛而髮落
多食苦脾氣不濡胃氣乃厚則皮槁而毛拔

26B

多食辛筋脉沮弛精神乃央則筋急而爪枯
五穀為食○五菓為助○五肉為益○五菜為充
氣味合和而食之則補精益氣
雖然五味調和食飲口嗜皆不可多也多者生疾少
者為益百味珎饌日有慎節是為上矣

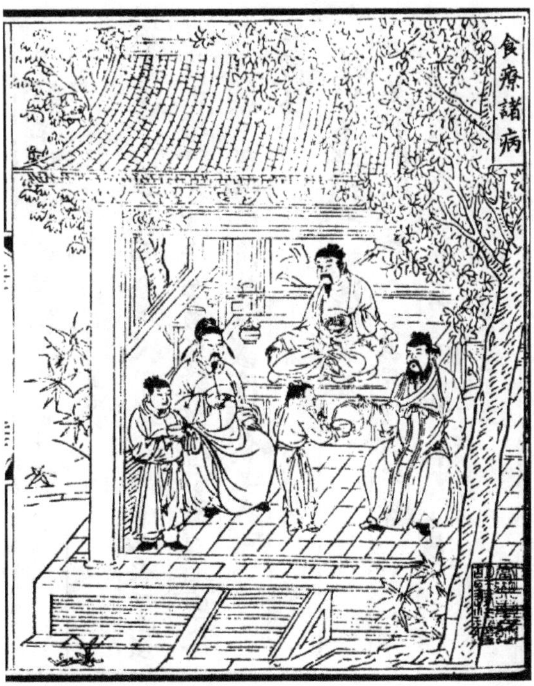

27A Medicinal Foods

27B

食療諸病

生地黄雞

治腰背疼痛骨髓虛損不能久立身重氣乏盜汗少食時復吐利

生地黄半斤 飴糖五兩 烏雞一枚

右三味先將雞去毛腸肚淨細切地黄與糖相和勻内雞腹中以銅器中放之復置甑中蒸炊飯熟成取食之不用鹽醋唯食肉盡却飲汁

羊蜜膏

治虛勞腰痛欬嗽肺痿骨蒸

28A

熟羊脂五兩 熟羊髓五兩 白沙蜜五兩煉淨

生姜汁一合 生黄地汁五合

右五味先以羊脂煎令沸次下羊髓又令沸次下蜜地黄生薑汁不住手攪微火熬數沸成膏每日空心温酒調一匙頭或作羹湯或作粥食之亦可

羊藏羹

治腎虛勞損骨髓傷敗

羊肝肚腎心肺各一具湯洗淨 牛酥一兩

胡椒一兩 蓽撥一兩 豉一合 陳皮二錢去白

良薑二錢 草菓兩箇 葱五莖

28B

右件先將羊肝等慢火煑令熟將汁濾淨和羊肝等幷藥一同入羊肚內縫合口令絹袋盛之再煑熟入五味旋旋任意食之

羊骨粥

治虛勞腰膝無力

羊骨一付全者搥碎 陳皮二錢去白 良薑二錢

草菓二箇 生薑一兩 塩少許

右水三斗慢火熬成汁濾出澄清如常作粥或作羹湯亦可

羊脊骨羹

29A

治下元久虛腰腎傷敗

羊脊骨一具全者搥碎 肉蓯蓉一兩洗切作片

草果三箇 蓽撥二錢

右件水熬成汁濾去滓入葱白五味作麵羹食之

白羊腎羹

治虛勞陽道衰敗腰膝無力

白羊腎二具切作片 肉蓯蓉一兩酒浸切

羊脂四兩切作片 胡椒二錢 陳皮一錢去白 蓽撥二錢

草果二錢

右件相和入葱白塩醬煑作湯入麵餺子如常作羹

29B

食之

猪腎粥

治腎虛勞損腰膝無力疼痛

猪腎一對去脂膜切 粳米三合 草果二錢

陳皮一錢去白 縮砂二錢

右件先将猪腎陳皮等煮成汁濾去滓入酒少許次下米成粥空心食之

枸杞羊腎粥

治陽氣衰敗腰脚疼痛五勞七傷

枸杞葉一斤 羊腎二對細切 葱白一莖

30A

羊肉半斤炒

右四味拌匀入五味煮成汁下米熬成粥空腹食之

鹿腎羹

治腎虛耳聾

鹿腎一對去脂膜切

右件於豆豉中入粳米三合煮粥或作羹入五味空心食之

羊肉羹

治腎虛衰弱腰脚無力

羊肉半斤細切 蘿蔔一箇切作片 草果一錢

30B

陳皮一錢去白 良薑一錢 蓽撥一錢 胡椒一錢

葱白三莖

右件水熬成汁入鹽醬熬湯下麵餜子作羹食之將

湯澄清作粥食之亦可

鹿蹄湯

治諸風虛腰脚疼痛不能踐地

鹿蹄四隻 陳皮二錢 草果二錢

右件煮令爛熟取肉入五味空腹食之

鹿角酒

治卒患腰痛暫轉不得

31A

鹿角新者長二三寸燒令赤

右件內酒中浸二宿空心飲之立效

黑牛髓煎

治腎虛弱骨傷敗瘦弱無力

黑牛髓半斤 生地黃汁半斤 白沙蜜半斤煉去蠟

右三味和勻煎成膏空心酒調服之

猯肉湯

治虛弱五藏邪氣

猯肉五斤煬洗淨 草果五箇 硇砂二錢 葱一握

陳皮一錢去白 良薑二錢 哈昔泥一錢即阿魏

31B

右件水一斗煮熟去草菓等次下胡椒二錢薑黄一錢醋五味調和勻空心食之

烏鷄湯

治虚弱勞傷心腹邪氣

烏雄鷄一隻撏洗淨切作塊子 陳皮一錢去白 良薑一錢

胡椒二錢 草菓二箇

右件以葱醋醬相和入瓶内封口令煮熟空腹食

醍醐酒

治虚弱去風濕

醍醐一盞

32A

右件以酒一盃和勻溫飲之效驗

山藥飥

治諸虚五勞七傷心腹冷痛骨髓傷敗

羊骨五七塊帶肉 蘿蔔一枚切作大片 葱白一莖

草果五箇 陳皮一錢去白 良薑一錢 胡椒二錢

硇砂二錢 山藥二斤

右件同煮取汁澄清濾去粗麵二斤山藥二斤煮熟研泥搜麵作飥入五味空腹食之

山藥粥

治虚勞骨蒸久冷

32B

羊肉一斤去脂膜爛煑熟研泥 山藥一斤煑熟研泥

右件肉湯內下米三合煑粥空腹食之

酸棗粥

治虛勞心煩不得睡卧

酸棗仁一椀

右用水絞取汁下米三合煑粥空腹食之

生地黃粥

治虛弱骨蒸四肢無力漸漸羸瘦心煩不得睡卧

生地黃汁一合 酸棗仁水絞取汁二盞

右件水煑同熬數沸次下米三合煑粥空腹食之

33A

椒麵羹

治脾胃虛弱久患冷氣心腹結痛嘔吐不能下食

川椒三錢炒為末 白麵四兩

右件同和勻入塩少許於豆豉作麵條煑羹食之

蓽撥粥

治脾胃虛弱心腹冷氣疞痛妨悶不能食

蓽撥一兩 胡椒一兩 桂五錢

右三味為末每用三錢水三大碗入豉半合同煑令熟去滓下米三合作粥空服食之

良薑粥

33B

治心腹冷痛積聚停飲

高良薑半兩為末 粳米三合

右件水三大椀煎高良薑至二椀去滓下米煮粥食之效驗

吳茱萸粥

治心腹冷氣衝脇肋痛

吳茱萸半兩水洗去涎焙乾炒為末

右件以米三合一同作粥空腹食之

牛肉脯

治脾胃久冷不思飲食

34A

牛肉五斤去脂膜切作大片 胡椒五錢 蓽撥五錢

陳皮二錢去白 草果二錢 縮砂二錢 良薑二錢

右件為細末生薑汁五合葱汁一合塩四兩同肉拌勻淹二日取出焙乾作脯任意食之

蓮子粥

治心志不寧補中強志聰明耳目

蓮子一升去心

右件煮熟研如泥與粳米三合作粥空腹食之

雞頭粥

治精氣不足強志明耳目

34B

雞頭實三合

右件煮熟研如泥與粳米一合煮粥食之

雞頭粉羹

治濕痺腰膝痛除暴疾益精氣強心志耳目聰明

雞頭磨成粉 羊脊骨一付帶肉熬取汁

右件用生薑汁一合入五味調和空心食之

桃仁粥

治心腹痛上氣咳嗽胷膈妨滿喘急

桃仁三兩湯煮熟去尖皮研

右件取汁和粳米同煮粥空腹食之

35A

生地黃粥

治虛勞瘦弱骨蒸寒熱往來咳嗽唾血

生地黃汁二合

右件煮白粥臨熟時入地黃汁攪匀空腹食之

鯽魚羹

治脾胃虛弱泄痢久不瘥者食之立效

大鯽魚二斤 大蒜兩塊 胡椒二錢 小椒二錢

陳皮二錢 縮砂二錢 蓽撥二錢

右件葱醬塩料物蒜入魚肚內煎熟作羹五味調和令匀空心食之

35B

炒黃麵

治泄痢腸胃不固

白麵一斤炒令焦黃

右件每日空心温水調一匙頭

乳餅麵

治脾胃虛弱赤白泄痢

乳餅一箇切作豆子樣

右件用麵拌煑熟空腹食之

炙黃鷄

治脾胃虛弱下痢

36A

黃雌雞 隻撏淨

右以鹽醬醋茴香小椒末同拌勻刷雞上令炭火炙乾焦空腹食之

牛妳子煎蓽撥法

貞觀中太宗苦於痢疾衆醫不効問左右能治愈者當重賞時有術士進此方用牛妳子煎蓽撥服之立瘥

猯肉羹

治水腫浮氣腹脹小便澀少

猯肉一斤細切 葱一握 草果三箇

36B

右件用小椒豆豉同煑爛熟入粳米一合作羹五味調匀空腹食之

黃鴨鷄

治腹中水癖水腫

黃鴨鷄一隻挦淨 草果二錢 赤小豆一升

右件同煑熟空心食之

青鴨羹

治十腫水病不瘥

青頭鴨一隻退淨 草果五箇

右件用赤小豆半升入鴨腹内煑熟五味調空心食

37A

蘿蔔粥

治消渴舌焦口乾小便數

大蘿蔔五箇煑熟絞取汁

右件用粳米三合同水并汁煑粥食之

野鷄羹

治消渴口乾小便頻數

野雞一隻挦淨

右入五味如常法作羹臛食之

鵓鴿羹

治消渴飲水無度

37B

白鵓鴿一隻切作大片

右件用土蘇一同煮熟空腹食之

鷄子黄

治小便不通

鷄子黄一枚生用

右件服之不過三服熟亦可食

葵菜羹

治小便癃閉不通

葵菜葉不以多少洗擇淨

右煮作羹入五味空腹食之

38A

鯉魚湯

治消渇水腫黄疸脚氣

大鯉魚一頭 赤小豆一合 陳皮二錢去白

小椒二錢 草果二錢

右件入五味調和匀煮熟空腹食之

馬齒菜粥

治脚氣頭面水腫心腹脹滿小便淋澀

馬齒菜洗淨取汁

右件和粳米同煮粥空腹食之

小麥粥

38B

治消渴口乾

小麥淘淨不以多少

右以煮粥或炊作飯空腹食之

驢頭羹

治中風頭眩手足無力筋骨煩痛言語蹇澀

烏驢頭一枚撏洗淨　胡椒二錢　草果二錢

右件煮令爛熟入豆豉汁中五味調和空腹食之

驢肉湯

治風狂憂愁不樂安心氣

烏驢肉不以多少切

39A

右件於豆豉中爛煮熟入五味空心食之

狐肉羹

治驚風癲癇神情恍惚言語錯謬歌笑無度

狐肉不以多少及五臟

右件如常法入五味煮令爛熟空心食之

熊肉羹

治諸風脚氣痹痛不仁五緩筋急

熊肉一斤

右件於豆豉中入五味葱醬煮熟空腹食之

烏鷄酒

39B

治中風背強舌直不得語目睛不轉煩熱

烏雌雞一隻撏洗淨去腸肚

右件以酒五升煮取酒二升去滓分作三服相繼服
之汁盡無時爇葱白生薑粥投之蓋覆取汁

羊肚羹

治諸中風

羊肚一枚洗淨 粳米二合 葱白數莖 豉半合

蜀椒去目閉口者炒出汗三十粒 生薑二錢半細切

右六味拌匀入羊肚內爛煮熟五味調和空心食之

葛粉羹

40A

治中風心脾風熱言語蹇澀精神昏憒手足不遂

葛粉半斤搗取粉四兩 荊芥穗一兩 豉三合

右三味先以水煮荊芥豉六七沸去滓取汁次將葛
粉作索麵於汁中煮熟空腹食之

荊芥粥

治中風言語蹇澀精神昏憒口面喎斜

荊芥穗一兩 薄荷葉一兩 豉三合 白粟米三合

右件以水四升煮取三升去滓下米煮粥空腹食之

麻子粥

治中風五藏風熱語言蹇澀手足不遂大腸滯澀

40B

冬麻子二兩炒去皮研 白粟米三合 薄荷葉一兩

荆芥穗一兩

右件水三升煮薄荷荆芥去滓取汁入麻子仁同煮

粥空腹食之

惡實菜即牛蒡子又名鼠粘子

治中風燥熱口乾手足不遂及皮膚熱瘡

惡實菜葉嫩肥者 酥油

右件以湯煮惡實葉三五升取出以新水淘過布絞

取汁入五味酥點食之

烏驢皮湯

41A

治中風手足不遂骨節煩疼心燥口眼面目喎斜

烏驢皮一張燖洗淨

右件蒸熟細切如條於豉汁中入五味調和勻煮過

空心食之

羊頭膾

治中風頭眩羸瘦手足無力

白羊頭一枚燖洗淨

右件蒸令爛熟細切以五味汁調和膾空腹食之

野豬臛

治久痔野雞病下血不止肛門腫滿

41B

野猪肉二斤細切

右件煮令爛熟入五味空心食之

獺肝羹

治久痔下血不止

獺肝一付

右件煮熟入五味空腹食之

鯽魚羹

治久痔腸風大便常有血

大鯽魚一頭新鮮者洗淨切作片 小椒二錢為末 草果一錢為末

右件用葱三莖煮熟入五味空腹食之

42A
When Taking Drugs

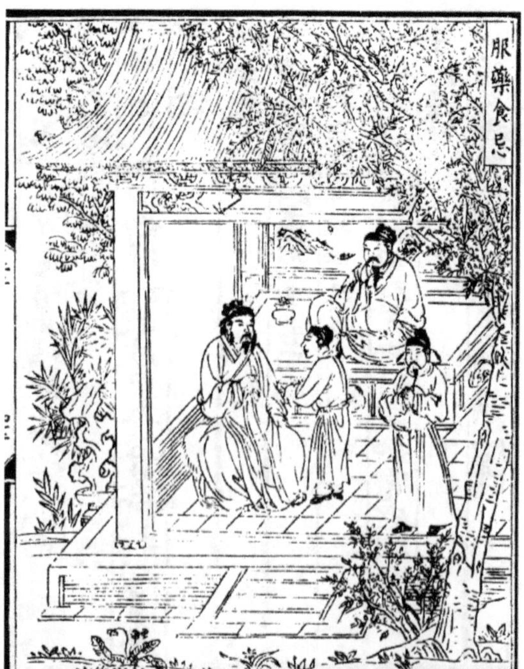

42B

服藥食忌

但服藥不可多食生芫荽及蒜雜生菜諸滑物肥猪肉犬肉油膩物魚膾腥羶等物及忌見喪尸產婦淹穢之事又不可食陳臭之物

有朮勿食桃李雀肉胡荽蒜青魚等物

有藜蘆勿食狸肉

有巴豆勿食蘆笋及野猪肉

有黃連桔梗勿食猪肉

有地黃勿食蕪荑

有半夏菖蒲勿食飴糖及羊肉

43A

有細辛勿食生菜

有甘草勿食菘菜海藻

有牡丹勿食生胡荽

有商陸勿食犬肉

有常山勿食生葱生菜

有空青朱砂勿食血 凡服藥通忌食血

有茯苓勿食醋

有鱉甲勿食莧菜

有天門冬勿食鯉魚

凡久服藥通忌

43B

未不服藥又忌滿日
正五九月忌巳日
二六十月忌寅日
三七十一月忌亥日
四八十二月忌申日

44A
Benefits
and
Harm

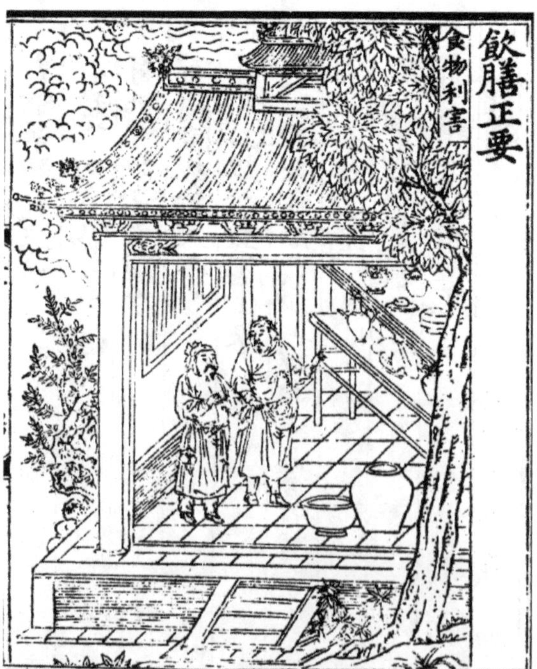

44B

食物利害

蓋食物有利害者可知而避之

麵有䴵氣不可食　生料色臭不可用
漿老而飯溲不可食　煮肉不變色不可食
諸肉非宰殺者勿食　諸肉臭敗者不可食
諸腦不可食　凡祭肉自動者不可食
猪羊疫死者不可食　曝肉不乾者不可食
馬肝牛肝皆不可食　兔合眼不可食
燒肉不可用桑柴火　獐鹿麋四月至七月勿食
二月內勿食兔肉　諸肉脯忌米中貯之有毒

45A

魚餒者不可食　羊肝有孔者不可食
諸鳥自閉口者勿食　蟹八月後可食餘月勿食
鰕不可多食無鬚及腹下丹黃之白者皆不可食
臘月脯腊之屬或經雨漏所漬虫鼠嚙殘者勿食
海味糟藏之屬或經濕熱變損日月過久者勿食
六月七月勿食鴈　鯉魚頭不可食毒在腦中
諸肝青者不可食　五月勿食鹿傷神
九月勿食犬肉傷神　十月勿食熊肉傷神
不時者不可食　諸果核未成者不可食
諸果落地者不可食　諸果虫傷者不可食

45B

桃杏雙仁者不可食　蓮子不去心食之成霍亂
甜瓜雙蒂者不可食　諸瓜沉水者不可食
蘑菇勿多食發病　榆仁不可多食令人瞑
菜着霜者不可食　櫻桃勿多食令人發風
葱不可多食令人虛　芫荽勿多食令人多忘
竹笋勿多食發病　木耳赤色者不可食
三月勿食蒜昏人目　二月勿食蓼發病
九月勿食着霜瓜　四月勿食胡荽生狐臭
十月勿食椒傷人心　五月勿食韮昏人五藏

46A
Food
Conflicts

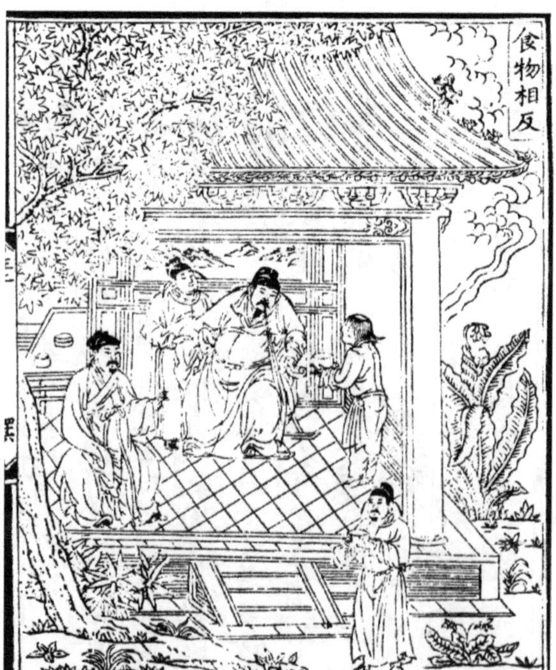

46B

食物相反

蓋食不欲雜雜則或有所犯知者分而避之

馬肉不可與倉米同食

馬肉不可與蒼耳薑同食

猪肉不可與牛肉同食

羊肝不可與椒同食傷心

兎肉不可與薑同食成霍亂

羊肝不可與猪肉同食

牛肉不可與栗子同食

羊肚不可與小豆梅子同食傷人

47A

羊肉不可與魚膾酪同食

猪肉不可與芫荽同食爛人腸

馬妳子不可與魚膾同食生癥瘕

鹿肉不可與鮠魚同食

麋鹿不可與鰕同食　麋肉脂不可與梅李同食

牛肝不可與鮎魚同食生風

牛腸不可與犬肉同食

鷄肉不可與魚汁同食生癥瘕

鵪鶉肉不可與猪肉同食面生黒

鵪鶉肉不可與菌子同食發痔

47B

野鷄不可與蕎麵同食生虫
野鷄不可與胡桃蘑菰同食
野鷄卵不可與葱同食生虫
雀肉不可與李同食　鷄子不可與鼈肉同食
鷄子不可與生葱蒜同食損氣
鷄肉不可與兎肉同食令人泄瀉
野鷄不可與鯽魚同食
鴨肉不可與鼈肉同食
野鷄不可與猪肝同食
鯉魚不可與犬肉同食

48A

野雞不可與鮎魚同食食之令人生癩疾
鯽魚不可與糖同食　鯽魚不可與猪肉同食
黄魚不可與蕎麵同食
蝦不可與猪肉同食損精
蝦不可與糖同食　蝦不可與鷄肉同食
大豆黄不可與猪肉同食
粟米不可與葵菜同食發病
小豆不可與鯉魚同食
楊梅不可與生葱同食
柹梨不可與蟹同食　李子不可與鷄子同食

48B

棗不可與蜜同食　李子菱角不可與蜜同食
葵菜不可與糖同食　生葱不可與蜜同食
萵苣不可與酪同食　竹笋不可與糖同食
蓼不可與魚膾同食　莧菜不可與鼈肉同食
韮不可與酒同食　苦苣不可與蜜同食
莚不可與牛肉同食生癥瘕
芥末不可與兔肉同食生瘡

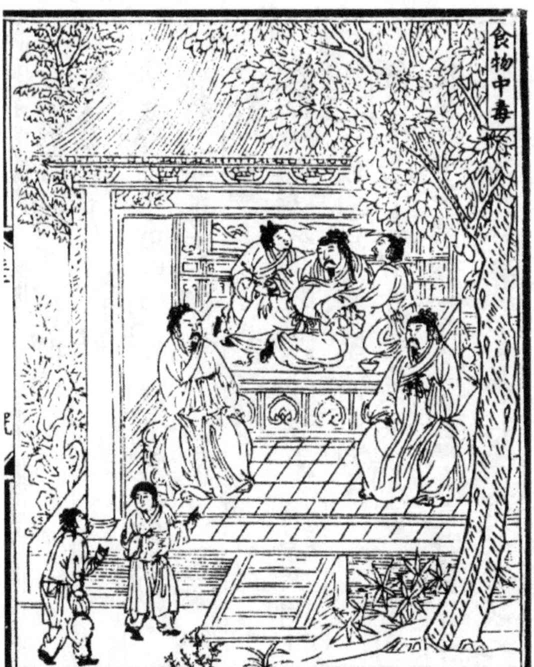

49A
Poisons
In Food

49B

食物中毒

諸物品類有根性本毒者有無毒而食物成毒者有雜合相畏相惡相反成毒者人不戒慎而食之致傷腑臟和亂腸胃之氣或輕或重各隨其毒而爲害隨毒而解之

如飲食後不知記何物毒心煩滿悶者急煎苦參汁飲令吐出或煑犀角汁飲之或苦酒好酒煑飲皆良

食菜物中毒取鷄糞燒灰水調服之或甘草汁或煑葛根汁飲之胡粉水調服亦可

50A

食瓜過多腹脹食塩即消

食蘑菰菌子毒地漿水解之

食菱角過多腹脹滿悶可暖酒和薑飲之即消

食野山芋毒土漿解之

食豚中毒煑粟穰汁飲之即解

食諸雜肉毒及馬肝漏脯中毒者燒猪骨灰調服或芫荽汁飲之或生韮汁亦可

食牛羊肉中毒煎甘草汁飲之

食馬肉中毒嚼杏仁即消或蘆根汁及好酒皆可

食犬肉不消成䐜脹口乾杏仁去皮尖水煑飲之

50B

食魚膾過多成蟲瘕大黃汁陳皮末同塩湯服之
食蟹中毒飲紫蘇汁或冬瓜汁或生藕汁解之乾
蒜汁蘆根汁亦可
食魚中毒陳皮汁蘆根及大黃大豆朴消汁皆可
食鴨子中毒煑秫米汁解之
食鷄子中毒可飲醇酒醋解之
飲酒大醉不解大豆汁葛花椹子柑子皮汁皆可
食牛肉中毒猪脂煉油一兩每服一匙頭温水調
下即解
食猪肉中毒飲大黃汁或杏仁汁朴消汁皆可解

51A
Animal Transformations

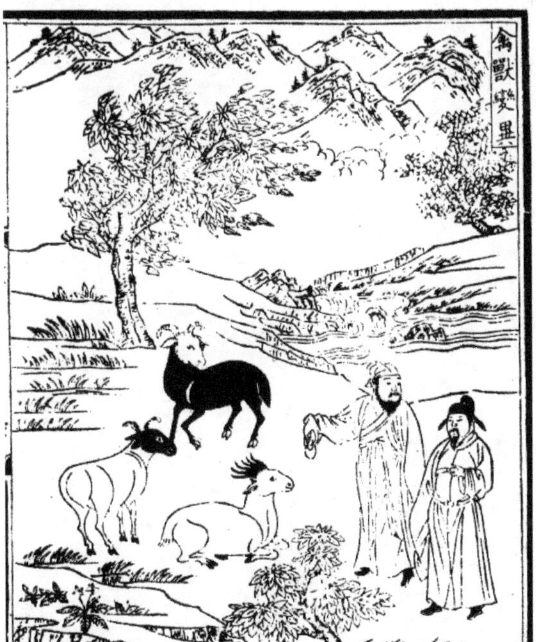

51B

禽獸變異

禽獸形類依本體生者猶分其性質有毒無毒者况異像變生豈無毒乎倘不慎口致生疾病是不察矣

獸岐尾　馬蹄夜目　羊心有孔　肝有青黑

鹿豹文　羊肝有孔　黑雞白首　白馬青蹄

羊獨角　白羊黑頭　黑羊白頭　白鳥黃首

羊六角　白馬黑頭　鷄有四距　曝肉不燥

馬生角　牛肝葉孤　蟹有獨螯　魚有眼睫

蝦無鬚　肉入水動　肉經宿暖　魚無腸膽腮

肉落地不沾土　魚目開合及腹下丹

JUAN 2

* * *

TRANSLATION

[*Juan* Two]

[1A] [Illustration Caption:] Various Hot Beverages and Concentrates[1]

Various Hot Beverages and Concentrates:

[1B] [96.] Cassia[2] Syrup

It produces saliva and stops thirst, augments *qi*, and harmonizes the center. It eliminates dampness and expels retention of fluid. Sprouting ginger (three *jin*; take the juice), boiled water (two *dou*), red China root (three *liang*; remove skin and make a fine powder), cassia (three *liang*; remove skin and make a fine powder), finely ground yeast (half a *jin*), apricot kernels (100 nuts; blanch in boiling water, and remove the skin and tips; grind fresh to make a mash), malted wheat (half a *jin*; make into a powder), crystallized honey (three *jin*; refine).

[For] ingredients, use the aforementioned medicinals, the honey and the water and combine together evenly. Put into a clean crockery pot. Close up the mouth with several layers of oiled paper and seal well with mud. [Allow to ferment, when fermentation is finished] leave for three days in an ice cellar and it will be ready. [To drink] strain with floss silk. Put the [strained] slush into water. Drink during the hot months.

[97.] Cassia-Garuwood Syrup

---

[1] This selection of recipes for drinks, syrups, and electuaries combines Chinese medical formulations, all fairly simple ones, with Near Eastern jams, conserves, and sweet syrups. The recipes are self-explanatory. Most are soothing and tonic. Presumably that was what the courtiers felt they needed.

[2] Cassia: mistranslated "cinnamon," is the bark of *Cinnamomum cassia*, native to southern China and a very common Chinese spice. Cinnamon is *C. zeylanicum* of Sri Lanka. Its taste and appearance is distinct and the traditional medical values quite different. The volatile oils of cassia and cinnamon are different too.

It eliminates dampness and expels retention of fluid. It brings forth saliva, controls thirst and accords *qi*.

[**2A**] Purple perilla[3] leaves [*Perilla frutescens* var. *crispa*] (one *liang*; cut up), garuwood (three *qian*; cut up), black Chinese apricots (one *liang*; take the meat), granulated sugar (six *liang*).

[For] the four ingredients use five or six bowls of water. Boil down to three bowls. Strain and remove the dregs. Add one *sheng* of Cassia Syrup. Combine into a syrup and drink.

[98.] Lichee[4] Paste

It brings forth saliva, controls thirst and gets rid of irritation.

Black Chinese apricots (half a *jin*; take the meat), cassia (10 *liang*; remove the skin and cut up), crude granulated sugar (26 *liang*), musk deer musk (one-half *qian*; grind up), juice of sprouting ginger (five *liang*), cooked honey (14 *liang*).

[For] ingredients [*i.e.*, black Chinese apricots and cassia] use one *dou*, five *sheng* of water. Boil down to half. Strain, remove dregs. Add the crude granulated sugar, and the juice of sprouting ginger. Boil again and get rid of the sediment. After it has become clear and settled for a short time, add the musk deer musk and mix together evenly. Allow to settle completely. Drink on a regular basis as desired.

[99.] Oriental Flowering Apricot [*Prunus mume*][5] Pellet

---

[3] Perilla (*Perilla frutescens* = *P. ocimoides*): *zisu* 紫蘇, "purple fresh," is a small purple annual herb with edible spinach-like leaves and small oil-rich seeds. Perilla leaves are still an important food and medicine in East Asia. The oil contains slight amounts of a poison that damages the lungs, but was a major oil in early East Asia. Leaves and seeds have both been held to have high medicinal value. The plant is common and well known in China, Japan, and Korea. The leaves are often pickled, stir-fried, roasted, or otherwise prepared. They form a common accompaniment to meat and other foods. Hu discusses several species, and considers the major cultivated one to be *P. maxima,* and regards the name *P. frutescens* as a synonym of a separate cultivated species, *P. crispa*. Most authors combine these as *P. frutescens.*

[4] No lichees are used in this recipe. It is a northern imitation of the real thing.

[5] Flowering apricot: The oriental flowering apricot is usually mistranslated "plum" or "gage" or "greengage" in Western Sinological literature although botanists and nursery men use the correct term. The oriental flowering apricot is similar to the Western apricot (*Prunus armeniaca*) but bears smaller, sour fruits. It is part of a subgenus that is very different from that of the plums within the vast and diverse genus *Prunus,* while the greengage is a variety of European plum, bearing no resemblance to

[**2B**] It brings forth saliva and controls thirst. It counteracts and transforms liquor poisons, and gets rid of dampness.

Black [i.e. fresh] oriental flowering apricots (one and one-half *liang;* take the meat), salted oriental flowering apricots (one and one-half *liang*; take the meat), dried Chinese quinces (one and one-half *liang*; finely ground), purple perilla leaves (one and one-half *liang*), liquorice[6] (one *liang*; heat dry), sandalwood (three *qian*), musk deer musk (one *qian;* grind up).

Make a fine powder of ingredients. Add the musk deer musk and combine evenly. [Use] crude granulated sugar and make into a pellet as large as a crossbow pellet. Whenever one consumes a pellet, let dissolve in the mouth.

[100.] Red Currant Puree (Drink in Place of Grape Wine)

It brings forth saliva and controls thirst. It warms the essence and augments *qi*.

Red currants ["northern schisandra"][7] (one *jin*; clean the meat), purple perilla leaves (six *liang)*, ginseng (four *liang*; remove the green shoots and cut up), crude granulated sugar (two *jin*).

---

the *mei*. Plums abound in China, and the confusion caused by this misidentification is far from trivial. There is no reason not to borrow Chinese *mei* as a good English word. The *mei* is the most popular Chinese flower. It blooms in January or February, often with snow on its branches. The flowers are large, range from white through pink to reddish, and are strongly carnation-scented. They even flavor the snow lying on them. It is melted for brewing tea by connoisseurs. The tree's indifference to weather makes it a symbol for the Daoist, and the sage. It is also long-lived and resilient, embodying those qualities in symbolism. The flowers, like those of the peach, also symbolize fertility and sex; venereal disease is politely "*mei* sickness." Of more concern here is the sour fruit. It is an excellent relish or snack when pickled. It can be salted and dried, often with flavorings such as liquorice, or it is pickled in brine, producing *suanmei* 酸梅, "sour *mei*." It is also made into a syrup. All of these have medicinal values, focally cooling and useful in "bringing down *qi*" and otherwise doing what the *YSZY* says they do. The flavorings contribute their own values; liquorice, for example, is harmonizing and soothing. The syrup often figures in Chinese medicinal compounds. See E. N. Anderson, "Flowering Apricot: Environmental Practice, Folk Religion, and Daoism," in N. J. Girardot, James Miller, and Liu Xiaogan, eds., *Daoism and Ecology: Ways within Cosmic Landscape* (Cambridge, MA, 2001), 157-84.

[6] Liquorice: important plant of the bean family, native to north China. It is the great harmonizer, emollient, evener-out, and soother of side effects in Chinese medicine, but dangerous in large quantities. It is a Mongol gathered plant (*shikher üvs*).

[7] This "northern schisandra" is the "red currant," a common Mongolian gathered food. The same Mongolian name also applies to the fruit of *Schisandra chinensis*.

[For] ingredients use two *dou* of water. Boil down to one *dou*. Strain and remove dregs. Let clear. Drink when one likes.

[101.] Ginseng Puree (Drink in Place of Liquor)

[3A] It accords the *qi*, opens the diaphragm, controls thirst and brings forth saliva.

Korean ginseng (four *liang*; remove green shoots and cut up), prepared mandarin orange peel (one *liang*; remove the white), purple perilla leaves (two *liang*), crude granulated sugar (one *jin*).

[For] ingredients use two *dou* of water. Boil down to one *dou*. Remove the dregs. Let clear. Drink when one likes.

[102.] Immortal's Tsangshu [*Atractylodes chinensis* and other *A.* spp] [Seed] Puree

It gets rid of all *qi* that is not proper. It warms spleen and stomach before a meal and promotes the digestion of drink and food. It wards off pestilence and eliminates cold-wetness evil.

Tsangshu (one *jin* of seeds; soak for three days, slice with a bamboo knife. Dry over a fire and make into a fine powder), fennel (two *liang*; roast and make into a fine powder), liquorice (two *liang*; roast and make into a fine powder), white flour (one *jin*; roast), dried jujubes (two *sheng*; dry over a fire and make into a fine powder), salt (four *liang*; roast).

Mix ingredients together evenly. Take a little each day on an empty stomach in boiling water.

[103.] Apricot Frost Puree

[3B] It harmonizes and accords lung *qi*, benefits the diaphragm, and cures coughing.

Millet grains (five *sheng*; roast. Make a flour), apricot kernels (two *sheng*; remove the skin, tips and bran. Roast and grind up), salt (three *liang*; roast).

Mix ingredients together evenly. Take two *qian* dissolved in boiling water each day on an empty stomach. Add a little cream.[8] It is all the better.

---

[8] The text says "cheese" but cream is apparently meant in the following recipe.

[104.] Chinese Yam [*Dioscorea opposita*][9] Puree

It augments for deficiency, increases *qi*, warms the center and moistens the lungs.

Chinese yams (one *jin*; cook until done), millet grains (half a *sheng*; roast. Make a flour), apricot kernels (two *jin*; roast until overdone. Remove the skin and tips. Cut up into grains).

Take two *qian* of ingredients [*i.e.*, millet grains and apricot kernels] dissolved in boiling water each day on an empty stomach. Add a little liquid butter, and [the cooked] Chinese yams to taste.

[105.] "Four Harmonies Puree"

It cures chill pain of the abdomen, and disharmony of spleen and stomach.

White flour (one *jin*; roast), sesame [seeds] (one *jin*; roast), fennel (two *liang*; roast), salt (one *liang*; roast).

[**4A**] Make all ingredients into a fine powder. Take a little each day on an empty stomach in boiling water.

[106.] Jujube [*Zizyphus jujuba* and other *Z.* spp][10] and Ginger Puree

---

[9] Chinese yam: *shanyao*, "mountain medicine," referring to any wild or semi-wild *Dioscorea* species of China. They are of various health values, but much sought after as a drug of the superior class. A large number of pharmacologically active compounds has been isolated from yams by modern biochemistry. Yams are nourishing as well as being valued for medical conditions. Related yams are important foods in Japan and worldwide. And old name for Chinese yam is *shuyu* 薯蕷.

Dioscorea is the genus of true yams, vines of the lily family. In the United States, the word "yam" is used for large sweet-potatoes, and other roots are called "yam" in other areas. The word "yam" is borrowed from a west African word for *Dioscorea* spp.

[10] Jujubes: several species of *Zizyphus* occur in China. *Z. sinensis* (= *Z. vulgaris*) is in cultivation, while *jujuba* is wild. There may be no valid difference between the two. The jujube fruit resembles the date, and is usually called "Chinese date" in English. The Chinese, in turn, call the date "foreign jujube," although the two trees are unrelated. The jujube is a genus within the buckthorn or mountain-lilac family and grows almost anywhere in the drier, but not desert parts of China. Jujube trees vary from small thorny bushes to medium-sized trees. Wild ones are the common scrub of desolate, eroded hills. Domesticated ones are the common door yard trees of the poorer households. Jujube trees are resistant to heat and drought, heavy rain, *etc.*, but ENA was once told in China that air pollution has damaged urban trees. Jujubes grow fast and sucker profusely. They soon reach bearing age, at which time they bear vast quantities of fruit ranging from 1 inch to 3 inches or more in length. Fruits may be red, brown or, specially, black. The fruit is a good source of vitamin C value and also has

It accords the stomach and promotes digestion of drink and food.

Sprouting ginger (one *jin*; cut into slices), jujubes (three *jin*; remove the pith; roast), liquorice (two *liang*; roast), salt (two *liang*; roast).

Make a fine powder of ingredients. Combine all ingredients together evenly. Take a little in boiling water each day on an empty stomach.

[107.] Fennel Puree

It cures asthenia of the store of primary energies, and chill pain of the middle abdomen.

Fennel (one *jin*; roast), Sichuan pagoda tree [*Melia toosendan*] fruits (one-half *jin*), prepared mandarin orange peel (one-half *jin*; remove the white), liquorice (four *liang*; roast), salt (one-half *jin*; roast).

---

some iron and other nutrients. Jujubes are recognized throughout China as a tonic food. In the North, jujubes may be the only source of vitamin C for the poor in many a North Chinese winter. Jujubes are also a valuable iron supplement when other sources fail, though its iron content is barely enough to be of help. Brown and, more especially, black jujubes are thought to build the body; red ones to build blood; sympathetic magic is obvious here. They are very commonly used as strengthening foods for convalescents, new mothers, and children. Gruel with jujubes is a traditional weaning food in poor families. It was often the only one. Jujubes are usually dried. They dry on the tree, without human intervention, and are often candied, sugared or cooked in honey and then dried. Sometimes they are repeatedly cooked and dried in honey or syrup till they become totally impregnated. These preserves may be flavored with liquorice or other healthful ingredients. Paste and syrup are made from jujubes. Cultivars are often thornless, forming a variety split off as *Jujub inermis* in the *ZYDCD*. Jujube wood is very hard and close-grained and is used for special purposes such as wood blocks for printing.

The jujube is of immense potential for world cultivation. Easiest to grow of all temperate-zone fruits and more nutritious than many of them, it is incomparably valuable for erosion control and reforestation as well as food. No household within its range need be without it, and it would be a uniquely valuable source of food and potential income for peasants in dry, rocky areas where little else grows. Several other species exist in many parts of the Old World, adapted to various local environments. Many superior cultivars of Chinese and other species are grown locally. We can think of no explanation for their small popularity outside North China, where they are by far the commonest fruit tree. The most likely explanation is that the true date has pre-empted the Western market. Jujubes are more nourishing than dates, and are not so sickly-sweet as sweet dates nor so dry and tough as "bread" dates.

Make ingredients into a fine powder. Combine together evenly. Each day take a little in boiling water on an empty stomach.

[4B] [108.] Puree for Stagnant *Qi*

It cures asthenia of the store of primary energies, abdomen pain, and obstructed listlessness of the diaphragm.

Apricot kernels (one *jin*; remove the skin, tips and bran; roast and grind up separately), fennel (four *liang*; roast), lesser galangal (one *liang*), cubebs [*Litsea cubeba*][11] (two *liang*; remove the white), prepared mandarin orange peel (two *liang*; remove the white), kueihua [*Osmanthus fragrans*] flowers (one-half *jin*), turmeric[12] (one *liang*), *muxiang* [root of *Vladimiria souliei* or *Saussurea lappa*] (one *liang*), liquorice (one-half *jin*), salt (one half *jin*).

Make a fine powder of ingredients. Take a little in boiling water on an empty stomach.

[109.] Oriental Flowering Apricot [*Prunus mume*] Puree

It cures heat of the center, dry sensation of the five centers,[13] acute diarrhea and vomiting syndrome, dry thirst, and failure of bodily fluids to pass.

Salted oriental flowering apricots (one *jin*), white sandalwood (four *liang*), liquorice (four *liang*), salt (one-half *jin*).

Make a fine powder of ingredients. Each dose is one *qian*. Add a little juice of sprouting ginger. Dissolve in boiling water.

---

[11] On cubebs see Schafer, 1963: 151, and O. W. Wolters, *Early Indonesia Commerce: A Study of the Origins of Srivijaya* (Ithaca, 1967), 233ff and *passim*. Cubebs are a medicinal in China, but a spice, and later a black pepper substitute elsewhere. In China, *Litsea cubeba* is a substitute for the real thing, *Piper cubeba*.

[12] Turmeric: probably native to south and southeast Asia where it is perhaps the most widely used spice, by weight. Usually the rhizome is dried and ground, but sometimes it is used fresh. It is not used much in China, except in curry recipes recently borrowed from the south. Like the other spices in this section, it is still held to be warming. It provides the dye for traditional Buddhist robes. It is confused terminologically with saffron in most of south and east Asia, but not as a culinary ingredient.

[13] These are the two palms, two soles and the heart.

[5A] [110.] Chinese Quince [*Chaenomeles sinensis*][14] Puree

It cures [evil] foot *qi* insensitivity, overstrained knee, chill numbness ache.

Chinese quinces (four pieces; steam cook. Remove the skin and grind, mashing up finely), crystallized honey (two *jin*; refine).

Combine the two listed ingredients together evenly. Put into a clean crockery pot and store. Take a little each day in boiling water on an empty stomach.

[111.] Detoxifying Dried Orange Peel Puree

It is used to cure intoxication that persists, vomiting and bile in the throat.

[Prepared] fragrant orange [*Citrus sinensis*] peel (one *jin*; remove the white.), prepared mandarin orange peel[15] (one *jin*; remove the white), sandalwood (four *liang*), kudzu flower (one-half *jin*), mungbean flower (one-half *jin*), ginseng (two *liang*; remove the green shoots), cardamom kernel (two *liang*), salt (six *liang*; roast).

Make a fine powder of ingredients. Each day take a little in boiling water on an empty stomach.

[5B] [112.] *Qatiq* Cakes

They bring forth saliva, and control thirst. They cure cough.

Qatiq (one *liang*, two *qian*), Korean ginseng (one *liang*; remove green shoots), acorus root (one *qian*; grind each to a fine powder), white *nabat* (three *liang*; powder. This is a kind of sugar).

[For] ingredients, use grape wine to make an emulsion with the *qatiq*. Combine evenly with the fine powders of other medicinals. Make a dose, press into a cake. Use one cake each time. Let it dissolve slowly in the mouth.

---

[14] Chinese quince: still a common medicinal food. The name *mugua* is used in south China for the papaya (*Carica papaya*) from the New World. Evidently it was first called the "foreign (or barbarian) quince," the "foreign" dropping off with time.

[15] The text uses a different word for prepared mandarin orange peel here for no apparent reason. Most likely Hu is simply copying out his source and using its terminology.

[113.] Cinnamon *Qatiq* Cakes

They bring forth saliva, and stop cough-caused-by-cold-evil.

Cinnamon (two *qian*; make a fine powder), *qatiq* (one *liang*, two *qian*), Korean ginseng (one *liang*; remove green shoots, make a fine powder), white *nabat* (three *liang*; powder).

[6A] [For] ingredients use rose-water to make an emulsion with the *qatiq*. Combine with the fine powders of other medicinals to make a dose. Use myrobalan [*Terminalia chebula*] oil. Cut out into cakes. Eat one cake each time. Let it dissolve slowly in the mouth.

[114.] *Tabilqa* Cakes

They make the head and eye clear, and benefit throat and diaphragm. They bring forth saliva, and stop thirst. They cure cough.

Tabilqa (two *qian*; finely powdered; the same as *caolongdan* [*Gentiana* spp], Korean ginseng (one *liang*, two *qian*; remove the green shoots and finely powder), white *nabat* (five *liang*; grind up).

[For] ingredients use *cicigina* (this is a northern *suanjueer*[16]) and decoct into an paste. Combine with medicinal powders to make a dose, cut into a cake. Eat one cake each time. Let it dissolve slowly in the mouth.

[115.] Fragrant Orange Aromatic Cakes

They extend the chest, and accord *qi*. They clean and benefit head and eye.

New fragrant orange peel (one *liang*; dry over a fire; remove white), garuwood (five *qian*), white sandalwood (five *qian*), grain-of-paradise[17] (five *qian*), **[6B]** cardamom kernel (five *qian*), cubebs (three *qian*), southern borax three *qian*; grind separately), baroos camphor [*Dryobalanops aromatica* resin] (one *qian*; grind

---

[16] *Suanjueer* usually refers to the tamarind. The leaves of the tamarind and *Potentilla anserina* do bear a superficial resemblance. But the *Suanjueer* of the text is probably to be understood as an equivalent of *Suanzao[er]*, *Zizyphus jujuba.* Note that this is given as an equivalent for *cicigina* later in the text.

[17] Grain-of-paradise: this is another of the large cardamoms, ultimately from Africa. The illustration in *juan* 3 seems to show *A. xanthioides*. *Shusha* is written differently there.

separately), musk deer musk (two *qian*; grind separately).

Make ingredients into a fine powder. Combine into a dose with liquorice paste and cut out into a cake. Eat one cake each time. Let it dissolve slowly in the mouth.

[116.] Cow Medullae Paste

It builds up essence, and the medullae. It strengthens sinew and bone, accords blood *qi*, lengthens the years, and augments longevity.

Solomon's seal [*Polygonatum cirrhifolium* or *P. multiflorum*] paste (five *liang*), Chinese foxglove [*Rehmannia glutinosa*] paste (three *liang*), Chinese asparagus [*Asparagus lucidus* or *A. cojinjinensis*] paste (three *liang*), oil from cow skull marrow (two *liang*).

[Of] ingredients take the Solomon's seal paste, the Chinese foxglove paste, and the Chinese asparagus paste and combine with the cow skull marrow oil quickly, using a silver spoon, and stirring without stopping the hand. Allow to solidify. Combine evenly into a paste. Every day take a spoonful dissolved in warm liquor on an empty stomach.

[7A] [117.] Chinese Quince Concentrate

Chinese quinces (10; remove the skin and stems, take the juice. Boil down until the liquid is gone), white granulated sugar (Ten *jin*; refine).

Boil ingredients together repeatedly and make into a concentrate.

[118.] Citron [including *Citrus medica*, also *C. medica* var. *sarcodactylis*][18] Concentrate

Citrons (20 pieces; remove the skin and take the meat), white granulated sugar (two *jin*; refine).

Boil ingredients together repeatedly and make a concentrate.

---

[18] Citron: medieval introduction from west and south Asia. This fruit is used in worship in the south, particularly the strangely shaped varieties known as "Buddha's hand" in Chinese. Their resemblance to a clenched fist of strange-shaped fingers makes them uncanny and allied to the sacred, and they partake of the reverence shown toward all citrus in the south.

[119.] Hazelnut Concentrate

Hazelnuts (100 pieces; take the cleaned meat), white granulated sugar (five *jin*; refine).

Boil ingredients together and make a concentrate.

[120.] Purple Perilla Concentrate

[**7B**] Purple perilla leaf (five *jin*), dried Chinese quince (five *jin*), white granulated sugar (ten *jin*; refine).

Boil ingredients together and make concentrate.

[121.] Kumquat [*Fortunella margarita*] Concentrate

Kumquats (50; remove the seeds and take the skin), white granulated sugar (three *jin*).

Boil ingredients together and make a concentrate.

[122.] Cherry [*Prunus pseudocerasus*][19] Concentrate

Cherries (50 *jin*; take the juice), white granulated sugar (24 *jin*; refine).

Boil ingredients together and make a concentrate.

[123.] Peach[20] Concentrate

---

[19] Cherry: the Chinese cherry, a different species from the Western, is a bit less sweet. They are often dried or honey-cured. The value of the cherry plant for complexion is still known. This, and anti-parasitic properties occasionally ascribed to the plant, may be related to the cyanogenic glycosides in the leaves and fruit kernels. These release quantities of prussic acid when the plant parts are crushed. Parasites and skin bacteria could be killed.

[20] Peach: the peach is native to China, where it occurs as a common scrubby tree on wild dryish mountains and in the uplands. It was domesticated in China at some very early date, most likely during the Neolithic. The peach is a symbol of fertility, because of the spectacular masses of red to pink flowers in spring and great quantities of rich, luscious fruit. The fruit is said to be shaped like the female genitalia, a resemblance that is remote enough to have been forced by a previous belief in the tree's feminine and fertile associations. The peach accumulates in Chinese culture many of the romantic and feminine associations that the rose has in the West. The peach is also a magical plant, presumably for the same reasons. Its ability to flower spectacularly and grow fast under harsh conditions shows it has a special *qi*. The wood is used to make fortune-telling blocks, apotropaic or lucky items. Twigs are used to repel evil. Branches in flower are used to decorate the house at Chinese New Year, to bring good

Large peaches (100; remove the skins, cut into slices and take the juice), crystallized honey (two *jin*; refine).

Boil ingredients together and make a concentrate.

[8A] [124.] Pomegranate[21] Syrup

Pomegranate seeds (10 *jin*; take the juice), white sugar (ten *jin*; refine).

Boil ingredients together and make a concentrate.

[125.] Rose [*Rosa laevigata* and other *Rosa* spp.] Hips[22] Concentrate

Rose hips (two *dou*; steam. When done remove the seeds; grind into a mash), crystallized honey (ten *jin*; refine).
Boil ingredients together and make a concentrate.

[126.] Red Currant *Sharba*[*t*]

Fresh northern red currants (ten *jin*; remove the seed. Immerse in

---

luck and keep away bad luck for the coming year. The Queen Mother of the West has a peach tree that bears peaches that confer long life, or immortality, to the eaters. The Spirit of Localities ("Earth God") is usually portrayed as an old man who is being presented with these fruits by young boys. Most educated Chinese, even today, know something of the Tao Yuanming 陶淵明 story of the fishermen who found and lost a paradise of flowering peach trees. This story evokes, and subtly compares or equates, mystical and sexual union in a thoroughly Daoist way. Peaches are, however, not much used specifically as medicine. They are much more familiar as a food, eaten at the crisp-ripe stage, when they are just beginning to color up. Westerners consider them "green," Chinese consider fully ripe peaches as "rotten." This taste probably arose from picking the fruit early to discourage pests and thieves. The graphic Chinese way of saying "do not act in an obviously suspicious way" is: "Do not adjust your hat in a peach orchard, or your shoes in a melon field."

21 Pomegranate (*Punica granatum*): an introduction from the West, grown today mainly as an ornamental, the fruit being incidental except in a few areas where the tree is well adapted. Being a Mediterranean and Near Eastern plant, it does not flourish in most of China. The womblike fruit filled with seeds is an emblem of fertility, as it is practically everywhere that pomegranates are long established. The plant, flower, and fruit are considered highly decorative, and the fruit's bright red color makes it auspicious, so it is widely grown in pots and gardens, and figured in art. The name can be punned with a Chinese phrase for "abundance of descendants."

22 One bit of evidence that the *YSZY* draws on Central Asia more than on the Near East is the lack of standard Near Eastern medicines. A Near Easterner would have emphasized the flower of rose, not the hips. The hips are rich in vitamin C, but it would not survive the cooking process.

water and take the juice), white granulated sugar (eight *jin*; refine).

Boil ingredients together and make a concentrate.

[127.] *Cicigina* (a kind of *Suanci* [*Ziziphus* spp.])

[**8B**] *Cicigina* (it does not matter whether a lot or a little is used; immerse in water; take the juice).

Boil ingredient down to a paste in a mica pot.

[128.] Pine Seed Oil

Pine seeds (it does not matter whether a lot or few are used; remove the skin; pound down into a mash).

Extract the juice from ingredient by "water pressing."[23] Boil down. Take the floating, clear oil and strain with cotton. Boil again and let clear.

[129.] Apricot Seed Oil

Apricot seeds (it does not matter whether a lot or a few are used; smash into fragments along with the skins).

Cook apricot seeds in water. Decoct, take the floating oil and strain with cotton. Boil again to make the oil.

[130.] Liquid Butter[24]

---

[23] That is, extract the pine seed oil much in the same way that soy milk is extracted in making *doufu* 豆腐, in this case by placing the wet seed mash into a sack and squeezing out the oil.

[24] Cow's butter: butter is still used in a small way in Chinese medicine, but is insignificant in China except among Inner Asian minority peoples. Among them, especially among the Tibetans, it is a staple food and can be a necessity of life, providing not only a rich calorie source but also a vitamin A source, an ointment for the terribly cold and dry air, a cooking oil, a lubricant and grease for equipment, a preservative, once turned to ghee by boiling the water out, after which it is an excellent seal for other foods, *etc.* The various types of butter discussed here represent stages in its progressive refinement and/or processing. The *Suyou* called for here is the crudest kind of butter, little more than thick congealed fat found floating on raw milk and subsequently rendered into a butter oil by boiling and most likely containing many impurities. A higher quality, churned butter is *mäskä*, while ghee is basically a butter oil with congealed fat carefully removed. In this case it is made from only the very best butter. Note that in some places in the *YSZY suyou* may actually mean cream. This is in part

Take the floating, congealed material from cow's milk. Boiled it becomes liquid butter.

[9A] [131.] Ghee

Take the very best liquid butter, something over a thousand *jin* in weight. After concentrating by boiling and straining, use a large crockery pot to store. During the winter months take that which is not congealed from the middle of the pot. This is called ghee.

[132.] *Mäskä* Oil

Take clean cow's milk. Without stopping the hand use a *qashiq* (this is a wooden implement for churning butter) and churn to get the floating congealment. This is *mäskä* oil. At present it is also called white liquid butter.

[133.] Chinese Matrimony Vine[25] Fruit Tea

[Take] five *dou* of Chinese matrimony vine fruits and scour in water to clean. Remove the floating chaff, dry over a fire. Use a white cloth tube to clean the fruits and remove the stems, calyxes,

---

due to the fact that Mongolian uses *tos*[*un*] in reference to either [boiled] butter, *e.g.*, *shar tos*[*un*] or cream, *tsötsgiyn tos*[*un*].

[25] Matrimony vine, otherwise known as Chinese wolfthorn or *gouqi* 枸杞, is a sprawling bushy plant, *Lycium chinense*, a close relative of the tomato and even closer to several American shrubs whose superb fruit was a staple food of American Indians. The fruits are essentially tiny tomatoes, though bitter and sour when fresh. The leaves are also used for food. Chinese species are among the richest sources of vitamins and minerals of any food ever tested anywhere in the world. They are especially valuable for vitamins A and C, the B vitamins except B12, iron, calcium, and certain trace minerals. As such, they were and are universally recognized in China as perhaps the finest of all general blood–building, strengthening, supplementing, and restorative medicines, used, *e.g.*, for women recovering from childbirth. The dried fruit, which loses most of its vitamin C value as it stores, is especially common and widespread. We have found the plant growing wherever Chinese have gone: pots on apartment windows in Hong Kong, tiny front–yards in central Los Angeles, isolated small towns in the American West. The references in the *YSZY* to supplementing in general exhaustion (read: malnutrition), thickening flesh, and strengthening *yang* are clear reference to the nutrient value. The dried berries are thus used in nutrient soups, teas, and other dishes, where they are well recognized as providing great nutritional benefit—they are considered prime *bu pin* 補品, "supplementing things" or "dietary supplements," basically equivalent to vitamin pills. They have recently become popular in some parts of the western world for the same reason, being often sold as "goji berries" from the Chinese name.

and black material. Choose only red and ripe fruits. First use Sparrow Tongue Tea to cleanse a stone roller. Do not use young tea buds. Then roll the matrimony vine fruit and make a fine powder. Use each day, on an empty stomach. Use **[9B]** a spoonful. Add liquid butter and mix evenly. Dissolve in warmed liquor. Boiling water can also be used. (Avoid eating it together with cream).

[134.] Jade Mortar Tea[26]

[Take] fifty *jin* of the best quality [tea], clean in a sieve tube. Take fifty *jin* of Sumen roasted rice and clean in a sieve tube. Combine uniformly together. Put into a jade mortar and grind. Make the tea.

[135.] Golden Characters Tea

This is a powdered tea that is made in Huzhou in Jiangnan and presented to the court.

[136.] Mr. Fan Tianshuai's Tea

This is a bud tea that is made by Qingyuan *lu* in Jiangzhe and presented to the court. It is absolutely superior in flavor and color to other teas.

[137.] Purple Shoots Sparrow Tongue Tea

After selecting and steaming new, tender shoots, make them into Purple Shoots Tea. The flavors of the Before Spring, Following Spring and Seeking for Spring **[10A]** varieties cannot compare with Purple Shoots Sparrow Tongue Tea.

[138.] *Nüxuer*[27] Tea

---

[26] "Tea," Chinese *cha*, usually refers to the leaves of *Camellia sinensis,* though (as in English) it can refer to any herbal infusion. Originally it had the latter meaning; in the Tang Dynasty the word became identified more and more with *C. sinensis*, then a rather exotic drink from the far southwest, but increasingly less so. By Song, it was a "necessity," though still expensive. It has grown steadily more popular, diverse, and accessible since, and has now spread worldwide. Various teas are believed to have various medicinal values, hence the many entries here, though details are few on their actual medical uses at the Yuan court. Interesting is that the range of teas discussed here exactly parallels the varieties of teas in common use at the time. The *YSZY* provides a snapshot of the tea usage of the time, including exotic Central Asian teas.

[27] See the discussion of this word in Lao, 1969: 407, Franke, 1970: 12. It is almost certainly related to Mongolian *tsuur* (MM: *boro chu'ur*, "gray *tsuur*?" or better *no-*

(It comes from the lands directly north. Its flavor is warming and sweet.)

[139.] Tibetan Tea

(It comes from Tibet. Its flavor is bitter and astringent. It is decocted using liquid butter.)[28]

[140.] Sichuan Tea

[141.] Rattan Tea

[142.] Kua Tea

(The above come from Sichuan.)

[143.] Swallow Tail Tea

(It comes from Jiangzhe and Jiangxi.)

[144.] Children's Tea [Catechu]

(It comes from Guangnan.)

[145.] Warm Mulberry Tea

(It comes from dark valleys.)

These various teas have flavors that are sweet and bitter, are slightly cooling, and lack poison. They get rid of accumulated evil heat and stop thirst. They benefit the urine, disperse food, and bring down *qi*. They make the intellect bright and reduce sleepiness.

[146.] Clear Tea

After first bringing water to a boil, strain. Put the tea buds in it. It will be steeped in a short while.

[147.] Roasted Tea

Use an iron cauldron; roast red. It is made by roasting *mäskä* oil, cow's milk, and tea buds together.

---

qo'a chu'ur, "green/leaf *chu'ur*?"), referring to *Dasiphora fructicosa*, a recent tea substitute, see Rinchen, 1979: 124.

[28] For a recipe see Rinjing Dorje, 1985: 53.

[10B] [148.] Orchid Paste

Stir together three spoonfuls of Jade Mortar Powdered tea, flour, and liquid butter to make the paste. Boil in water and take a little.

[149.] **Süttiken*

Add liquid butter to two spoonfuls of Golden Characters Powdered Tea and combine. Boil in water and take a little.

[150.] Fortified Broth

Put one spoonful of Jade Mortar Tea into a cup and grind up evenly. Use after boiling a hundred times [*i.e.*, repeatedly].

[151.] Aromatic Tea

Grind together finely white tea (one bag), sliced Baroos camphor (three *qian*), paiyao [*Millettia lasiopetala*] decoction (one-half *qian*), and musk deer musk (two *qian*). Make a congee using aromatic non-glutinous rice. Combine [all ingredients] into a dose. Press into a cake.

[11A] [152.] Spring Water

It is sweet and neutral, and lacks poison. It controls diabetes, regurgitation, and heat type dysentery. At present there is a Jade Spring in the Western Mountains. Its waters are sweet and delicate, and their flavor is superior to those of other spring waters.

[153.] Well Splendor Water

It is sweet and neutral and lacks poison. It is used to treat blood produced from the nine apertures of the body due to great fright [or convulsion]. The blood is stopped by spurting [Well Splendor Spring] water on the face [from the mouth]. It can also be used to bathe people's cataracts. It is put into liquor and into vinegar to prevent spoilage. This is what should be imbibed at dawn. At present the water used by the[29]

EMPEROR is taken, as a rule, from the Zhou Shop. The reason is that the

[29] Note that, as in the introduction to the *YSZY*, each mention of the emperor or empress, or of an imperial order, begins a new paragraph.

EMPEROR WUZONG [r. 1308-12] made a progress to the Liu Forest during the early Zhida Era [1308-12] to hunt using falcons. HE asked

THE EMPRESS to go with him to view the forest. Because of this

HIS path led past the Zhou Shop.
THE EMPEROR became thirsty, and longed for tea.

HE consequently ordered [Chang] *Buralgi* and the Dynastic Duke Jinjienüduoerzhi[30] to make tea. The [Dynastic] Duke personally visited various wells [**11B**] to choose water. The flavor of the water of only one well was extremely pure and sweet. He drew some and made tea.

THE EMPEROR praised the special nature of the tea's flavor. This is the tea regularly presented
By the Inner Palace to the

EMPEROR. Its flavor and color are both extraordinary.

THE EMPEROR consequently ordered the [Dynastic] Duke to build a Guanyin Temple where the well was, and a covered pavilion above the well. It was flanked with balustrades. A stone was inscribed to record the event. Subsequently the water used by the

EMPEROR must be taken daily from this well. Boiled water and tea made from the well's water are greatly superior to that made from other waters. Nearby there are other wells, but they are not as good as the Zhou Shop well. After the water has been boiled, it is always limpid and shining. Whenever like quantities are weighed, the Zhou Shop water is heavier than other waters [due to its mineral content].

[12A] [Illustration Caption:] Doses and Foods of the Beneficent Immortals

[30] Possibly Kun-rgya rdo-rje. The name is clearly Tibetan as was, most likely, Jinjienü himself. Note that his name is given in its full form here, and not in a Sinicized manner, as in the introduction. Chang Buralgi, on the other hand, is here called by what was clearly his Mongolian name. This passage is clear indication that both Jinjienü and Chang Buralgi had more than a passing role in the composition of the *YSZY*. This entire section of teas and drinks may be due to their influence.

[12B] Doses and Foods of the Beneficent Immortals

[154.] Mr. Tie Weng's Red Jade Paste[31]

This paste fills out the essence and is a tonic for the marrow. [It makes] the bowels transform. [It makes] the tendons and the ten-thousand spirits complete and full, the five viscera filled out in excess, marrow [substantial][32] and blood full, white hair become black. It reverses old age and restores youth. [It makes] the gait like a running horse. If it is taken repeatedly as the days advance, one will not starve if one does not eat for the entire day. It opens the way for a strong will. One can intone ten-thousand words a day. The spirit and knowledge will go to great heights. One will be without dreams or visions at night. If one takes the materials [of the paste] when one is not yet aged 27 *sui*, one can attain the age of 360 *sui*. If one takes it before the age of 45 *sui*, one can reach the age of 240 *sui*. If one takes it before the age of 63 *sui*, one can reach the age of 120 *sui*. If one takes it above the age of 64 *sui*, one can live to 100 *sui*. If ten doses are taken, it should suppress the passions, and if one cultivates secret merits, I think one could become an earth immortal. If one set of materials is divided into five portions, it can help the abscess diseases of five persons. If divided into ten portions, it can help the **[13A]** debility diseases of ten persons. When you compound it, wash your hair and body, perfect your heart, and do not frivolously show it to others:

Korean ginseng (24 *liang*; remove the shoots), fresh Chinese foxglove (16 *jin*; the juice), China root (49 *liang*; remove the black skin), crystallized honey (10 *jin*, refine).

[For] ingredients, grind the ginseng and China root finely. After using thin silk to strain the honey, take the natural juice of the Chinese foxglove. Do not use a copper or iron vessel to catch the juice when it is pounded. When finished remove the sediment. Take the medicinals and mix together evenly at one time. Put into a mica vessel, or a good porcelain pot and seal. Use 20 or 30 layers of clean paper to seal. Put [*i.e.*, sealed pot] into boiling water. Boil for three days and nights over a mulberry wood fire. When the mixture is removed from the fire, several layers of waxed pa-

---

[31] This recipe is taken from the *Hongshi ji yanfang* 洪氏集驗方. See Li's introduction in Hu Sihui, 1988: 141.

[32] This is Li's emendation from the original text.

per should be used to wrap the mouth of the pot. Put the pot into a well. When the pot has been submerged for a while to remove fire poison, take it out of the well and put it into the old boiled water. Boil for one day to bring out [get rid of] the water *qi* and then remove. Open the seal and take three spoonfuls. Put into three small cups and offer them to Heaven, Earth, and the hundred spirits. Burn incense, spread out the offerings and worship. Be very sincere and upright of spirit. Take a spoonful each day on an empty stomach, dissolved in liquor.

[13B] [155.] Earth Immortal Concentrate

It cures soreness and ache of waist and knee, and all chill illnesses of the abdomen. It causes the complexion to be pleasant and sleek, and the bone and marrow to be firm and solid. When one walks it will be like a running horse.

Chinese yams (one *jin*), apricot kernel (one *sheng*; blanch; remove the skin and tips), fresh cow's milk (two *sheng*).

[For] ingredients, take the apricot kernels and grind up finely. Add the cow's milk and Chinese yams. Mix together and press to get the juice. Use a new porcelain pot and seal tightly. Boil in water for a day. Each day take a spoonful dissolved in liquor on an empty stomach.

[156.] Golden Marrow Concentrate

It extends life and amplifies longevity. It replenishes the essence, and is a tonic for the marrow. If taken for a long time, white hair becomes black again. It counteracts old age and restores youth.

Chinese matrimony vine fruits (the quantity does not matter; select those that are red and ripe).

Soak ingredient in liquor without impurities for six days in the winter, and three days in the summer. Grind in a stoneware bowl, until [the fruits] are mashed **[14A]** finely. After that squeeze out the juice in a cloth bag. Reduce into a paste over a slow fire along with the liquor previously used to soak the fruits. Seal in a porcelain pot and store. Cook by boiling repeatedly. When taking a spoonful, on each occasion add a little liquid butter. Dissolve in warm liquor.

[157.] Chinese Asparagus[33] Paste

It gets rid of abdominal mass, wind-phlegm, depressive seizure, and infestation by the Three Worms. It eliminates pestilence, lightens the body, and amplifies *qi*. It makes a person able to withstand hunger. It lengthens the years and prevents aging.

Chinese asparagus (the quantity does not matter; remove the skin; remove the root hairs; clean).

Pulverize ingredient. Squeeze in a cloth to get the juice. After straining to clear the liquid, decoct into a paste over a slow fire using porcelain, or an earthenware pot, or any silver vessel. Take a spoonful each time, on an empty stomach, dissolved in warm liquor.

The Daoist Classic of the Eight Emperors [says:]

[**14B**] If you wish not to fear the cold, make a fine powder of Chinese asparagus and China root, and take. Take several times a day. When it is extremely cold one will sweat when wearing unlined clothing.

The *Baopuzi*[34] says:

Du Ziwei ate Chinese asparagus. He managed 80 wives, had 140 sons, and could travel 300 *li* a day.

The *Liexianzi*[35] says:

Zhisongzi ate Chinese asparagus. When his teeth fell out they grew in again. The fine hairs on his head grew in again.

The *Shenxian zhuan*[36] says:

Gan Shi was a man of Taiyuan. He took Chinese asparagus. He was among people for three hundred years.

---

33 Chinese Asparagus, *Asparagus cochinchinensis,* has recently been used for pains, sores, parasites, and similar conditions.

34 For an introduction to Ge Hong 葛洪, his life and work, See James R. Ware, *Alchemy, Medicine and Religion in China of A.D. 320, the Nei P'ien of Ko Hung* (New York, 1981).

35 On this work. also called the *Liexianzhuan* 列仙傳, see the discussion by Li in Hu Sihui, 1988: 144. The work is supposed to date from Eastern Han times but was apparently at least partially reworked during the Jin 晉 period.

36 On this work see Hu Sihui, *loc. cit*. It is attributed to Ge Hong.

The *Xiuzhen bizhi* says:

[**15A**] The spirit immortals took Chinese asparagus. After one hundred days they were pleasant and composed and had pleasant countenances. Those who were emaciated and infirm became strong. In three hundred days their bodies were light, and in three years they could travel as if flying.

The *Baopuzi* says:

Chuwenzi took Chinese foxglove for eight years. At night he was seen to shine. In his hand was a chariot [*i.e.*, heavy] crossbow.

The *Baopuzi* says:

Mr. Wen of Nanyang encountered anarchy and fled into the Hu Mountains. He was hungry and in difficulty. Some one told him to eat [tsang]shu [*Atractylodes* spp].[37] He consequently did not suffer from hunger. After a few years he returned to his village. His face and coloring were younger. His energy had returned fully.

The *Yaojing* says:

If you strongly wish to lengthen you life, you must take *shanjing*. This is tsangshu.

The *Paopuzi* says:

[**15B**] Renjizi took China root for 18 years. The Jade Woman accompanied him. He could conceal his appearance. He did not eat grains. A glow issued from his face.

The *Zhenzhong ji* of Sun the Adept[38] says:

If one takes China root for a long time, the hundred ailments will be eliminated within a hundred days. If one takes it twice a day, at night and in the morning, for two hundred days, the ghosts and spirits will be at your command. After taking it for four years, the Jade Woman will come and wait on you.

---

[37] See Li (Hu Sihui, 1988: 145) on *tsangshu* and its relatives in early times.

[38] This is Sun Simiao 孫思邈. See Li in Hu Sihui, 1988: 146.

The *Baopuzi* says:

The Lingyang Zhongzi took Chinese Senega [*Polygala sibirica* or *P. tenuifolia*] for 20 years. He had 30 sons. When he read a book he remembered and did not forget anything he read.

The *Zhushi jing* of the Tonghua Adept[39] says:

Shun used to climb Cangwu Mountain. He said that [it was because of] its *Jinyu xiangcao*. This is the same as wuchiapi [Acanthopanax] bark. One takes it to [**16A**] lengthen the years. Therefore it is said, it is better to have a handful of wuchiapi than gold and jade filling a cart. It is better to have one *jin* of burnet-bloodwort [*Sanguisorba officinalis*] than precious pearls bright as the moon. Formerly, Duke Ding of Lu's mother only took Wuchiapi Liquor so that she might attain long life. Persons such as Zhang Zisheng, Yang Shijian, Wang Shucai, and Yu Shiyan were all ancients who took Wuchiapi Liquor and their houses were not cut off. All attained an age of 300 years. They had 30 or 20 sons. The number of those who took Wuchiapi Liquor and attained longevity from one generation to the other has been extremely numerous.

The *Baopuzi* says:

Zhao Tazi took cassia for 20 years. Hair grew on the bottoms of his feet. he could travel 500 *li* a day. He had the strength to raise 1000 *jin*.

The *Liexian zhuan* [says:]

Wo Chuan ate pine seeds. He could travel by flying and move along like a running horse.

[16B] The *Shenxian zhuan* [says:]

Pine seeds; it does not matter if they are many or few. Grind them into a paste. Take on an empty stomach, dissolve a spoonful in warm liquor. If one takes three doses a day, one will not suffer from hunger or thirst. If you take doses for a long time, you will travel 500 *li* a day. Your body will be light, and your frame will be fortified.

The *Shenxian zhuan* [says:]

If you wish to cure the aches of the hundred joints, chronic wind defi-

[39] On this book see Hu Sihui, *loc. cit.*

ciency, and foot numbness pain, ferment pine knots into a liquor and take it. It has marvelous results.

The *Shenxian zhuan* [says:]

Pagoda tree fruits [*Sophora japonica*]: soak them thoroughly in a cow's gall bladder for 100 days. Dry them in the dark. Each day swallow a piece. In ten days the body will be light. In 20 days one's white hair will become dark again. In 100 days one will have communication with the spirits.

The *Shiliao*[40] says:

Chinese matrimony vine leaves can cause a person's sinews and bone to be strong. They get rid of wind, are a tonic and augment [*qi*], drive out *xulao* diseases,[41] and augment *yang* aspects. **[17A]** Collect the leaves in spring, summer or autumn. Collect the seed in winter. They can be eaten for a long time.

Taiqing zhu bencao [says:]

Collect 7 *fen*[42] of lotus flowers on the seventh day of the seventh month. Collect 8 *fen* of lotus root on the eighth day of the eighth Month. Collect 9 *fen* of lotus seed on the ninth day of the ninth Month. Dry them in the dark and eat them. They will prevent one from getting old.

The *Shiliao* says:

If kidney *qi* is deficient and weak, take fresh chestnuts, it does not matter how many. Let the wind dry them. Each day chew up thoroughly on an empty stomach. Slowly swallow three or five.

The "Story of How the Adept took Solomon's Seal and Became an Earth Immortal:"[43]

---

[40] This lost work survives only as quotations, was written by Meng Shen 孟詵 of Tang, and later revised by Zhang Ding 張鼎. See Li in Hu Sihui, 1988: 148.

[41] These are (Ou, 1982): "1. diseases caused by asthenia of the viscera; 2. consumptive disease."

[42] A *fen* is one one-hundredth of a *liang* or today .312 grams.

[43] A variant of this story can be found Ware, 1981: 194. See the discussion in Robert Campany, *To Live as Long as Heaven and Earth* (Berkeley, 2002), 21-22.

Formerly there was a gentleman of Linquan who mistreated his maid. His maid thereupon fled into the mountains. After being there a long time, she saw wild herb branches and leaves that were delightful. She then picked them and ate them. The taste was fine. From then on she regularly ate them. After a while [**17B**] she no longer felt hunger. She consequently felt light and fortified. At night she rested beneath a great tree. She heard the grasses move and thought that it was a tiger. She was afraid and climbed the tree to avoid it. When it became morning she descended to the ground again. Her body soared into space. Sometimes she was like a bird flying from the pinnacle of a peak. After several years her household was collecting firewood and saw her. They told her master. He sent people to catch her but they were unable. One day they encountered her below a sheer precipice. They hemmed her in on three sides with a net. Suddenly she leapt to the mountain peak. The master thought it uncanny. Someone said, how can this woman have the manner of an immortal, and *dao* bones? She must have taken numinous medicinals. Consequently they put out liquor and food, the most aromatic and fine-tasting of the five flavors, along the path on which she went back and forth. They looked to see if she ate them or not. She finally ate them. She consequently was unable to get away and they captured her. They asked her to set forth the cause of her condition. The herb that she said that she had eaten was Solomon's seal. Now you know that Solomon's seal extends the center and augments *qi*. It augments the five internal viscera, accords and attunes muscle and flesh, fills out bone and marrow, firms and strengthens sinew and bone, lengthens the years so that one does not get old, and makes the complexion and color bright and fresh. If the hair is white it makes it black again. When the teeth fall out they grow in again.

[18A] [158.] The Method for the Spirit Pillow

Wudi of Han (r. 140-87 BC) went on patrol in the east below Taishan. He saw an old man hoeing by the road. Above his back there was a white brilliance several *chi* tall. The emperor found it strange and questioned him as to whether or not he possessed Daoist arts. The old man replied saying: "Formerly, when I was 85 years old, I was decrepit and old, and on the verge of death. My head was white, and my teeth were falling out. There was a Daoist who instructed me to take jujubes, drink water, and completely avoid grains. He also made a spirit pillow method. There were 32 components of the method. Of these 32 components, 24 were good. They correspond to the 24 [seasonal varieties of] *qi*.[44] Eight were poisonous. They are proper to the 8 'winds.' Your servant became progressively younger. My black hair grew back again. The teeth that had fallen out appeared again. I could travel 300 *li* in a day. I think that your servant was then 180 years old. I was unable to abandon the world and enter the mountains. I was still fond of my sons and grandsons. I went back to eating grain. Another twenty years have passed, but I am still able to gain the power of the spirit pillow. I do not get any older as time passes." The Wudi saw that the old man's countenance and vigor were equal to those of any man of fifty or so. He made inquiries with the man's neighbors. They all said that the old man had spoken the truth. The emperor [**18B**] then received his method from him and made a pillow. However, the emperor was unable to follow the old man's method of stopping eating grain, and drinking water.

Recipe for the Spirit Pillow:

Take cypress wood from a mountain forest on the fifth day of the fifth month [and] the seventh day of the seventh month to make the pillow. It should be 1 *chi,* two *cun* long and 4 *cun* tall. The internal capacity should be 1 *dou,* 2 *sheng*. Make the covering of the red heart of the cypress. It should be 2 *fen* thick. Make sure that the wood goes together tightly. Also make sure it can be opened and closed. Also drill into the covering. Make three rows [of holes] in it. Each row should have 49 holes. There should be 147 holes altogether. Make each of them large as rice in its husk. Use the following medicinals:

[1.] *Xiongqiong* [*Conioselinum univittatum*] [fruit], [2.] *Danggui* [root of *Angelica sinensis*], [3.] Chinese angelica [root of *A. anomala* or *A. dahurica*], [4.] Magnolia [*Magnolia sprengeri*] flower, [5.] Forbes' wild ginger [*Asarum forbesii*], [6.] paishu [*Atractylodes macrocephala*] [rhizome], [7.] Chinese lovage [*Ligusticum sinense* or *L. jeholense*], [8.] Magnolia [*Magnolia sprengeri*] [bark], [9.] Chinese flower pepper, [10.] cinnamon, [11.] dried ginger, [12.] fangfeng [*Ledebouriella seseloides*], [**19A**] [13.] ginseng, [14.] balloon flower [*Platycodon grandiflorum*], [15.] *Cynanchum* Root, [16.] Seashore Vitex Fruits [*Vitex trifolia*], [17.] Broomrape, [18.] *Feilian* [herb or root of *Carduus crispus* and other *C.* spp], [19.] *Boshi* [fruit of *Biota orientalis*], [20.] Job's Tears [*Coix lacryma-jobi*], [21.] Tussilago Flower [*Tussilago far-*

[44] See the discussion in Hu Sihui, 1988: 151.

fara], [22.] *Boheng* [unidentified],[45] [23.] *Qinjiao* [*Aconitum* sp.],[46] [24.] *Miwu* [*Ligusticum chuanxiong*].

Altogether there are 24 substances. They are used to correspond to the 24 *qi*s.

[1.] *Wutou* [*Aconitum* sp., probably Chinese Aconite, *A. chinense*], [2.] Sichuan Aconite [*A. carmichaelii*], [3.] False hellebore [*Veratrum nigrum* or *V. maackii*] [root and rhizome], [4.] Chinese Honey-Locust [*Gleditsia sinensis*] [Fruit], [5.] *Wangcao* [*Illicium lanceolatum*], [6.] *Fanshi* [alunite, alum], [7.] Panhsia [*Pinellia ternata*] Rhizome, [8.] Chinese Wild ginger [*Asarum heterotropoides* or *A. sieboldii*].

These eight substances are poisonous. They are used to correspond to the eight 'winds.'

Take a *liang* of each of the aforelisted 32 substances. Break all apart into small pieces [using the teeth]. Arrange with the poisonous herbs on the top. Fill up the pillow. Use a bag to cover the pillow. After 100 days one's face will have a brilliance and sleekness. After one year all the various ailments in the body will be healed, and the body will be completely aromatic. After four years the white hair will become black again. The teeth will grow in again when they fall out. Ear and eye will be sharp and discerning. The spirit [**19B**] recipe is proven and mysterious. It should not be transmitted to the wrong person. Wudi asked Tongfang shuo about it. He replied saying: "Formerly Nulian transmitted it to Yuqing. Yuqing transmitted it to the Guang Chengzi. Guang Chengzi transmitted it to the Yellow Emperor. Recently, Chun, a Daoist of Gu City, slept on this medicine pillow for more than a hundred years and his hair is still not white. As for the origins of illness, they arise from the *yang* pulse. If one sleeps on this medicine pillow, I think that 'wind evils' cannot invade! Although the pillow is wrapped in a cloth, one must also repeatedly wrap it in a gauze bag. When one wants to sleep, all you have to do is remove the wrappings." The emperor ordered the old man to be given a roll of silk. The old man would not receive it and said: "What I have done for you, my Lord, is what a son would do for a father. The son understands the *Dao* in order to present it to the father.

[45] This may be a variety of Forbes' wild ginger.

[46] This name is normally a synonym for *shujiao* 蜀椒, Chinese flower pepper. We follow Ulrike Unschuld's suggestion based upon the *Bencao gangmu* here.

There is a duty not to receive gifts in such a case. Your servant would also not be one to sell the *Dao*! Just because your majesty likes the good, therefore I have presented it." The emperor then stopped [his plan of rewarding the old man], but still gave various herbs.

Food for Beneficent Immortals:

Sweetflag [*Acorus calamus*]: seek for sweetflag with nine joints. Dry in a cellar. After one hundred days grind into a powder. Take three times a day. If taken for a long time, it will make sensitive and bright [**20A**] the ear and the eye. It will increase the years and enhance longevity.

Food for Beneficent Immortals:

Sesame seeds: eaten they can eliminate all kinds of obstinate illnesses. If eaten for a long time they lengthen life, and make a person plump and strong. They lengthen the years and prevent one from getting old.

The *Baopuzi* [says:]

If you take Schisandra, after 16 years your facial color will be like jade. If you enter fire you will not be burnt. If you enter water you will not get wet.

The *Baopuzi* says:

Han Ju took sweetflag for 13 years. He sprouted hair on his body. He could read ten thousand words in a day. He was not cold [when] naked in winter. You should obtain sweetflag growing on rocks, with nine knots per *cun*. Sweetflag with purple flowers is still better.

The *Shiyi xinjing*[47] [says:]

[**20B**] Sacred lotus fruits have a sweet flavor, are neutral and lack poison. They are a tonic for the center, nourish *qi,* and clear the spirit. They eliminate the hundred illnesses. If one takes them for a long time, they cause a person to no longer thirst, and to be in a good state of health and look good.

---

[47] This is a lost work by Yin Gui 殷晷 of the Tang. See Hu Sihui, 1988: 154.

The *Rihuazi*[48] says:

Lotus and *Shilian*:[49] Remove the embryonic shoots [hearts]. If taken for a long time they make one joyful in the heart. They augment *qi* and stop thirst. They cure waist pain, leaking essence, and diarrhea.

The *Rihuazi* says:

Lotus Flower Stamens: if taken for a long time they strengthen the heart and augment color. They preserve a youthful appearance, and lighten the body.

The *Rihuazi* says:

Chinese Cornbind [*Polygonum multiflorum*] is sweet in flavor and lacks poison. If taken for a long time it strengthens sinew and bone. It augments the essence and marrow. It makes the hair black. It makes one have a son.

[21A] [Illustration Caption:] It is Beneficial to Eat Wheat in The Spring

[21B] What is Advantageous for the Four Seasons:[50]

Spring, three months: this means emerging and issuing forth. Heaven and Earth are altogether alive. The Ten-thousand-things avail of this to be luxuriant. One goes to sleep at night and arises early. One takes long walks in the palace. The hair is to be worn down the back loosely. This is to cause the intention to be on life. The intention should be on life, and not on killing; on giving, and not on taking; on rewards, and not on punishment. This is the way to accord with spring *qi*. This is the way to nurture life. To act contrary will wound the liver. In the summer it will become a cold transformation. Little will be retained for [summer] growth.

---

[48] This work is attributed to the Tang writer Da Ming 大明. See Hu Sihui, 1988: 155.

[49] Hu (1980) calls *Shilian Caesalpinia minas*, Snake Bramble seed, but the term is currently used to designate a number of similar plants. The identification here is thus uncertain.

[50] The bulk of this section, except for the summary at the end of each paragraph on the four seasons by Hu Sihui, is taken from the *Yellow Emperor's Inner Canon* (*Huangdi neijing, suwen, juan* 2). Compare the translation in Paul Unschuld, *Chinese Life Sciences, Introductory Readings in Classical Chinese Medicine*, (Taos, NM, 2005), 101-02.

The *qi* of spring is warming. It is beneficial to eat wheat to cool it. There cannot be a complete correspondence with the warmth. Warming drink and foods are prohibited, and hot clothing.

[22A] [Illustration Caption:] In the Summer it is Beneficial to Eat Pulses.

[**22B**] Summer, three months: this means flourishing and maturing. The *qi* of Heaven and Earth come together. The Ten-thousand-things luxuriate and bear fruit. One goes to sleep at night and arises early. One should not dislike the sun. This is to cause the intention to be without hate, to cause one's splendor to be mature, to cause the *qi* to attain outward flow, as if what one loves is outside [or away]. This is what corresponds to summer *qi*. This is the way to nurture a long life. To act contrary will wound the heart. In the autumn it will become malaria. Little will be retained for [autumn] gathering. There will be severe illness at the winter solstice.

Summer *qi* is heating. It is suitable to eat pulses to make it cold. There cannot be a complete correspondence with the heat. Warm drink and foods are prohibited, [as are] eating to satiation, swampy places, and damp clothing.

[23A] [Illustration Caption:] In Autumn it is beneficial to eat Sesame.

[**23B**] Autumn, three months: this means harvesting crops and weighing. The *qi* of Heaven is tending towards urgency, the *qi* of Earth towards brightness. One should go to bed and rise early, rising along with the rooster. This is to cause the intention to be peaceful and placid, to relax autumn harshness, and to receive and accumulate spirit *qi*. This is to cause the autumn *qi* to be in balance, without externalization of the will. This is to cause lung *qi* to be clear. This is what corresponds to autumn *qi*. This is the way to nurture gathering. To act contrary will wound the lungs. In the winter it will become food leakage.[51] Little will be retained for [winter] harboring.

Autumn *qi* is drying. One should eat sesame to moisten the dryness. Cold drink and foods, and cold clothing are prohibited.

[51] Today this is "watery diarrhea with indigested food." See Ou, 1982: 214.

[24A] [Illustration Caption:] In Winter it is Beneficial to Eat Panicled Millet.

[**24B**] Winter, three months: this means closing and harboring. The water is frozen, and the earth cracked [with the cold]. There should be no disturbance of *yang* influences. One goes to bed early, and arises late. One must wait for the brightness of the day. This causes the intention to become as suppressed; as hidden; as if there is a private concern; as if one has already obtained one's desire. One gets rid of cold and seeks heat, not allowing it to leak out through the skin, causing the amassed *qi* to be stolen. This is what corresponds to winter *qi*. This is the way to nurture harboring. To act contrary wounds the kidneys. In the spring it turns into syncope accompanied by flaccidity. Little will be retained for [spring] coming to life.

Winter *qi* is cold. One should eat panicled millet to regulate the cold with its heating nature. Hot drink and foods, warm clothing dried at the fire are prohibited.

[25A] [Illustration Caption:] Overindulgence in the Five Flavors

[25B] Overindulgence in the Five Flavors[52]

Sour and astringent are to gather together. If too much is eaten the bladder is blocked. It gives rise to dysuria.

Bitter and dry are to make firm. If too much is eaten then the triple burner is closed up. If gives rise to vomiting.

Acrid flavors produce hot vapor. If too much is consumed then it rises up into the lungs. The blood and the constructive and protective *qi* will not be seasonal and the heart will become hollow [*qi* deficient].

Salty flavors cause discharge through vomiting. If too much is eaten then the flow is outside into the blood vessels. The stomach becomes exhausted, the throat dry, and one contracts diabetes.

Sweet flavors [make] weak and inadequate. If too much is eaten the stomach becomes soft and slow, and worms pass. Therefore there is abdominal flatulence, and a pressing in the chest.

Acridity moves the *qi*. If one has a *qi* ailment one should not eat too much acridity.

---

[52] Much of this section is directly borrowed or adapted from the food sections of the *Qian jin beiji fang* of Sun Simiao although other sources have been used as well, as indicated below.

Salt moves the blood. Those with blood ailments should not eat too much salt.

Bitterness moves the bones. Those with bone ailments should not eat too much bitterness.

Sweetness moves the flesh. Those with flesh illness should not eat too much sweetness.

[26A] Sourness moves the tendons. Those with tendon illness should not eat too much sourness.

It is prohibited for those with liver illnesses to eat acridity. It is suitable to eat things such as non-glutinous rice, beef, musk mallow, and jujube.

It is prohibited for those with heart illnesses to eat salt. It is suitable to eat things such as beans [other than soybeans], dog meat, plums, and leeks.

It is prohibited for those with spleen illnesses to eat sour foods. It is suitable to eat things such as soybeans, pork, chestnuts, and pulses.

It is prohibited for those with lung illnesses to eat bitter food. It is suitable to eat such things as wheat, mutton, apricots, and shallots.

It is prohibited for those with kidney illnesses to eat sweet foods. It is suitable to eat such things as yellow glutinous millet, chicken, peaches, and onions.

If one eats too much sour food, liver *qi* thereupon collects and the spleen *qi* is cut off. There will be thickenings of the flesh and splitting of the lips.[53]

If one eats too much salt, bone *qi* becomes exhausted and short. The *qi* of the fat is cut through. The blood vessels then congeal, and the face changes color.[54]

If one eats too much sweet food, the heart *qi* will become full rapidly, the color become black, and kidney *qi* will be out of balance. The bones will then be painful, and the hair fall out.[55]

---

[53] This passage is adapted from the *Yellow Emperor's Inner Canon*. See Li in Hu Sihui, 1988: 165.

[54] This passage is adapted from the *Yellow Emperor's Inner Canon*. See Hu Sihui, *loc. cit.*

[55] This passage is adapted from the *Yellow Emperor's Inner Canon*. See Hu Sihui, 1988: 166.

If one eats too much bitter food, lung *qi* will not be moist, and stomach *qi* will be full. The skin will then become dried and withered, and the hair will come out.[56]

[26B] If one eats too much acrid food, sinew and blood vessels will become injured and slack. The essence and spirit will then be finished. The sinews will then be anxious, and the feet withered.[57]

The Five Grains are to be made [staple] food.

The Five Fruits are to be assistance.

The Five Meats are to augment.

The Five Vegetables are to fill up.

If *qi* and flavors are harmonized and the food eaten, it will then be a tonic for the essence, and augment *qi*.[58]

However, even if the five flavors are flavored [evenly], and the mouth wishes to eat and drink, one cannot eat large amounts of any food. If too much is eaten it gives rise to illness. Small amounts augment. Rare delicacies of the hundred flavors, and careful moderation daily, that is the best thing.

[27A] [Illustration Caption:] Foods that Cure the Various Illnesses.

[27B] Foods that Cure the Various Illnesses:[59]

---

[56] This passage is adapted from the *Yellow Emperor's Inner Canon.* See Hu Sihui, *loc. cit.*

[57] This passage is adapted from the *Yellow Emperor's Inner Canon.* See Hu Sihui, 1988: 167.

[58] This is another quote from the *Yellow Emperor's Inner Canon.* See Hu Sihui, *loc. cit.*

[59] Foods that Cure the Various Illnesses: most are simpler forms of dishes in the first section, adapted to specific medical ingredients. They are attempts to make things like fox and otter palatable, rather than gourmet fare. The fish and chicken recipes are still familiar, in almost identical forms, in today's Chinese medical cuisine. They are excellent eating. Being simpler and less spicy than the recipes in *juan* 1, they require first-rate ingredients.

Note that this section is much more Chinese than the first two recipe sections in the *YSZY* (see discussion in Chapter 2). The first section is overwhelmingly Near Eastern and Central Asian. The second is primarily Chinese, but with a long section of Near Eastern jams and preserves, and other exotic delicacies. This final section is almost entirely Chinese in execution and medical indications, except for the inevitable sheep recipes, and even they have primarily Chinese flavorings. A very few others could be

[159.] Sprouting Chinese Foxglove Chicken[60]

It treats pain of the back and loins, deficiency and injury of bone and marrow, inability to stand upright for long periods, heaviness of body and *qi* shortage, night sweating and lack of appetite, and occasional vomiting and dysentery.

Sprouting Chinese foxglove (half a *jin*), sweetmeats (five *liang*), and black chicken (one).

[Of the] ingredients first take the chicken, pluck, remove the giblets and clean. Cut up finely. Combine the Chinese foxglove and the sugar together evenly. Put the mixture inside the intestinal cavity of the chicken. Put it into a copper pot. Then put the copper pot into a cauldron and steam. When the dish has been cooked completely, remove the chicken and eat. Do not use salt or vinegar. Eat the meat. When it is gone also drink the broth.

[160.] Lamb Honey Paste

It treats *xulao* diseases, waist pain (lumbago), coughing, withered lung, and hectic fever due to *yin* deficiency.

[**28A**] Cooked sheep's fat (five *liang*), cooked sheep's marrow (five *liang*), crystallized honey (five *liang*; refine), juice of sprouting ginger (one *he*), juice of sprouting Chinese foxglove (one *he*). [Of] ingredients, first decoct the sheep's fat and bring to a boil. Then add the sheep's marrow. Bring to a boil again, then add the honey and [sprouting] Chinese foxglove and sprouting ginger juice. Stir constantly. Slowly simmer and bring repeatedly to a boil over a small fire to make a paste. Take a spoonful dissolved in warm liquor every day on an empty stomach. Or make it into a soup or a congee and eat it. This is also acceptable.

---

from anywhere, such as the wheat gruel, originally Near Eastern, but only because wheat itself came from there to China.

Honey, which features in these recipes, is used in Chinese medicine as a cooling, soothing, harmonizing ingredient.

[60] For the following medicinal recipes, compare the translation by Gwinner in Gwinner, 1988: 81-108. Chinese foxglove, *Rehmannia glutinosa,* is an extremely common and important herbal drug in the Chinese pharmacopoeia. The root is usually used, but the sprout (as here) is important too, for bleeding, heat, and related conditions needing a "cooling" influence.

[161.] Sheep Entrails Gruel

It treats consumptive disease damage to the kidney, and damage to bone and marrow.

Sheep's liver, stomach, kidney, heart and lung (one each; wash in hot water), cow's [milk] cheese (one *liang*), black pepper (one *liang*), long pepper[61] (one *liang*), salted fruits (one *he*), prepared mandarin orange peel (two *qian*; remove white), lesser galangal (two *qian*), tsaoko cardamom (two), onions (five "stalks").

[**28B**] [Of] ingredients, first take the sheep entrails and boil slowly until done over a slow fire. Take the juice and strain clean. Combine with sheep entrails [other than the stomach] and herbs, and stuff everything into the sheep's belly. Sew up the opening. Put into a thin silk bag. Boil again. When done add five spices. Eat regularly as desired.

[162.] Sheep Bone Congee

It treats *xulao* diseases and debility of waist and knee.

Sheep's bones (an entire set; broken up), prepared mandarin orange peel (one *qian*; remove white), lesser galangal (two *qian*), tsaoko cardamom (two), fresh ginger (one *liang*), salt (a little).

Decoct ingredients into a juice over a slow fire in three *dou* [of water]. Strain. When the liquid has cleared, make a congee in the conventional way. It is also possible to make a soup from the bones.

[163.] Sheep's Spine Gruel

[**29A**] It treats a condition of chronic lower burner primordial *qi* deficiency, and damage to waist and kidney.

Sheep's spine (one complete; broken up), broomrape (one *liang*; wash and cut into slices), tsaoko cardamom (three), long pepper (two *qian*).

Boil ingredients in water into a juice. Filter and remove the dregs.

---

[61] Long pepper resembles black pepper, but the tiny seeds are in a thin head. It is less flavorful and more piquant than black pepper, and therefore was replaced by chiles when these were introduced from the New World in the 16th century. Often the chiles even took over the name formerly used for long pepper (as in Bahasa Indonesia *lada*). It survives today only as a rare medicinal plant.

Add spring onions, and five spices. Make a flour gruel. Eat.

[164.] White Sheep Kidney Gruel

It treats *xulao* diseases, degeneration of the *yang* ways, and debility of waist and knee.

White sheep's kidney (two; cut into slices), broomrape (one *liang*; soak in liquor and cut), sheep's fat (four *liang*; cut into slices), black pepper (two *qian*), prepared mandarin orange peel (one *qian*; remove white), long pepper (two *qian*), tsaoko cardamom (one *qian*).

Combine ingredients. Add spring onions, salt and sauce, and boil into a soup. Add flour *qizi*. Make into a gruel in the normal way [**29B**] and eat.

[165.] Pig Kidney Congee

It cures kidney *xulao* damage, debility and ache of waist and knee.

Pig kidney (one, remove fatty tissue and slice), non-glutinous rice (three *ho*), tsaoko cardamom (three), prepared mandarin orange peel (one *qian*; remove white), grain-of-paradise (two *qian*).

[Of] ingredients, first take the pig kidney, the prepared mandarin orange peel *etc.* and boil to make a juice. Strain and remove the dregs. Add a small amount of liquor. Then add the rice to make a congee. Eat on an empty stomach.

[166.] Chinese Matrimony Vine Fruit and Sheep's Kidney Congee

It cures *yang qi* degeneration, ache of waist and foot, the five kinds of impairments and the seven wounds.

Chinese matrimony vine fruits (one *jin*), sheep's kidney (two; finely cut up), spring onions (one stalk), [**30A**] mutton (half a *jin*; roast).

Combine four ingredients evenly. Add the five spices and boil down into a juice. Add rice and decoct into a congee. Eat on an empty stomach.

[167.] Deer's Kidney Gruel

It cures kidney deficiency and deafness.

Deer's kidney (one; remove the fatty tissue and slice).

Surround ingredient with fermented black beans. Add three *he* of non-glutinous rice and boil [into a] congee. A gruel could also be made. Add the five spices. Eat on an empty stomach.

[168.] Mutton Gruel

It cures kidney deficiency failing and debility of waist and foot.

Mutton (half a *jin*; cut up finely), Chinese radish (one; cut into slices), tsaoko cardamom (one *qian*), **[30B]** prepared mandarin orange peel (one *qian*; remove white), lesser galangal (one *qian*), long pepper (one *qian*), black pepper (one *qian*), spring onions (three).

Boil ingredients in water to make a juice. Add salt and sauce and boil into a broth. Add wheat flour *qizi*. Eat. It can also be eaten by taking clear soup and making into a congee.

[169.] Deer Feet Soup

It cures the various wind deficiencies, ache of waist and foot and inability to walk.

Deer feet (four pair), prepared mandarin orange peel (two *qian*), tsaoko cardamom (two *qian*).

Boil ingredients until thoroughly cooked. Take the meat and add the five spices. Eat on an empty stomach.

[170.] Deer Horn Liquor

It cures lumbago pain due to strain and acute back spasm.

[31A] Deer horn (young horn, two to three *cun* in length; roast red).

Soak ingredient in liquor for two nights. Drink on an empty stomach. It is effective immediately.

[171.] Black Ox Marrow Decoction

It cures kidney asthenia, bone damage and fatigue from wasting.

Black ox marrow (half a *jin*), juice of sprouting Chinese foxglove (half a *jin*), crystallized honey (half a *jin*; roast; remove wax).

Combine three ingredients. Decoct into a paste. Dissolve in liquor and take on an empty stomach.

[172.] Fox Meat Soup

It cures asthenia and evil *qi* of the five viscera.

Fox meat (five *jin*; wash in boiling water), tsaoko cardamom (five), grain-of-paradise (two *qian*), onions (one handful), prepared mandarin orange peel (one *qian*; remove white), lesser galangal (two *qian*), *kasni* (one *qian*; same as *angwa* [asafoetida]).

[**31B**] Boil ingredients in one *dou* of water until done. Remove the tsaoko cardamom, *etc.* Then add two *qian* of black pepper, one *qian* of turmeric, vinegar and the five spices. Flavor evenly. Eat on an empty stomach.

[173.] Black Chicken Soup

It cures asthenia internal impairment caused by overstrain, and evil *qi* of chest and abdomen.

Black chicken (one; pluck, clean and cut up into small pieces), prepared mandarin orange peel (one *qian*; remove white), lesser galangal (one *qian*), black pepper (two *qian*), tsaoko cardamom (two).

Combine ingredients with onions, vinegar, and sauce and put into a jug. Seal the mouth. Let boil until done. Eat on an empty stomach.

[174.] Ghee Liquor

It cures asthenia and removes wind-wetness.

Ghee (one bowl).

[**32A**] Mix ingredient with a cup of liquor and drink warm. It is proven effective.

[175.] Chinese Yam *Tuo*[62]

[62] Note that this word also occurs in Turkic as the name of a sour batter drink. See Appendix 2.

It cures the various deficiencies, the five kinds of impairments and the seven kinds of wounds, cold ache of chest and abdomen, and damage to bone and marrow.

Sheep's bone (five to seven chunks; meat attached), Chinese radish (one; cut into large slices), spring onions (one), tsaoko cardamom (five), prepared mandarin orange peel (one *qian*; remove white), lesser galangal (one *qian*), black pepper (two *qian*), grain-of-paradise (two *qian*), Chinese yams (two *jin*).

Boil ingredients together and take the juice. Clarify. Strain and remove the gross parts. Cook two *jin* of flour and two *jin* of Chinese yams. When done grind up into a mash. Apply flour to make the *tuo*. Add the five spices and eat on an empty stomach.

[176.] Chinese Yam Congee

It cures *xulao* diseases, and chronic chill of hectic fever due to *yin*-deficiency.

[**32B**] Mutton (one *jin*; remove fat and membrane; roast until cooked and grind into a paste), Chinese yams (one *jin*; cook thoroughly and grind into a paste).

Add three *he* of rice to meat broth containing ingredients. Boil into a congee. Take on an empty stomach.

[177.] Sour Jujube Congee

It cures asthenia of the viscera, vexation and insomnia.

Sour jujubes (a bowl).

Use water for ingredient, twist [in a bag] and obtain the juice. Add three *he* of rice. Boil into a congee. Take on an empty stomach.

[178.] Sprouting Chinese Foxglove Congee

It cures asthenia of hectic fever due to *yin*-deficiency, general fatigue, gradual emaciation, and vexation causing insomnia.

Sprouting Chinese foxglove juice (one *he*), sour jujubes ([use] water, twist [in a bag] and obtain the juice; two wine cups [full]).

Decoct ingredients together by boiling in water. Bring to a boil several times. Then add three *he* of rice. Cook into a congee. Take on an empty stomach.

[33A] [179.] Chinese Flower Pepper Dough Gruel

It cures asthenia of spleen and stomach, chronic chill *qi*, pain of chest and abdomen stagnation, and vomiting and inability to keep down food.

Chinese flower pepper (three *qian*; roast and make into a powder), flour (four *liang*).

Mix ingredients together uniformly. Add a little salt. Make flour dough strips on fermented black beans.[63] Boil into a Gruel and eat.

[180.] Long Pepper Congee

It cures asthenia of spleen and stomach, intense chill-*qi* pain of chest and abdomen, and inability to eat due to obstructed listlessness.

Long pepper (one *liang*), black pepper (one *liang*), cassia (five *qian*).

Make a fine powder of ingredients. Use three *qian* for each three large cups of water. Add half a *he* of fermented black beans. Boil together until cooked. Remove the dregs. Add three *he* of rice and make a congee. Eat on an empty stomach.

[181.] Lesser Galangal Congee

[**33B**] It cures chill pain of chest and abdomen, abdominal mass indigestion.

Lesser galangal (half a *liang*; make into fine powder), non-glutinous rice (three *he*).

[For] ingredient [*i.e.*, the galangal] use three large cups of water. Boil the lesser galangal down to two cups. Remove the dregs. Add the rice, boil into a congee and eat. It is of proven efficacy.

[182.] Evodia[64] Fruit Congee

It cures chilled *qi* perversity of chest and abdomen, [and] rib pain.

---

[63] Perhaps the pepper dough and fermented black beans are to be combined.

[64] *Evodia rutaecarpa* has been used for a vast range of conditions, including magical medicine; an old folktale found in Li Shizhen 李時珍, *Bencao gangmu* 本草綱目 (*jiao dian ben* 校點本), (32, 2, 1861) tells of a man who tied sacks of *evodia* to his arms and those of his family, fled to the hills, and thus escaped a supernatural blight that killed his livestock instead of the humans.

Evodia fruits (half a *liang*; wash with water and remove the effusion. Dry, roast and make fine a powder).

Make ingredient into a congee with three *he* of rice. Eat on an empty stomach.

[183.] Dried Beef

It cures chronic chill of spleen and stomach, compulsive drinking and eating.

[**34A**] Beef (five *jin*; remove fat and membrane, cut up into large strips.), black pepper (five *qian*), long pepper (five *qian*), prepared mandarin orange peel (two *qian*; remove white), tsaoko cardamom (two *qian*), grain-of-paradise (two *qian*), lesser galangal (two *qian*).

Make a fine powder of ingredients. Combine evenly with the meat, five *ho* of sprouting ginger juice, one *he* of onion juice, four *liang* of salt. Let sit for two days, remove meat and dry over a fire until dried. Eat as desired.

[184.] Lotus Seed Congee

It cures disrepose of heart and will. It supplements the center and strengthens the will. It makes ear and eye quick and sharp.

Lotus seeds (one *sheng*; remove hearts).

Cook ingredient. When done grind up into a paste-like substance. Make a congee with three *he* of non-glutinous rice. Eat on an empty stomach.

[185.] Euryale Fruits Congee

It cures insufficiency of primary vitality *qi*. It strengthens the will. It makes sharp ear and eye.

Euryale fruits (three *he*).

[**34B**] Cook ingredients. When done grind up into a paste-like substance. Boil into a congee with one *he* of non-glutinous rice. Eat.

[186.] Euryale Fruits Gruel Powder

It cures arthralgia chiefly caused by wetness-evil, pain of waist and knee. It gets rid of sudden, violent illnesses. It increases primary vitality *qi* and strengthens heart and will. It makes ear and eye quick and sharp.

Euryale fruits (grind into a powder), sheep's spine (one set, with meat. Decoct. Take the juice).

[For] ingredient use one *he* of juice of sprouting ginger. Add the five spices. Flavor evenly. Eat on an empty stomach.

[187.] Peach Seed Congee

It cures pain of chest and abdomen, abnormal-rising-of-lung-*qi*-cough, obstruction filling up of the diaphragm, and rapid respiration.

Peach seeds (three *liang*; cook in broth. When done remove the ends and skin. Grind).

Take the juice of the ingredient, combine with non-glutinous rice and make into congee. Eat on an empty stomach.

[35A] [188.] Sprouting Chinese Foxglove[65] Congee

It cures *xulao* disease wasting away, hectic fever, alternating episodes of chills and fevers, and coughing up of blood.

Juice of sprouting Chinese foxglove (two *he*).

Boil a white congee of ingredient. When it is nearly done add the juice of sprouting Chinese foxglove and combine evenly. Eat on an empty stomach.

[189.] Bream Gruel

It cures asthenia of spleen and stomach, leaking diarrhea from which one does not recover for a long time. If it is eaten there is immediate effect.

Large bream (two *jin*), large garlic (two chunks), black pepper

---

[65] Chinese foxglove, *Rehmannia glutinosa,* is a common and important medicine in the Chinese pharmacopoeia. The root is usually used, but the sprout (as here) is important too, for bleeding, heat, and related conditions needing a "cooling" influence.

(two *qian*), Chinese flower pepper (two *qian*), prepared mandarin orange peel (two *qian*), grain-of-paradise (two *qian*), long pepper (two *qian*).

[Of] ingredients put onions, sauce, salt, spices, and garlic into the intestinal cavity of the fish and decoct. When done make a gruel. [Add] the five spices. Flavor evenly. Eat on an empty stomach.

[35B] [190.] Roasted Yellow Flour

It cures leaking diarrhea and looseness of intestine and stomach.

White flour (one *jin*; roast, scorch yellow).

Each day take a spoonful of ingredient mixed with warm water on an empty stomach.

[191.] Cheese Flour

It cures asthenia of spleen and stomach, and reddish and whitish leaking diarrhea.

Cheese (one; cut up into bean-sized pieces).

Mix ingredient with flour and cook. When done eat on an empty stomach.

[192.] Broiled Yellow Chicken

It cures asthenia-weakness of spleen and stomach diarrhea.

[36A] Yellow hen (one; pluck and clean).

[Of] ingredients,[66] combine together evenly: salt, sauce, vinegar, fennel, fine Chinese flower pepper powder. Brush onto the chicken. Roast until dry and scorched on coals. Eat on an empty stomach.

[193.] Method for Cow's Milk Decocted Long Pepper

During the Zhenguan period [of Tang, 627-50], Taizong [r. 627-50] was suffering from dysentery. The various doctors were unable to treat it successfully. The emperor asked his courtiers [saying] that whoever could cure the disease would be heavily rewarded. At that time there was a gentlemen with special ability

[66] The text of this recipe is defective.

who advanced this method. He employed cow's milk to decoct long pepper. The emperor took it. It was immediately beneficial.

[194.] Chinese Badger Meat Gruel

It cures edema, surface *qi* syndrome, abdominal distension, and difficulty in urination.

Chinese badger meat (one *jin*; cut up finely), onions (a handful), tsaoko cardamoms (three).

[**36B**] Cook ingredients together using Chinese flower pepper and fermented black beans. When overcooked add one *he* of non-glutinous rice and make a gruel. Flavor evenly with the five spices. Take on an empty stomach.

[195.] Yellow Hen

It cures abdomen water indigestion and edema.

Yellow hen (one; pluck and clean), tsaoko cardamom (two *qian*), adzuki beans ["Red Small Beans"][67] (one *sheng*).

Cook ingredients together. When done eat on an empty stomach.

---

[67] Adzuki Bean (*Vigna angularis*): here *chi xiaodou*, modern *hongdou* 紅豆, "red bean." This name, in modern south China at least, includes the rice bean, *Phaseolus calcaratus* Roxb., but the *YSZY* surely means the Adzuki.

The adzuki bean is the original bean of China, the original *tou* 豆. It has probably been known since far back in the Neolithic. With the coming of the soybean, the smaller adzuki became the *xiaodou* 小豆, "small bean." Then came other small beans such as the mung, and the adzuki's red color became more distinctive. Now several species of beans with red forms are known, and terminological confusion has not been sorted out. Contrary to the *YSZY*, modern folk belief holds adzukis to be heating, apparently solely because of their red color (see under mung bean). They are often made into a porridge sweetened with sugar and used to heat the body on cold days. Warming it certainly is, in the physical sense at least, whatever may be true of the effect on *qi*.

Other color forms of adzuki are known, which can result in such confusing names as *bo hongdou* 白紅豆, "white red bean." The English name is borrowed from the Japanese.

Sources: G. W. Herklots, *Vegetables in Southeast Asia* (London, 1977); (for *V. calcarata*) Frank M. Sachs, "A Literature Review of *Phaseolus angularis*–The Adsuki Bean," *Economic Botany* 31 (1977): 1: 9-15.

[196.] Green[-headed] Duck [Male Mallard] Gruel

It cures the ten water swelling illnesses from which one does not recover.

Green-headed duck (one, skin and clean), tsaoko cardamoms (five).

[For] ingredient put half a *sheng* of adzuki beans into the intestinal cavity of the duck. Cook. When done flavor with the five spices. Eat on an empty stomach.

[37A] [197.] Chinese Radish Congee

It cures diabetes, scorched tongue and dry mouth and frequent urination.

Large Chinese radish (five; cook. When done twist [in a bag] to get the juice).

[As] ingredients take three *he* of non-glutinous rice and water and combine with the juice. Boil into a congee. Eat.

[198.] Pheasant Gruel

It cures diabetes and dry mouth and frequent urination.

Pheasant (one; pluck and clean).

[To] ingredient add the five spices according to the normal method. Make a gruel-meat broth. Eat.

[199.] Pigeon Gruel

It cures diabetes and excessive drinking of water.

[**37B**] White pigeon (one; cut up into large slices).

Cook ingredient with **tosu[n]* [fat, grease]. When done eat on an empty stomach.

[200.] Egg Yolk

It cures urine that does not pass.

Egg yolk (one; use fresh).

Take ingredient. Do not take more than three times. It can also be eaten cooked.

[201.] Chinese Mallow[68] Gruel

It cures urine which is retained and does not pass.

Mallow leaves. (It does not matter if they are many or few. Wash, select and clean.)

Boil ingredient into a gruel. Add the five spices. Eat on an empty stomach.

[38A] [202.] Carp Soup

It cures diabetes and edema, jaundice and [evil] foot *qi*.

Large carp (one), adzuki beans (one *he*), prepared mandarin orange peel (two *qian*; remove white), Chinese flower pepper (two *qian*), tsaoko cardamom (two *qian*).

[To] ingredients add the five spices and flavor evenly. Cook. When done eat on an empty stomach.

[203.] Purslane [*Portulaca oleracea*][69] Congee

It cures [evil] foot *qi*, edema of head and face, swelling of chest and abdomen, and dripping discharge of urine.

Purslane. (Wash clean. Take the juice.)

Boil ingredient into a congee combined with non-glutinous rice. Eat on an empty stomach.

[204.] Wheat Congee

[**38B**] It cures diabetes and dry mouth.

Wheat. (Scour clean. It does not matter if a lot or little is used.)

Boil ingredient into a congee. It can perhaps also be steamed as cooked food. Eat it on an empty stomach.

[205.] Donkey's Head Gruel

It cures apoplexy-vertigo, debility of hand and foot, annoying pain

---

68 Mallow: *Malva* spp. were a major vegetable in early China. The leaves are strongly diuretic and are still widely used for this purpose. They are also, like the leaves of Chinese matrimony vine, exceptionally high in vitamins and minerals.

69 Purslane: *Portulaca oleracea* is another cooling, diuretic, highly nutritious herb.

of extremities, and trouble in speaking.

Black donkey's head (one; remove hair and wash clean), black pepper (two *qian*), tsaoko cardamom (two *qian*).

Cook ingredients until overcooked. Add the five spices in fermented black bean juice. Flavor with the spices. Flavor evenly. Eat on an empty stomach.

[206.] Donkey's Meat Soup

It cures wind mania and depression and pacifies heart *qi*.

Meat of a black donkey. (The quantity does not matter. Cut up.)

[**39A**] Cook ingredient until overcooked in fermented black beans. When done add the five spices. Eat on an empty stomach.

[207] Fox[70] Meat Gruel

It cures infantile convulsion epilepsy, spiritual confusion, indistinct speech, and inappropriate [unmeasured] singing and laughing.

Fox meat. (The quantity does not matter. Include organ meat.)

[To] ingredient add the five spices according to regular method. Cook until overcooked. When done eat on an empty stomach.

[208.] Bear Meat Gruel

It cures the various winds, [evil] foot *qi* numbness-insensitivity, and five-flaccidities tendon and muscle spasms.

Bear meat (one *jin*).

[To] ingredient add the five spices [to the bear meat] in fermented black beans. [Add] onions and sauce. Cook. When done eat on an empty stomach.

---

[70] Fox: *Vulpes vulpes,* the Eurasian red fox, is associated with magic and demons, and its meat is thus properly used for trances, fits, metal ailments, and other conditions that appear uncanny. Li Shizhen (*Bencao gangmu* 51, 2, 2878) notes that the name is homonymous with the Chinese word for "lonely," and that the fox is indeed solitary.

[209.] Black Chicken Liquor

[**39B**] It cures apoplexy, paralysis and inability to speak, rigidity of the pupil of the eye, and fever accompanied by restlessness.

Black hen (one; pluck and wash clean. Remove the entrails).

Cook with ingredient five *sheng* of liquor. Take [reduce to] two *sheng* of liquor. Remove the dregs. Divide into three doses. Take one after the other. If the juice is exhausted and there is no time [to make more], decoct a gruel of green onions and sprouting ginger, and add it [to what is left]. Again take the juice.

[210.] Sheep's Stomach Gruel

It cures the various apoplexies.

Sheep's stomach (one; wash clean), non-glutinous rice (two *he*), green onions (several), salted fruits (half a *he*), Chinese flower pepper [Sichuan Pepper] (Remove the closed up corns, roast to bring out the juice; 30 corns), sprouting ginger (two *qian* and a half. Cut up finely).

Combine six ingredients evenly and put inside the sheep's stomach. Cook until overcooked. When done, flavor with the five spices. Eat on an empty stomach.

[211.] Kudzu Starch Gruel

[**40A**] It cures apoplexy, wind-heat of heart and spleen, indistinct speech, mental confusion, and hand and foot which do not obey.

Kudzu starch (half a *jin*; pound to get four *liang* of the starch), *Schizonepeta tenuifolia* herb (one *liang*), salted fruits (three *he*).

[Of] the three ingredients, first use water to boil the *S. tenuifolia* herb and the salted fruits. Bring to a boil six or seven times. Remove the dregs and take the juice. Then take the kudzu starch and make large rope noodles. Cook in the juice. When done, eat on an empty stomach.

[212.] *Schizonepeta tenuifolia* Congee

It cures apoplexy, indistinct speech, mental confusion and deviation of mouth and face.

S. tenuifolia herb (one *liang*), field mint leaves (one *liang)*, salted fruits (three *he*), white millet seeds (three *he*).

Use four *sheng* of water [for] ingredients and cook down to three *sheng*. Remove the dregs. Add the grain and boil into a congee. Eat on an empty stomach.

[213.] Hemp Seed Congee

It cures apoplexy, wind-heat of the five viscera, indistinct speech, hand and foot which do not obey, and obstruction of the large intestine.

[**40B**] Hemp seeds [*Cannabis sativa*] (two *liang*; roast; remove the skins and grind up), white millet grains (three *he*), field mint leaves (one *liang*), *Schizonepeta tenuifolia* herb (one *liang*).

[Of] ingredients, boil the field mint and *S. tenuifolia* herb in three *sheng* of water. Remove the dregs and take the juice. Add the hemp seed piths and boil everything together into a congee. Eat on an empty stomach.

[214.] Burdock. (This is *niupangzi*. Another name is *shuzhan zi*.)

It cures apoplexy, mouth dryness due to dryness-heat evil, and hand and foot which do not obey as well as skin herpes.

Burdock [*Arctium lappa*] leaves (tender and thick), liquid butter.

[For] ingredients use broth to boil three to five *sheng* of Burdock leaves. Remove and after washing with fresh water, squeeze in a cloth to get the juice. Add the five spices and a little liquid butter and eat.

[215.] Black Donkey Skin Soup

[**41A**] It cures apoplexy, hand and foot which do not obey, joint irritation pain, heart dryness-evil, deviation of eye and mouth, face and mouth and eyeball.

Black donkey's skin (one sheet; remove hair, wash clean).

Steam ingredient. When cooked cut up finely into lengthwise strips. Add the five spices in fermented black bean juice. Flavor evenly. After cooking, eat on an empty stomach.

[216.] Sheep's Head Hash

This cures apoplexy, vertigo, emaciation, and debility of hand and foot.

White sheep's head (one; pluck and wash clean.)

Steam ingredient until overcooked. When done cut up finely. Use five spices juice. Flavor hash evenly. Eat on an empty stomach.

[217.] Wild Pig Meat Broth

It cures recto-anal fistula, bleeding piles, bleeding which will not stop and rectum swelling.

[**41B**] Wild pig meat (two *jin*; cut up finely).

Cook ingredient until overcooked. When done add the five spices. Eat on an empty stomach.

[218.] Otter Liver Gruel

It cures recto-anal fistula, and bleeding which will not stop.

Otter liver (one).

Cook ingredient. When done add five spices. Eat on an empty stomach.

[219.] Bream Soup

It cures recto-anal fistula, fresh blood-stool, and chronic blood in the stool.

Large bream (one; young and fresh; wash clean and cut up into strips), Jinese flower pepper (two *qian*; make a fine powder), tsaoko cardamom (one *qian*; make a fine powder).

[For] ingredients use three onion bulbs. Cook. When done add the five spices. Eat on an empty stomach.

[42A] [Illustration Caption:] Food Avoidances When Taking Medicines

[42B] Food Avoidances When Taking Medicines

If one is taking medicine one cannot eat a lot of sprouting coriander, as well as garlic, miscellaneous fresh vegetables, and various slippery things, fat pork, dog meat, extremely oily and rich things, fish hash, rank-smelling foods, *etc.* One should even avoid seeing corpses, women in labor, and filthy things. One also cannot eat stale and smelly things.

If one has [taken] tsangshu [*Atractylodes* spp.], one must not eat peaches, plums, sparrow [small bird] meat, coriander, garlic, green fish,[71] etc.

If one has [taken] false hellebore, one must not eat orang-outang meat.

If one has [taken] croton beans, one must not eat edible shoots of young reeds and wild pig meat.

If one has [taken] golden thread [or] balloon flower, one must not eat pork.

If one has [taken] Chinese foxglove, one must not eat [prepared] stinking elm.

If one has [taken] panhsia [or] sweetflag, one must not eat sweetmeats and mutton.

[**43A**] If one has [taken] Chinese wild ginger, one must not eat fresh vegetables.

If one has [taken] liquorice, one must not eat *songcai*,[72] and seaweed [*Sargassum fusiforme* or *S. pallidum*].

If one has [taken] tree peony, one must not eat sprouting coriander.

If one has [taken] poke root, one must not eat dog meat.

If one has [taken] Chinese quinine [*Dichroa febrifuga*], one must not eat onions and fresh vegetables.

If one has [taken] hollow malachite or cinnabar, one must not eat blood. (Whenever one takes medicine, one must universally avoid eating blood.)

If one has [taken] China root, one must not eat vinegar.

If one has [taken] turtle, one must not eat *xiancai* [edible greens of *Amaranthus* spp.]

If one has [taken] Chinese asparagus, one must not eat carp.

[71] This is probably *Mylopharyngodon piceus*.
[72] This is a kind of cabbage, probably *Brassica chinensis*.

General prohibitions for those taking medicines for long periods of time:

[**43B**] Do not take medicines on *wei* days [*i.e.*, days in the cycle of 60 containing the element *wei*]. Also avoid days of the full moon.

Avoid the *siu* day when it is the first day of the fifth and ninth lunar months.

Avoid the *yin* day during the second, sixth and tenth lunar months.

Avoid the *hai* day during the third, seventh and eleventh lunar months.

Avoid the *shen* day during the fourth, eighth and twelfth lunar months.

[44A] [Illustration Caption:] Benefits and Harmfulness of Foods

Benefits and Harmfulness of Foods

Now foodstuffs have those which are beneficial and those which are harmful. One can know and avoid them.

If flour has a stinking smell, it cannot be eaten.

If fresh ingredients are [dis]colored and stink, they cannot be eaten.

If broth is old and food is watery, it cannot be eaten.

If one boils meat and it does not change color, it cannot be eaten.

If the various meats are not slaughtered, they should not be eaten.

If the various meats smell and are spoiled, they cannot be eaten.

The various brains cannot be eaten.

Any sacrificial meat which moves on its own cannot be eaten.

Pigs and sheep which die of epizootics cannot be eaten.

Dried meat which is still damp cannot be eaten.

Neither horse's liver nor cow's liver can be eaten.

A hare with closed eyes cannot be eaten.

One cannot use a mulberry wood fire for roasting meat.

Roebuck, deer and tailed-deer should not be eaten between the fourth and seventh months.

Hare meat should not be eaten during the second month.

Avoid storing various meats' jerkies in rice. There is poison.

[**45A**] putrid fish cannot be eaten.

If a sheep's liver has a hole in it, it cannot be eaten.

The various birds which have closed their own mouths should not be eaten.

Crabs can be eaten after the eighth month. They should not be eaten during the remaining months of the year.

One should not eat lots of shrimp. All those lacking hair, or with pills in the intestines, or which become white when boiled, cannot be eaten.

During the twelfth lunar month, things such as dried and salted meats should not be eaten if they have absorbed moisture due to leaking rain, or if they have been chewed and damaged by insects and rodents.

Things such as marine delicacies and pickled preserves, if they have spoiled due to been exposed to moisture or heat, and if they are old, they should not be eaten.

During the sixth and seventh months one must not eat wild geese.

Carp heads cannot be eaten. The poison is in the brain.

Any livers which are green cannot be eaten.

One should not eat deer in the fifth month; it wounds the spirit.

One should not eat dog meat during the ninth month; it wounds the spirit.

One should not eat bear meat during the tenth month; it wounds the spirit.

One cannot eat anything which is not in season.

Whenever fruit kernels have turned into dust, they cannot be eaten.

When the various fruits have fallen to the ground, they cannot be eaten.

When the various fruits have been damaged by insects, they cannot be eaten.

[**45B**] If a peach has two pits, it cannot be eaten.

If one does not remove the heart of a lotus seed, and eats it, it will give rise to *huoluan*.[73]

If a musk melon has two peduncles, it cannot be eaten.

The various cucurbits which have absorbed a lot of water cannot be eaten.

One cannot eat a lot of **möög* mushrooms. They give rise to illness.

A lot of elm seed cannot be eaten. It causes a person to be unable to open the eyes.

If a vegetable is covered by a frost, it cannot be eaten.

Lots of cherries should not be eaten. They cause a person to have a fit.

A lot of onions cannot be eaten. They cause a person to be deficient.

One should not eat a lot of coriander. It causes a person to be very forgetful.

A lot of bamboo shoots should not be eaten. It gives rise to illness.

Red-colored tree fungus cannot be eaten.

One should not eat garlic in the third month. It confuses a person's eyes.

One should not eat smartweed in the second month. It gives rise to illness.

In the ninth month one should not eat a melon which has been exposed to a frost.

One should not eat coriander [leaves] in the fourth month. It produces odor from the armpits.

One should not eat pepper in the tenth month. It wounds a person's heart.

One should not eat leeks in the fifth month. It confuses a persons five viscera.

[46A] [Illustration Caption:] Foodstuffs which mutually conflict

[46B] Foodstuffs Which Mutually Conflict

When one eats one should not wish for [too much] variety. If there is

---

[73] The conventional translation of *huoluan*, which Ou, 1982 calls "diseases characterized by acute diarrhea and vomiting" (246), is cholera. This is appropriate only relatively late in Chinese history and not during the fourteenth century.

[too much] variety then there will be what violates. The one in the know separates his foods [eats them separately] and avoids this.

Horse meat cannot be eaten together with granary rice.

Horse meat cannot be eaten with cocklebur [*Xanthium sibiricum*] or with ginger.

Pork cannot be eaten together with beef.

Sheep's liver cannot be eaten together with pepper. It wounds the heart.

Hare meat cannot be eaten together with ginger. It creates *huoluan.*

Sheep's liver cannot be eaten together with pork.

Beef cannot be eaten together with chestnuts.

Sheep's stomach cannot be eaten together with small beans [or] flowering apricot [fruits]. It wounds a person.

[**47A**] Mutton cannot be eaten together with fish hash [or] cream.

Pork cannot be eaten with coriander. It rots a person's bowels.

Mare's milk cannot be eaten together with fish hash. It produces obstruction of the bowels.

Venison cannot be eaten together with catfish.

Tailed-deer cannot be eaten together with river shrimps.

Tailed-deer fat cannot be eaten together with flowering apricot and plums.

Beef liver cannot be eaten together with sheatfish. It gives rise to wind.

Beef stomach cannot be eaten together with dog meat.

Chicken meat cannot be eaten together with fish stock [juice]. It produces obstruction of the bowels.

Quail meat cannot be eaten together with pork. The face will turn black.

Quail cannot be eaten together with *Agaricus* mushrooms. It produces hemorrhoids.

[**47B**] Pheasant cannot be eaten together with buckwheat flour. It produces vermin.

Pheasant cannot be eaten together with peaches or **möög* mushrooms.

Pheasant eggs cannot be eaten together with onions. It produces vermin.

Meat of sparrows [*i.e.*, small birds] cannot be eaten together with plums.

Eggs cannot be eaten together with turtle meat.

Eggs cannot be eaten together with onions and garlic. It harms the *qi*.

Chicken meat cannot be eaten together with hare meat. It causes one to have diarrhea.

Pheasant cannot be eaten together with bream.

Duck meat should not be eaten together with turtle meat.

Pheasant meat cannot be eaten together with pork liver.

Carp cannot be eaten together with dog meat.

[**48A**] Pheasant cannot be eaten together with sheatfish. If it is eaten it causes one to develop depression.

Bream cannot be eaten together with sugar.

Bream cannot be eaten together with pork.

Yellow fish[74] cannot be eaten together with buckwheat flour.

Shrimp cannot be eaten together with pork. It harms the essence of life.

Shrimp cannot be eaten together with sugar.

Shrimp cannot be eaten together with chicken meat.

Soybean sprouts cannot be eaten together with pork.

Panicled millet cannot be eaten together with mallow leaves. It produces illness.

Small beans cannot be eaten together with carp.

Chinese myrica [fruits] cannot be eaten together with onions.

Persimmons and Chinese pears cannot be eaten together with crab.

---

[74] *Huangyu* here may be maigre or more likely sturgeon. A "yellow fish" could also be a "yellow" carp.

Plums cannot be eaten together with eggs.

[**48B**] Jujubes cannot be eaten together with honey.

Plums [and] water chestnuts cannot be eaten together with honey.

Mallow leaves cannot be eaten together with sugar.

Fresh onions cannot be eaten together with honey.

Lettuce cannot be eaten together with cream.
Bamboo shoots cannot be eaten together with sugar.

Smartweed cannot be eaten together with fish hash.

Xiancai [edible greens of *Amaranthus* spp, *Chenopodium* spp, *etc.*] cannot be eaten together with turtle meat.

Leeks cannot be eaten together with liquor.

Sonchus greens [*Sonchus* spp] cannot be eaten together with honey.

Shallots cannot be eaten together with beef. It gives rise to obstruction of the bowels.

Ground mustard cannot be eaten together with hare meat. It produces sores.

[49A] [Illustration Caption:] Poisons in Foodstuffs

Poisons in Foodstuffs

Among the various substances there are those which are fundamentally poisonous by nature. There are those which lack poison but are poisonous when cooked. There are various substances which are sensitive to one another, which react to one another, and which counter one another and form poisons. If people do not practice control and restraint, and eat them, it will result in wounding of the internal organs and disordering of abdomen and stomach *qi*. Some [poisonings] are not serious, others severe. Each damages according to the nature of the poison contained [in the substance]. They must be countered according to the poison.

If one has already eaten or drunk and does not know what the poison is, [and there is] vexation and a feeling of dull listlessness, one should immediately decoct shrubby sophora juice, drink it and induce vomiting. Or one can boil rhinoceros horn juice and drink it. Or one can boil bitter liquor [vinegar] and "good liquor"[75] and drink it. All these things are good.

If one eats poisonous vegetables, one should take chicken excrement and roast into an ash and take dissolved in water. One can also take liquorice juice. Or one can boil kudzu root juice and drink it. It is also possible to blend and take white lead ["Iranian Powder"] water.

[**50A**] If one eats an excessive amount of melon, [and there is] abdominal distension. If one eats salt it will then be assimilated.

If one eats **möög* mushroom or *Agaricus* mushroom and is poisoned, "earth broth"[76] will form a counter.

If one eats an excessive amount of water chestnuts, [and there is] abdominal distension and a feeling of dull listlessness, one can warm liquor and drink it combined with ginger. It will then be assimilated.

If one eats wild taro [*Colocasia antiquorum*] and is poisoned, earth broth will form a counter to it.

If one eats gourd and is poisoned, boil panicled millet stalks juice and drink it. The poison will then be countered.

If one eats the various meats and is poisoned, including when one is poisoned from eating horse liver or wet dried meat, roast pig bone ash and take it blended. Also possible would be drinking coriander juice or juice of fresh leeks.

If one eats beef or mutton and is poisoned, decoct liquorice juice and drink it.

If one eats horse meat and is poisoned, it will be assimilated if one chews apricot kernel. Both reed root juice and "good liquor" are possible.

If one eats dog meat, and it is not digested and gives rise to intestinal distension or dryness of the mouth, blanch in water apricot kernels after removing the skin and tips and drink.

[**50B**] If one eats too much fish hash, it gives rise to vermin accumulation.[77] Combine rhubarb juice and ground mandarin orange peel with

---

[75] This phrase, if it does not refer to distilled liquor, may be an attempt to translate Mongolian *sayin darasun*, "good wine (or liquor)."

[76] See the discussion by Li in Hu Sihui, 1988: 208. This is basically a clay filtered water.

[77] On this parasitic infestation of the stomach see Li in Hu Sihui, 1988: 208.

salt broth and drink.

If one eats crab and is poisoned, drink purple perilla juice. Also winter melon juice or fresh sacred lotus juice will counter it. Also possible are dry garlic juice and reed root juice.

If one eats fish and is poisoned, mandarin orange peel juice, reed root and rhubarb, soybeans, and Glauber's salt's juice are all possible.

If one eats duck and is poisoned, boil glutinous millet grain juice and it will counter it.

If one eats chicken and is poisoned, one can drink a good wine vinegar and counter it.

If one drinks liquor, is extremely tipsy and it is not countered, soybean juice, common kudzu, mulberry seeds, and orange peel juice are all possible.

If one eats beef and is poisoned, [prepare] one *liang* of pork lard and each time take a spoonful dose. If dissolved in warm water the poison will then be countered.

If one eats pork and is poisoned, drink rhubarb juice or apricot kernel juice or Glauber's salts juice. All can counter it.

[51A] [Illustration Caption:] Animal Transformations

[51B] Animal Transformations

The forms of animals are various. Each grows according to its bodily form. In addition animal natures are divided into poisonous and non-poisonous varieties. Also, strange transformations take shape. These would not be without poison. If one is then not cautious it will result in one becoming ill. This is not to look into things, I think.

An animal with a jutting tail.

A horse with "night eye" [*i.e.*, white-spot-marked] hooves.[78]

A sheep whose heart has a hole.

A liver which is colored green-black.

A deer which is spotted like a leopard.

A sheep whose liver has a hole.

[78] See the discussion in Hu Sihui, 1988: 210.

A black chicken with a white head.

A white horse with green hooves.

A sheep with only one horn.

A white sheep with a black head.

A black sheep with a white head.

A white bird with a yellow head.

A sheep with six horns.

A white horse with a black head.

A chicken with four spurs.

Meat dried in the sun which is not dry.

A horse which grows a horn.

A sheep with a liver which has only one lobe.

A crab which has only a single claw.

A fish which has eyelashes.

A shrimp which lacks hair.

Meat which moves when put into water.

Meat which is warm through the night.

A fish which is without bowels, a gall bladder or gills.

Meat which falls to the ground but to which dirt does not adhere.

Fish eyes which open and close, and pills in the abdomen.

JUAN 3

* * *

CHINESE TEXT

忽思慧
飲膳正要卷三

四部叢刊續編子部: 1A-20A , 21A-24B, 25B-26B, 27B-28B, 30B, 31B- 32B, 33B, 37B-40A, 41A-46B, 47B, 51A-53B, 54B-58A, 59A

中國古代版畫叢刊: 20B, 25A, 27A, 34B-37A, 40B, 58B

中國古代版畫叢刊(元殘卷): 29A-30A, 31A, 33A, 34A, 47A, 48A-50B, 54A

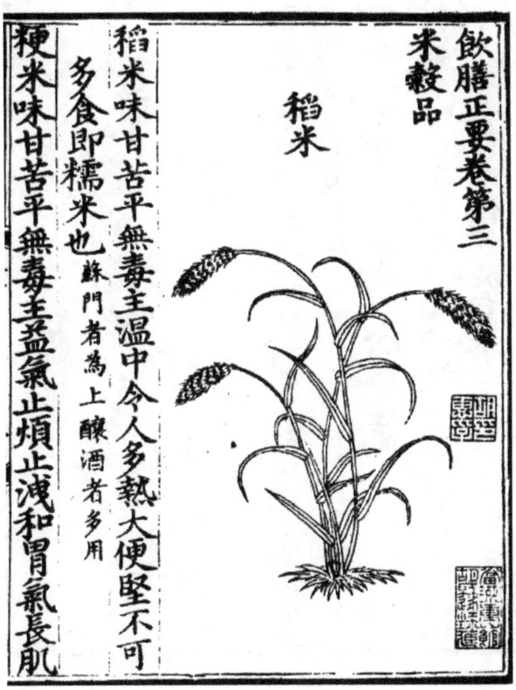

飲膳正要卷第三

米穀品

稻米

稻米味甘苦平無毒主温中令人多熱大便堅不可多食即糯米也蘇門者為上釀酒者多用

粳米味甘苦平無毒主益氣止煩止洩和胃氣長肌

1A
Paddy
Rice

1B
Foxtail
Millet

肉即今有數種[香粳米 雪裹白][匾子米 香子米]香味尤勝諸粳
米搗碎取其圓淨者為圓米亦作渴米

粟米

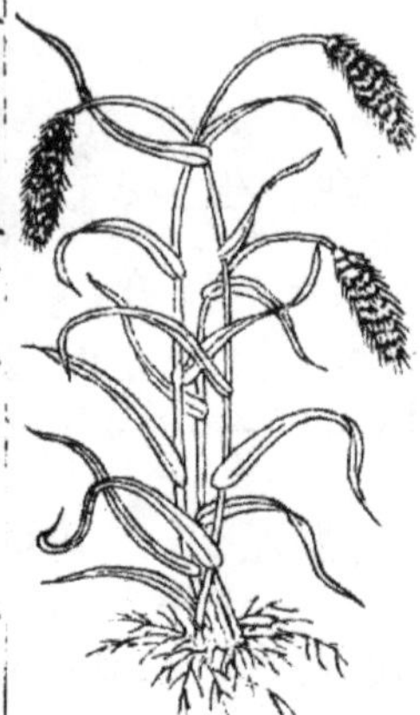

粟米味鹹微寒無毒主養腎氣去脾胃中熱益氣陳
者良治胃中熱消渴利小便止痢唐本注云粟類
多種顆粒細如粱米搗細取匀淨者為淅米

2A
Millet

粱米

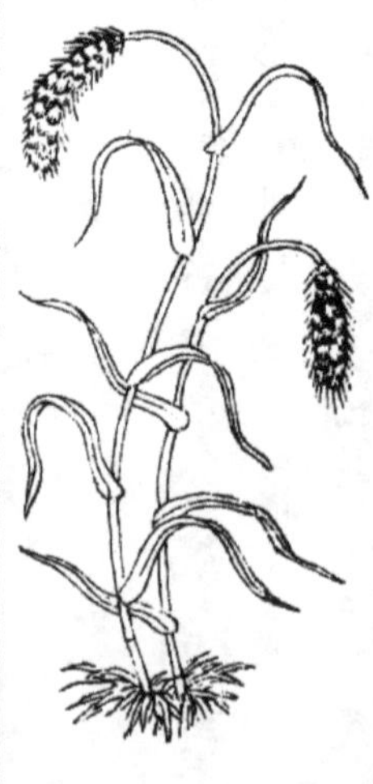

青粱米味甘微寒無毒主胃痺中熱消渴止洩痢益
氣補中輕身延年
白粱米味甘微寒無毒主除熱益氣
黃粱米味甘平無毒主益氣和中止洩唐本注云穗
大毛長穀米俱麄於白粱

2B Panicled Millet

黍米

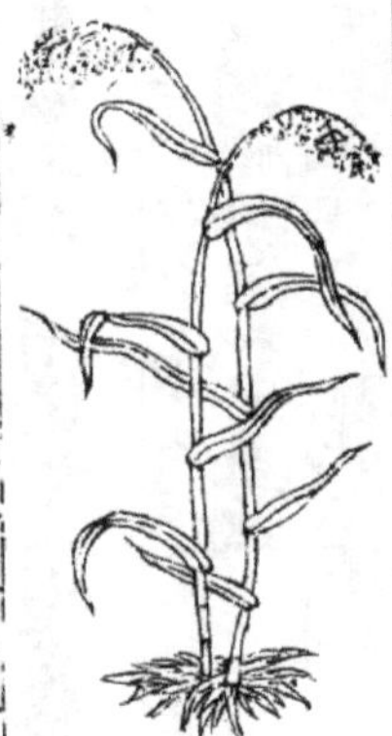

黍米味甘平無毒主益氣補中多熱令人煩久食昏
人五藏令人好睡肺病宜食
丹黍米味苦微溫無毒主欬逆霍亂止煩渴除熱
穄米味甘無毒主益氣補不足關西謂之糜子米亦
謂穄米古者取其香可愛故以供祭祀
河西米味甘無毒補中益氣顆粒硬於諸米出本地

3A Mung Beans

菉荳

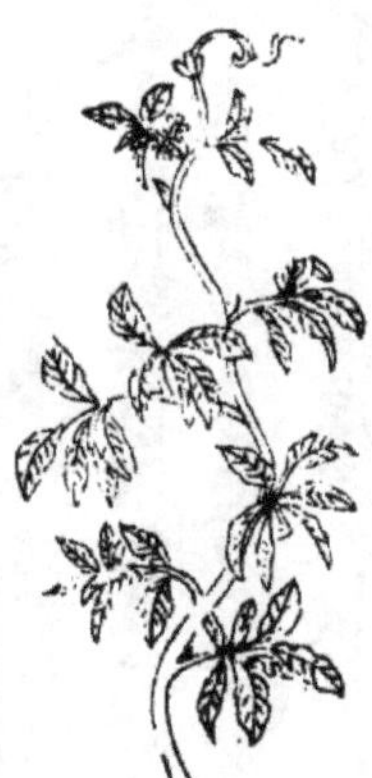

菉荳味甘寒無毒主丹毒風疹煩熱和五藏行經脉
白豆味甘平無毒調中暖腸胃助經脉腎病宜食
大豆味甘平無毒殺鬼氣止痛逐水除胃中熱下瘀
血解諸藥毒作豆腐即寒而動氣
赤小豆味甘酸平無毒主下水排膿血去熱腫止瀉
痢通小便解小麥毒

3B
Chickpeas

回回豆子

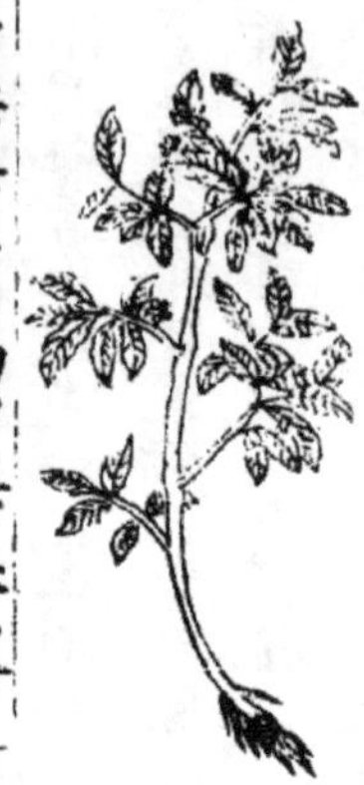

回回豆子味甘無毒主消渴勿與鹽煮食之出在回
回地面苗似豆今田野中處處有之
青小豆味甘寒無毒主熱中消渴止下痢去腹脹産
婦無乳汁爛煮三五升食之即乳多
豌豆味甘平無毒調順榮衛和中益氣
扁豆味甘微温主和中葉主霍亂吐下不止

4A
Wheat

小麥

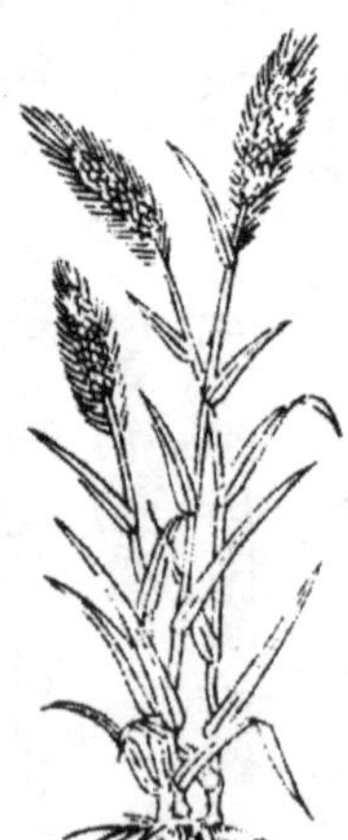

小麥味甘微寒無毒主除熱止煩燥消渴咽乾利小
便養肝氣止痛唾血
大麥味鹹温微寒無毒主消渴除熱益氣調中令人
多熱為五穀長藥性論云能消化宿食破冷氣
蕎麥味甘平寒無毒實腸胃益氣力久食動風氣令
人頭眩和猪肉食之患熱風脫人鬚眉

4B
Sesame

芝麻

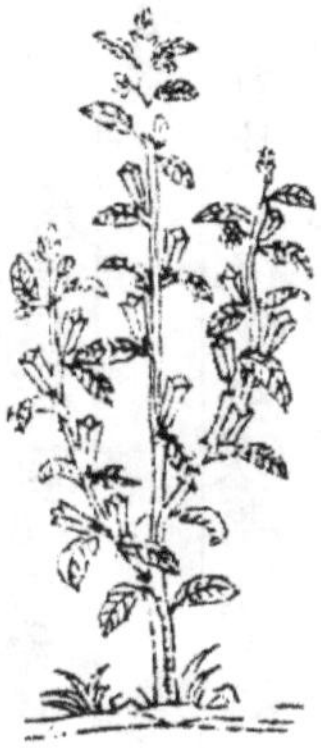

白芝麻味甘大寒無毒治虛勞滑腸胃行風氣通血脉去頭風潤肌膚食後生噉一合與乳母食之令子不生病

胡麻味甘微寒除一切痼疾久服長肌肉健人油利大便治胞衣不下脩真秘旨云神仙服胡麻法久服面光澤不飢三年水火不能害行及奔馬

5A
Malt Sugar

餳味甘微溫無毒補虛乏止渴去血建脾治嗽小兒誤吞錢取一斤漸漸盡食之即出

Honey

蜜味甘平微溫無毒主心腹邪氣諸驚癇補五藏不足氣益中止痛解毒明耳目和百藥除衆病

Leaven

麴味甘大暖療藏府中風氣調中益氣開胃消食補虛冷陳久者良

Vinegar

醋味酸溫無毒消癰腫散水氣殺邪毒破血運除癥塊堅積醋有數種酒醋桃醋麥醋葡萄醋棗醋米醋為上入藥用

Soy sauce

醬味鹹酸冷無毒除熱止煩殺百藥熱湯火毒殺一切魚肉菜蔬毒豆醬主治勝麵醬陳久者尤良

5B

Fermented Black Beans
豉味苦寒無毒主傷寒頭痛煩燥滿悶

Salt
鹽味鹹溫無毒主殺鬼蠱邪疰毒傷寒吐胷中痰癖
止心腹卒痛多食傷肺令人咳嗽失顏色

Liquor
酒味苦甘辣大熱有毒主行藥勢殺百邪通血脉厚
腸胃潤皮膚消憂愁多飲損壽傷神易人本性酒
有數般唯醞釀以隨其性
虎骨酒以酥炙虎骨擣碎釀酒治骨節疼痛風
疰冷痹痛
枸杞酒以甘州枸杞依法釀酒補虛弱長肌肉
益精氣去冷風壯陽道

6A

地黃酒以地黃絞汁釀酒治虛弱壯筋骨通血
脉治腹內痛
松節酒仙方以五月五日採松節剉碎煮水釀
酒治冷風虛骨弱脚不能履地
茯苓酒仙方依法茯苓釀酒治虛勞壯筋骨延
年益壽
松根酒以松樹下撅坑置瓮取松根津液釀酒
治風壯筋骨
羊羔酒依法作酒大補益人
五加皮酒五加皮浸酒或依法釀酒治骨弱不

6B

能行走久服壯筋骨延年不老
膃肭臍酒治腎虛弱壯腰膝大補益人
小黃米酒性熱不宜多飲昏人五藏煩熱多睡
葡萄酒益氣調中耐飢強志酒有數等有西番
者有哈剌火者有平陽太原者其味都不及
哈剌火者田地酒最佳
阿剌吉酒味甘辣大熱有大毒主消冷堅積去
寒氣用好酒蒸熬取露成阿剌吉
速兒麻酒又名撥糟味微甘辣主益氣止渴多
飲令人膨脹生痰

7A
Ox

獸品

牛

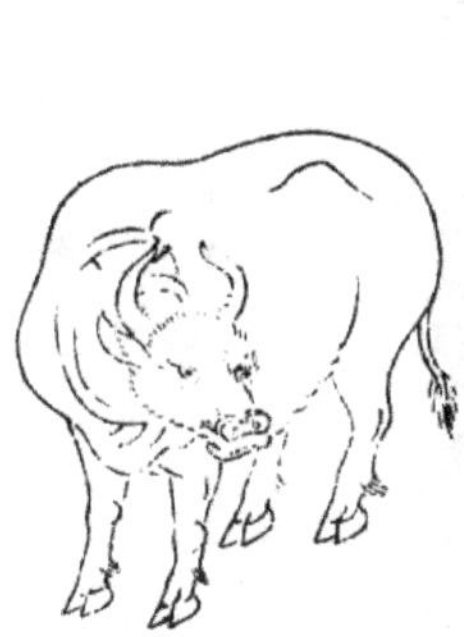

牛肉味甘平無毒主消渴止㖟泄安中益氣補脾胃
○牛髓補中填精髓○牛酥涼益心肺止渴嗽潤
毛髮除肺痿心熱吐血○牛酪味甘酸寒無毒主
熱毒止消渴除胷中虛熱身面熱瘡○牛乳腐微

7B
Sheep

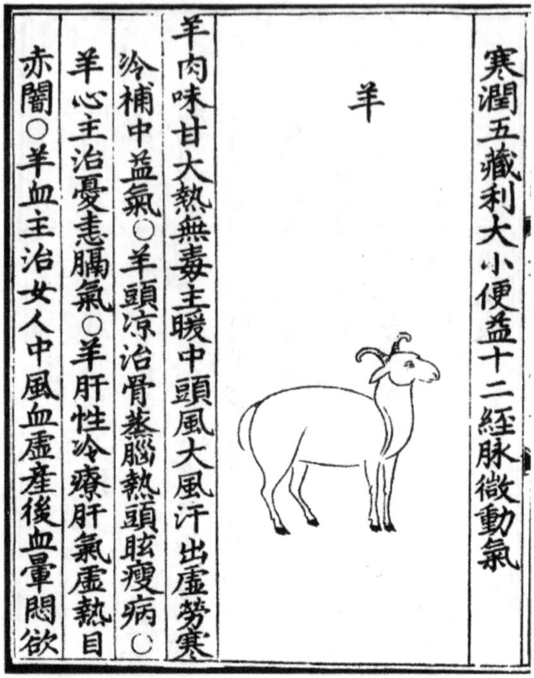
寒潤五藏利大小便益十二經脉徵動氣
羊
羊肉味甘大熱無毒主暖中頭風大風汗出虛勞寒
冷補中益氣○羊頭涼治骨蒸腦熱頭眩瘦病○
羊心主治憂恚膈氣○羊肝性冷療肝氣虛熱目
赤闇○羊血主治女人中風血虛產後血暈悶欲

8A
Gazelle

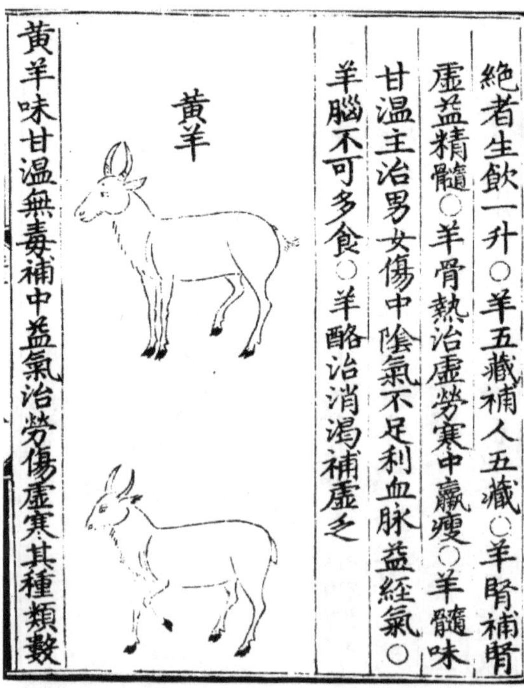
絶者生飲一升○羊五藏補人五藏○羊腎補腎
虛益精髓○羊骨熱治虛勞寒中羸瘦○羊髓味
甘溫主治男女傷中陰氣不足利血脉益經氣○
羊腦不可多食○羊酪治消渴補虛乏
黃羊
黃羊味甘溫無毒補中益氣治勞傷虛寒其種類數

8B
Goat

等成群至於千數白黃羊生於野草內黑尾黃羊
生於沙漠中能走善卧行走不成群其腦不可食
髓骨可食能補益人煮湯無味
山羊味甘平無毒補益人生山谷中

羖䍽

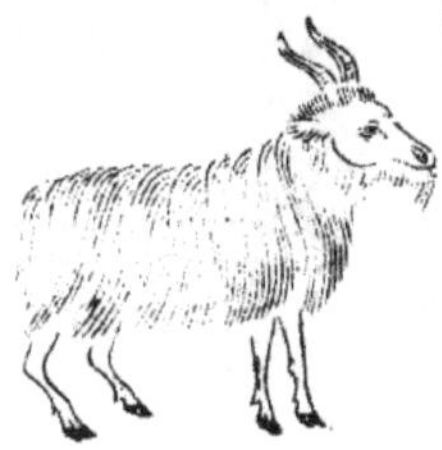

羖䍽味甘平無毒補五勞七傷溫中益氣其肉稍腥

9A
Horse

馬

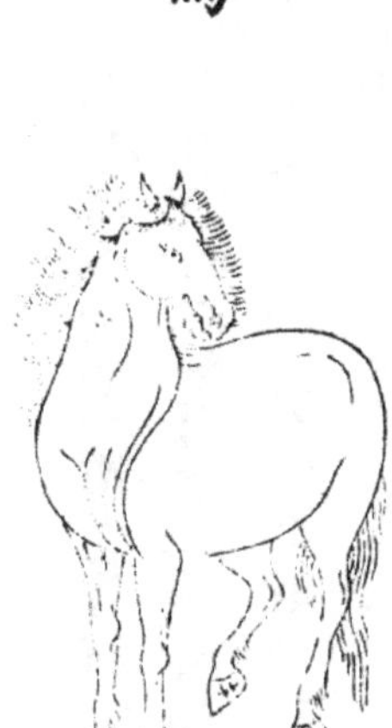

馬肉味辛苦冷有小毒主熱下氣長筋骨強腰膝壯
健輕身○馬頭骨作枕令人少睡○馬肝不可食
○馬蹄白者治婦人漏下白崩赤者治婦人赤崩
○白馬莖味鹹甘無毒主傷中脉絕強志益氣長
肌肉令人有子能壯盛陰氣○馬心主喜忘○馬

9B
Wild
Horse

肉內有生黑墨汁者有毒不可食白馬多有之

馬乳性冷味甘止渴治熱有三等一名升堅一名晃禾兒一名窓兀以升堅爲上

野馬

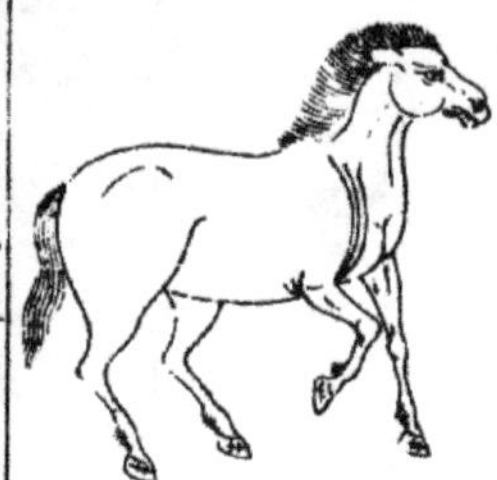

野馬肉味甘平有毒壯筋骨與家馬肉頗相似其肉落地不沾沙然不宜多食

10A
Elephant

象

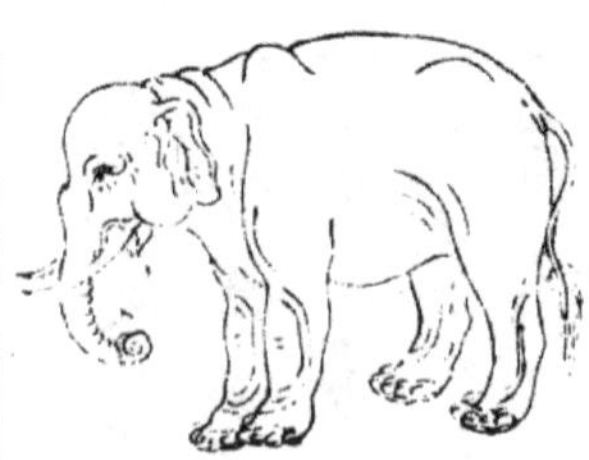

象肉味淡不堪食多食令人體重胷前小橫骨令人能浮水身有百獸肉皆有分段惟鼻是本肉○象牙無毒主諸鐵及雜物入肉刮取屑細研和水傅瘡上即出

10B
Camel

駞

駞肉治諸風下氣壯筋骨潤皮膚療一切頑麻風痺肌膚緊急惡瘡腫毒○駞脂在兩峯內有積聚者酒服之良○駞乳係愛刺性温味甘補中益氣壯筋骨令人不飢

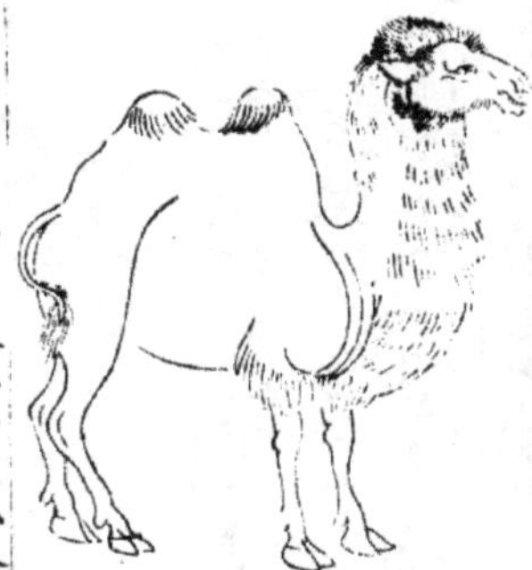

11A
Wild
Camel

野駞

野駞味甘温平無毒治諸風下氣壯筋骨潤皮膚○駞峯治虛勞風有冷積者用葡萄酒温調峯子油服之良好酒亦可

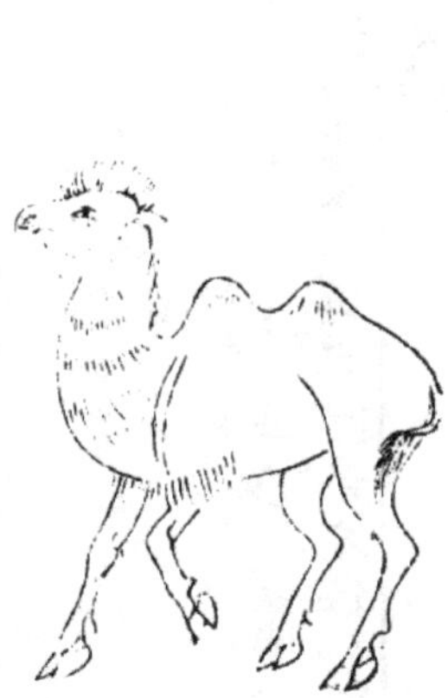

11B
Bear

熊

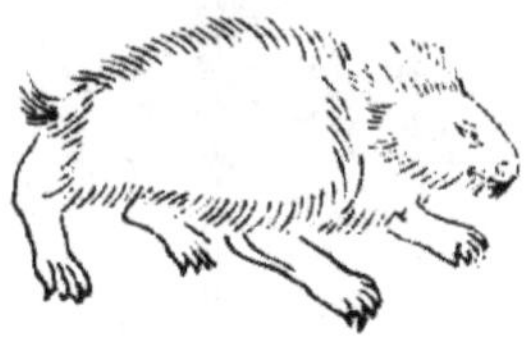

熊肉味甘無毒主風痺筋骨不仁若腹中有積聚寒熱羸瘦者不可食之終身不除○熊白涼無毒治風補虛損殺勞虫○熊掌食之可禦風寒此是八珍之數古人最重之○十月勿食之損神

12A
Donkey

驢

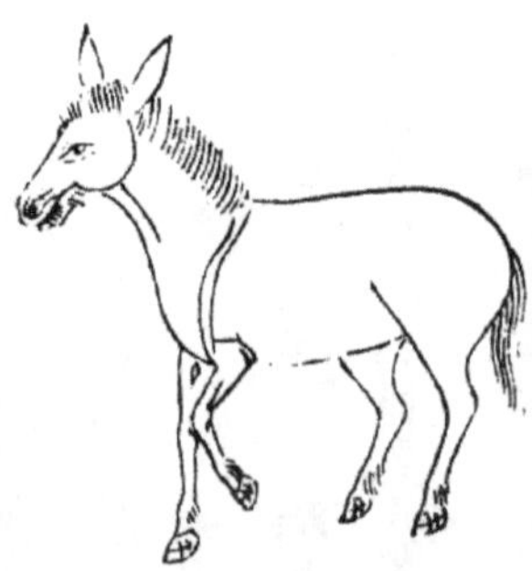

驢肉味甘寒無毒治風狂憂愁不樂安心氣解心煩頭肉治多年消渴煮食之良烏驢者尤佳○脂和烏梅作丸治久瘧

野驢性味同比家驢鬃尾長骨格大食之能治風眩

12B Sika Deer

麋

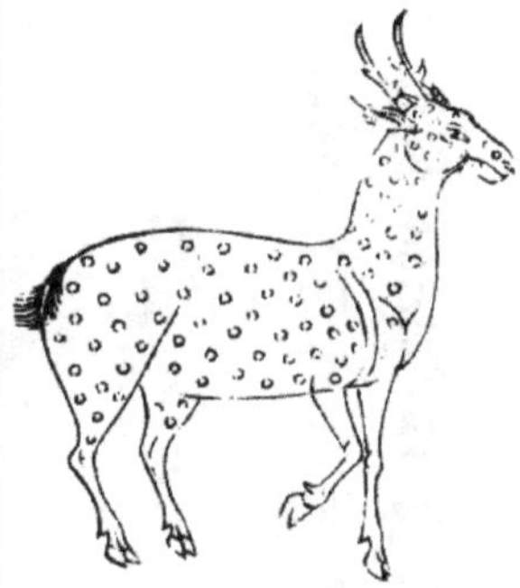

麋肉味甘温無毒益氣補中治腰脚無力不可與野雞肉及蝦生菜梅李果實同食令人病○麋脂味辛温無毒主癰腫惡瘡風痺四肢拘緩通血脉潤澤皮膚○麋皮作靴能除脚氣

13A Red Deer

鹿

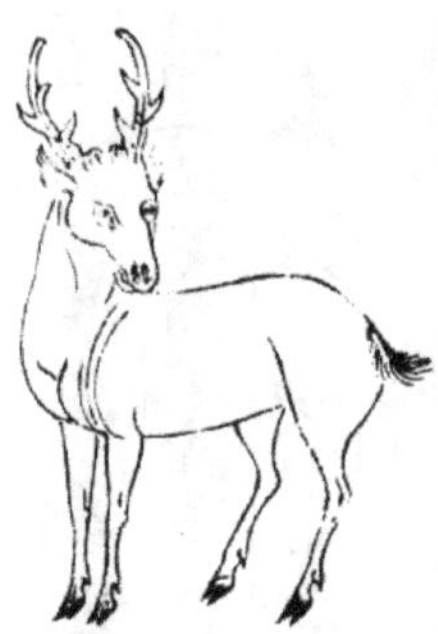

鹿肉味甘温無毒補中強五藏益氣○鹿髓甘温主男女傷中絶脉筋急欬逆以酒服之○鹿頭主消渴夜夢見物○鹿蹄主脚膝疼痛○鹿腎主温中補腎安五藏壯陽氣○鹿茸味甘微温無毒主漏下惡血寒熱驚癇益氣強志補虛羸壯筋骨○鹿

13B
River
Deer

角徵鹹無毒主惡瘡癰腫逐邪氣除小腹血急痛
腰脊痛及留血在陰中

麞

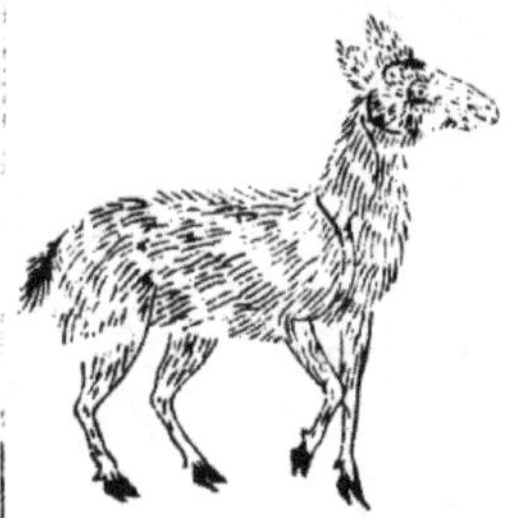

麞肉温主補益五藏日華子云肉無毒八月至臘月
食之勝羊肉十二月以後至七月食之動氣道家
多食言無禁忌也

14A
Dog

犬

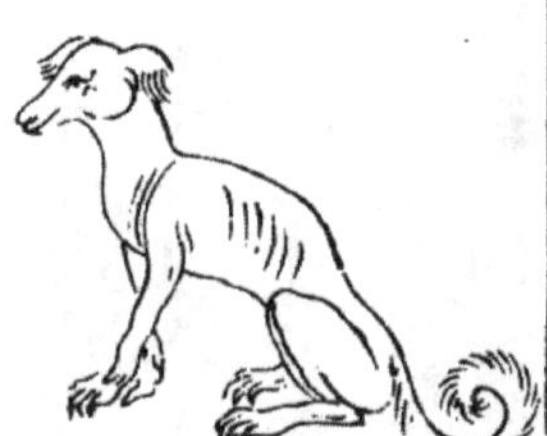

犬肉味鹹温無毒安五藏補絶傷益陽道補血脉厚
腸胃實下焦填精髓黄色犬肉尤佳不與蒜同食
必頻損人九月不宜食之令人損神○犬四脚蹄
煑飲之下乳汁

14B
Pig

猪

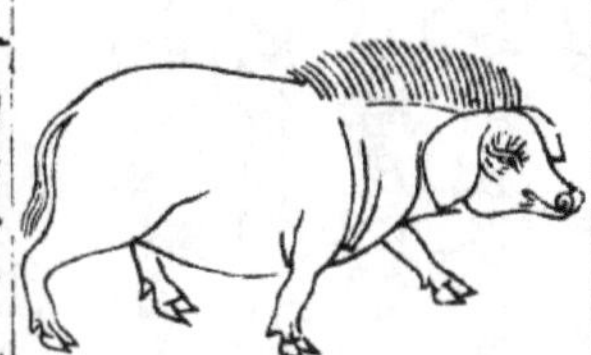

猪肉味苦無毒主閉血脉弱筋骨虚肥人不可久食動風患金瘡者尤甚○猪肚主補中益氣止渴○猪腎冷和理腎氣通利膀胱○猪四蹄小寒主傷撻諸敗瘡下乳

15A
Wild
Boar

野猪

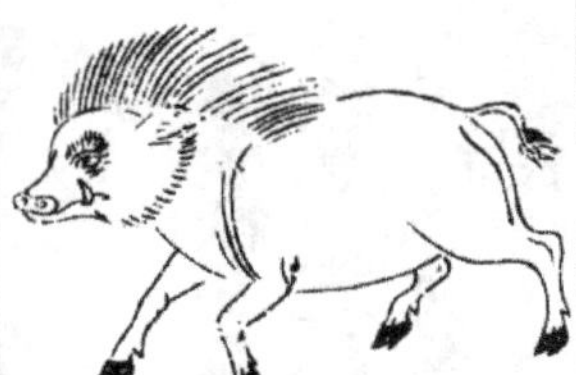

野猪肉味苦無毒主補肌膚令人虛肥雌者肉更美冬月食橡子肉色赤補人五藏治腸風瀉血其肉味勝家猪

江猪味甘平無毒然不宜多食動風氣令人體重

15B
Otter

獺

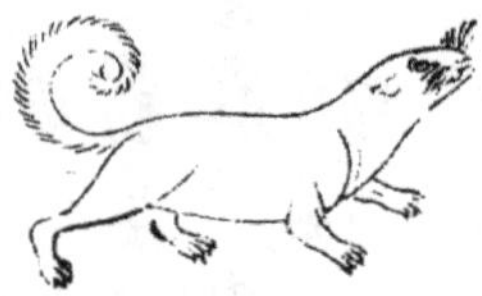

獺肉味醎平無毒治水氣脹滿療溫疫病諸熱毒風
欬嗽勞損不可與兎同食○獺肝甘有毒治腸風
下血及主疰病相染○獺皮飾領袖則塵垢不著
如風沙翳目以袖拭之即出又魚刺鯁喉中不出
者取獺爪爬項下即出

16A
Tiger

虎

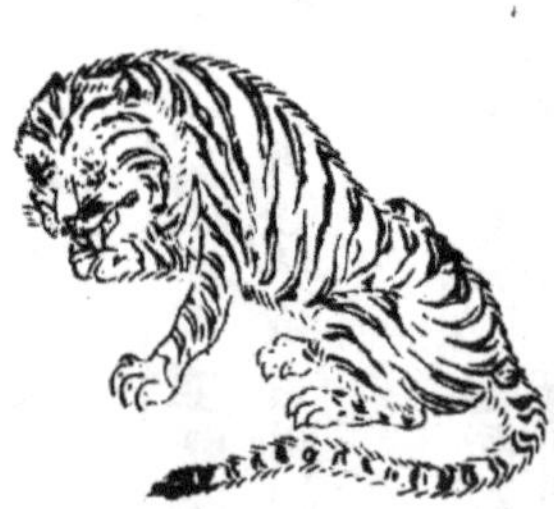

虎肉味醎酸平無毒主惡心欲嘔益氣力食之入山
虎見則畏辟三十六種魅○虎眼睛主瘧疾辟惡
止小兒熱驚○虎骨主除邪惡氣殺鬼疰毒止驚
悸主惡瘡鼠瘻頭骨尤良

16B
Leopard

豹

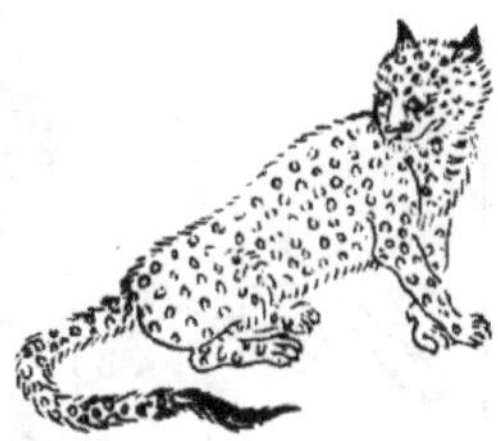

豹肉味酸平無毒安五藏補絶傷壯筋骨強志氣久
食令人猛健忘性麁踈耐寒暑正月勿食之傷神
唐本注云車駕鹵簿用豹尾取其威重為可貴也
土豹腦子可治腰疼

17A
Pere
David's
Deer

Musk
Deer

麞

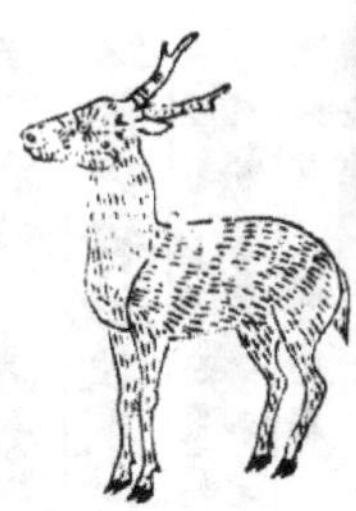

麞子味甘平無毒補益人

麂

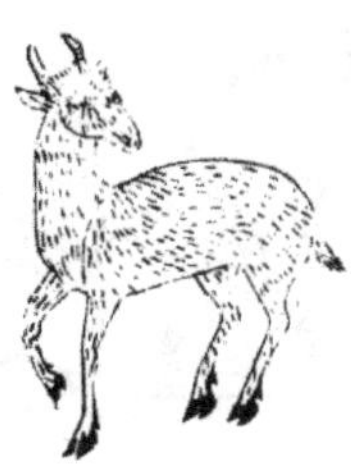

麂肉味甘平無毒主五痔多食能動人痼疾

17B
Muntjac
Deer

Fox

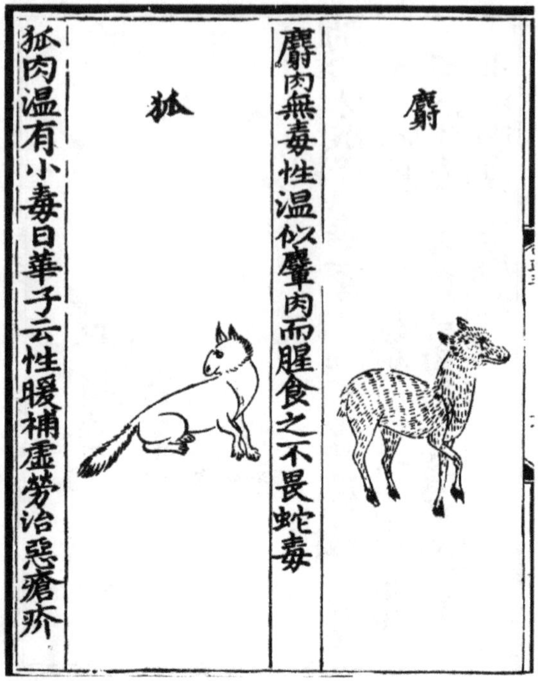

18A
Rhino-
ceros

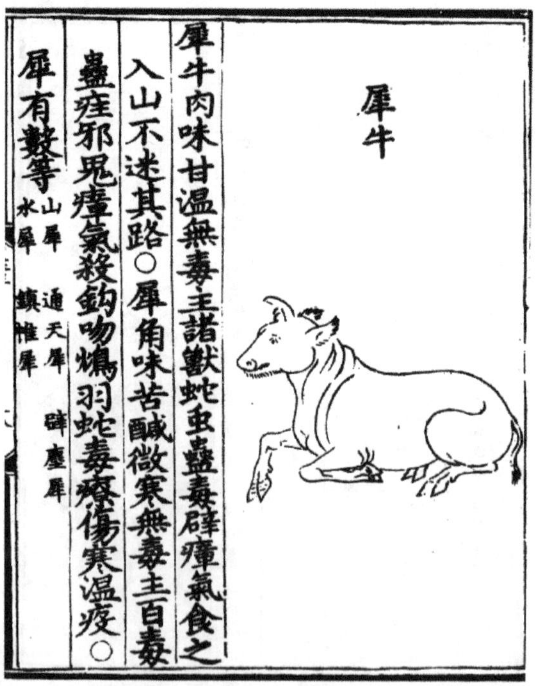

18B
Wolf

狼

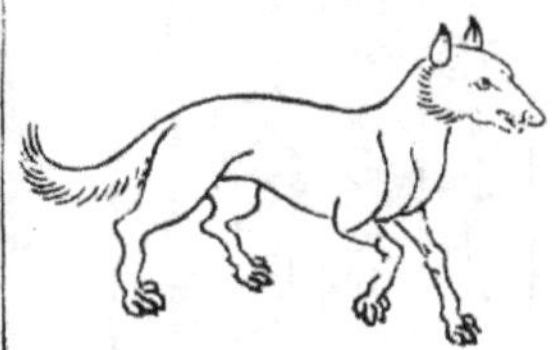

狼肉味鹹性熱無毒主補益五藏厚腸胃填精髓腹
有冷積者宜食之味勝狐犬肉○狼喉嗉皮熟成
皮條勒頭去頭痛○狼皮熟作番皮大暖○狼尾
馬胷堂前帶之辟邪令馬不驚○狼牙帶之辟邪

19A
Hare

兔

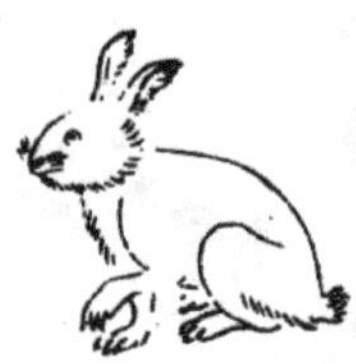

兔肉味辛平無毒補中益氣不宜多食損陽事絕血
脉令人痿黃不可與薑橘同食令人患卒心痛姙
娠不可食令子缺唇二月不可食傷神○兔肝主
明目○臘月兔頭及皮毛燒灰酒調服之治産難
胞衣不出餘血不下

19B
Tarba-aan

塔剌不花

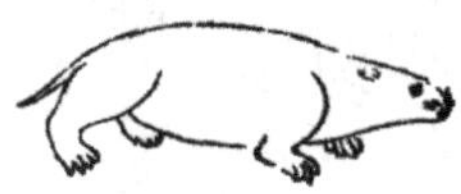

塔剌不花一名土撥鼠味甘無毒主野雞瘻瘡煑食之宜人生山後草澤中北人掘取以食雖肥煑則無油湯無味多食難克化微動氣○皮作番皮不濕透甚暖○頭骨去下頦肉令齒全治小兒無睡懸之頭邊即令得睡

20A
Badger

Wild
Cat

獾

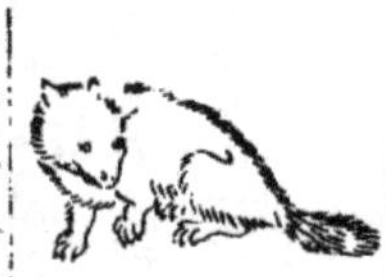

獾肉味甘平無毒治上氣欬逆水腹不差作羹食良

野貍

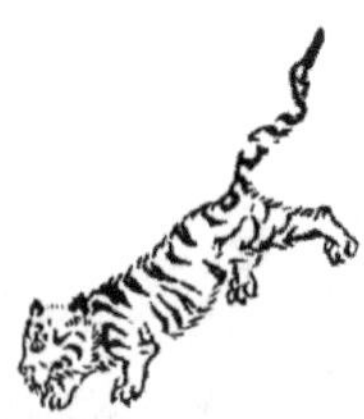

野貍味甘平無毒主治鼠瘻惡瘡頭骨尤良

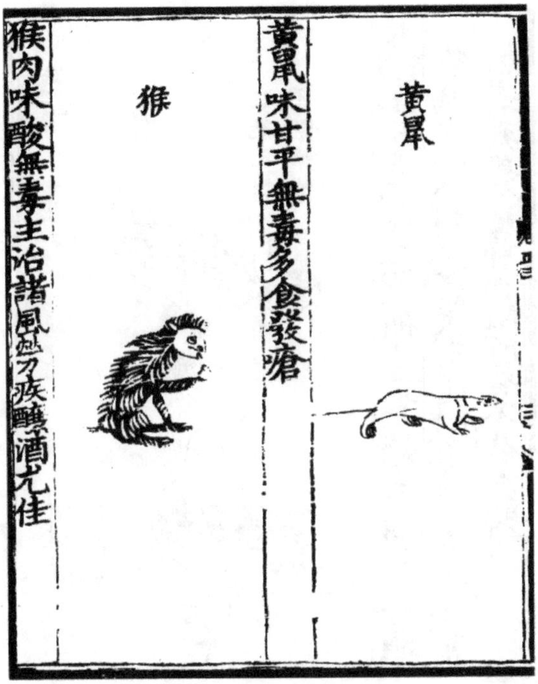

黃鼠
黃鼠味甘平無毒多食發瘡
猴
猴肉味酸無毒主治諸風勞及釀酒尤佳

20B
Weasel

Monkey

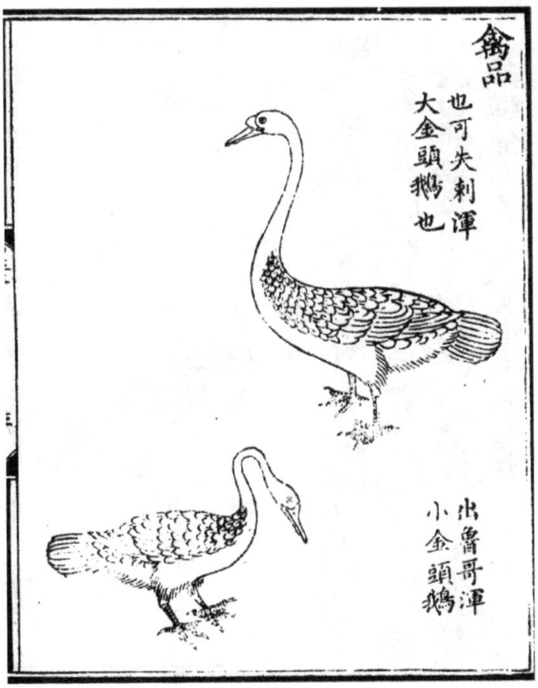

21A
Whooper
Swan

Tundra
Swan

21B
Mute
Swan

Variega-
ted
Swan

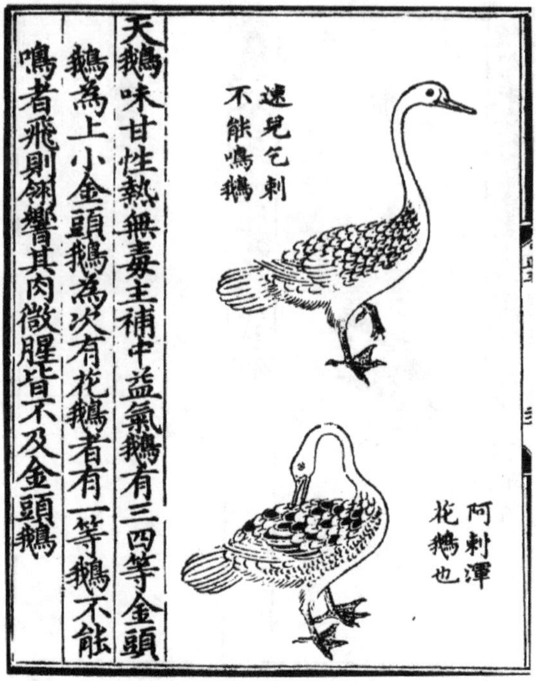

天鵝味甘性熱無毒主補中益氣鵝有三四等金頭鵝為上小金頭鵝為次有花鵝者有一等鵝不能鳴者飛則翎響其肉微腥皆不及金頭鵝

22A
Swan-
goose

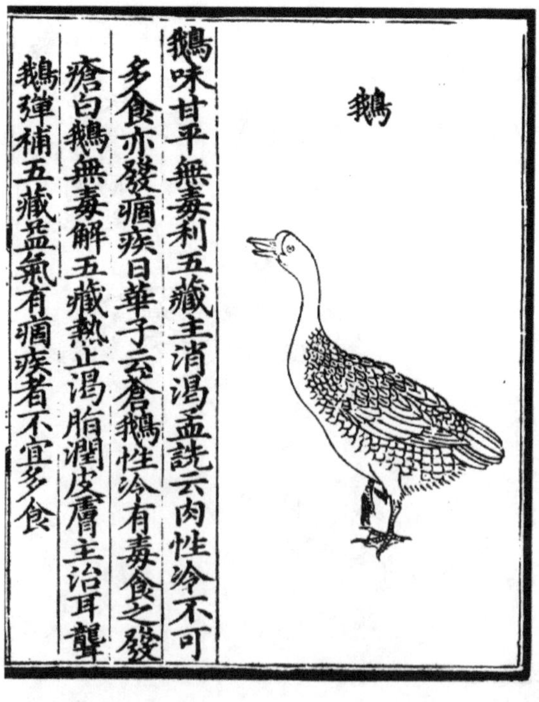

鵝味甘平無毒利五臟主消渴孟詵云肉性冷不可多食亦發痼疾日華子云蒼鵝性冷有毒食之發瘡白鵝無毒解五臟熱止渴脂潤皮膚主治耳聾彐鵝弹補五臟益氣有痼疾者不宜多食

22B
Wild
Goose

鴈

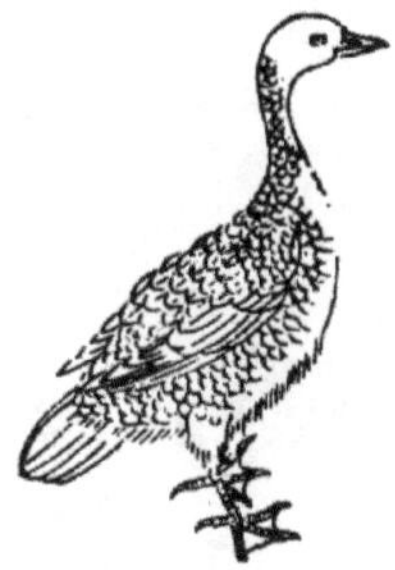

鴈味甘平無毒主風攣拘急偏枯氣不通利益氣壯筋骨補勞瘦鴈骨灰和米泔洗頭長髮○鴈膏治耳聾亦能長髮○鴈脂補虛羸令人肥白○六月七月勿食鴈令人傷神

23A
Cranes

嶋[illegible]

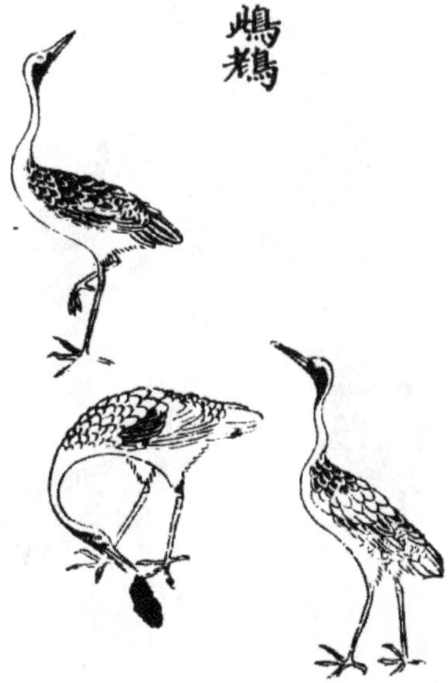

23B
Curlew

鴜鵝味甘溫無毒補中益氣食之甚有益人炙食之味尤美然有數等白鴜鵝黑頭鴜鵝胡鴜鵝其肉皆不同○髓味甘美補精髓

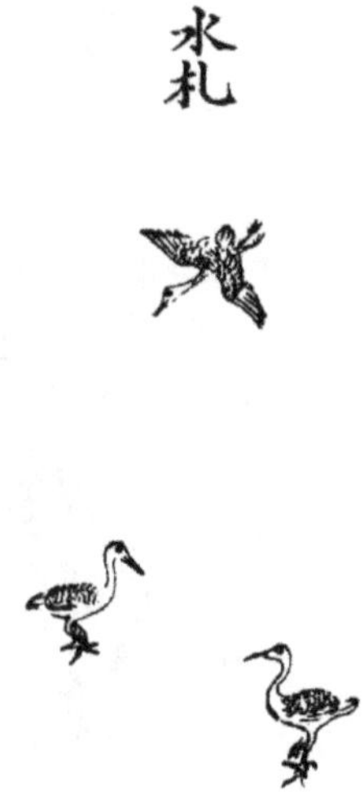

水札味甘平無毒補中益氣宜炙食之甚美

24A
Chicken

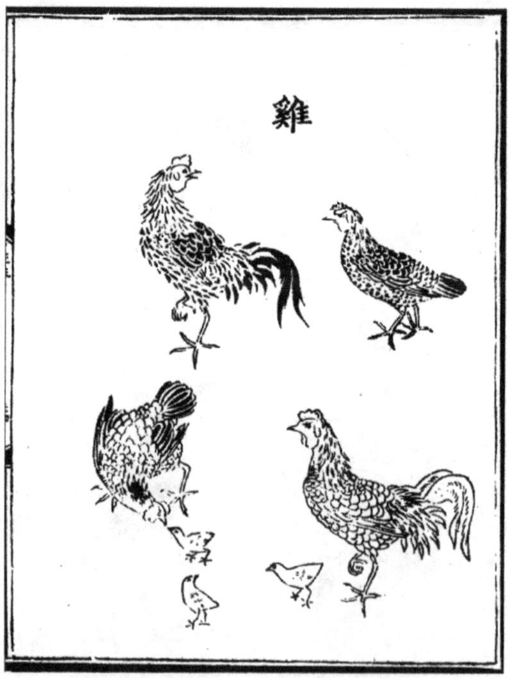

24B

丹雄鷄味甘平微溫無毒主婦人崩中漏下赤白補
虛溫中止血○白雄鷄味酸無毒主下氣療狂邪
補中安五藏治消渴○烏雄雞味甘酸無毒主補
中止痛除心腹惡氣虛弱者宜食之○烏嶋雞味
甘溫無毒主風寒濕痺五緩六急中惡腹痛及傷
折骨疼安胎血瘀乳難○黃嶋鷄味酸平無毒主
傷中消渴小便數不禁腸澼洩痢補五藏先患骨
熱者不可食○鷄子益氣多食令人有聲主産後
痢與小兒食之止痢日華子云鷄子鎭心安五藏
其白微寒療目赤熱痛除心下伏熱止煩滿欬逆

25A
Pheasant

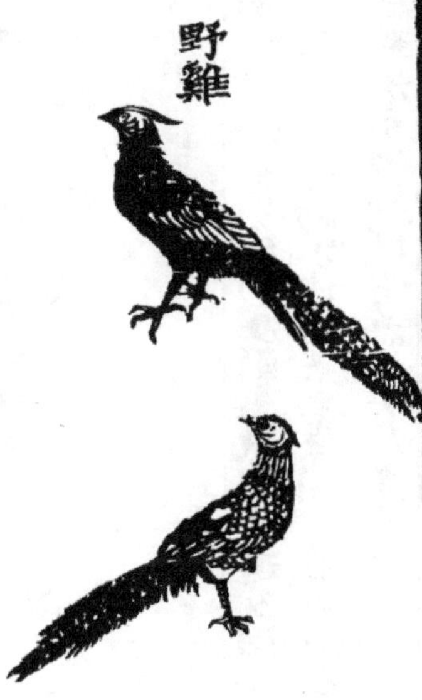

野鷄味甘酸微寒有小毒主補中益氣止洩痢久食
令人瘦九月至十一月食之稍有益他月即發五
痔及諸瘡亦不可與胡桃及菌子木耳同食

25B
Wild
Phea-
sant

山鷄

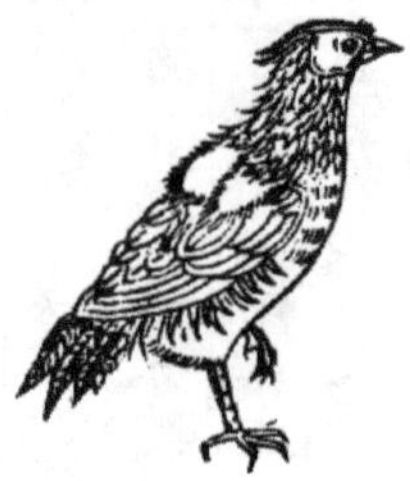

山雞味甘溫有小毒主五藏氣喘不得息者如食法服之然久食能發五痔與蕎麥麵同食生蟲今遼陽有食雞味甚肥美有角鷄味尤勝諸鷄肉

26A
Mallard

Pintail

鴨

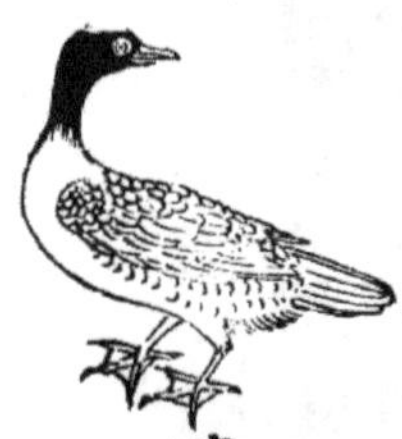

速速兒

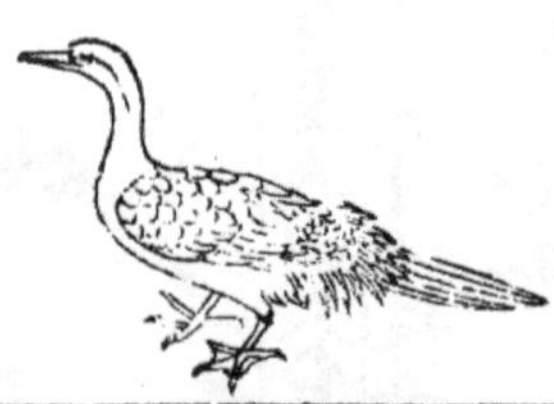

鴨肉味甘冷無毒補內虛消毒熱利水道及治小兒熱驚癇○野鴨味甘微寒無毒補中益氣消食和胃氣治水腫綠頭者為上尖尾者為次

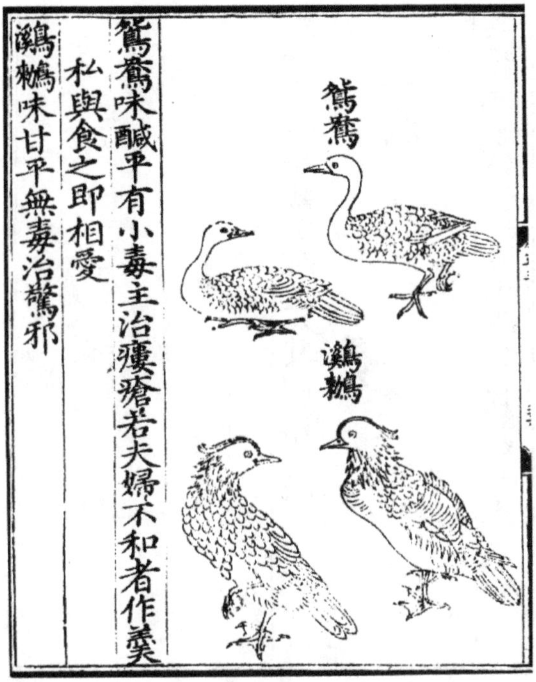
鴛鴦
鸂鶒
鴛鴦味鹹平有小毒主治瘻瘡若夫婦不和者作羹
私與食之即相愛
鸂鶒味甘平無毒治驚邪

26B
Mandarin Duck

Tufted Duck

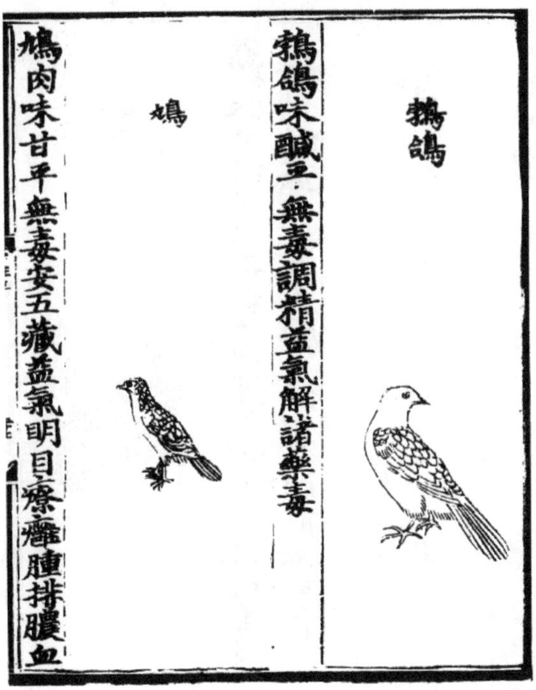

27A
Pigeon

Dove

27B
Bustard

Crow

鳵

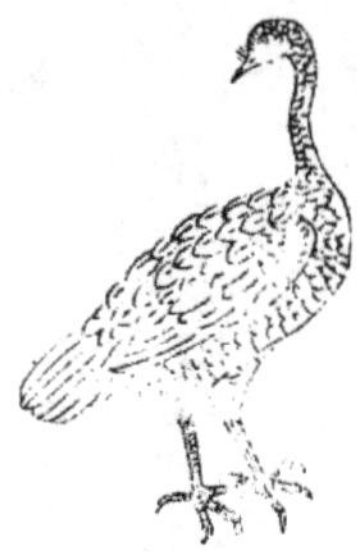

鳵肉味甘平無毒補益人其肉麤味美

寒鴉

寒鴉味酸鹹平無毒主瘦病止欬嗽骨蒸羸弱者

28A
Quail

Sparrow

鵪鶉

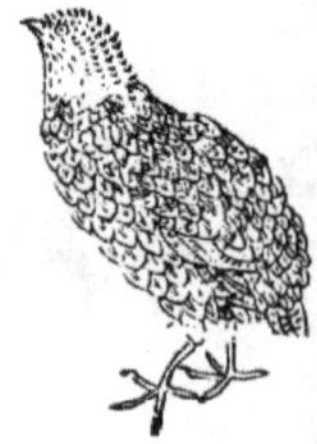

鵪鶉味甘溫平無毒益氣補五藏實筋骨耐寒暑消結熱酥煎食之令人肥下焦四月以前未可食

雀

28B

雀肉味甘無毒性熱壯陽道令人有子冬月者良
蒿雀味甘溫無毒食之益陽道羨於諸雀

29A
Carp

Golden
Carp

魚品

鯉魚

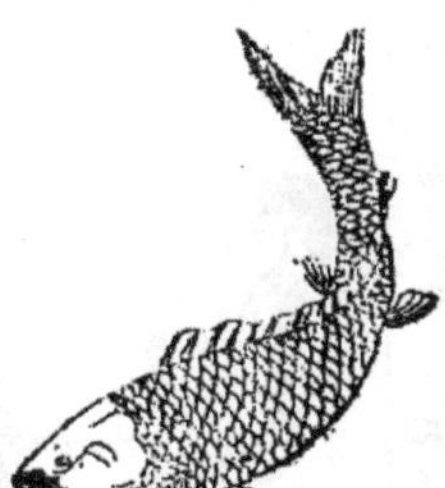

鯉魚味甘寒有毒主欬逆上氣黃疸止渴安胎治水
腫脚氣天行病後不可食有宿癥者不可食

鯽魚

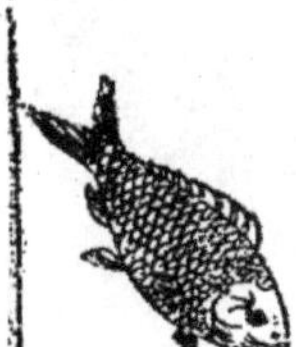

29B
Bream

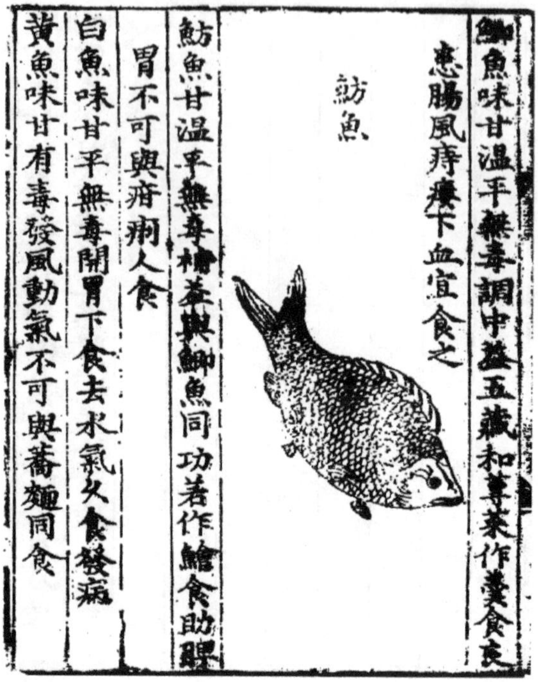

鯽魚味甘溫平無毒調中益五藏和蓴菜作羹食良
患腸風痔瘻下血宜食之

魴魚

魴魚甘溫平無毒補益與鯽魚同功若作鱠食助脾
胃不可與病痢人食

白魚味甘平無毒開胃下食去水氣久食發病

黃魚味甘有毒發風動氣不可與蕎麵同食

30A
"Green
Fish"

Sheat-
fish

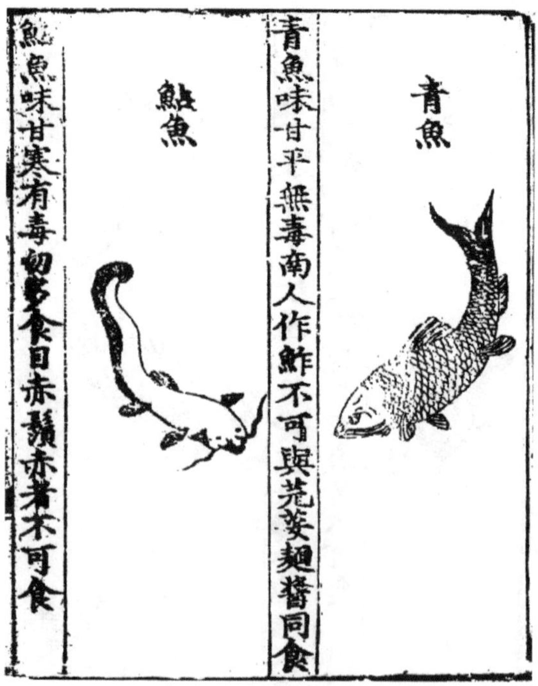

青魚

青魚味甘平無毒南人作鮓不可與芫荽麵醬同食

鮎魚

鮎魚味甘寒有毒勿多食目赤鬚赤者不可食

30B
Sawfish

沙魚

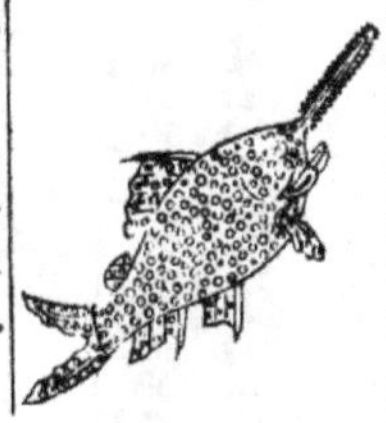

沙魚味甘醎無毒主心氣鬼疰蠱毒吐血
鱓魚味甘平無毒主濕痺天行病後不可食
鮑魚味腥臭無毒主墜蹶踠折瘀血痺在四肢不散
者及治婦人崩血不止
河豘魚味甘溫主補虛去濕氣治腰脚痔等疾
石首魚味甘無毒開胃益氣乾而味鹹者名為鮝

31A
Siberian
Sturgeon

阿八兒忽魚

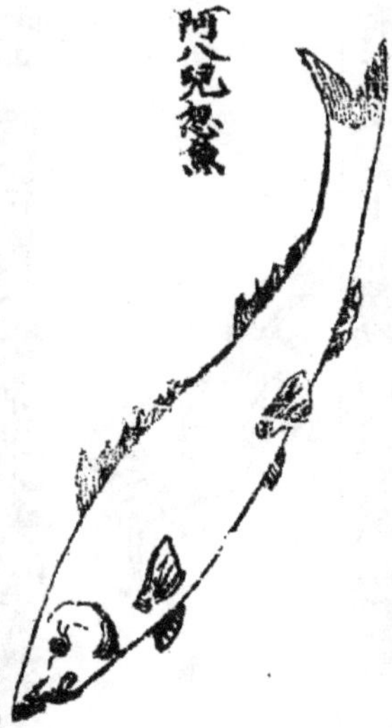

阿八兒忽魚味甘平無毒利五藏肥美人多食難尅
化○脂黃肉麄無鱗骨止有脆骨○胞可作膘膠
甚粘膘與酒化服之消破傷風其魚大者有一二
丈長一名鱘魚又名鱣魚生遼陽東北海河中

31B
Chinese
Sturgeon

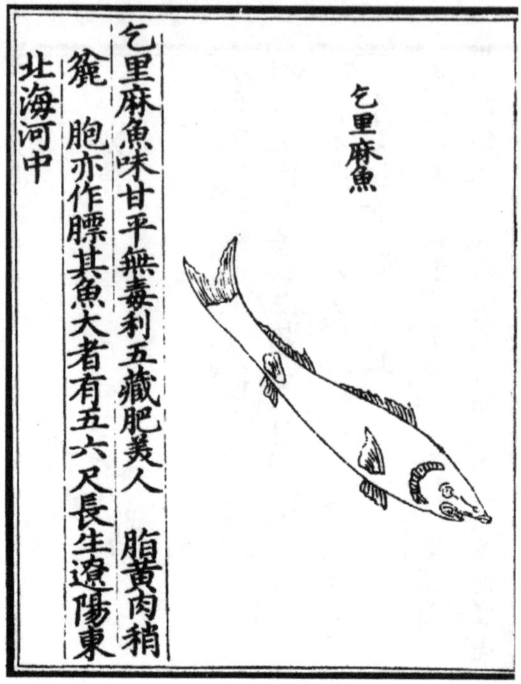
乞里麻魚

乞里麻魚味甘平無毒利五藏肥美人　脂黄肉稍
麄　胞亦作膘其魚大者有五六尺長生遼陽東
北海河中

32A
Turtle

Crab

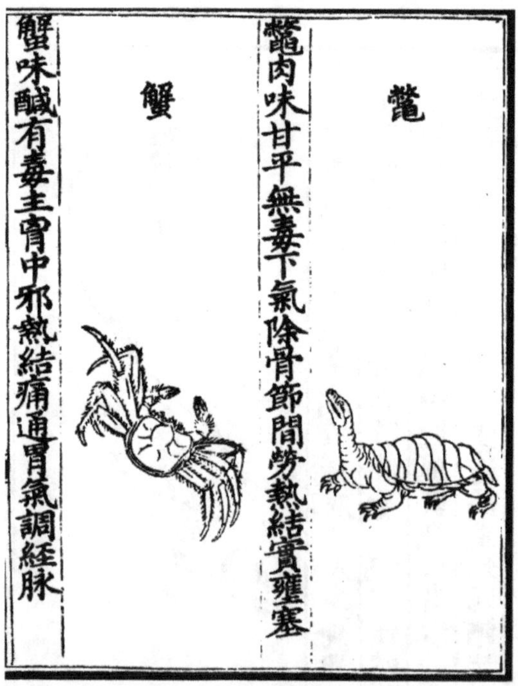
鼈

鼈肉味甘平無毒下氣除骨節間勞熱結實壅塞

蟹

蟹味鹹有毒主胷中邪熱結痛通胃氣調經脉

32A
Shrimp

蝦

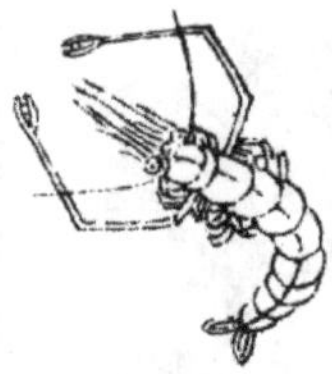

蝦味甘有毒多食損人無鬚者不可食

螺味甘大寒無毒治肝氣熱止渴解酒毒

蛤蜊味甘大寒無毒潤五藏止渴平胃解酒毒

蝟味苦平無毒理胃氣實下焦

蚌泠無毒明目止消渴除煩解熱毒

鱸魚平補五藏益筋骨和腸胃治水氣食之宜人

33A
Peach

Pear

果品

桃

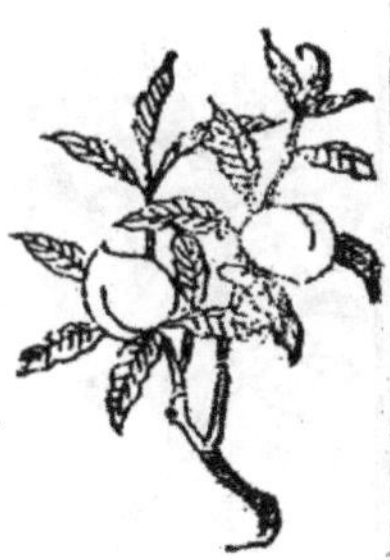

桃味辛甘無毒利肺氣止欬逆上氣消心下堅積除

卒暴擊血破癥瘕通月水止痛○桃仁止心痛

梨

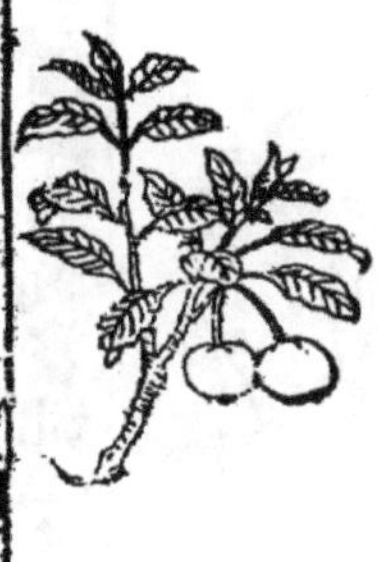

33B
Persimmon

Quince

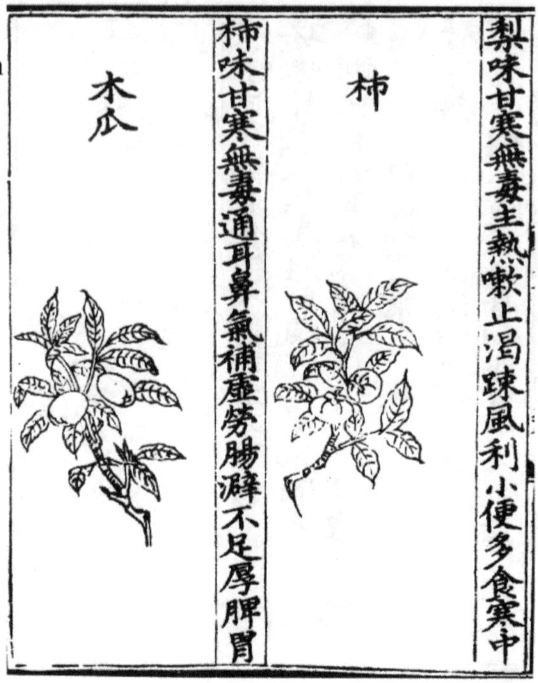
梨味甘寒無毒主熱嗽止渴疎風利小便多食寒中

柿

柿味甘寒無毒通耳鼻氣補虛勞腸澼不足厚脾胃

木瓜

34A
Flowring
Apricot

Japanese
Plum

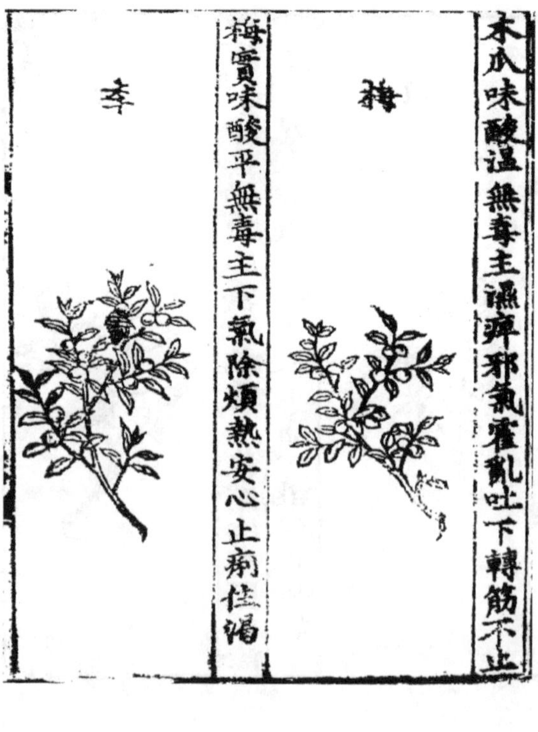
木瓜味酸温無毒主濕痺邪氣霍亂吐下轉筋不止

梅

梅實味酸平無毒主下氣除煩熱安心止痢住渴

李

34B Prinsepia

Pomegranate

李子味苦平無毒主僵仆瘀血骨痛除痼熱調中

柰

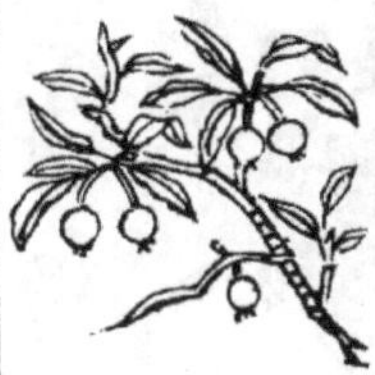

柰子味苦寒多食令人腹脹病人不可食

石榴

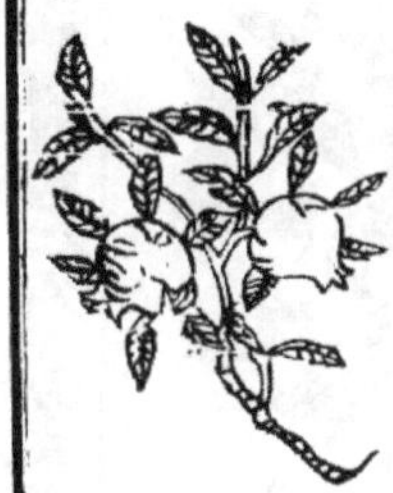

35A Crab Apple

Apricot

石榴味甘酸無毒主咽渴不可多食損人肺止漏精

林檎

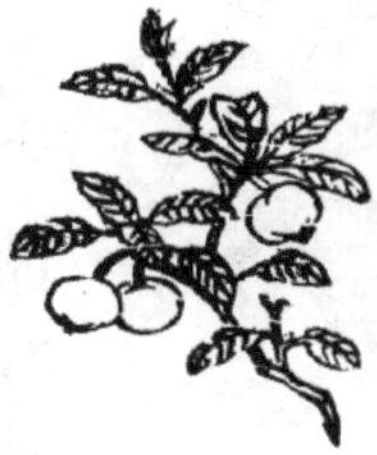

林檎味甘酸温不可多食發熱澀氣令人好睡

杏

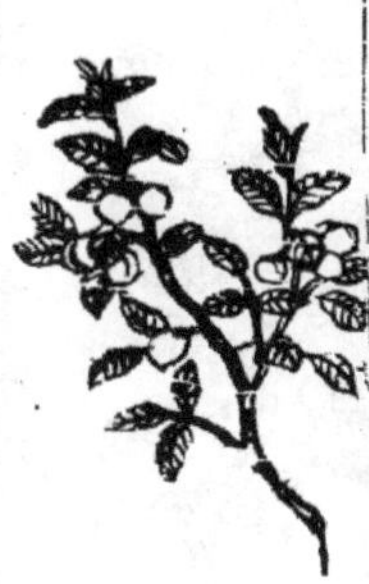

35B
Mandarin
Orange

Tangerine

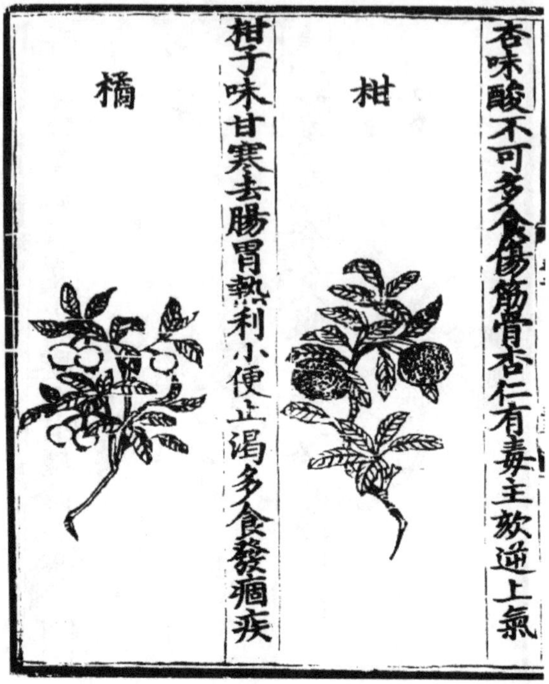

杏味酸不可多食傷筋骨杏仁有毒主欬逆上氣

柑

柑子味甘寒去腸胃熱利小便止渴多食發痼疾

橘

36A
Sweet
Orange

Chestnut

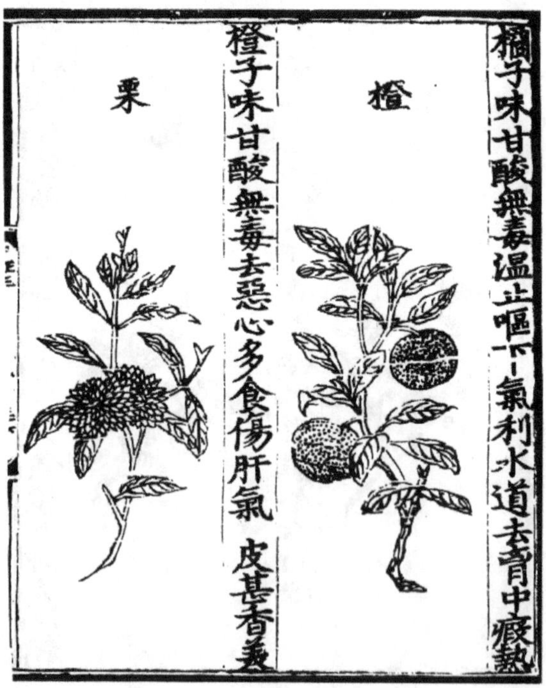

橘子味甘酸無毒溫止嘔下氣利水道去胷中瘕熱

橙

橙子味甘酸無毒去惡心多食傷肝氣 皮甚香美

栗

36B
Jujube

Cherry

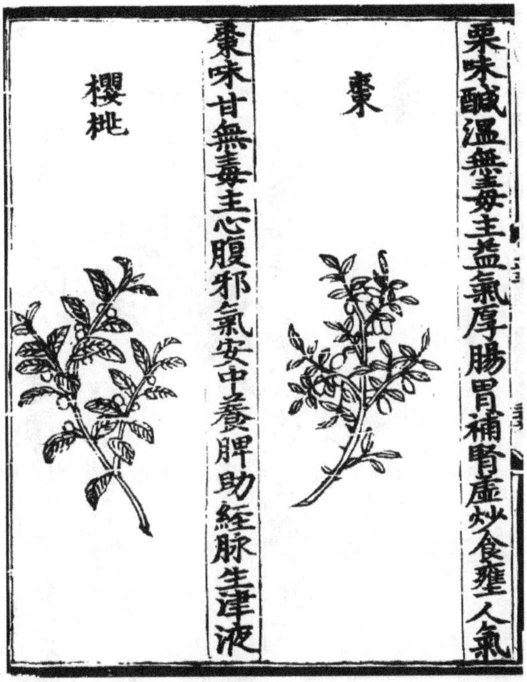

栗味鹹溫無毒主益氣厚腸胃補腎虛炒食壅人氣

棗

棗味甘無毒主心腹邪氣安中養脾助經脉生津液

櫻桃

37A
Grapes

Walnut

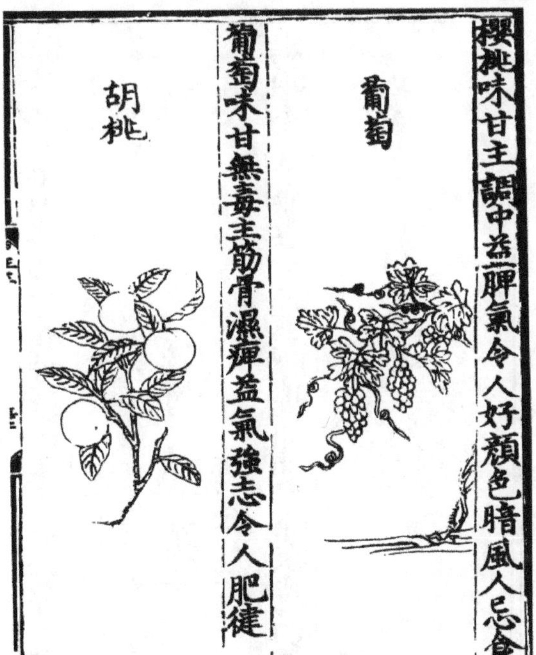

櫻桃味甘主調中益脾氣令人好顏色暗風人忌食

葡萄

葡萄味甘無毒主筋骨濕痺益氣強志令人肥健

胡桃

37B
Pine
Nuts

Lotus
Seeds

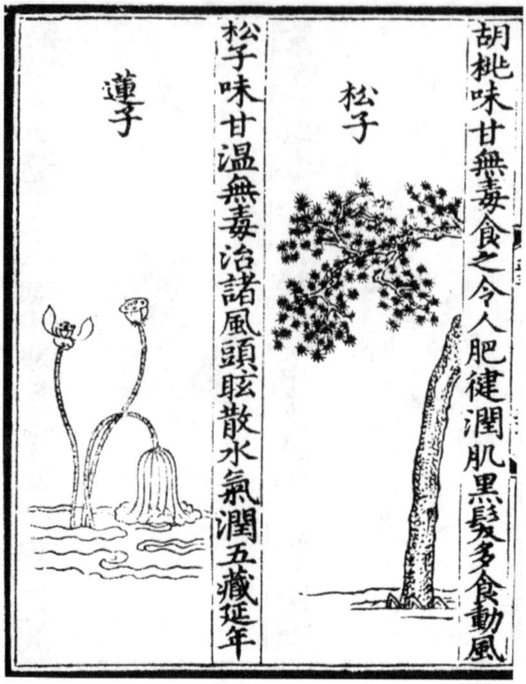

胡桃味甘無毒食之令人肥健潤肌黑髮多食動風

松子

松子味甘溫無毒治諸風頭眩散水氣潤五藏延年

蓮子

38A
Euryale
Fruits

Trapa
Fruits

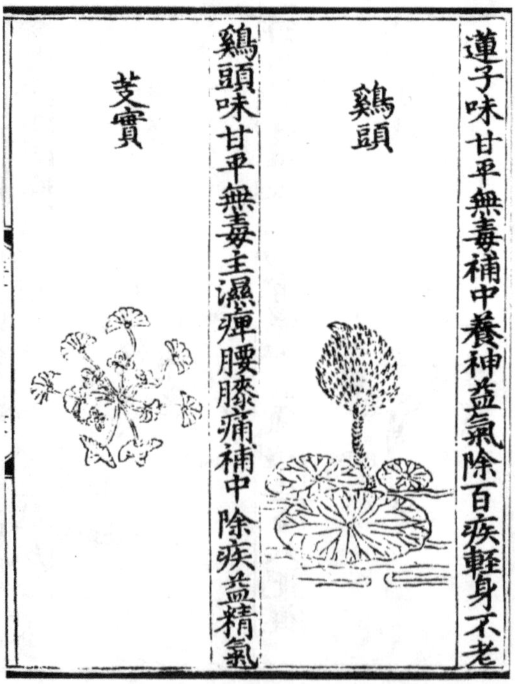

蓮子味甘平無毒補中養神益氣除百疾輕身不老

鷄頭

鷄頭味甘平無毒主濕痺腰膝痛補中除疾益精氣

芰實

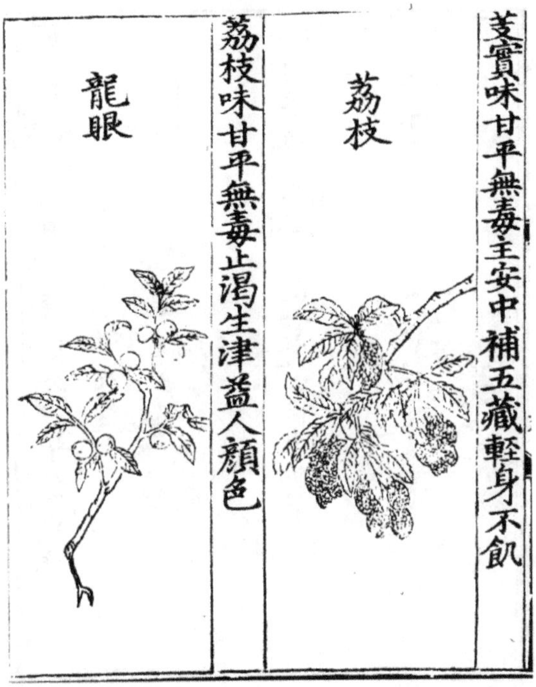

芰實味甘平無毒主安中補五藏輕身不飢

荔枝

荔枝味甘平無毒止渴生津益人顏色

龍眼

38B
Lichee

Longan

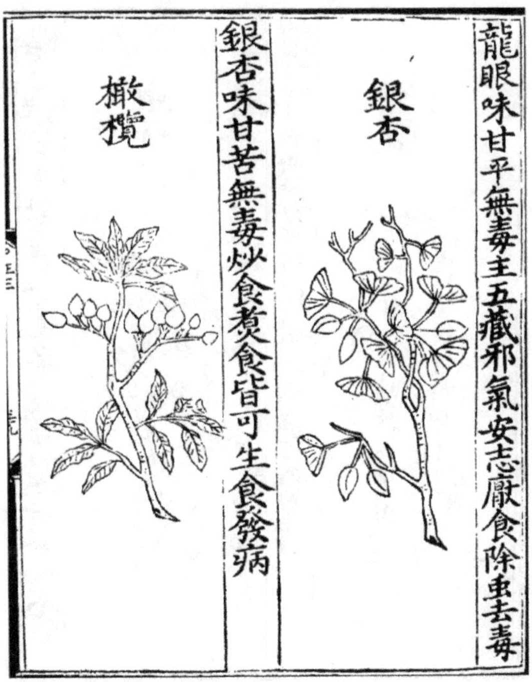

龍眼味甘平無毒主五藏邪氣安志厭食除蟲去毒

銀杏

銀杏味甘苦無毒炒食煮食皆可生食發病

橄欖

39A
Gingko
Fruits

Chinese
Olives

39B
Myrica

Hazelnuts

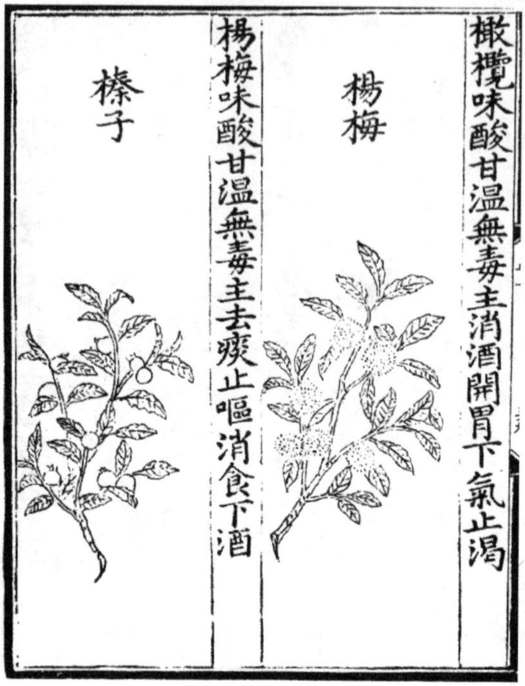

橄欖味酸甘温無毒主消酒開胃下氣止渴

楊梅

楊梅味酸甘温無毒主去痰止嘔消食下酒

榛子

40A
Torreya
Nuts

Sugar
Cane

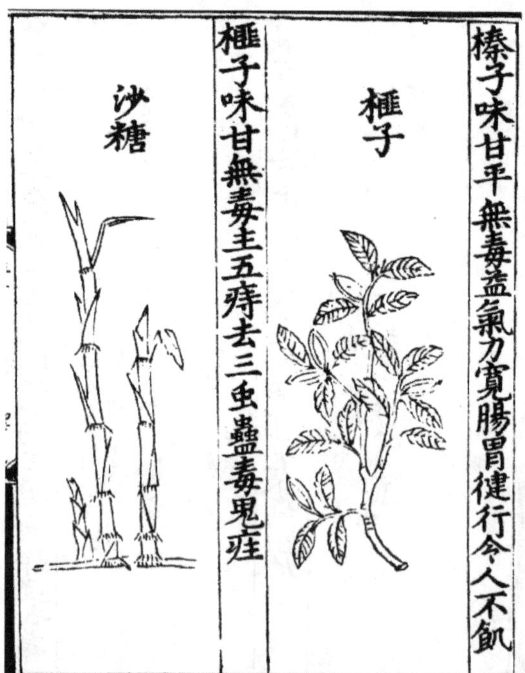

榛子味甘平無毒益氣力寬腸胃健行令人不飢

榧子

榧子味甘無毒主五痔去三虫蠱毒鬼疰

沙糖

40B Sweet Melon

Water-Melon

沙糖味甘寒無毒主心腹熱脹止渴明目即甘蔗汁熬成沙糖

甜瓜

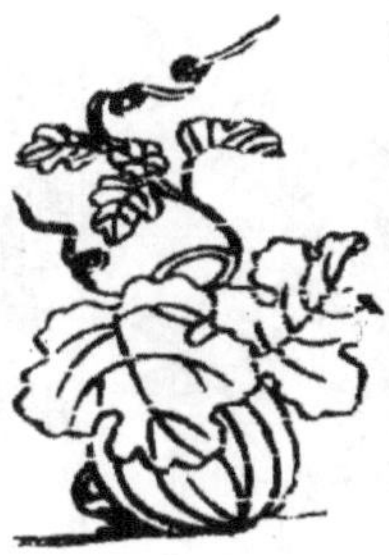

甜瓜味甘寒有毒止渴除煩熱多食發冷病破腹

西瓜

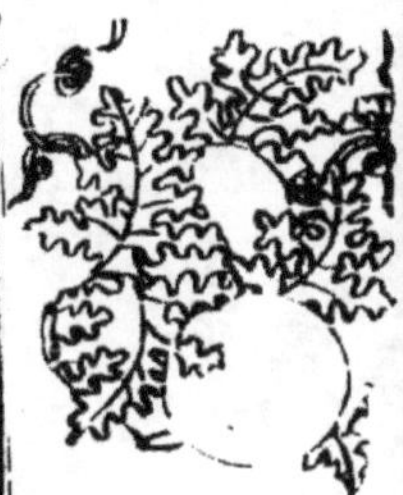

41A Sour Jujube

Apricot Red

西瓜味甘平無毒主消渴治心煩解酒毒

酸棗

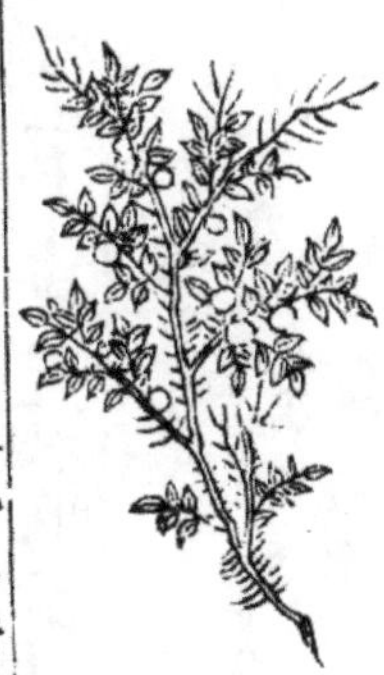

酸棗味酸甘平無毒主心腹寒熱邪結氣聚除煩

海紅

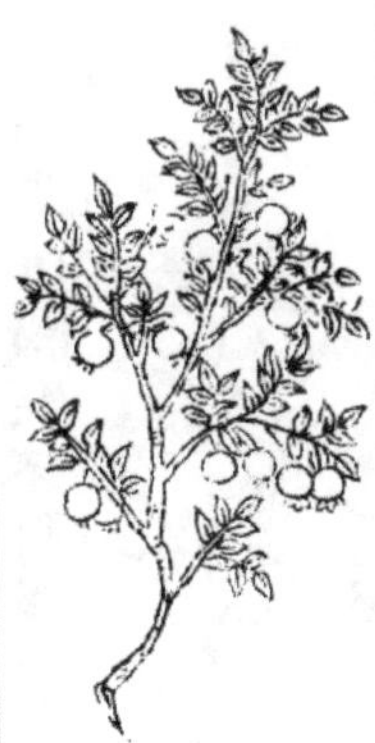

41B
Citrons

Acorns

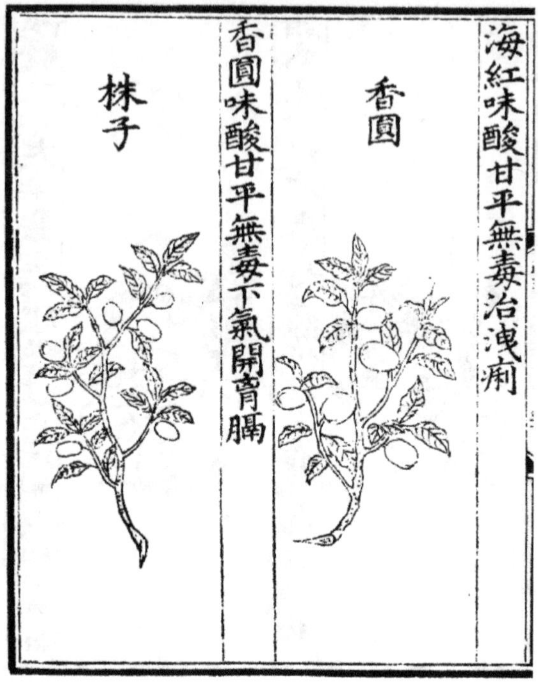
海紅味酸甘平無毒治洩痢

香圓

香圓味酸甘平無毒下氣開胷膈

株子

42A
Apple

Almond

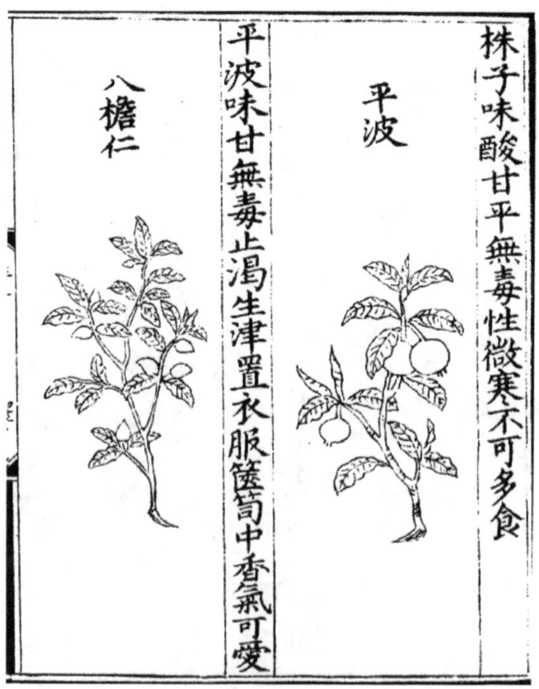
株子味酸甘平無毒性微寒不可多食

平波

平波味甘無毒止渴生津置衣服篋笥中香氣可愛

八檐仁

42B Pistachio

八檐仁味甘無毒止欬下氣消心腹逆悶其果出回回田地

必思荅

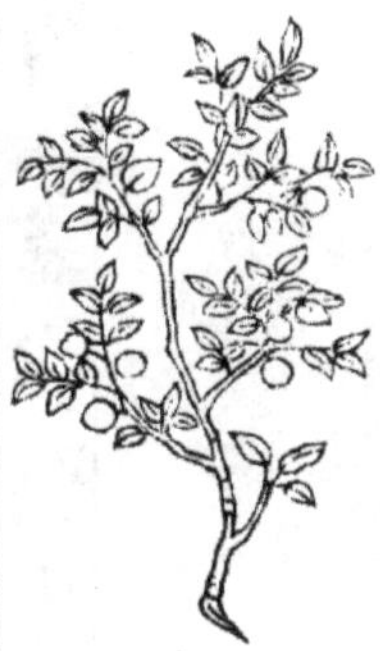

必思荅味甘無毒調中順氣其果出回回田地

43A Mallow

Swiss Chard

菜品

葵菜

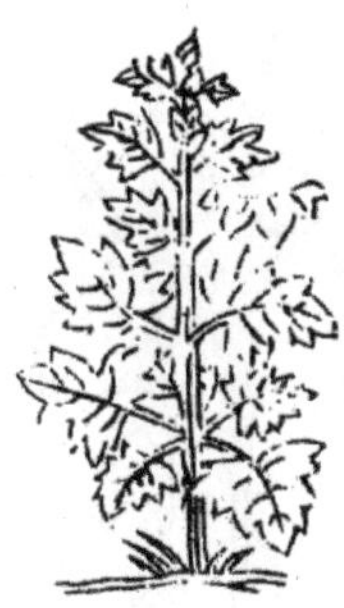

葵菜味甘寒平無毒爲百菜主治五藏六府寒熱羸瘦五癃利小便療婦人乳難

蔓菁

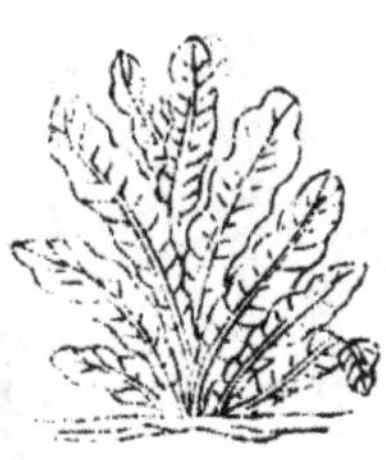

43B
Cilantro

Mustard

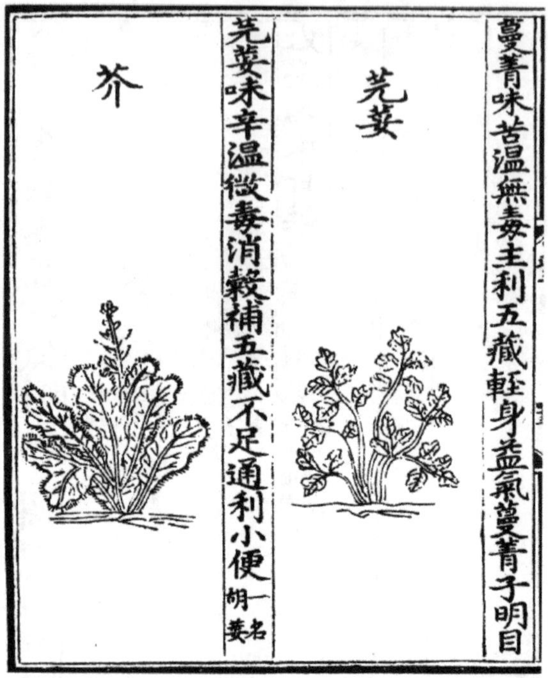

蔓菁味苦温無毒主利五藏輕身益氣蔓菁子明目

芫荽

芫荽味辛温微毒消穀補五藏不足通利小便一名胡荽

芥

44A
Chinese
Onions

Garlic

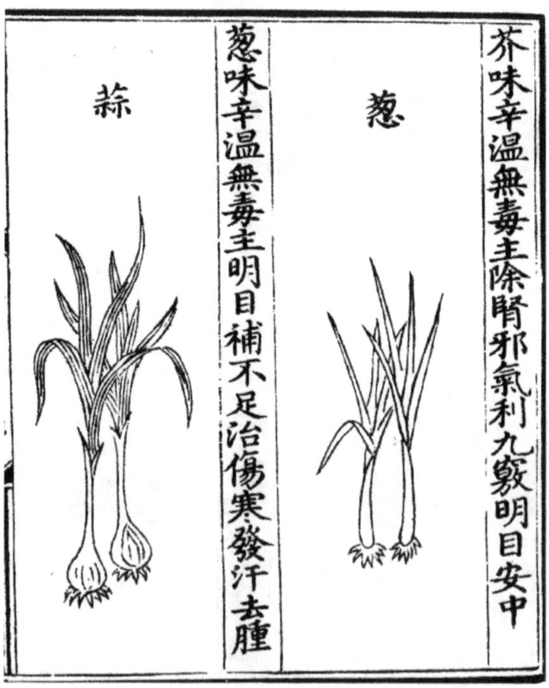

芥味辛温無毒主除腎邪氣利九竅明目安中

葱

葱味辛温無毒主明目補不足治傷寒發汗去腫

蒜

44B Chinese Chives

Winter Melon

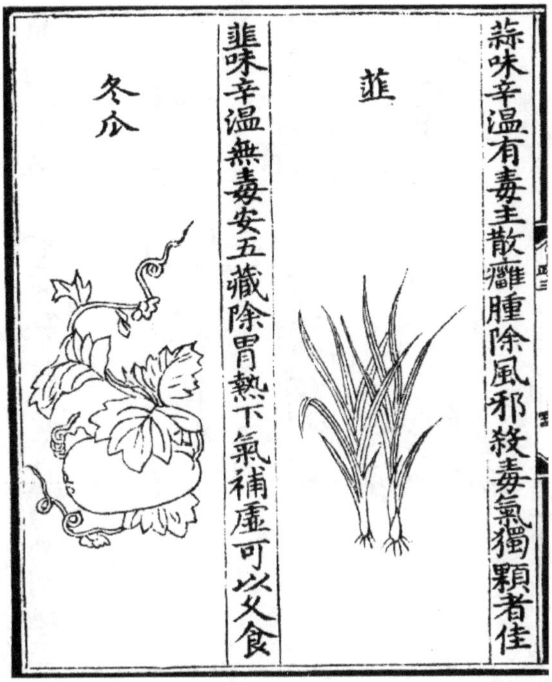

蒜味辛溫有毒主散癰腫除風邪殺毒氣獨顆者佳

韭

韭味辛溫無毒安五藏除胃熱下氣補虛可以久食

冬瓜

45A Cucum-ber

Radish

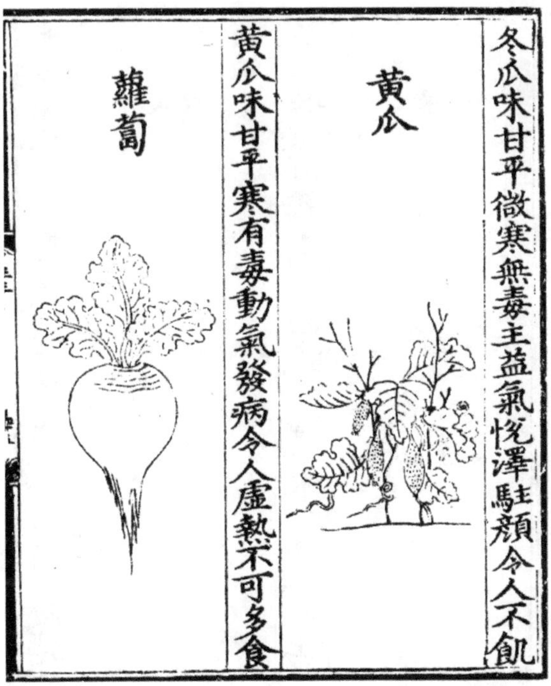

冬瓜味甘平微寒無毒主益氣悅澤駐顏令人不飢

黃瓜

黃瓜味甘平寒有毒動氣發病令人虛熱不可多食

蘿蔔

45B
Carrot

Tian-jing Vegetable

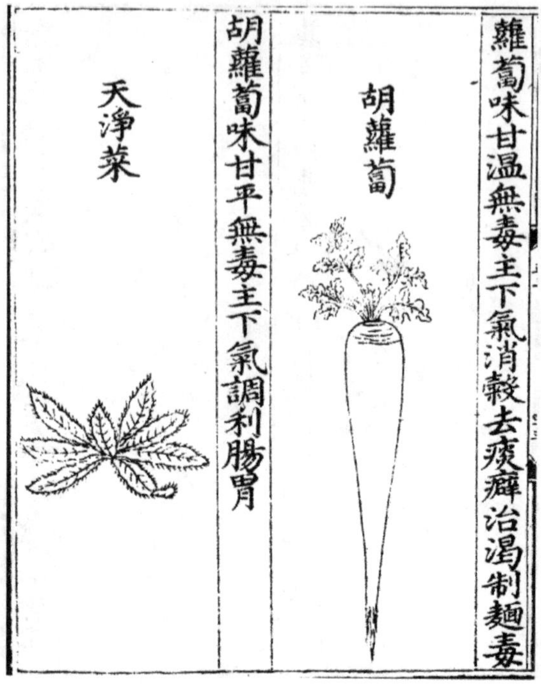

46A
Bottle Gourd

Pickling Melon

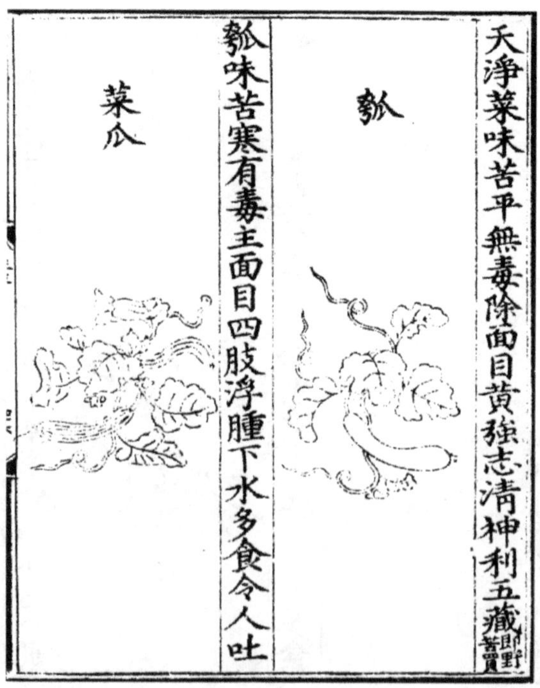

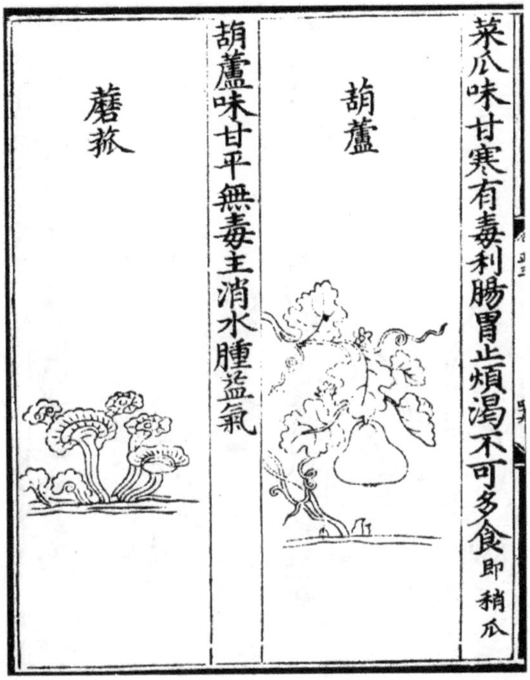

菜瓜味甘寒有毒利腸胃止煩渴不可多食即稍瓜

葫蘆

葫蘆味甘平無毒主消水腫益氣

蘑菰

46B
Pear-Shaped Bottle Gourd

Möög
Mushrooms

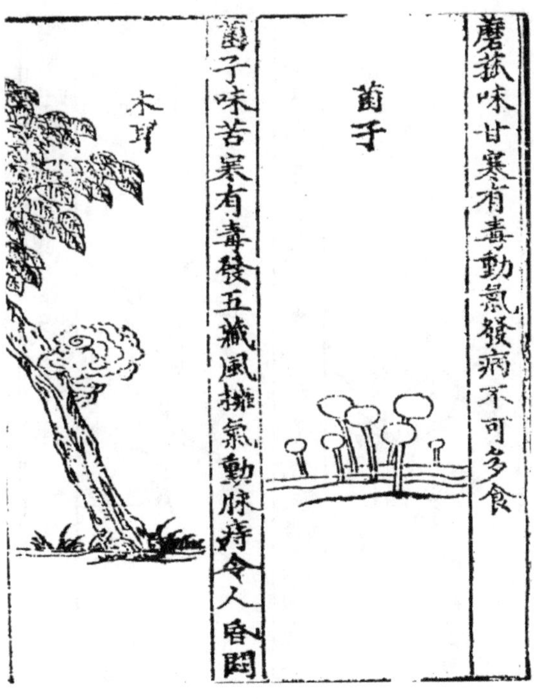

蘑菰味甘寒有毒動氣發病不可多食

菌子

菌子味苦寒有毒發五藏風擁氣動脉痔令人昏悶

木耳

47A
Junzi
Fungi

Tree Ears

47B
Bamboo Shoots

Cattail Shoots

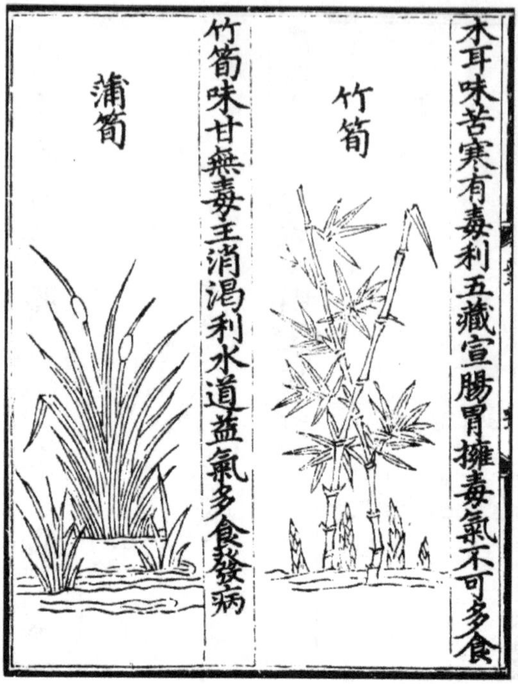

木耳味苦寒有毒利五藏宣腸胃擁毒氣不可多食

竹筍

竹筍味甘無毒主消渴利水道益氣多食發病

蒲筍

48A
Lotus Rhizome

Yam

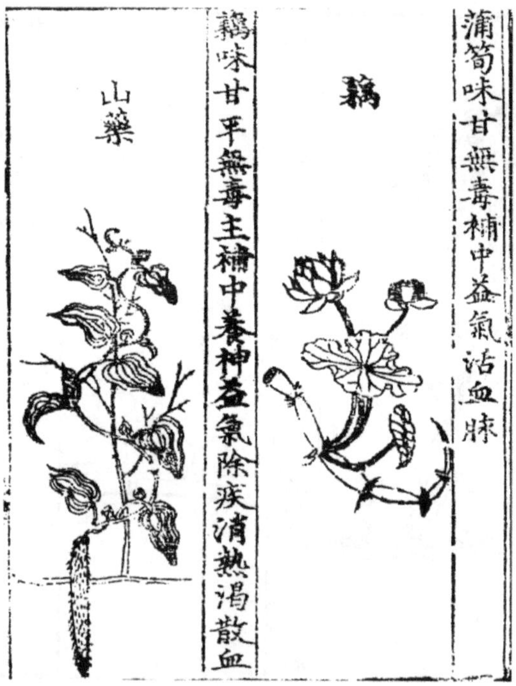

蒲筍味甘無毒補中益氣活血脈

藕

藕味甘平無毒主補中養神益氣除疾消熱渴散血

山藥

48B
Taro

Lettuce

山藥味甘溫無毒補中益氣治風眩止腰痛壯筋骨

芋

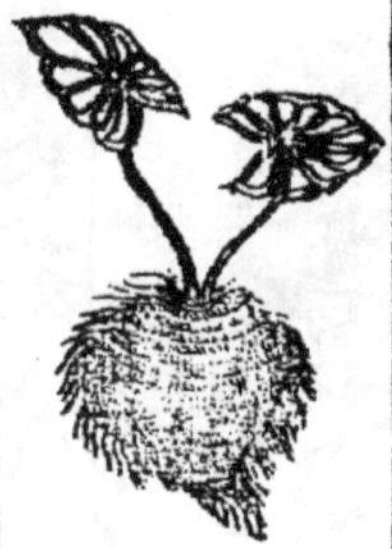

芋味辛平有毒寬腸胃充肌膚滑中野芋不可食

萵苣

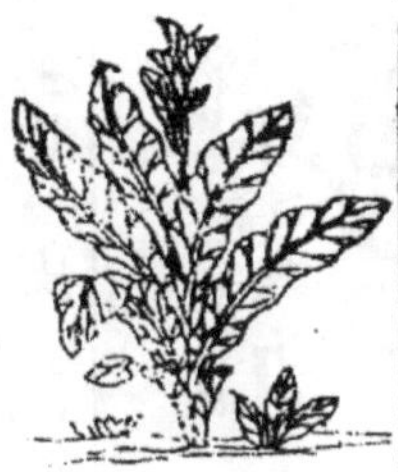

49A
Bokchoy

Chrysanthemum Greens

萵苣味苦冷無毒主利五藏開胷膈擁氣通血脉

白菜

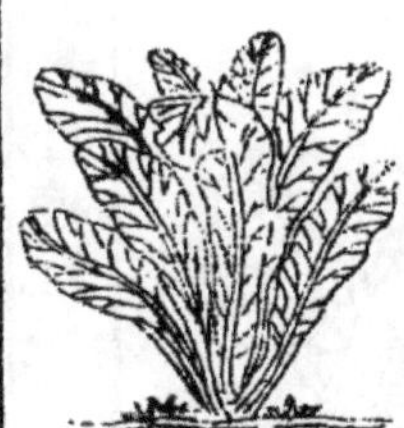

白菜味甘温無毒主通利腸胃除胷中煩解酒渴

蓬蒿

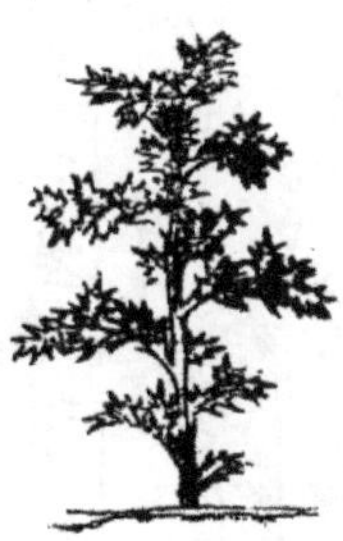

49B
Eggplant

Amaranth

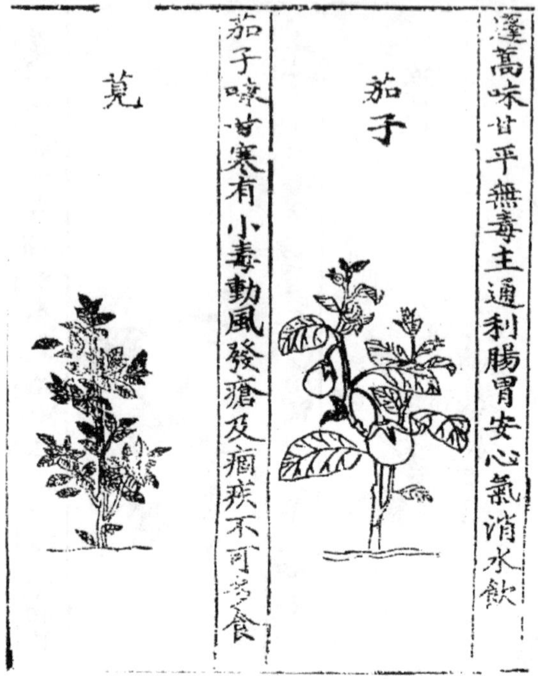

蓬蒿味甘平無毒主通利腸胃安心氣消水飲

茄子

茄子味甘寒有小毒動風發瘡及痼疾不可多食

莧

50A
Oil
Rape

Spinach

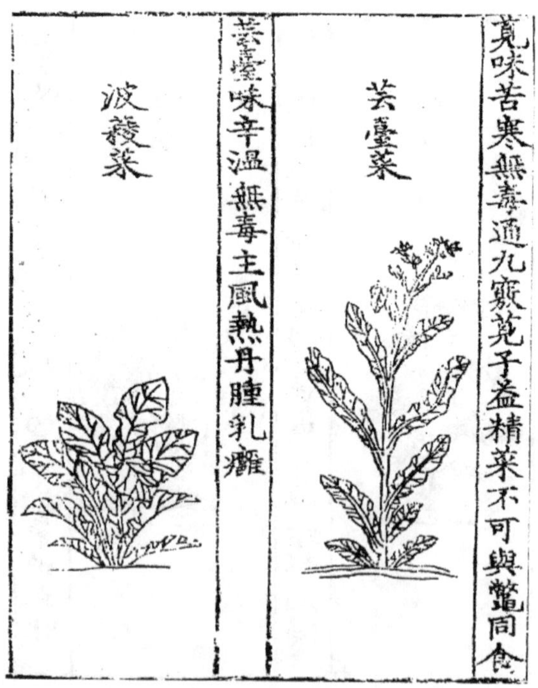

莧味苦寒無毒通九竅莧子益精菜不可與鼈同食

芸薹菜

芸薹味辛溫無毒主風熱丹腫乳癰

波薐菜

50B
Sugar
Beets

Basil

波薐味甘冷微毒利五藏通腸胃熱解酒毒 附赤根

莙薘菜

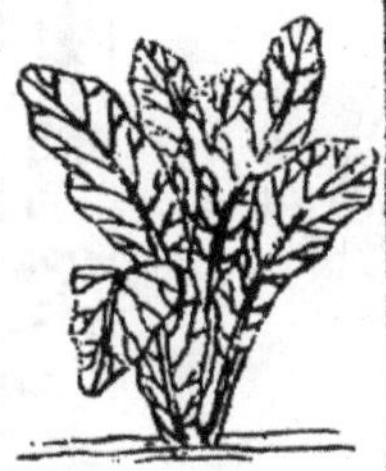

莙薘味甘寒無毒調中下氣去頭風利五臟

香菜

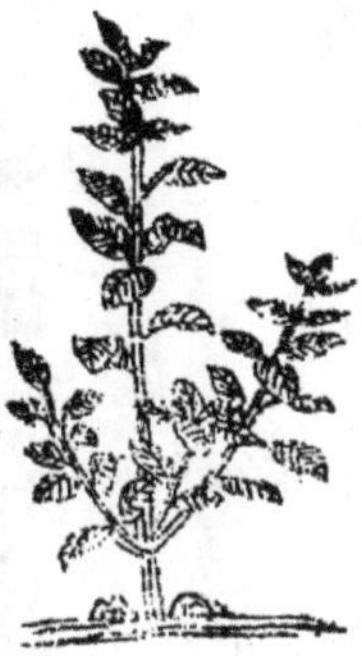

51A
Smart-
weed

Purslane

香菜味辛平無毒與諸菜同食氣味香辟腥

蓼子

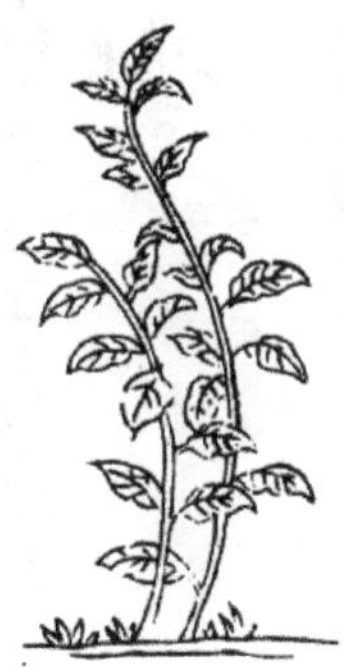

蓼子味辛溫無毒主明目溫中耐風寒下水氣

馬齒菜

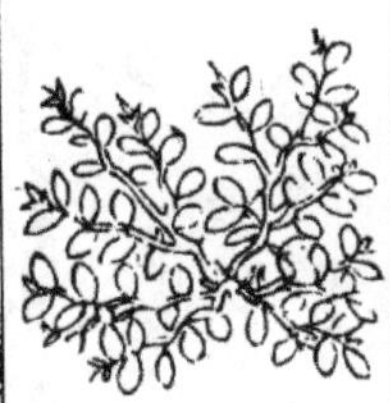

51B
Unknown
Fungus

Shallot

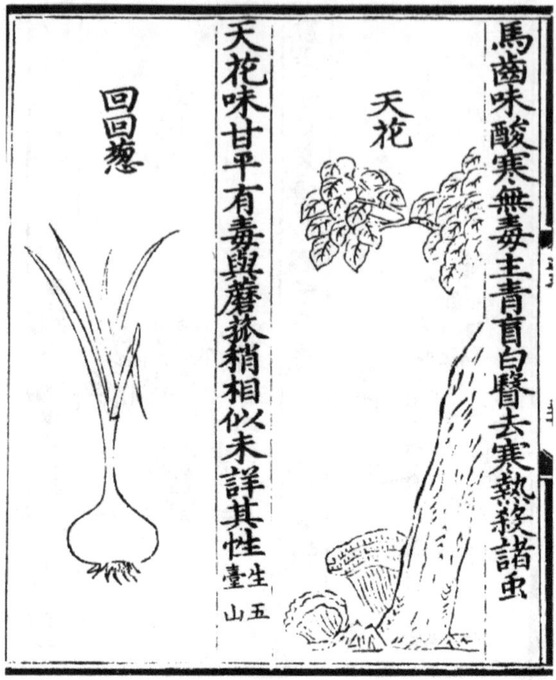

馬齒味酸寒無毒主青盲白瞖去寒熱殺諸虫

天花

天花味甘平有毒與蘑菰稍相似未詳其性 生五臺山

回回葱

52A
Chinese
Artichoke

Elm
Seeds

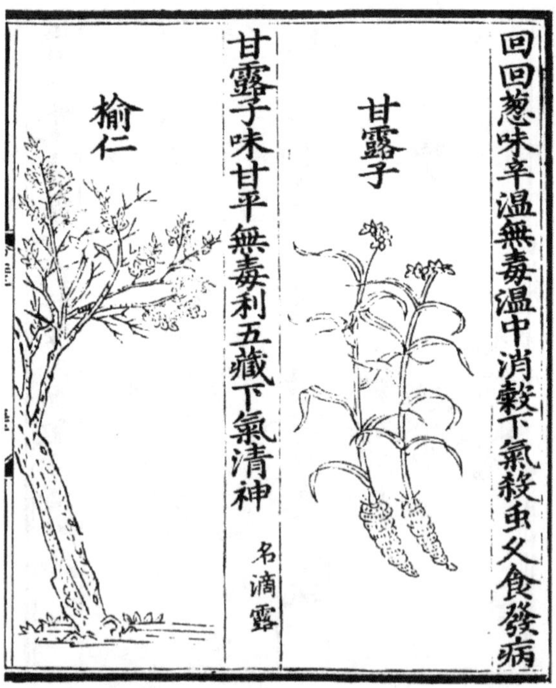

回回葱味辛溫無毒溫中消穀下氣殺虫久食發病

甘露子

甘露子味甘平無毒利五藏下氣清神 名滴露

榆仁

52B
Rape

Sugar
Beet

榆仁味辛溫無毒可作醬甚香美能助肺氣殺諸虫

沙吉木兒

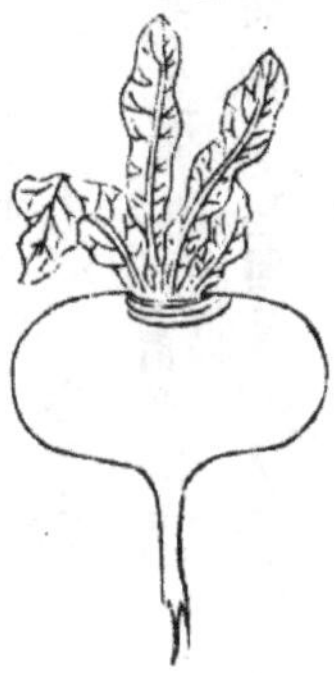

沙吉木兒味甘平無毒溫中益氣去心腹冷痛即蔓菁根

出莙達兒

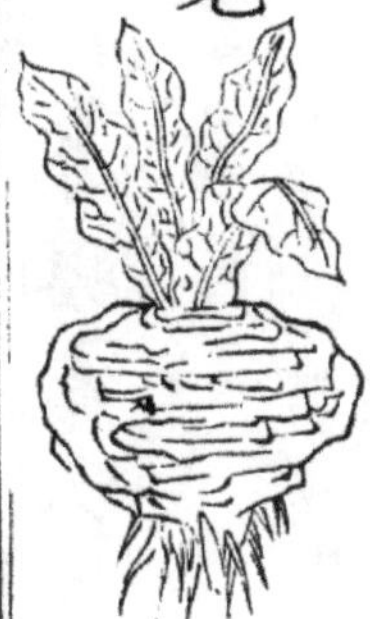

53A
Lily Root

Seaweed

出莙達兒味甘平無毒通經脉下氣開胷膈即莙薘根也

山丹根

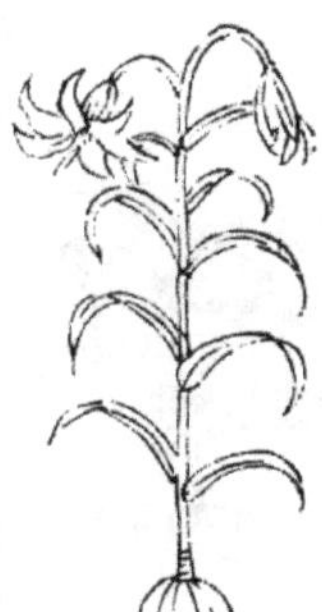

山丹根味甘平無毒主邪氣腹脹除諸瘡腫一名百合

海菜

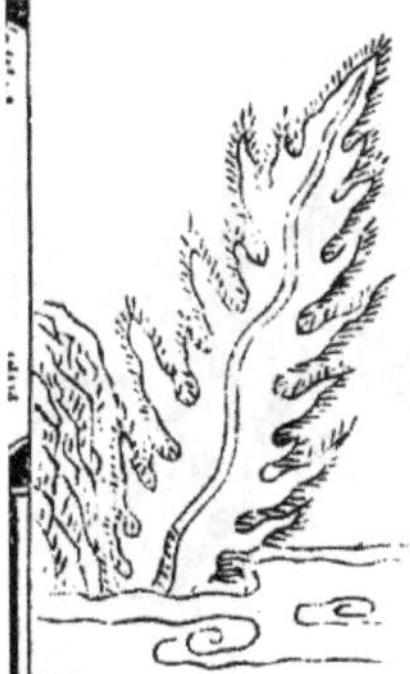

53B
Bracken

海菜味鹹寒微腥無毒主癭瘤破氣核癰腫勿多食

蕨菜

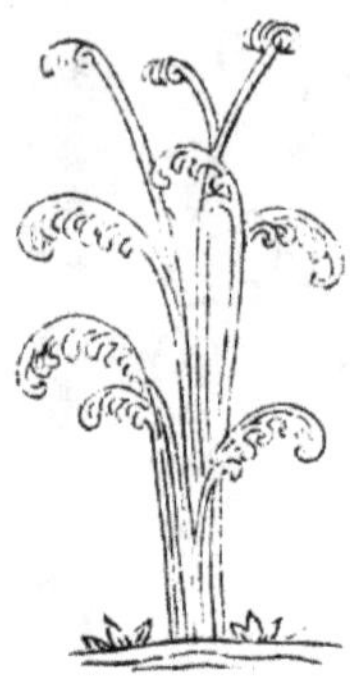

蕨菜味苦寒有毒動氣發病不可多食

薇菜味甘平無毒益氣潤肌清神強志

苦買菜味苦冷無毒治面目黄強力止困可傅諸瘡

水芹味甘平無毒主養神益氣令人肥健殺藥毒療

女人赤沃

54A
Pepper

Flower
Pepper

料物性味

胡椒

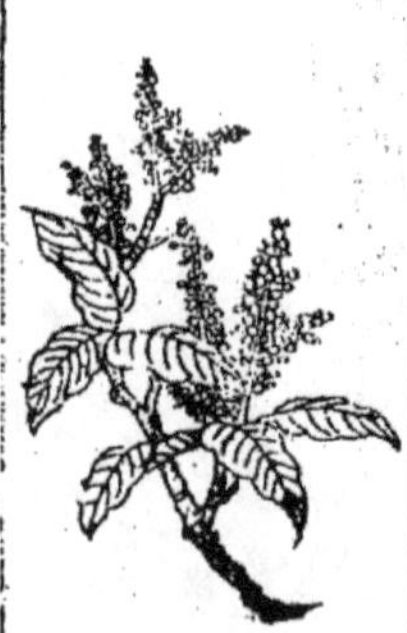

胡椒味辛温無毒主下氣除臟腑風冷去痰殺肉毒

小椒

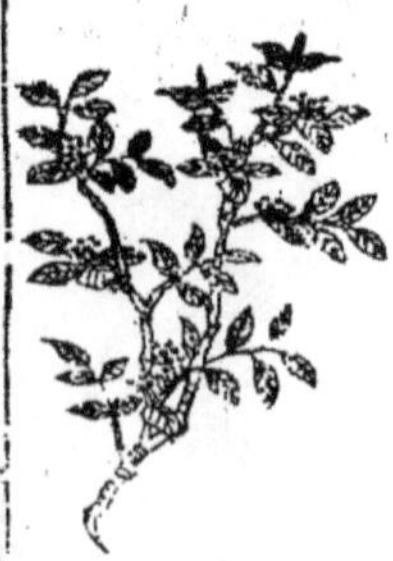

小椒味辛熱有毒主邪氣欬逆温中下冷氣除濕痹

54B
Lesser
Galangal

Fennel

良薑

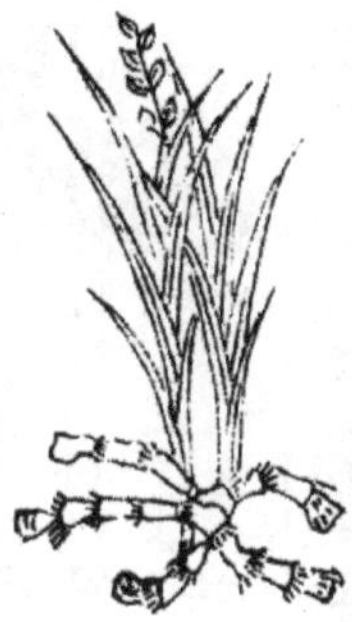

良薑味辛温無毒主胃中冷逆霍亂腹痛解酒毒

茴香

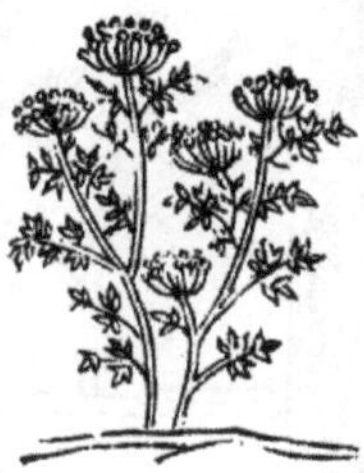

茴香味甘温無毒主膀胱腎經冷氣調中止痛住嘔

55A
Cumin

Mandarin
Peel

蒔蘿

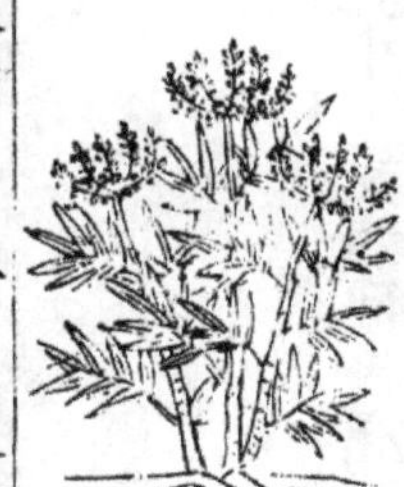

蒔蘿味辛温無毒建脾開胃温中補水藏殺魚肉毒

陳皮

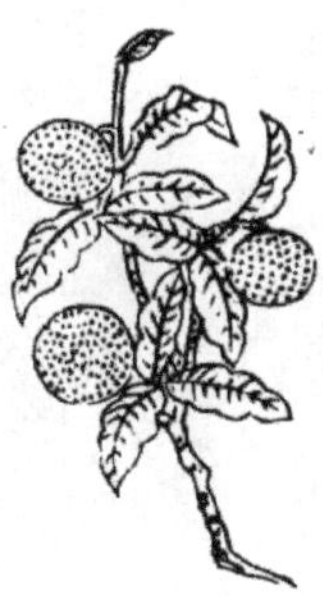

陳皮味甘平無毒止消渴開胃氣下痰破冷積

55B
Tsaoko

Cassia

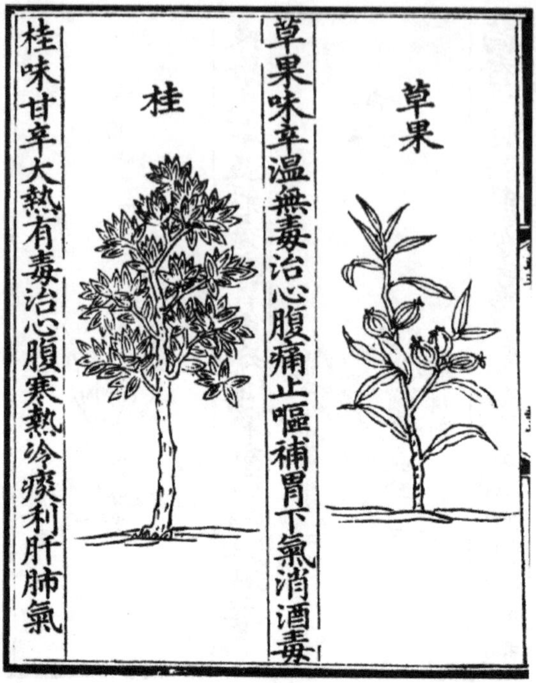
草果

草果味辛温無毒治心腹痛止嘔補胃下氣消酒毒

桂

桂味甘辛大熱有毒治心腹寒熱冷痰利肝肺氣

56A
Turmeric

Pippali

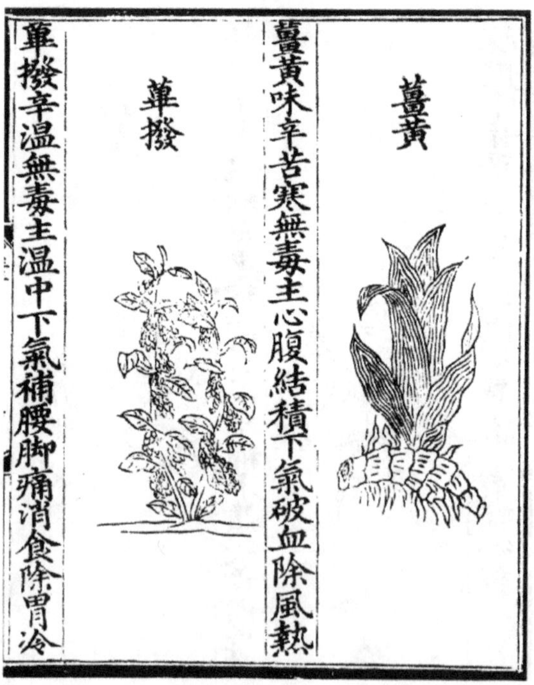
薑黃

薑黃味辛苦寒無毒主心腹結積下氣破血除風熱

蓽撥

蓽撥辛温無毒主温中下氣補腰脚痛消食除胃冷

56B
Grain-of-Paradise

Cubebs

縮砂

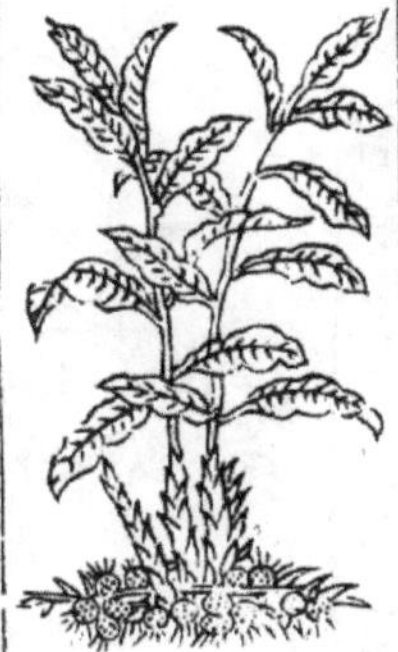

縮砂味辛温無毒主虛勞冷瀉宿食不消下氣

蓽澄茄

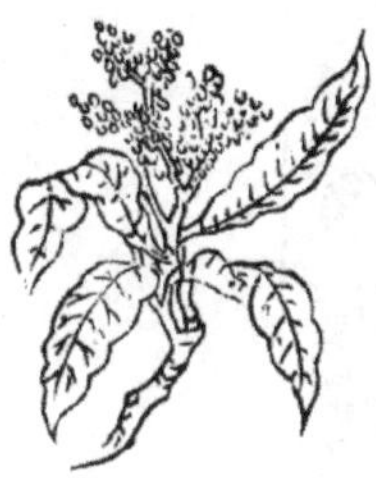

蓽澄茄味辛温無毒消食下氣去心腹脹令人能食

57A
Liquorice

Coriander

甘草

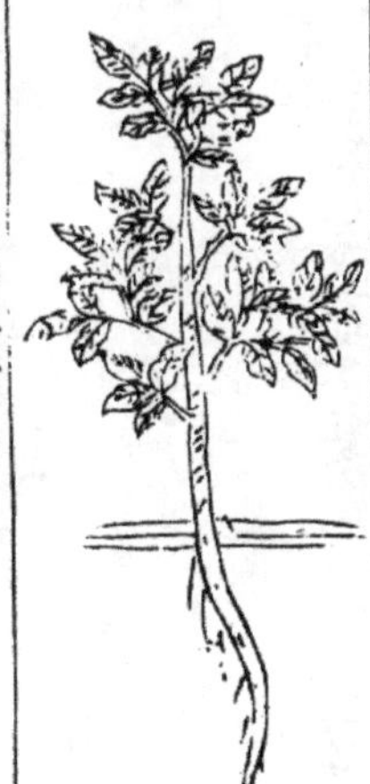

甘草味甘平無毒和百藥解諸毒

芫荽子

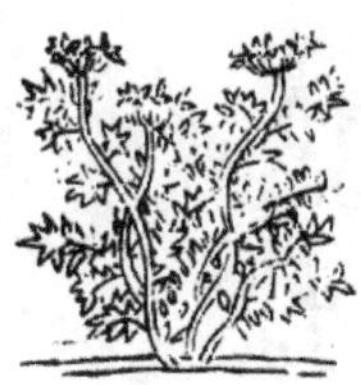

芫荽子辛温無毒消食治五藏不足殺魚肉毒

57B Dried Ginger

Fresh Ginger

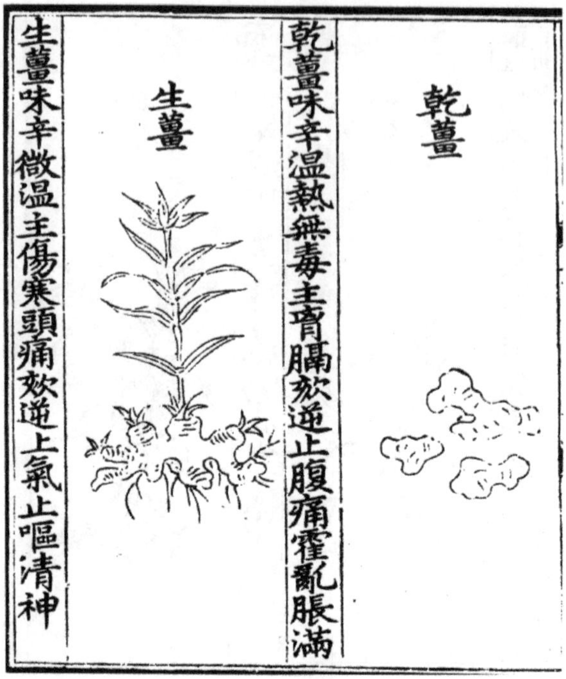
乾薑

乾薑味辛温熱無毒主胷膈欬逆止腹痛霍亂脹滿

生薑

生薑味辛微温主傷寒頭痛欬逆上氣止嘔清神

58A Schisandra

Fenugreek

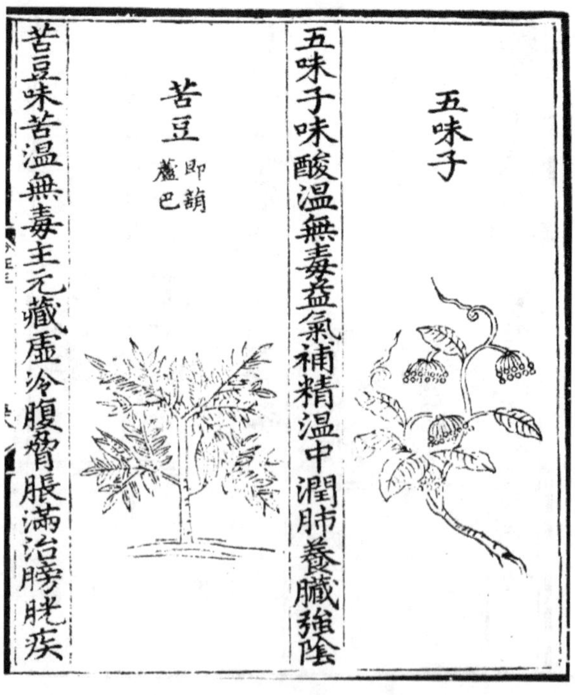
五味子

五味子味酸温無毒益氣補精温中潤肺養臟強陰

苦豆 即葫蘆巴

苦豆味苦温無毒主元藏虛冷腹脅脹滿治膀胱疾

紅麴味甘平無毒建脾益氣温中淹魚肉內用
黑子兒味甘平無毒開胃下氣燒餅內用極香美
馬思荅吉味苦香無毒去邪惡氣温中利膈順氣止
痛生津解渴令人口香生回回地面云是極香種類
咱夫蘭味甘平無毒主心憂鬱積氣悶不散久食令
人心喜即是回回地面紅花未詳是否
哈昔泥味辛温無毒主殺諸虫去臭氣破癥瘕下惡
除邪解蠱毒即阿魏
穩展味辛温苦無毒主殺虫去臭其味與阿魏同又
云即阿魏樹根淹羊肉香味甚美

58B
Red
Yeast

Poppy
Seeds

Mastajhi

Za'faran

Kasni

Anguzhad

胭脂味辛温無毒主產後血運心腹絞痛可傅遊腫
梔子味苦寒無毒主五內邪氣療目赤熱利小便
蒲黃味甘平無毒治心腹寒熱利小便止血疾
回回青味甘寒無毒解諸藥毒可傅熱毒瘡腫

飲膳正要卷第三

59A
Saf-
flower

Zhizi

Cattail
Pollen

"Muslim
Green"

JUAN 3

* * *

TRANSLATION

[*Juan* Three]

[1A] Grain Foods

[Illustration Caption:] Paddy Rice[1]

Paddy Rice is sweetish-bitter in flavor, neutral, and lacks poisons. It is good for warming the center. It makes one very heated and consti-

---

[1] Rice (*Oryza sativa*): may have been cultivated in and around the Yangtse Valley by 8000 BC. See An, 1989; Chang Te–tzu, 1989; MacNeish and Libby, 1995; Chang, 1999; Liu 2004; Tracey Lu, "The Origin and Dispersal of Agriculture and Human Diaspora in East Asia," in *The Peopling of East Asia: Putting Together Archaeology, Linguistics and Genetics,* edited by Laurent Sagart, Roger Blench, and Alicia Sanchez-Mazas, eds. (London 2005), 51-62; Jiang and Liu 2006. Both currently common types, short–grained "japonica and long–grained "indica," were grown by the Hemudu 河姆渡 Culture before 5000 BC. Cultivated rice is part of a complex of annual and perennial "species" that cross freely. It is always grown as an annual when cultivated. Rice was probably domesticated from perennial or annual stock growing in ponds, sloughs, and marshy areas wet in summer and dry in winter. Its center of growth and variation is in south China and nearby. Several domestication sites have been proposed. Present evidence points to the lower Yangtse. Rice may also have been domesticated in Thailand and India. Rice cultivation spread rapidly and had become a basis of agriculture in east and south China well before 4000 BC. By 2000 BC it was widely cultivated throughout east, south, and southeast Asia.

Rice is normally grown irrigated, in paddies. It otherwise produces low yields, even with abundant rainfall. For this reason rice is primarily grown in China south of the Huai River and the northern limits of the Yangtse drainage, where water is abundant.

Cultivated Chinese rices respond well to fertilizer and careful water control. They are adapted to the lengths of summer days and local climatic conditions. Thousands of ecotypes exist. There are color varieties and the Chinese distinguish between forms which become sticky when cooked, due to a form of starch amylose, and those which do not. The former are called "glutinous," not strictly correctly.

Rices also vary in flavor and scent. Most East Asian rice has a minimum of taste. Other rices have pronounced nutlike flavors, e.g., the famous "jasmine" rice of Thailand. Important worldwide is basmati rice, preferred in the Arab and Iranian worlds, in Pakistan and northwest India. The *YSZY* stresses "scented" rice in several places.

Today rice is daily grain, is used as rice gruel, as soft food for infants and convalescents, for brewing, and for vinegar, and other industrial uses. It provides a substrate for a variety of yeasts and other cultivated microorganisms. See Hu Shiu-ying, 2004.

pated. Too much should not be eaten. This is the same as *nomi*. (***Sumen*** [*i.e.*, Indonesian **paddy rice**] is best. It is often used to make liquor).

Non–Glutinous Rice is sweetish–bitter in flavor, neutral and lacks poison. It is good for increasing *qi.* It controls irritation and leaking [of *qi*. It harmonizes stomach *qi* and thickens muscle **[1B]** and flesh. There are various varieties at present. (**Aromatic Non–glutinous Rice**, **Tablet Rice**, **Snow–white–interior Rice**, **Aromatic Rice**) These varieties are superior to [plain] non-glutinous rices in aroma and flavor. [Non-glutinous rice can be milled and the kernel washed to make polished rice. This is also called **Dried rice**.

[Illustration Caption:] Foxtail Millet[2]

Foxtail Millet is salty in flavor, slightly cooling and lacks poison. It is good for nourishing kidney *qi*. It removes [evil] heat of spleen and stomach. It increases *qi*. Old [Foxtail Millet is best. It is used to regulate [evil] heat of the stomach, and excessive thirst. It benefits urination and controls leaking dysentery. The *Tangben zhu*[3] says: "There are many varieties of Foxtail Millets. The kernels are fine like *Liangmi* ["Millet"]. The Uniform washed grains obtained from fine millet are *zhemi*."

[Illustration Caption:] Millet

[2A] Green Millet is sweetish in flavor, slightly cooling and lacks poison. It is good for [evil] heat–diabetes–stomach–stagnation. It controls dysentery, increases *qi*, and supplements the center. It lightens the body and lengthens the years.

White Millet is sweetish in flavor, slightly cooling, and lacks poison. It is used to expel heat and increase *qi*.

---

[2] Foxtail millet is one of many small-seeded grain grains called "millet." Wild foxtail millet was domesticated in ancient Mexico, but abandoned when maize appeared. (The same process is ongoing in China. Maize, appearing in the seventeenth century, is replacing millet.) Foxtail millet was domesticated by 8000 BC (Chang 1999: 44-45; Liu 2004; Liu Xinli, Harriet V. Hunt, and Martin K. Jones. "River Valleys and Foothills: Changing Archaeological Perceptions of North China's Earliest Farms," *Antiquity* 83 (2009): 82-95; Lu 2005; Sagart et al. 2005) and panic millet (*Panicum* spp.) at least by 6000-6500 BC (Bellwood 2005:21). The earliest center of millet agriculture was around the Wei 渭 River (the Peiligang 裴李崗 culture).

[3] These are notes by Su Jing 蘇敬 in the Tang dynasty *Xinxiu bencao* 新修本草.

Yellow Millet is sweetish in flavor, neutral and lacks poison. It is used to increase *qi*. It harmonizes the center. It controls leaking [of *qi*]. The *Tangben zhu* says: "The ears are as long as a long hair. The grains and the kernels are coarser than those of white millet."

[2B] **Panicled Millet** is sweetish in flavor, neutral and lacks poison. It is good for increasing *qi* and supplements the center. It is very heating and makes people irritated. If eaten for a long period of time, it dulls the five viscera. It makes one sleep well. It may be beneficially eaten for lung ailments.

Red Panicled Millet is bitter in flavor, slightly warm and lacks poison. It is good for cough and *huoluan*. It controls excessive thirst. It expels heat.

[Illustration Caption:] *Ji* Panicled Millet

***Ji* Panicled Millet** is sweetish in flavor and lacks poison. It is good for increasing *qi* and supplements for insufficiency. In Guanxi [i.e., Northwest China] it is called *mizi* grain. It is also called *ji* grain. In ancient times it was highly esteemed for its aroma. Thus it was used as a sacrificial offering.[4]

****Qamh*** ["Hexi grain," durum wheat, *Triticum durum*] is sweetish in flavor and lacks poison. It supplements the center and increases *qi*. The kernels are harder than other grains. It comes from Hexi.

[3A] [Illustration Caption:] Mung Beans[5]

Mung Beans are sweetish in flavor, cooling, and lack poison. They

[4] S*hu* 黍,Glutinous, panicled millet, is even said to include a character for religious sacrifice as part of its phonetic.

[5] Mung Beans (*Vigna mungo*), *ludou*: these golden–green beans are native to India and perhaps southeast Asia. They may have come in with Champa rice during Song. Mung beans resist drought and grow almost anywhere, prefering warm climates.

Dry, Mung beans are usually cooked into a porridge. Often sweetened with sugar it is used as a cooling tea. Mung beans are also used to make *fensi* 粉絲, "pea-starch noodles" in English. The starch is separated in a boiling process, and made into a gelatinous, translucent mass. Noodles are hand–cut or the starch forced through a colander. Today mung beans are the source of most bean or "pea" sprouts. Mung bean sporouts are generally preferred to coarser sprouts of the soybean.

Mung beans are "cooling" because of their "cool" color. Red beans are heating.

are good for red poisoning,[6] rubella, and fever accompanied by restlessness. They harmonize the five internal organs and move the [blood in the] blood vessels.

White Beans[7] are sweetish in flavor, neutral and lack poison. They adjust the center, warm the bowels, and aid the blood vessels. They may be beneficially eaten for kidney diseases.

Soybeans[8] are sweetish in flavor, neutral and lack poison. They decrease demon *qi*,[9] control pain and drive out water. They expel [evil]

---

[6] This is "Inflammatory disease characterized by redness of skin" (Ou, 1982: 41).

[7] *Bodou* may be cowpeas (dried seeds of *Vigna sinensis*), if not soybeans. The cowpea is usually eaten in China only as a green vegetable, pod and all, under the name *changdou* 長豆 , "long bean." With other bean pods it can also be known as *doujiao* 豆角, "bean horn, bean pod." In English it is "yard–long bean." The cowpea, at least this variety, is native to China and widespread. Hu Shiu-ying (2005: 488-89) separates the yard-long bean *Vigna sinensis* from the cowpea *Vigna unguiculata*.

[8] Soybean (*Glycine max*): *dadou* 大豆, and other names, referring to color varieties probably the case with the "white beans" above. Prior to the development of technology to ferment them or extract curd, soybeans were of little importance and considered a plebeian crop, typical of Spartan conditions. This is due to the nutritional disadvantages of unprocessed soybeans, apparently understood since early times. When boiled and eaten, for example, phytic acid, primarily in the seed coat, combines with minerals and niacin in the diet, rendering those nutrients in the beans more or less unavailable to human digestion. Other compounds tie up protein, iodine, and other nutrients. Fermentation destroys most of the phytic acid. Bean curd manufacture gets rid of the phytic acid and other unfortunate chemicals in the waste water.
Fermented soybean products appeared in late Zhou. First were *doushi* 豆豉, "fermented black beans," now used mainly in Cantonese cooking but once general articles of diet. To make *doushi*, soybeans are boiled, then pickled. A mixed fungal fermenting agent blackens and preserves. Next came fermented pastes called *jiang* 醬 and soy sauce, now *douyou* 豆油, "bean oil." Originally thinned *jiang*, or liquids produced in fermenting beans were used, but true soy sauce is made by the fermentation of boiled soybeans and wheat flour using *Aspergillus*, *Mucor*, *Rhizopus* and other fungi. Today herbs or other substances are added as antibiotics or to add flavor. Many varieties are known. Localities and firms pride themselves on distinctive bean oils. Paralleling the use of wheat flour to produce soy sauce was the development of *mian shi jiang* 面豉醬, "flour bean sauce," still important. A variant *tianmianjiang* 甜面醬, "sweet flour paste," is based on soybeans, flour and pea flour, with malt, sugar, and various other flavorings added, most recently, chilies. On fermented soy products see H. T. Huang, *Science and Civilisation in China*, vol. 6, *Biology and Biological Technology*, pt. 5, *Fermentations and Food Science* (Cambridge, 2000); Christine M. Du Bois, Chee-Beng Tan, and Sidney Mintz. eds. *The World of Soy*. (Urbana, 2008); Charles V. Piper and William J. Morse, *The Soybean* (New York, 1923).

[9] See the discussion of this syndrome by Li (Hu Sihui, 1988: 225).

heat of the stomach, bring down blood stasis,[10] and counteract the poisons of various drugs. They are made into *doufu*.[11] [*Doufu*] is cooling and moves the *qi*.

Adzuki Beans [Red Small Beans, *Vigna angularis*] are sweetish-sour in flavor, neutral and lack poison. They are good for bringing down water [*i.e.*, reducing swelling]. They clear out pus and blood, remove flatulence due to evil heat, and control leaking dysentery. They make the urine pass and counteract wheat toxicity.

[3B] [Illustration Caption:] Chickpeas ["Muslim Beans," *Cicer arietinum*][12]

Chickpeas are sweetish in flavor and lack poison. They are good for diabetes. They should not be eaten boiled with salt. They come from the Muslim areas. The sprouts are like [those of other] beans. Today they are found here and there among fields and waste lands.

---

[10] This includes "stagnated blood and extravasated blood" (Ou 1982: 235).

[11] *Doufu*–making was invented around Han (legend associates it with Han prince Liu An 劉安) but was uncommon until later. Cheese– and curd–making of China's Medieval Altaic neighbors may have been an influence.

Doufu is made by soaking soybeans, grinding soaked beans finely in water, boiling the resulting slurry, and precipitating it with gypsum or other coagulant. The result is usually dried, pressed in cheesecloth between boards, and cut into cubes. It is about 87% water, 7% protein, and 6% starch and oil. By–products include the "skin," *doufu pi* 豆腐皮, skimmed off and dried. It is high in protein and useful in a vegetarian diet. Hulls, starch grains, and other solids (*okara*, from Japanese) are usually fed to animals. The water, "whey," can be drunk but is usually discarded. Oil and much of the starch goes with it. Boiled "milk" can be drunk without coagulating the curd. Bean curd coagulated and left in the milk is eaten, usually sweetened, as *doufu hua* 豆腐花, "bean curd flowers." It can be pressed and dried into *doufu gan* 豆腐乾, "dry bean curd." It is also processed in other ways, including freezing. Fermentation products include *chou doufu* 臭豆腐, "stinking bean curd." It deserves its name. Many specialized bean curd and bean curd skin products are used in Buddhist vegetarian cooking. On *Doufu* see William Shurtleff and Akiko Aoyagi, *The Book of Tofu* (Berkeley, 1975). The invention of Doufu marked the emergence of the soybean as a major crop.

[12] The chickpea, *Cicer arietinum*, a typical legume of the Mediterranean, has been cultivated there at least since the eighth or ninth millennium. Later its cultivation spread to southern Europe and India, where chickpea–based *dal* is a staple, and more recently to the New World and Africa. The crop requires a Mediterranean climate and has never flourished in China, except, if the *YSZY* is to be believed, in a few outlying areas occupied by "Muslims." Thus it is called "Muslim Bean." On the chickpea see N. W. Simmonds, *Evolution of Crop Plants* (London and New York, 1976), 157–9.

Green Small Beans [*Vigna radiata*] are sweetish in flavor, cooling, and lack poison. They are good for stagnation of heat-evil in the center diabetes. They control diarrhea and remove abdominal distension. If a mother has no milk after giving birth, 3-5 *sheng* can be eaten boiled until overdone. Milk will then be abundant.

Garden Peas [*Pisum sativum*][13] are sweetish in flavor, neutral, and lack poison. They adjust the constructive and protective *qi* and harmonize the center and increase *qi*.

Hyacinth Beans [*Dolichos purpureus*][14] are sweetish in flavor and slightly warming. They are good for harmonizing the center. The leaves are good for uncontrolled vomiting of *huoluan*.

[Illustration Caption:] Wheat [*Triticum aestivum*][15]

---

[13] Pea: *wandou*, "creeping bean," with various variant writings.

This and the field pea (*Pisum arvense*) appeared in China just before Yuan. Peas were more important in old China than generally realized. Some were grown for dried peas. Other special varieties had edible pods, our "snow peas." Pea tendrils are widely considered the choicest of all fresh vegetables. These are the growing tips with the quintessential form of a crisp, succulent texture when stir–fried, even if little taste.

[14] Dolichos or hyacinth bean: *biandou*, "flat bean." *Bian*, "side; having sides," refers to flattened members of sects whose other members are roundish.

The dolichos or hyacinth bean has been long grown in China. Many varieties exist, and wild forms abound. The green pod and dry beans are both edible, but inferior to other beans. It grows under poor conditions and is resistant to heat and drought. The dolichos bean is normally South Chinese. It must have been strange to the Yuan court.

This discussion omits the broad bean (*Vicia faba*), *candou* 蠶豆, "silkworm bean," earlier *hudou* 胡豆, "Iranian bean." It may be lumped with the chickpea or the pea, another "Iranian bean." See Laufer, 1919: 305–8. The broad bean replaced the soybean in West China. It is made into sprouts, bean starch noodles, bean oil, and especially *doubanjiang* 豆辦將, also made of soybeans. *Doubanjiang* is very important in West China, known for spicy food. It is blazing hot from chilies and strongly flavored with garlic and/or Chinese Flower pepper. Broad beans cause an acute, usually fatal breakdown of red blood cells in individuals, common in malarial regions, genetically susceptible due to low blood levels of glucose–6–phosphate–dihydrogenase. Females with this condition die as embryos. Only males survive to be killed by favism, a major cause of death in old China. See Solomon Katz and J. Schall, "Favism and Malaria: A Model of Nutrition and Biocultural Evolution" (unpublished paper).

[15] Wheat: *xiaomai*, "small wheat", or *lai* 來, in the early texts.

At the time of Buck's survey (Buck, 1937) wheat was found growing in every province, although marginal in the far south. By 1977–80, average annual per capita wheat consumption in China was 62 kg, 103 kg in the United States. See United Nations, Food and Agriculture Organization, *Ceres* 13 (1981): 4: 11–12. In China, wheat was providing about one–fifth to one–fourth of total calories.

[4A] **Wheat** is sweetish in flavor, slightly cooling and lacks poison. It is good for expelling heat and controlling fidgetiness, diabetes, and dry throat. It benefits the urine and nourishes liver *qi* and controls pain and blood spitting.[16]

Barley [*Hordeum vulgare*] is salty-warm in flavor, slightly cooling and lacks poison. It is good for diabetes, expels heat, increases *qi* and harmonizes the center. It makes people very heated and is the best of

---

The worldwide trend is for hard red wheats to be grown in the North and softer, whiter ones in the South. This seems also true of China although we know little about Chinese wheat varieties and their distribution in the past. Wheat has been important in Tibet at low altitudes, more important in Xinjiang, where the Uighurs and others are part of the wheat–based culinary culture of West Asia. The Mongols of the fourteenth century were more familiar with sorghum and millet than with wheat, but the Iranians and Turks serving them could scarcely have imagined life without wheat bread. It was available, judging by *YSZY* recipes and its popularity may have been growing.

Wheat is the most important crop in the world, in terms of tonnage grown, the number of people using it as starch staple, and variety of uses. Even in China, stereotypically rice–eating, wheat is about half as important as rice. It is far more important in the North. Wheat is not particularly hardy or versatile, nor is it widely adapted. Wheat does extremely well only in temperate grasslands or steppe environments. Until recent advances it was not particularly productive. It owes its popularity and its worldwide prestige mainly to its gluten, a special protein vital for bread and noodle–making.

Hard red wheat, common in North China, has up to 63.5 grams of protein per pound. It is close behind oats, with the most protein, and ahead of foxtail millet. Red wheats usually have less, amounts similar to soft white wheats with just over 40 grams per pound. Brown rice has only 34 grams per pound, 30 when milled. *Proso* millet is the only Chinese grain competing with the best red wheats, but foxtail is comparable with the general run of wheat. About two grams of protein are lost in milling.

Wheat protein is of good quality. Chinese doctors have long recognized its benefits. Like most grains, wheat is low in lysine and methionine, although a combination with soybean protein adds lysine, yielding a protein value approaching that of muscle meat.

[16] The medicinal qualities described here reflect the vitamin and mineral content of wheat. Unmilled wheat is a good source of B vitamins, found in the outer coats and germ, although this is lost in milling. Thiamin is almost 90% depleted in fine white flours. Enriching restores it but the process is new. With the B vitamins go several mineral nutrients. Iron is around 15 mg per pound in the whole grain, but only around 4 mg in white flour. For Western diets, wheat is not usually a major source of protein, vitamins, and minerals, but it is in China. Grain may provide over 90% of calories. Workers in Beijing around 1920 knew that they needed less wheat flour than corn flour to do a day's work, but needed more wheat flour than millet–soybean meal, tracking protein content accurately. See Sydney Gamble and J. S. Burgess, *Peking: A Social Survey*, New York: Doran, 1921. Another problem is the phytic acide abundant in wheat bran. It forms tight chemical bonds with metal nutrients and with niacin, preventing their digestion. Leavening neutralizes all or most of the acid.

the five grains. The *Yaoxing lun* says: "It can digest old food retained in the stomach and intestines[17] and destroy chill *qi*."

Buckwheat [*Fagopyrum esculentum* and *F. tataricum*][18] is sweetish in flavor, neutral–cooling and lacks poison. It fills out the bowels and increases *qi* force. If eaten for a long time it excites wind *qi*. It makes a person dizzy in the head. If eaten with pork one contracts evil heat wind. It makes beard and eyebrows fall out.

[4B] [Illustration Caption:] Sesame Seeds[19]

"White" Sesame Seeds are sweetish in flavor, very cooling and lack poison. They regulate *xulao* diseases and smooth the bowels. They move [*i.e.*, disperse] wind *qi* and makes blood pass in the blood vessels. They remove head wind[20] and make the flesh sleek. Eat a mouthful of the raw seeds after meals. Give them to wet nurses to eat. They prevent the child from falling ill.

"Iranian" Sesame Seeds[21] are sweetish in flavor and slightly cooling. They expel all obstinate illnesses. If eaten for a long time they thicken muscle and flesh and firm a person's oils. They benefit excretion and regulate retention of afterbirth. The *Xiuzhen mizhi* says: "[As for the]

---

17 According to Ou, 1982: *sushi bing* is a "syndrome with prolonged retention of food in the stomach and intestines" (204).

18 Buckwheat, *qiaomai*: Used as a grain, buckwheat is a pseudo–cereal, the seed of a member of the family *Polygonaceae*, and not the *caryopsis* of a grass. The most important species is *esculentum*. The other, *tataricum*, is low–yielding and used under conditions too harsh for *esculentum*. Both species are native to the mountains of Central Asia and were domesticated there, in historic times or shortly before. They have always been essentially confined to these mountains, except for extensions in historic times west via Russia. Buckwheat is a minor crop in the world, important only in Central Eurasia, China, and Korea and is often grown as a summer crop in rotation with winter barley. The mountain Yi of Sichuan crop both species of buckwheat, often alternating with other crops, and once ate buckwheat cakes as a staple; these survive, but rice is replacing the buckwheat (Stevan Harrell, personal communcation to ENA, 2008). In Manchuria and West China buckwheat is used as the Yi do, or as noodles made by pushing dough through a sieve into boiling water, done to dough without gluten and the ability to hold together. Buckwheat is a least choice Chinese food. *Tataricum* is bitter and *esculentum* may be also. This bitter principle is of dubious health value, and probably explains bad effects of buckwheat eating noted in the *YSZY*.

19 Sesame (*Sesamum indicum*): *zhima*, "*zhi* hemp, sesame," also called *youma* 油麻, "oil hemp." Sesame seeds are an ancient Near Eastern crop, probably late in coming to China. Their value as a nutritional source is still widely recognized.

20 Ou, 1982: 60: "recurrent headache."

21 "Iranian sesame seeds" are probably the black ones, judging from indicated uses.

method according to which immortals take Iranian sesame seeds: after they have taken them for a long time their faces are radiant. They are not hungry for three years. They cannot be harmed by water or fire. When they walk they overtake horses."

[5A] Malt–Sugar[22] is sweetish in flavor and slightly warming and lacks poison. It supplements for exhaustion, controls thirst and removes blood. If fortifies the spleen and regulates coughing. If a small child has mistakenly swallowed a coin, a *jin* should be obtained and gradually consumed. The coin will then come out.

Honey[23] is sweetish in flavor, neutral, slightly warming and lacks poison. It is good for evil *qi* of chest and abdomen and the various fright convulsions.[24] It supplements for insufficiency *qi* of the five viscera. It augments the center and controls pain. It counteracts poisons, makes ear and eye sharp, harmonizes the hundred drugs, and expels the host of illnesses.

Yeast[25] is sweetish in flavor and very warming. It heals apoplexy *qi* of the viscera. It adjusts the center and augments *qi*. It opens the belly and disperses food. It supplements for deficiency chill. Old yeast is best.

---

22 Malt sugar can be made from any grain. It is mostly maltose, different from sucrose in physiological effects. It is used in China medicinally, and in cooking .

23 Honey is still important in Chinese medicine and widely used, more medicine than food. Cooked at a high heat, its taste is quite different from the raw or pasteurized honey of the West. It is still considered warming and a general tonic, detoxifier, and harmonizer. Different honeys are not noted, but poisonous honeys are avoided.

24 According to Ou, 1982: 201, *jingxian* can refer to: "1. epilepsy induced by terror; 2. convulsion."

25 Yeast cultures are maintained primarily for brewing. H. T. Huang's meticulous research has sorted out the varieties of yeasts and other fungi used in Chinese foodstuffs (Huang 2000). Brewer's yeast is extremely nourishing. It is the richest of all B vitamin sources. It is especially valuable for its high content of vitamin B12, otherwise known only in animal foods and in other yeast and fungal foods. Strict vegetarians (vegans) depend on it. Chinese vegetarians had the many fungal ferments in soy sauce, soybean paste, and so forth, but must have found yeast to have a beneficial effect. The very warming effect noted in the *YSZY* may refer to the yeast's ability to cure anemia, a focal "cold" disease, which can be caused by lack of vitamin B12.

Vinegar[26] is sour in flavor, warming and lacks poison. It disperses carbuncle swelling and edema. It decreases evil poisons and destroys postpartum faintness. It expels obstructions of the bowels and impacted stool. There are various kinds of vinegar: (**Liquor Vinegar, Peach Vinegar, Wheat Vinegar, Grape Wine Vinegar**. **Rice Vinegar** is the best and is used medicinally.)

Sauce is salty in flavor, chilling and lacks poison. It expels heat and controls irritation. It decreases the heat of medicine and soup fire poison. It decreases all fish, meat, and vegetable poisons. **Soybean sauce** is superior to **Wheat sauce** for dietary and medicinal use. Old sauce is better.[27]

[5B] **Salted Bean Relish**[28] is bitter in flavor, cooling, and lacks poison. It is good for exogenous febrile diseases, headache, fidgetiness [with a feeling of] fullness in the chest.

Salt[29] is salty in flavor, warming and lacks poison. It is good for decreasing demon vermin [parasites], evil-possession-poison, exogenous febrile disease, and for bringing up accumulation of phlegm of the thorax center. It controls sudden chest and abdomen pain. If too much is eaten it wounds the lungs. It causes one to cough and lose color.

Liquor is bitter-sweet and piquant in flavor. It is very heating and has poison. It is good for enhancing the effects of drugs. It decreases the hundred evils [pathologies] and makes blood pass in the blood vessels. It fills up the bowels and enriches the skin. It disperses melancholy. If too much is drunk it harms the life span and wounds the spirit. It changes a person's nature. There are many kinds of liquor. Each sort is brewed specially:[30]

---

[26] Vinegar: it is odd that vinegar is regarded here as warming. Sour, watery, low–calorie foods are usually considered cooling today.

[27] Wheat sauce is fermented flour paste, possibly with bean mash added. Inoculation is with a starter including *Aspergillus* (Huang, 2000), *Rhizobium* and other fungi.

[28] Salted bean relish: this is modern *doushi*, already discussed under soybeans.

[29] Salt is little used in modern Chinese medicine.

[30] Except for grape wine and fruit drinks, Chinese liquor is brewed from grain. The medicinal liquors described in the *YSZY* are tinctures produced by steeping the various objects in liquor, adding them to the grain mash during fermentation, as descriptions make clear. Not implied is that pine sap and pine knots were fermented into liquor themselves. Lamb liquor is mutton in local vodka. Tiger bone liquor is distilled grain alcohol with a tiny bit of powdered tiger bone. There is a vast variety of similar tinc-

Tiger Bone Liquor: It is brewed from ground, roasted tiger bone. It regulates arthralgia, wind fixation[31] and chill numbness pain.

Wolfthornberry [*i.e.*, the fruit of the Chinese Matrimony Vine] **Liquor:** It is fermented according to a recipe with Ganzhou berries. It supplements for asthenia and thickens flesh. It augments vital *qi*, removes chill wind and strengthens *yang* paths.

[6A] **Chinese Foxglove Liquor:** It is fermented from the juice squeezed from foxglove [root]. It regulates asthenia, strengthens joint and bone, makes the blood pass, and regulates pain in the abdomen.

Pine Knot [*Pinus* spp] **Liquor**: [According] to a Daoist recipe the pine knots are collected on the fifth day of the fifth month, ground up, boiled in water and fermented into liquor. It regulates chill wind exhaustion, bone weakness, and inability to stand.

China Root [*Poria cocos*] **Liquor:** [In a] Daoist recipe the China root is fermented into a liquor according to a special method. It regulates *xulao* diseases, strengthens joint and bone, lengthens the

---

tures and cordials. The Chinese know that an alcohol extract of a drug may have properties different from a water extract. "Pine knot liquor" could also be translated "tincture of pine knots." Today, tincture of iodine is "iodine *jiu.*"

In classical times, *jiu* was beer or ale, made from millet, especially sticky or "glutinous" varieties. Other grains could sometimes be substituted, including rice.

Given the universal distribution of rice beer in Southeast Asia, we may assume that it has been in South China since the Neolithic. Anyone who left rice porridge sitting around the house for a couple of days inadvertently created it, and control of the process was not far behind. *Tapai* (Malay rice beer) is rice mashed boiled with water and inoculated with a starter, old *tapai* or a bit of yeast saved from earlier brewing. It is a thick porridge tasting like beer-flavored cream of wheat. It is strained and many rice beers are drunk with straws, with gratings to prevent clogging. In China, *jiu* is strained and bottled, but minority groups still offer thick beer similar to tapai.

Various herbs were added during brewing, often for their antibiotic properties, why hops were added to beer. The bitterness has become an acquired taste. In the West many herbs were used but hops proved most effective. The Chinese instead developed superior brewing techniques, gradually dispensing with herbs. The West differentiated ale, brewed with a yeast rising to float on the mash, and beer, bottom–fermented. Some *jiu* had top–fermentation. The *Qimin yaoshu* refers to "floating ants," *i.e.*, ant–sized particles of yeast, observed during fermentation but the Chinese did not bother about different strains of yeast. *Jiu* seems to have been both top– and bottom–fermented. A typical Chinese starter has brewer's yeast (*Saccharomyces cerevisiae*) but also other yeasts as well, even fungi such as *Aspergillus*.

[31] On this syndrome see Li in Hu Sihui, 1988: 243.

life span, and augments longevity.

Pine Root Liquor: Place a jar in a hole below a pine tree. Collect the pine root sap and ferment it into a liquor. It regulates wind and strengthens joint and bone.

Lamb Liquor:It is made according to a special method.[32] It greatly supplements and augments a person.

***Acanthopanax* Bark Liquor**: [This is] tincture of *Acanthopanax* Bark or *Acanthopanax* Bark fermented into liquor according to a special method. It regulates bone weakness [causing] [**6B**] inability to walk. If taken for a long time it strengthens joint and bone and lengthens the years so that one does not age.

***Olnul* "Navel"**[33] [penis and testes of *Callorhinus ursinus* or *Phoca vitulina*] **Liquor:** It regulates kidney asthenia, strengthens waist and knee, and greatly supplements and augments a person.

"Small Coarse Grain"[34] Liquor: It is heating by nature. It is not beneficial to drink a lot. It confuses the five viscera, [makes one] miserable with fever and very sleepy.

Grape Wine: It augments *qi*, accords the center, [makes one] able to bear hunger, and energizes the will. There are several kinds of wine: there is Tibetan Wine, there is Qaraqojha Wine, there is Wine of Pingyang and of Taiyuan. Their flavor is not as good as that of the Qarakhoja Wine. *_Tngri_ Wine is the best [Qarakhoja Wine].[35]

---

[32] The "special method" was probably the modern one of simply steeping lamb meat a distilled vodka (see Anderson 1988). Lamb Liquor is also used as tonic and restorative, the easily available heme iron in the meat being evidently of value. It has been used for malaria, the effect being presumably to build up the blood.

[33] *Wunaqi* is from Korean *olnul*, "seal," plus Chinese *qi*, "navel." Seal genitalia are still used as indicated, and may be found dried or in tincture in Chinese drugstores. The seal is thought especially potent and its genitalia, with those of deer, the best restorers of health and vigor to the "loins." They are not aphrodisiacs *per se*; they improve sexual performance by improving health in the whole genito–urinary system, not by actual mechanical stimulation or irritation in the manner of yohimbine or Spanish fly. The value is more magical: male seals and deer can service many females.

[34] Small coarse grain here may be sorghum, used in brewing by the Chinese probably from late Tang or Five Dynasties on. The liquor was quite probably a *gaoliang*.

[35] Grapes and grape wine came to China during Former Han, among the crops associated with explorer and traveler Zhang Qian. It was extremely popular in Tang.

***Arajhi* Liquor [Brandy]**[36] is sweetish in flavor and piquant. It is very heating and has great poison. It is good for dispersing chill hard accumulation. It removes cold *qi*. Good wine is distilled to procure a dew. This is the *Arajhi*.

Sürmä* Liquor**: It is also called ****Boza. It is slightly sweet and piquant in flavor. It is good for augmenting the *qi* and controlling thirst. If too much is drunk it makes a person fat and produces phlegm.

[7A] Animal Products:

[Illustration Caption:] Ox

Beef[37] is sweetish in flavor, neutral, and lacks poison. It is good for diabetes. It controls leaking [of *qi*] due to retching, tranquilizes the center, augments *qi*, and supplements the stomach.

Beef Medullae[38] supplement the center and fill out the vital medullae.

Cow's Milk Cheese[39] is cooling. It augments the heart and lungs, controls thirst [and] cough, makes the hair sleek, and expels with-

---

[36] Distillation was known in China from late Han and spread throughout Asia. Technically distilled Chinese grain *jiu* is vodka, unaged distilled grain liquor. If aged, it becomes "whiskey." In Chinese, it is known as *sanshao* 三燒 ("three times roasted", *i.e.*, three times distilled) and by various other names. One old name, *shaojiu* 燒酒, corresponds closely to English "brandy" (German *Branntwein*, "burned wine"). Mao-tai 茅台 the most familiar sort, made from glutinous millet or sorghum and distilled up to nine times. Distilled drinks are known as *araq* (*alachi*) widely in Asia.

[37] Beef: The cow, native to West Asia and Europe, reached China as a domestic animal by 2500 BC, following other Near Eastern domesticates. See Yuan Jing and Rod Campbell, "Recent Archaeometric Research on 'the Origins of Chinese Civilisation.'" *Antiquity* 83 (2009): 96-109. Beef was little eaten in China and not at all in Japan because the cow is so useful as a draft animal that one should not treat it as mere food. This may come from Indian cow–reverence but see also Vincent Gossaert, *L'interdit du boeuf en Chine. agriculture, éthique et sacrifice* (Paris, 2005). The meat is considered warming. See H. Epstein, *Domestic Animals of China* (London, 1969).

[38] Beef "medullae" can be spinal cord, marrow, and similar parts. Spinal cord is implied in modern usage. Spinal cord of cow is a popular dish of the Hakka who were, until recently, too poor to pass up any meat source out of idealistic reverence.

[39] Cow Cheese is not eaten by Chinese, but cheese is made from the milk of smaller livestock in Central Asia. The Baghlan area of Afghanistan produces pleasant cheddar–like cow and sheep cheese similar to what the Mongol court knew.

ered lung[40] and heart heat blood–spitting.

Cow's Milk Cream is sweetish-sour in flavor, cooling, and lacks poison. It is good for intense evil heat. It controls diabetes and expels asthenic heat in the thorax and body and face heat sores.

Cow's Milk Curds[41] are slightly **[7B]** cooling. They enrich the five viscera, benefit urination and excretion, augment the 20 chief blood vessels, and slightly move the *qi*.

[Illustration Caption:] Sheep

Mutton[42] is sweetish in flavor, very heating and lacks poison. It is good for warming the center, head wind, severe wind producing sweat, *xulao* cold-evil, supplements the center and augments *qi*.

Sheep's Head is cooling. It regulates hectic fever due to *yin* deficiency, brain heat, vertigo and emaciation.

---

[40] Ou, 1982: "Consumptive pulmonary disease due to deficient *yin*" (132).

[41] Cow's Milk Curds: this refers primarily to yogurt but rennet–coagulated or otherwise coagulated milk was known. Yogurt is still eaten throughout west, central, and south Asia. It is an important Chinese food in parts of the mountain west, such as the plateau of Yunnan where it has been spread by Tibeto–Burman peoples and Mongol settlers. Dairy products and yogurt were much more important in Medieval China, due to Central Asian influence. Following the fall of Yuan, nationalist reaction and a desire for self–sufficiency led to general Chinese rejection of Central Asian goods and ways. Meanwhile, the decline of Indian influence, religion, trade, *etc.*, throughout Southeast Asia led to decline of dairy product use from South China southward. Yogurt persists as a rare and fascinating survival among the Batak and Minangkabau peoples of the mountains of Sumatra. It is made from water buffalo milk, richer than cows' and producing a product much like pot cheese. Otherwise the decline of dairy use in Eastern Asia was virtually universal and total. Westernization has now led to a reversal. Yogurt is again sold in Beijing. Western visitors add their desires to those of both minority and Han peoples from China's west. It is not used in Chinese medicine, but has significance in traditional healing in India and Central Asia. Sabban, 1986, gives the history of milk products in China. See also Paul Wheatley, "A Note on the Extension of Milking Practices into Southeast Asia during the First Millennium AD," *Anthropos* 60 (1965): 577–90, and Luo Feng, "A History of the Production and Consumption of Milk Products in the North of China: an Archaeological and Ethnological Enquiry," *Journal of Chinese Dietary Culture* 4 (2008): 115-178.

[42] Sheep: Sheep were domesticated in the Near East and spread from there. It now seems less likely that sheep were domesticated independently in China. Its sheep are of an strain found all across Asia then and now (Jing and Campbell, 2009).

The meat is still regarded as especially heating and nourishing. These animals abound in north and west China but are less known in the south. They are the mainstay of all pastoral peoples in China. Nothing special need be said of the dairy products.

Sheep's Heart is used to regulate diaphragm *qi* of depression and rage.

Sheep's Liver is chilling in nature. It treats liver *qi* deficiency heat and conjunctivitis impaired vision.

Sheep's Blood is good for regulating female apoplexy and blood deficiency. In cases of postpartum faintness and a pressing [chest sensation] **[8A]** that is extreme, one *sheng* is drunk fresh.

The Five Viscera of Sheep supplement the five viscera of people.

Sheep's Kidneys supplement kidney asthenia and augment the vital *medullae*.

Sheep's Bone is heating. It controls *xulao* diseases and cold–evil attack emaciation.

Sheep's Medullae are sweetish in flavor and warming. They are good for regulating male and female wounding of the center and insufficiency of *yin qi*. They benefit the blood vessels and augment essential *qi*.

Sheep's Brain: A lot should not be eaten.

Sheep's Milk Cream regulates diabetes and supplements for exhaustion.

[Illustration Caption:] Gazelle [Two varieties are shown.][43]

Gazelle [meat] is sweetish in flavor, warming, and lacks poison. it supplements the center and augments *qi*. It regulates internal impairment caused by overstrain and deficiency-cold.[44] There are numerous **[8B]** varieties of gazelle. They form herds of up to several

---

[43] Gazelle: the "yellow sheep" of the text is focally the dseiran antelope *Procapra gutturosa*, here probably intended by the "black–tailed yellow sheep" so that *huang-yang* here is probably generic for antelopes. The "white yellow sheep" seems to be the Central Asian gazelle. Note reference to "several varieties." These animals once lived in enormous herds, but are now almost exterminated by hunting, except in isolated regions. Buddhism, with its ethic of non–violence, protected them in Tibet and Mongolia. It did not eliminate hunting, but led the hunters to be fewer and less bloodthirsty than they might have been. Chinese settlement and Communist anti–religious sentiment has allowed mass slaughter and very rapid declines in recent decades. There is no conceivable reason why the brain of the antelope should not be eaten, and we are presumably dealing with some local taboo here.

[44] Ou, 1982: "Cold–syndrome due to *yang*–deficiency" (194).

thousand.

The White Gazelle [probably Przewalsky's Gazelle, *Procapra picticaudata*] lives in the open steppe.

The Black–Tailed Gazelle [the Dseiren Antelope] lives in the desert. It can move fast. It is good at lying down [and keeping cover]. It does not travel in herds. Its brain cannot be eaten. The medullae and bone can be eaten. It can supplement and augment people. The broth lacks flavor.

[The Meat of the] Blue Sheep [*Pseudois nayaur*][45] is sweetish in flavor, neutral, and lacks poison. It supplements and augments people. It lives in mountain valleys.

[Illustration Caption:] The Goat[46]

Goat [*Capra sp.*] [**Meat**] is sweetish in flavor, neutral and lacks poison. It supplements [for] the five kinds of impairments[47] and the seven kinds of wounds. It warms the center and augments *qi*. The meat is somewhat rank.

[9A] [Illustration Caption:] Horse[48]

Horse Meat is acrid–bitter in flavor, chilling and has a small amount

---

45 Normally *shanyang*, "mountain sheep," is "goat," but not here. This *shanyang* is described as living "in mountain valleys" and is here placed just after the gazelles. The blue sheep resembles the gazelle in behavior, and size, and is strictly confined to high altitude valleys. It was probably more common in Mongol times than today, when it is rare. In Mongolian the blue sheep is "mountain goat (*yangir yamaa*)," probably the reason for the confusion.

46 Chinese glosses to the *Secret History* define *guli*, equivalent to Middle Mongolian *eshik*, as a "goat less than one year old." The goat is common livestock in Central Asia and throughout China.

47 Ou, 1982: These are: "1. Disorders of the five solid organs; 2. five kinds of impairments caused by overstrain" (20).

48 Horse: the horse was domesticated before 3000 BC as a food source, for meat and milk. Later it was used to draw vehicles, including chariots. Riding did not become common in the West until around 1000 BC, and was later in China. The horse first became important there in Shang times to draw chariots, introduced from Central Asia. The horse has attracted a disproportionate share of odd medical beliefs including some listed here. The *BCGM* includes many more. On early chariots from Central Asia see M.A. Littauer and J. H. Crouwel. "The Origin of the True Chariot." *Antiquity*, 70: 270, 1996, 934-39. See also Robert Drews, *Early Riders, the Beginnings of Mounted Warfare in Asia and Europe* (New York and London, 2004).

of poison. It is good for heat that brings down *qi*. It thickens joint and bone, energizes waist and knee and builds up a light body.

If a **Horse's Skull** is made into a pillow, it makes a person need little sleep.

Horse's Liver[49] cannot be eaten.

White Horse's Hooves controls the profuse, sudden leucorrhagia of women.

Red of a Horse's Hooves controls the sudden reddish discharge of women.

The Penis of a White Stallion is salty–sweetish in flavor and lacks poison. It is good for wounded center [and] pulse rapidity. It energizes the will and augments *qi*. It thickens flesh and causes one to have a child. It can strengthen and make profuse *yin qi*.

Horse's Heart is good for depression.

There is **Horse [9B] Meat Which Produces an Ink–Black Juice**. It has poison and cannot be eaten. White horses often have it.

[Fermented] Mare's Milk[50] is chilling by nature and sweetish in flavor. It controls thirst and regulates heat. There are three grades: (one kind is called ***Chige'en***. One kind is called ***Qongqor***. One kind is called ****Caqa'an***.) *Chige'en* is considered the best.

[Illustration Caption:] Wild Horse [*Equus przewalskii*][51]

---

[49] The belief that horse liver was poisonous was universal in old China. It is stated in such a matter–of–fact way and so generally in early texts, *e.g.*, from the Zhou Dynasty, that we cannot dismiss it as error. The liver concentrates poisons. Perhaps the horses of old North China were eating some plant or plants that were toxic to humans but not to horses, and the liver concentrated the toxin. The black–juiced meat noted as poisonous in the *YSZY* may be of similar danger, but it sounds more like necrosed tissue. Horse meat is relatively rich in glycogen and tastes somewhat sweet.

[50] Horse milk is high in lactose and tastes quite sweet. This is what allows it to be fermented successfully. Yeast lives on sugar. Cow's milk cannot be fermented without added sugar, and few have thought it worth doing. Fermented mare's milk, usually known by its Turkic name kumiss, was staple food for Central Asian nomads and is still widely drunk in Inner Asia. It was extremely popular in North, especially Northwest China from Wei through Tang. Countless poems refer to it, and Chinese from the Yangtse valley were fond of teasing Northerners about this "barbarian" custom.

[51] Przewalsky's horse is a survival of the wild form of the species, ancestral to the domestic horse.

Wild Horse Meat is sweetish in flavor, neutral, and has poison. It strengthens joint and bone. It is very similar to the meat of a domestic horse. If the meat falls to the ground it does not pick up dirt. However, it is not beneficial to eat a lot.

[10A] [Illustration Caption:] Elephant[52]

Elephant Meat is insipid in flavor and is not palatable. If much is eaten it makes one heavy in the body. The small transverse bone at the front of the thorax causes one to be able to float on water. On the body of the elephant is the meat of the hundred animals. Each has is portion. Only the trunk is real elephant meat.

Elephant Tusk lacks poison. It is good for various metals and other objects which have entered the flesh. One shaves off a fragment and grinds it up finely. It is placed on the wound combined with water. The object will then come out.

[10B] [Illustration Caption:] Camel[53]

Camel [Bactrian Camel] **Meat** controls the various winds and brings down *qi.* It strengthens joint and bone and makes the skin sleek. It treats all chronic numbness, migratory arthralgia, tightness of muscle and skin, malignant boils, and swelling poison.

> **Camel Fat** is found in the two humps where it is accumulated in layers. It is best taken in tincture.
>
> **[Fermented] Camel's Milk** (A kind of *airaq*)[54] is warming by nature and sweetish in flavor. It supplements the center and augments *qi.* It strengthens joint and bone. It renders a person free from hunger.

---

[52] Elephant: elephants occurred throughout China in the Pleistocene, and in Shang times as far north as Central China. By Yuan they were reduced to the southern border areas and obviously very poorly known to the writers of the *YSZY*! On the elephant in China see now Mark Elvin, *The Retreat of the Elephants: An Environmental History of China* (New Haven, 2004).

[53] Camel: the Bactrian camel is a common domesticate throughout north and northwest China. Wild ones occur in Xinjiang. Medical benefits are still held to accrue to camel parts. See now Matt Walker, "Wild Camels 'Genetically Unique'," BBC Earth News, 22 July, 2009.

[54] Fermented camel's milk is better known by its Turkic name of *shubat.*

[11A] [Illustration Caption:] Wild Camel[55]

Wild Camel [Meat] is sweetish in flavor, warming, neutral, and lacks poison. It regulates the various winds and brings down *qi*. It strengthens joint and bone and makes the skin sleek.

> **[Wild] Camel Hump** controls *xulao* disease wind. If one is suffering from chill accumulation, warm grape wine is used to make a tincture of wild camel hump oil. It is effective when taken. "Good Liquor" can also be used.

[11B] [Illustration Caption:] Bear[56]

Bear [*Ursus arctos* and other spp] **Meat** is sweetish in flavor and lacks poison. It is good for migratory arthralgia and insensitivity of muscles and joints. If there is abdominal mass or cold–hot emaciation [Bear Meat] should not be eaten. It will not be expelled for one's whole life.

> **Bear Fat** is cooling and lacks poison. It controls wind and supplements for deficiency. It destroys exhausting parasites.[57]

> **Bear's Paw**:[58] If one eats bear's paw one can withstand wind and cold. This is one of the rarities. Ancient people greatly treasured it.

> **Bear's Paw of the Tenth Lunar Month** cannot be eaten. It harms the spirit.

[12A] [Illustration Caption:] Donkey[59]

---

[55] The illustration shows what appears to be a dromedary but with two humps. This could be an error but it could also be an attempt to show a hybrid camel, popularly bred during the era, particularly among the Turkic peoples of Central Asia. On the importance of hybred camels see Richard W. Bulliet, *Cotton, Climate, and Camels in Early Islamic Iran, a Moment in World History* (New York, 2009).

[56] Bear: in addition to *Ursus arctos*, the Himalayan or Tibetan black bear (*Selenarctos thibetanus*) occurs in the Himalayas and the mountains of West China and once occurred at least locally throughout most of the Eighteen Provinces. On bears see also Laurence Delaby, *L'Ours, l'autre de l'homme* (Paris, 1980).

[57] See the discussion of this syndrome by Li (Hu Sihui, 1988: 268–9).

[58] Bears' Paws, one of the Eight Rarities of ancient Chinese conspicuous consumption, are popular with Native Americans and others who know their game meats.

[59] Donkey: the Donkey, a native of North Africa, was domesticated very early in the West. It reached China at a late and uncertain time.

Donkey Meat is sweetish in flavor, cooling, and lacks poison. It controls wind mania and chronic depression. It tranquilizes heart *qi* and counteracts [heart] vexation.

[Donkey] Head Meat controls chronic diabetes. It is best eaten boiled. [The Head Meat] of a black donkey is better.

If **[Donkey] Fat** is combined with *Prunus mume* into a pill it controls chronic malaria.

Kulan [*Equus hemionus*] **[Meat]** has the same nature and flavor as [Donkey Meat]. The Kulan's mane and tail are longer than those of the domestic donkey. Its bones are large.[60] If eaten, [Kulan Meat] can control dizziness due to wind–evil.

[12B] [Illustration Caption:] Sika Deer[61]

Sika Deer Venison is sweetish in flavor, warming, and lacks poison. It augments *qi* and supplements the center. It controls fatigue of waist and leg. It cannot be eaten together with pheasant meat and shrimp, fresh vegetables, plums, and fruits and nuts. It makes one sick.

Sika Deer Fat is acrid in flavor, warming and lacks poison. It is good for carbuncle swelling, malignant boils, migratory arthralgia, and spasms of the limbs. It makes the blood pass and makes the skin sleek and glossy.

Sika Deer Skin is made into boots. It can expel [evil] foot *qi*.

[13A] [Illustration Caption:] Red Deer[62]

Red Deer Venison is sweetish in flavor, warming and lacks poison. It supplements the center, energizes the five internal organs, and augments *qi*.

---

60 Kulan wild ass: the Asian replacement of the donkey, it is larger, faster, and wilder. It has been domesticated without much success. It has the advantages of neither horse nor donkey and the disadvantages of both. Wild kulan still occur.

61 *Mi* is normally *Elaphurus davidianus*, Pere David's Deer. The illustration is clearly a Sika Deer *Cervus nippon*. Deer meat is still considered medicinal. Deer genitalia are a favorite restorative for the genital system. Older men consume great quantities. As with seal genitalia, the deer penes and testes improve the health of the system, rather than being "aphrodisiacs." Sika Deer have been domesticated and are farmed in North China. Other deer are locally kept. Pere David's Deer is extinct in China but have been preserved on a game park in England. They zoo animals in China.

62 Here *lu* = *malu* 馬鹿. The identification is from the illustration.

Red Deer Medullae are sweetish in flavor, warming, and lack poison. They are good for wounded center in males and females, cut–off pulse, tendon and muscle spasms, and cough. They are taken in liquor.

Red Deer Head is good for diabetes and nightmares.

Red Deer's Hoof is good for pain of the leg or knee.

Red Deer Stag's Penis [includes testicles, urethra and kidneys] is good for warming the center and supplementing the kidneys. It tranquilizes the five viscera and strengthens *yangqi*.

Red Deer Velvet is sweetish in flavor, slightly warming, and lacks poison. It is good for profusely flowing extravasated blood, and cold-hot infantile convulsions. It augments *qi*, energizes the will, supplements for deficiency emaciation, and strengthens joint and bone.

Red Deer [13B] Horn is slightly salty and lacks poison. It is good for malignant boils and carbuncle swelling. It drives out evil *qi* and expels lower abdomen blood acute pain, pain along the spinal column, and retained blood situated within *yin*.

[Illustration Caption:] River Deer

River deer [*Hydropotes inermis*] **Venison** is warming. It is good for supplementing and augmenting the five viscera. The *Rihuazi* says: "The venison lacks poison. If it is eaten from the eighth to the twelfth lunar month, the venison is superior to mutton. If eaten from the twelfth month to the seventh month, it moves *qi*. It is much eaten by Taoists. They say that there is no prohibition against eating it."

[14A] [Illustration Caption:] Dog[63]

Dog Meat is salty in flavor, warming and lacks poison. It tranquilizes

---

[63] Dog: the domestic dog is known from earliest Neolithic China, by 8000 BC. It presumably was ancient then. East Asian dogs are close to wolf ancestors. Dogs may have been domesticated there but may also have been domesticated in the Near East. Dog meat is a standard warming and strengthening food, consumed in quantities in winter in south China. Islam and more general westward influences have now led to the disappearance of dog–eating in north China. Today, black is the choice of color for a dog; black dog meat is more warming and strengthening than other dog meats. Guinness Stout, "black dog" in Chinese, partakes of this reputation.

the five viscera, supplements for extreme abuse, and augments the *yang* ways. It supplements the pulse, fills out the bowels, makes ample the lower burner and fills in the vital medullae. The meat of a **Yellow Dog** is better. [Dog meat] cannot be eaten with garlic. It will injure a person. It is not advantageous to eat dog meat during the ninth lunar month. It causes one to harm the spirit.

If the **Four Paws of a Dog** are boiled and [the broth] drunk, it brings down milk.

[14B] [Illustration Caption:] Pig[64]

Pig Meat is bitter in flavor and lacks poison. It is good for obstructed pulse. It weakens joint and bone. Persons with depletion fat (puffiness) should not eat pork for an extended time. It moves wind. It is even worse for those suffering from wounds caused by metal weapons.

Pig Suet is good for supplementing the center and augmenting *qi*. It stops thirst.

Boar Kidney [*etc.*] is chilling. It harmonizes and orders kidney *qi* and penetrates and benefits the bladder.

The **Four Hooves of a Pig** are somewhat cooling. They are good for whip or cudgel injuries and infected wounds, and bring down milk.

[15A] Wild Boar

Wild Boar Meat is bitter in flavor and lacks poison. It is good for supplementing flesh. It causes one to put on depletion fat. The meat of

---

[64] Pig: by 6000 BC pigs were domested in China and were being fed millet husks and waste (Jing and Flad 2002; Liu 2004). This is about as early as domestic pigs are found in the Near East; they were independently domesticated in both places. Around 5500 BC, people, pigs, and dogs in central north China suddenly shifted toward eating a lot more C4 plants, i.e. millets; before that they were eating mostly C3 plants, i.e. wild foods (Jing and Campbell 2009). The reference is to the type of carbon-fixing metabolism. The vast majority of temperate-zone plants use the C3 pathway to fix carbon into nutrients. A few grasses use C4: millets and maize. The latter, of course, was not to reach China for another 9000 years or so. See also Greger Larson, et al, "Worldwide Phylogeography of Wild Boar Reveals Multiple Centers of Pig Domestication." *Science* 307 (2005): 1618-1621, and Sarah M. Nelson, "Pigs in the Hongshan Culture," in Sarah M. Nelson ed., *Ancestor for the Pigs: Pigs in Prehistory* (Philadelphia, 1998), 99-107. Pork is of course *the* meat of China, but not of the non–Han peoples of Inner Asia except among the Tungus groups of Manchuria.

the female is better. It eats acorns in the winter months. The meat is red. It supplements a person's five viscera and regulates bowel wind leaking blood.[65] The flavor of the meat is superior to that of the domestic pig.

Yangtse Porpoise[66] ["River Pig;" *Delphinus delphis*] [**Meat**] is sweetish in flavor, neutral, and lacks poison. However, it is not advantageous to eat a lot. It moves wind *qi* and makes a person's body heavy.

[15B] [Illustration Caption:] Otter[67]

Otter [*Lutra lutra*] **Meat** is salty in flavor, neutral, and lacks poison. It regulates swelling due to retention of fluid and treats pestilence, various intense evil heat winds, and cough internal impairment. It cannot be eaten along with rabbit.

> **Otter Liver** is sweetish in flavor and has poison. It regulates bowel wind producing blood [*i.e.*, fresh–bloody stool] and is good for *zhu* [possession] illness contagions.[68]
>
> If **Otter skin** is used to decorate collar and sleeves, dirt does not adhere. If wind blown dirt enters the eye, it comes out if wiped with [the otter skin decorated] sleeve. If a fish bone sticks in the throat, one rubs below the neck with otter [skin]. The fish bone will come out.

[16A] [Illustration Caption:] Tiger[69]

Tiger [presumably the Manchurian variety] **Meat** is salty–sour in flavor, neutral, and lacks poison. It is good for nausea and augments *qi*

---

65 See the discussion by Li (Hu Sihui, 1988: 279).

66 Yangtse porpoise: fairly common until recently, this animal was eaten mainly for medicine. The name probably confounds other fresh–water *Cetacea* notably the now extinct white–flag dolphin (*Lipotes vexillifer*) of Dongting 洞庭 Lake.

67 Otter: the fine soft fur of the otter is noted here. The prescription about the fish bone seems to be sympathetic magic.

68 See the discussion in Li, 1988: 281.

69 Tiger: the tiger has attracted more magical beliefs than any other wild Asian animal, because of size and ferocity. Tiger is still of the utmost medicinal value as a strength–builder and tonic, but the raw material is hard to get due to virtual extermination. We have heard that "tiger balm" uses defunct zoo and circus specimens, and that the dilution is extreme, a single bone having to do for many, many gallons, or even thousand gallons, of medicine. In Yuan times there was a better tiger/human ratio. On tiger decline see Robert Marks, *Tigers, Rice, Silk and Silt* (New York, 1998).

force. If one eats tiger meat and enters the mountains the tigers will be afraid when they see you. It wards off the 36 kinds of *mei* demons.[70]

Tiger Eyes are good for intermittent fevers [*i.e.*, of malaria] and for warding off evil. They control the heat convulsions of children.

Tiger Bones are good for expelling evil and pathological *qi*. They decrease demon-possession poison and control agitation. They are good for malignant boils and scrofula. The head bones are best.

[16B] [Illustration Caption:] Leopard[71]

[Snow] Leopard Meat is salty in flavor, neutral, and lacks poison. It tranquilizes the five viscera and supplements extreme abuse. It strengthens joint and bone and energizes emotion *qi*. If eaten for a long time, it causes one to be fierce and violent, rough and coarse in nature, and able to endure cold and heat. It should not be eaten during the first lunar month. It wounds the spirit. The *Tangben zhu* says: "The leopard's tail is used as an imperial insignia when the emperor rides in a carriage. It makes it all the more imposing."

The **Brain of the Local Leopard** [possibly *Felis nebulosa*] can regulate waist pain [lumbago].

[17A] [Illustration Caption:] Pere David's Deer [*Elaphurus davidianus*][72]

Pere David's Deer [Venison] is sweetish and neutral and lacks poison. It supplements and augments a person.

[Illustration Caption:] Musk Deer

Musk Deer [*Moschus moschiferus]* **Venison** lacks poison. It is good for the five kinds of hemorrhoids. If too much is eaten it can excite a person's obstinate illnesses.

---

[70] That is, demons causing otherwise unexplained illnesses. See Li in Hu Sihui, 1988: 283.

[71] The Chinese term for leopard usually refers to *Felis pardus*, but the illustration clearly shows the Snow Leopard *Felis uncia*. Leopard: as with tiger, and other animals, sympathetic magic is evident here.

[72] The identification is from the illustration. It seems to clearly show Pere David's deer.

[17B] [Illustration Caption:] Muntjac Deer

Muntjac Deer [*Muntiacus reevesi]* **Venison** is sweetish in flavor, neutral, and lacks poison. It is warming by nature. It has rank smell like River Deer Venison. If it is eaten, one does not fear snake poison.

[Illustration Caption:] Fox

Fox Meat is warming and has a small amount of poison. The *Rihuazi* says: "[Its] nature is warming. It supplements for *xulao* diseases and controls malignant boils and itching."

[18A] [Illustration Caption:] Rhinoceros[73]

Rhinoceros Meat is sweetish in flavor, warming, and lacks poison. It is good for the poisons of the various animals, snakes, and noxious creatures. It wards off *changqi*.[74] If you eat it and enter the mountains you do not lose your way.

> **Rhinoceros Horn** is bitter–salty in flavor, slightly cooling, and lacks poison. It is good for the hundred poisons, *gu* possession, evil spirits, and *changqi*. It destroys hook, lip, venom, feather, and serpent poisons. It heals exogenous febrile diseases and pestilence. There are various kinds of rhinoceroses:[75] **(Mountain Rhi-**

---

[73] A two–horned Sumatran variety appears to be illustrated. Rhinoceros: present in ancient China and no doubt still in the far south during Yuan, the rhinoceros is now extinct there and most other places due to the enormous value placed on its horn by the Chinese. Surviving rhinos are subject to heavy poaching. Note that the "aphrodisiac" value, so dear to Western journalistic accounts of this trade, is not even mentioned by the *YSZY*. Rhino horn strengthens and tones the body, including the sexual system, but is far more than a mere excuse for a reporter's obscene jests. Its poison–destroying function, which is purely mythical, was far more important in its popularity at least in early times as the *YSZY* shows.

[74] Ou, 1982: "1. pathogens causing infectious diseases; 2. malaria" (247). See also Li in Hu Sihui, 1988: 290.

[75] Today three species of Asian rhinoceroses are recognized: the one–horned Indian rhinoceros, *Rhinoceros unicornis*, the two–horned Sumatran *R. sumatrensis* and the one–horned Java rhinoceros, *R. sondaicus*. Two species are now confined to the islands of Southeast Asia, but all three were once common on the Asian mainland. *R. sumatrensis* was common as recently as the last century, and in extreme south China at least as late as Tang times. The illustration of the *YSZY*, not drawn from life, clearly shows *R. sumatrensis*. *R. sumatrensis,* with perhaps the Indian or even Javan species, was found in the mountains of Southwest China probably as late as Yuan times, even later in Assam and Burma. There are also reports of single–horned rhinoceroses in the Lingnan area from Medieval times. Thus the five kinds of rhinoceroses listed here

noceros, the ***Tongtian*** **Rhinoceros**, the **Pichen Rhinoceros**, the **Water Rhinoceros**, the **Zhenwei Rhinoceros**.)

[18B] [Illustration Caption:] Wolf[76]

Wolf Meat is salty in flavor, heating in nature, and lacks poison. It is good for supplementing and augments the five viscera. It fills up the bowels and fills out the essential air medullae. If there is chill accumulation, it is beneficial to eat it. The flavor is superior to that of fox or dog meat.

Wolf's Throat Skin can be tanned into a hide. If wound around the head it removes headache.

Wolf's Skin can be tanned and made into a *fanpi*.[77] It is very warm.

Wolf's Tail: If hung before the breast of a horse, it wards off evil influence and makes the horse unafraid.

Wolf's Tooth is worn to ward off evil influence.

[19A] [Illustration Caption:] Hare[78]

Hare Meat is bitter in flavor, neutral and lacks poison. It supplements the center and augments *qi*. It is not advantageous to eat a lot. It harms *yang* elements and cuts off the pulse. It causes one to [show] flaccidity yellow. It cannot be eaten with ginger and oranges. It causes one to contract sudden chest pains. A pregnant woman should not eat rabbit. It causes the child to have a hare–lip. It cannot be eaten in the second

---

may have some basis in thirteenth to fourteenth century distributions. For example, the Zhenwei rhinoceros is most likely a one–horned, probably Javan variety from the Yunnan borderlands, where Zhenwei is located. Schafer is probably correct in seeking to identify the Tongtian variety with the "Great One–Horned Indian Rhinoceros." See Edward Schafer, *The Golden Peaches of Samarkand* (Berkeley, 1963), 83. Of the others, the "Mountain Rhinoceros" may be a memory of the two–horned variety of south and southeast China, a "wild" ("mountain") variety rather than zoo rhinoceroses from tribute expeditions. For the two other varieties may be more mythological than real. The "Water Rhinoceros," for example, may be the south Chinese variety (water spirit) of the dragon rather than the rhinoceros *per se*. In the same manner, Pichen, a semi–mythical island where rhinoceroses and elephants abound, may stand for all island varieties of the rhinoceros. See Schafer, 1963: 83–4 and notes.

[76] Wolf: wolves are now very rare in China. This is clearly a Mongolian food.

[77] Literally, "foreign barbarian skins." This may be a defective transcription of Turkic *yapinci*, a kind of raincoat. On the word see Doerfer, 1963-197: IV, 50-52.

[78] Probably *Lepus tolai* or *Lepus mandschuricus*. This is often considered cooling.

lunar month. It wounds the spirit.

Hare Liver is good for eye brightness.

If the **Head and Hair of a Hare of the twelfth lunar month** are roasted to ash and taken in liquor, it will control birth difficulty, failure of the placenta to descend, and blood stasis which will not descend.

[19B] [Illustration Caption:] *Tarbaqa[n]*

Tarbaqa[n] [*Marmota bobak]* (One name is *tubo* rodent) [**Meat**] is sweetish in flavor and lacks poison. It is good for pheasant sores. If eaten boiled, it benefits a person. The *Tarbaqa[n]* lives beyond the mountains in the grasses and swamps. The Northern people [= The Mongols] dig them out and capture them to eat. Although they are fat, they make no oil when boiled. The broth lacks flavor. If too much is eaten it is difficult to accomplish transformation. It excites the *qi* slightly.

[Tarbaqan] **Skin** can be made into a *fanpi*. It does not allow water to penetrate and is very warm.

[Tarbaqan] **Head Bones**, after the neck meat is pulled down and removed, make the teeth perfect and control the sleeplessness of small children. If hung next to the [child's] head it will then be able to sleep.

[20A] [Illustration Caption:] Badger[79]

Badger [*Meles meles*] **Meat** is sweetish in flavor, neutral, and lacks poison. It regulates cough due to abnormal rising of lung–energy and extreme retention of fluid. It is good eaten as a broth.

[Illustration Caption:] Wildcat[80]

Wildcat [Meat] is sweetish in flavor, neutral, and lacks poison. It is

---

[79] Badger: native but uncommon in Central Asia and north China.

[80] Wildcat: the illustration shows a small tiger–like animal. It could be any local wildcat including *Felis euptylura*, also *F. manul* or *F. margarita*. The leopard cat (*Felis bengalensis*) is found throughout most of China but not in the Inner Asian parts. If this distribution was true also in the thirteen and fourteenth centuries *Felis bengalensis* was less likely to be the animal encountered and hunted by the Mongols.

good for regulating scrofula and infected boils.

[Wildcat] Skulls are still better.

[20B] [Illustration Caption:] Weasel[81]

Weasel [Meat] is sweetish in flavor, neutral, and lacks poison. If too much is eaten it produces sores.

[Illustration Caption:] Monkey[82]

Monkey Meat is salty in flavor and lacks poison. It is good for regulating the various wind asthenia illnesses. It is best when fermented into a liquor.

[21A] Birds

[Illustration Caption:] *Yeke siraqun qun* means Greater Golden–Headed Swan [Whooper Swan, *Cygnus cygnus*].

[Illustration Caption:] *Qarlaq qun* means Lesser Golden–Headed Swan [Tundra Swan, *Cygnus columbianus*].

[21B] [Illustration Caption:] **Surqyl* means Mute Swan [*Cygnus olor*].

[Illustration Caption:] *Alaq qun* means Variegated Swan.[83]

Swan [Meat] is sweetish in flavor, heating by nature, and lacks poison. It is good for supplementing the center and augmenting *qi*. There are three or four kinds of swans:

The Golden–Headed Swan is best.

The Lesser Golden–Headed Swan[84] is next best.

---

[81] Weasel: several small species of *Mustela* occur in the relevant areas.

[82] Monkey: focally the rhesus macaque (*Macaca mulata*), but there are many monkey species in China. Probably any one will do.

[83] The "variegated swan" seems most likely to be an immature swan of any of the other species. This would explain why the text refers to "three or four forms." The Mongols most likely hunted swans only during certain seasons of the year when many were still in an immature or darker winter plumage on the lakes of Central Asia.

[84] Both the whooper and tundra swans are exceedingly rare in China proper, but not uncommon in Mongolia and well known in Siberia and other northern areas. They do not figure in Chinese knowledge or medicine, and we have here a clear Mongol presence. The "golden neck" of the whooper swan is due to staining of the white feathers by iron in the acidic, boggy waters of the swans' subarctic and arctic home lakes.

There is the **Variegated Swan.**

There is one kind of **Swan that is Unable to Call** [= Mute Swan]. When it flies the wings echo. Its meat is slightly rank.
All are inferior [in flavor] to the Golden-Headed Swan.

[22A] [Illustration Caption:] Oriental Swangoose [*Anser cygnoides*][85]

Oriental Swangoose [**Meat**] is sweetish in flavor, neutral, and lacks poison. It benefits the five viscera. It is good for diabetes. *Meng Shen* says: "The Meat is chilling in nature. A lot should not be eaten. It also causes obstinate illnesses." The *Rihuazi* says: "The green oriental swangoose: It is chilling in nature and has poison. If eaten it causes sores. The white swangoose lacks poison. Its [meat] counteracts the heat of the five viscera and stops thirst."

[Oriental Swangoose] Fat makes the skin sleek and is good for regulating deafness.

[Oriental Swangoose] Droppings supplement the five viscera and augment *qi*. If one has an obstinate illness, too much should not be eaten.

[22B] [Illustration Caption:] Wild Goose[86]

Wild Goose [*Anser* spp., primarily *A. albifrons albifrons* and *A. indi-*

---

[85] Goose: the Chinese swangoose is the domestic goose of East Asia, a quite different species from that of Europe (*Anser anser*). Wild ones breed in Northern Manchuria and in Mongolia.

[86] Wild goose: A single–word character, distinct from the character for "goose," covers wild geese in Chinese. Nesting commonly in Mongolia is the bar–headed goose (*Anser indicus*). No species breeds in China proper, but millions once wintered there. In China the wild goose is a symbol of transience and homeless wandering, the birds' wild, lonely cries is often mentioned in poetry. Certainly there are few more evocative sounds, and Native Americans too immortalized wild geese and their cries. In India the bird is a symbol for the soul, which appears from nowhere in the human body and departs, at death, we know not where. The Sanskrit term, *hamsa*, is cognate with Latin *anser* and English "goose," *cf.*, German *gans*. Known throughout the entire Northern Hemisphere from China to Ireland and the American Indians is the story of the man who saw wild geese, or similar water–birds, taking off their clothes and becoming beautiful maidens. He captured one feather cloak and thus obtained the woman, keeping her as his wife until one day she regained the cloak and disappeared into the sky. The story's universal popularity is easily understood by anyone who has ever lost a love, or watched geese disappear into the sky in spring.

cus] [**Meat**] is sweetish in flavor, neutral, and lacks poison. It is good for paralytic spasms, hemiplegia, and *qi* that will not pass through and benefit. It augments *qi* and strengthens joint and bone. It supplements [for] wasting weakness.

When **Wild Goose Bone Ash** is combined with rice and used to wash the head, it makes the hair long.

Wild Goose Grease regulates deafness. It can also make the hair long.

Wild Goose Fat supplements for wasting away. It makes one white and fat.

Wild goose [**meat**] cannot be eaten in the sixth and seventh lunar months. It causes a person to wound the spirit.

[23A] [Illustration Caption:] Cranes[87]

[23B] Crane [**Meat**] is sweetish in flavor, warming, and lacks poison. It supplements the center and augments *qi*. If eaten it greatly augments a person. If eaten broiled its flavor is still better. However, there are various kinds:

The "White Crane" [the Siberian crane, *Grus leucogeranus*],[88] **The "Black–Headed Crane"** [the black–necked crane, *Grus nigrocollis*], The "**Iranian Crane"** [probably the common crane, *Grus grus*]. Their meat is all different.

Crane Medullae are sweet in flavor and delicate. They supplement the essential air medullae.

[Illustration Caption:] Eurasian Curlew [*Numenius arquata*][89]

Eurasian Curlew [**Meat**] is sweetish in flavor, neutral, and lacks poi-

---

87 Three varieties are illustrated exhibiting slight differences. The illustrations do not appear be specifically of the species named in the text below, although the "black–headed crane" appears to have been the immediate model for the artist.

Cranes: cranes are avian symbol of longevity and Taoist wisdom. They are shown in art with other symbols of extended life, such as pines and bamboos. Tame cranes were once kept at Taoist retreats. Crane meat is widely used medicinally. Today, herons and egrets are lumped with cranes and used for treating illnesses and supernatural conditions. Cranes have now become vanishingly rare.

88 But none of the illustrations shows an all–white crane.

89 Kököluu (Hu Sihui, 1982: 261) calls this the Eurasian Curlew, *üker zarag*, "ox zarag," in Khalkha. Possibly other shorebirds have been lumped under the same name.

son. It supplements the center and augments *qi*. It is beneficial eaten broiled. It is very tasty.

[24A] [Illustration Caption:] Chickens[90]

[24B] Red Rooster [Meat] is sweetish in flavor, neutral, and slightly warming. It lacks poison. It is good for female metrorrhagia and bloody mucus spotting. It supplements for deficiency and warms the center. It stops blood.

White Rooster [Meat] is salty in flavor and lacks poison. It is good for bringing down *qi*. It heals mania evil,[91] supplements the center, tranquilizes the five viscera, and regulates diabetes.

Black Rooster[92] **[Meat]** is sweetish–salty in flavor and lacks poison. It is good for supplementing the center and stopping pain. It expels evil *qi* of chest and abdomen. It is beneficial for those suffering from asthenia to eat it.

Black Hen [Meat] is sweetish in flavor, warming, and lacks poison. It is good for wind-cold wetness type of arthralgia, the five slownesses,

---

90 Domestic fowl: the common "chicken" was domesticated in South China or Southeast Asia. By at least 4000 BC, it had spread north to central China where it was not native but where its bones become common in Neolithic sites. Wild red jungle fowl, the wild form of the domestic fowl, still occur in the southern border. Probably it was more widespread in early times, but even with the more favorable climate of the Neolithic it could not have occurred naturally as far north as the earliest bones, so evidently it spread from even earlier taming in the south. Wild jungle fowl tame themselves; they like human company and become as tame as barnyard fowl if tolerated. Perhaps deliberate breeding of chickens began with their northward spread from their homeland. Chicken is the appropriate festive dish for ordinary celebrations, and a part of larger feasts too. This has been part of the Chinese code of manners for a good three millennia, and probably twice that long. Chicken is the standard warming and restorative food for, *e.g.*, rebuilding strength in convalescents and in women after childbirth. The supreme virtue of chicken soup as a cure–all is recognized in most of Asia. Chinese grandmothers are as dedicated to the cult as Jewish ones.

Widely in East and Southeast Asia, chickens are known as *kai* or derivatives thereof (including Mandarin *ji*). This may be a Thai word, borrowed from the ancestors of the Thai possibly along with domesticated chickens.

91 See the explanation by Li (Hu Sihui) 1988: 308.

92 The black poultry noted in the *YSZY* are possibly the strange race found in extreme southwest China and neighboring Southeast Asia. This has a dark plumage and also grayish or black bones. It lays bluish eggs. Transported to South America as a curiosity by early explorers, it sired the Araucanian breed. Non–Han peoples of southwest China use "black bone" like Europeans use "blue blood."

and the six rapidities, abdomen pain due to attack by pestilent factors, and ache of broken bones. It tranquilizes the womb.

[Black Hen] Blood heals milk difficulty.

Yellow Hen [Meat] is salty in flavor, neutral, and lacks poison. It is good for a wounded center, diabetes, frequent incontinence of urine, dysentery, and leaking diarrhea. It supplements the five viscera. Those formerly suffering from bone heat should not eat it.

Eggs augment *qi*. If a lot is eaten it makes one produce a sound [*i.e.*, cluck].[93] They are good for postpartum diarrhea. If given to small children to eat they stop diarrhea. The *Rihuazi* says: "Eggs guard the heart and tranquilize the five viscera. The white is slightly cooling. It cures acute conjunctivitis inflammation. It expels insidious heat-evil of the upper abdomen. It controls a feeling of fullness in the chest and cough."

[25A] [Illustration Caption;] Pheasant [*Phasianus colchicus*][94]

Pheasant [**Meat**] is sweetish-sour in flavor, slightly cooling, and has a small amount of poison. It is good for supplementing the center and augments *qi*. It controls leaking diarrhea. If eaten for a long time it causes emaciation. If eaten from the ninth to the eleventh lunar months it will augment slightly. If eaten during other months it causes one to suffer from the five hemorrhoids and various sores. It also cannot be eaten with walnuts, *Agaricus* mushrooms, and tree ears.

[25B] [Illustration Caption:] Wild Pheasant[95]

The Wild Pheasant's [**Meat**] is sweetish in flavor, warming, and has a small amount of poison. It is good for those suffering from dyspnea of the five viscera that is not alleviated, if consumed [in soup] according to a recipe. If eaten for a long time, however, it can produce the

---

93 Note the delightful line that people who eat too many eggs come to sound like chickens, a typical example of the sympathetic magic often seen in the *YSZY*.

94 Pheasant: Probably all pheasants are conflated under this name, "wild chicken," as today. Pheasants, like other wild game birds, are considered very strengthening.

95 The identity of this bird is uncertain. The illustration seems to show a Koklass Pheasant, *Pucrasia macrolopha,* but the tail is too short and markings are wrong. The species illustrated also seems to show the feathered nostrils characteristic of the *Tetraonidae,* suggesting that the *shanji* is a ptarmigan or grouse rather than a pheasant. If so, it may be the Hazel grouse, *Tetrastes bonasia,* a popular Mongolian game bird. Probably any short–tailed montane game bird would be called *shanji*.

five hemorrhoids. If eaten with buckwheat flour it gives rise to vermin.

At present there is the **Food Fowl**[96] [the Manchurian variety of the chicken][97] in Liaoyang. The flavor [of the meat] is rich and fine.

There is the **Eared Fowl** [another variety of the Manchurian Chicken].[98] The flavor [of its meat] is far superior to that of any other fowl.

[26A] [Illustration Captions:] [Mallard] Duck [*Anas platyrhynchos*]; *Suqsur [*A. acuta*, the common pintail][99]

Duck Meat is sweetish in flavor, chilling, and lacks poison. It supplements for interior deficiency, disperses poison heat and benefits the water ways. It also regulates the heat-evil convulsion fits of children.

Wild Duck[100] **Meat** is sweetish in flavor, slightly cooling, and lacks poison. It supplements the center and augments *qi*. It disperses food, harmonizes abdomen *qi* and regulates edema. **The "Duck with the Green Head"** [*i.e.*, the male mallard] is the best. **The "Duck with the Pointed Tail"**[101] [common pintail] is next.

[26B] [Illustration Caption:] The Mandarin Duck [*Aix galericulata*][102]

[Illustration Caption:] Tufted Duck [*Aythya fuligula*][103]

---

96 Food Fowl, Eared Fowl: nothing much can be said. The Eared Fowl could be the Eared Pheasant (*Crossoptilon spp*), species of which occur widely in China.

97 See Bernard E. Read, *Chinese Materia Medica:* part VI: *Avian Drugs* (Peiping, 1932), #268.

98 *Ibid.*

99 The illustration shows a Mallard, *Anas platyrhynchos,* now called *yeya* 野鴨, "wild duck," and ancestor of the domestic duck now called *ya* 野.

Ducks in general: the domestic duck of China comes from wild mallard stock, a local domesticate of uncertain age. All Old World domestic ducks may derive from it, or western Eurasia may also have domesticated the mallard. The Muscovy duck is a New World bird domesticated by South American Indians which has spread to China.

100 Today the mallard is called *yeya,* "Wild" or "Steppe Duck," but the illustration here is a common pintail, even called by its Mongolian name.

101 Note Hu Sihui's obvious confusion about the Chinese names of these ducks. Here he uses new descriptions to make his varieties abundantly clear.

102 The illustrations have been switched. The upper, labeled *yuanyang* is a badly drawn tufted duck. Below, labeled *xiji* (tufted duck), is a mandarin duck pair.

103 See Read, 1932: #260.

Mandarin Duck [**Meat**] is salty in flavor, neutral, and has a small amount of poison. It is good for regulating running sores. If a woman is unwilling, a soup is made and eaten privately with her, [the man and the woman] will then fall in love.

Tufted Duck [**Meat**] is sweetish [in flavor], neutral, and lacks poison. It regulates convulsion evil.

[27A] [Illustration Caption:] Pigeon[104]

Pigeon [**Meat**] is salty in flavor, neutral, and lacks poison. It adjusts the essential [air] and augments *qi*. It counteracts the poison of the various drugs.

[Illustration Caption:] Dove

Dove Meat is sweetish in flavor, neutral, and lacks poison. It pacifies the five viscera and augments *qi*. It makes the eye bright and heals tumorous swellings. It clears out pus and blood [in the stool].

[27B] [Illustration Caption:] Great Bustard [*Otis tarda*][105]

Great Bustard [**Meat**] is sweetish in flavor, neutral, and lacks poison. It supplements and augments a person. The meat is coarse but the flavor is fine.

[Illustration Caption:] Collared Crow [*Corvus torquatus*][106]

Collard Crow [**Meat**] is sour–salty in flavor, neutral, and lacks poison. It is good for emaciation illnesses. It controls cough and hectic fever due to *yin* deficiency and emaciation weakness.

[28A] [Illustration Caption:] Common Quail [*Coturnix cotur-*

---

[104] Pigeon (*Columba* spp) and Dove (small *Columbidae* various spp): regarded today as nourishing and strengthening.

[105] Great Bustard: now very rare, but a game bird whose meat is nourishing and strengthening. The high iron content, high digestibility and high protein value of wild bird meats produce effects on health well recognized by villagers and doctors alike.

[106] This bird is still called by this name, that is, "cold crow," or perhaps "crow of cold weather," but the collared crow is not especially tolerant of cold, as crows go. The illustration resembles the similar white–winged magpie *Cissopica whiteheadi* more closely than the collared crow. Perhaps *hanya* referred to both birds.

***nix*]**[107]

Common Quail [Meat] is sweetish in flavor, warming–neutral, and lacks poison. It augments *qi* and supplements the five viscera. It fills out joint and bone and [makes one][108] able to endure cold and heat. It disperses accumulated heat. If eaten fried crisp, it causes one to become fat in the lower burner. It cannot be eaten before the fourth lunar month.

[Illustration Caption:] Sparrows[109]

[28B] Sparrow Meat is sweetish in flavor and lacks poison. It is heating by nature. It strengthens *yang* ways and causes one to have children. Those of the winter months are best.

Bunting[110] [*Emberiza* spp, probably including *E. spodocephala*] **[Meat]** is sweetish in flavor, warming, and lacks poison. If eaten it augments *yang* ways. It is the tastiest small bird meat.

[29A] [Fish]

[Illustration Caption:] Carp [*Cyprinus carpio*][111]

---

107 Eastern Quail: still used commonly as a digestible, highly nutritious strengthening food. Quail eggs are regarded as excellent too.

108 The text is somewhat abbreviated here.

109 Sparrow: the term covers any small bird. Most common and obvious is the Eurasian tree sparrow (*Passer montanus*), which seems to be the bird. It is still used as a medicinal food. Winter birds are best because they fatten for migration and for cold weather, and eat many seeds and grain. In summer they are lean from feeding young, and eat many insects and other foods that make the meat less desirable.

110 Buntings: Still used as indicated here. Very popular as food in south China, but now rare due to overhunting, cultivation of habitat, and the anti–sparrow campaign of the 1950s. This was intended to save grain, but instead it led to an outbreak of the insect pests that sparrows eat. Many species of bunting occur. Few would bother to make terminological distinctions within the genus or between it and closely related genera, though the food quality does lead to a relatively strong sense of sparrows and "buntings" as against other small birds.

111 Carp (*Cyprinus carpio*): is the commonest and most widespread Chinese food fish. This species has been domesticated for thousands of years. Serious fish culture already existed by the end of Zhou and may have arisen in that dynasty, though it could also go back to the Neolithic. The Chinese seem to be the only people to have invented fish cultivation with actual domestication, as opposed to simple pond–rearing. The idea spread from China to the West quite early, along with the carp, although Roman traditions may have combined with those imported from China. Carp

Carp is sweetish in flavor, cooling, and lacks poison. It is good for coughing–bringing up *qi* (asthmatic coughing), and for jaundice. It controls thirst and tranquilizes the womb. It regulates edema and evil foot *qi*. It should not be eaten after a contagious ailment. Those with chronic asthma cannot eat it.

[Illustration Caption:] Golden Carp [*Carassius auratus*][112]

[29B] **Golden Carp** is sweetish in flavor, warming–neutral, and lacks poison. It adjusts the center and augments the five viscera. If eaten as a soup with *Brasenia schreberi* it is good. It is beneficial to eat for those suffering from intestinal wind [producing fresh–bloody stool] and bleeding hemorrhoids complicated by anal fistula.

[Illustration Caption:] Chinese Bream [*Megalobrama terminalis*][113]

Chinese Bream is sweetish [in flavor], warming–neutral, and lacks poison. It supplements and augments much like golden carp. If eaten as a meat hash it helps the spleen and stomach. Should not be given as food to a person who has infantile malnutrition complicated by dysentery.

"White Fish" [possibly *Erythroculter ilishaeformis*] is sweetish in flavor, neutral, and lacks poison. It opens the stomach and brings down food. It removes retention of fluid in the body. If eaten for a long time it causes illness.

---

have been introduced throughout the world and have succeeded too well, driving out the more choice local fish in many areas. They are especially fitted to survive in human–altered waters by their millennia of artificial selection. They are still used as a health–bringing food in China, to say nothing of their symbolic value. Y*u* 魚 means both "fish" and "abundance," and there is the more specific legend that carp which leap up the falls of the Yellow River become dragons. Therefore leaping carp have long symbolized examination candidates, a symbolism no less compelling in today's frantic educational rat–race than in the old days of the Imperial "examination hell."

112 Goldfish: this fish has long been domesticated in China and has spread throughout the world with occasionally unfortunate effect. Koi carp and some other brilliantly colored carp are of the preceding species, but most fancy cultivated carp are of this present one.

113 Bream; white fish: little can be said of north Chinese fish discussed here. Standard current medical works give contemporary beliefs and findings. There has, however, been no in–depth study of the place of these fish in folk culture.

"Yellow Fish"[114] [in south China *Pseudosciaenia crocea*] is sweetish in flavor and has poison. It brings forth wind and moves q*i*. It cannot be eaten with buckwheat flour.

[30A] [Illustration Caption:] "Green Fish" [probably *Mylopharyngodon pictus*][115]

"Green Fish" is sweetish in flavor, neutral, and lacks poison. Southerners make salt fish condiment [out of it]. It cannot be eaten with coriander and wheat soy sauce.

[Illustration Caption:] Sheatfish [*Parasilurus asotus*][116]

Sheatfish is sweetish in flavor, cooling, and has poison. A lot should not be eaten. Sheatfish with red eyes and red whiskers cannot be eaten.

[30B] [Illustration Caption:] Sawfish [*Pristis cuspidatus*][117]

Sawfish is sweetish–salty in flavor, and lacks poison. It is good for chest *qi* demon possession [tuberculosis], worm poison [tympanites due to parasitic infection], and blood spitting.

---

[114] The "yellow fish" here is certainly not *Pseudosciaenia crocea*; the term applies, throughout China, to whatever local fish is yellower than the others.

[115] The "green fish" is certainly some cultivated carp, if not *Mylopharyngodon* then something very close. Several carp, (noble carp, *Aristichthys nobilis*; grass carp, *Ctenopharyngodon idellus;* bighead carp; and this species, the black carp) are domesticated and raised together widely in China. They complement each other, using different resources in the pond, such as grass, algae, or snails.

[116] Sheatfish: this gigantic catfish occurs in North China, but nothing appears in the literature beyond standard medical remedies.

[117] Sawfish: *shayu*, "sand fish," means different things in different parts of China. In the south, for instance, it means any shark. The illustration's identification is probably confirmed by the text here. The sawfish is believed, at least by Chinese fishermen known to ENA, to be the most powerful of all fish. It is very widely regarded as magically potent, and it is often offered in temples. Small ones are hung up, mummifying in the temple. Large ones have their saws cut off and preserved as good luck charms. South Chinese fishermen do not kill it if they can avoid doing so, and usually avoid eating it, believing that disaster can result from so using a supernaturally powerful animal. It is believed throughout China that anything huge and unusual has a great deal of *qi* and possibly a magical or uncanny power. Fish such as the sawfish and sturgeon, huge and strikingly anomalous compared with "normal" fish, are thus revered.

Mud Eel[118] [various genera including *Anguilla*] is sweetish in flavor, neutral, and lacks poison. It is good for arthralgia chiefly caused by wetness–evil. It should not be eaten after a contagious ailment.

Baoyu[119] [primarily abalone, *Haliotis* spp, may include other shellfish] is rancid in flavor and lacks poison. It is good for fractures of the ankle and twisting of the legs due to falls, and blood stasis numbness of the four limbs that will not disperse. It also regulates women's flooding that will not stop.

Puffer[120] [*Fugu* spp] is sweetish in flavor, warming. It is good for supplementing for deficiency. It removes wetness-evil and regulates waist, foot, and hemorrhoid diseases.

Sciaenid Fish[121] [*Pseudosciaena* sp.] is sweetish in flavor and lacks poison. It opens the stomach and augments *qi*. Dried it has a salty taste. It is called *hou* [when dried].

[31A] [Illustration Caption:] *Abarqu* Fish [Siberian Sturgeon, *Huso dauricus*][122]

---

118 Eels: the commonest are *Anguilla* spp, which breed at sea but run up rivers to spend most of their life in muddy marshes and slow waters. They are captured and raised in ponds in enormous quantities. Taiwan has developed a major export market. In Japan the eel is so popular that whole restaurants devote themselves entirely to eel cookery. The Chinese also do a great many things with the rich, meaty flesh of the eel. Many other species of eel, less choice as food, occur in fresh and salt water.

119 Abalone: now an extremely popular and high–priced food, the abalone has been fished to near extinction in China, and huge supplies are imported from the rest of the world. Shellfish of similar texture and flavor, such as the South American conch, *Concholepas concholepas*, are becoming popular substitutes. Slow–growing, abalones are easily fished out of a given area, and have been from most of their range. In England they are so rare that their English name, *ormer*, has been forgotten. The Californian Indian name borrowed via Spanish has become their modern designation. "Abalone" is one of very few words that now survive from a native Californian language. The Chinese name, meaning "wrapped or packaged fish," is apt.

120 Puffer: the Chinese do not make a macho cult of eating the puffer whose liver contains tetrodotoxin, one of the most potent poisons. South Chinese fishermen report that the puffer tastes very unspecial, being coarse and poorly flavored. We take this on faith. Japanese love of puffers appears to be due to the romance and risk involved.

121 Sciaenid Fish: this could be almost any fish. A large variety of sciaenid and other fast oceanic fish occurs off China. It is doubtful whether the writers of the *YSZY* familiar with Inner China knew what fish occurred off the coasts.

122 Sturgeon: another fish believed to have supernatural powers, the sturgeon is regarded as a kind of dragon because of its anatomy and barbels. These resemble the

Siberian Sturgeon is sweetish in flavor, neutral, and lacks poison. It benefits the five viscera and makes a person fat and beautiful. If a lot is eaten it will be difficult to undergo transformation.

[Siberian Sturgeon] Fat is yellow.

The Meat is coarse and lacks scales. For bones it only has cartilage.

[Siberian Sturgeon] Bladder can be made into a thick glue. It is very sticky. If the glue is made into a tincture and taken it disperses and overcomes common cold.

The largest Siberian Sturgeon are 1–2 *chang* long. (One name is *xinyu*, another name is *zhanyu*.)[123] It lives in the oceans and rivers north and east of Liaoyang.

[31B][Illustration Caption] *Qilam* Fish [Chinese Sturgeon, *Acipenser sinensis*]

Chinese Sturgeon is sweetish in flavor, neutral, and lacks poison. It benefits the viscera. It makes a person fat and beautiful.

[Chinese Sturgeon] Fat is yellow.

The Meat is somewhat coarse.

[Chinese Sturgeon] Bladder can be made into a glue.

The largest Chinese Sturgeons are 5–6 *chi* long. They live in the oceans and rivers north and east of Liaoyang.

[32A] [Illustration Caption:] Softshelled Turtle [*Amyda sinensis*]

Softshelled Turtle Meat is sweetish in flavor, neutral, and lacks poison. It brings down *qi*. It expels impairment heat within bone and joint, and congestion and obstruction.

---

tendrils about the face of Chinese dragons in art. The accounts of sturgeons in the *YSZY* are realistic and accurate. Size, cartilaginous bones, bladder glue, and habitat, *etc.*, are covered as thoroughly as in many modern ichthyology texts.

[123] B. E. Read, Chinese *Materia Medica,* part IX, *Scaly and Scaleless Fish* (Peiping, 1939), 66ff, says that the names *xin* and *zhan* here given as applying to the Siberian sturgeon actually are names for the Chinese sturgeon.

[Illustration Caption:] Crab [usually *Eriocheir sinensis*][124]

Crab is salty in flavor and has poison. It is good for heat–evil congestion pain in the thorax. It makes stomach *qi* pass through and adjusts the chief blood vessels.

[32B] [Illustration Caption:] Shrimp[125]

The **Shrimp** is sweetish in flavor and has poison. If too much is eaten it harms a person. Shrimp without whiskers should not be eaten.

Sea Snail is sweetish in flavor, very cooling, and lacks poison. It regulates liver *qi* heat. It controls thirst and counteracts liquor poison.

Trough Shells [including *Mactra quadrangularis*] are sweetish in flavor, very cooling, and lack poison. They make the five viscera moist. They control thirst and settle the stomach. They counteract liquor poison.

Wei [unidentified][126] are bitter in flavor, neutral, and lack poison. They order stomach *qi* and make ample the lower burner.

Fresh Water Mussels are chilling and lack poison. They brighten the eye and control diabetes. They expel irritation and counteract intense evil heat.

The Prickly Sculpin [*Lateolabrax japonicus*] is neutral. It supplements the five viscera, augments joint and bone, harmonizes the abdomen, and regulates retention of fluid in the body. It benefits a per-

---

[124] Crabs: many species, varieties and conditions of crabs occur in China, each with its own medical value.

[125] Shrimp: shrimp are today believed to be heating and wetting to the body, and the idea that too many are harmful persists. They are said to exacerbate venereal disease. Among fishermen, this leads to ribald teasing if anyone passes up the shrimps at dinner. One reason is that shrimps and other shellfish can produce dramatic allergic reactions. The reactions are not to the shrimp but to tiny food organisms they have consumed. In his experiences eating Chinese *crustacea*, ENA once turned a brilliant red for a few hours, and occasionally developed huge but transient welts and skin eruptions. Itchiness is also recognized. In Malay folk medicine, "itchiness" occupies a place similar to "poison" in Chinese medical literature. It refers focally to allergic reactions. See Carol Laderman, *Wives and Midwives*, Berkeley: 1984).

The other water animals in this chapter are too poorly identified to comment on.

[126] This normally means hedgehog (see Li in Hu Sihui, 1988: 346), but not here.

son to eat it.

[33A] [Fruits]

[Illustration Caption:] Peach [*Prunus persica*]

The **Peach** is acrid-sweet in flavor and lacks poison. It benefits lung *qi* and controls coughing bringing up *qi* (asthmatic coughing). It disperses hard accumulation of the upper abdomen, expels sudden severe throbbing [palpitation] of the blood, and destroys obstructions of the bowels. It causes the menses to pass and controls pain.

Peach Kernel: It controls chest pain.[127]

[Illustration Caption:] Chinese Pear [*Pyrus* spp]

[33B] **Chinese Pears**[128] are sweetish in flavor, cooling, and lack poison. They are good for heat–type cough, control thirst and dissipate wind. They benefit the urine. If too many are eaten they [result in] cold–evil [damage to] the center.

[Illustration Caption:] Persimmon [*Diospyros kaki*][129]

Persimmons are sweetish in flavor, cooling, and lack poison. They cause ear and nose *qi* to pass, and supplement for *xulao*, bloody stool insufficiency. They make the stomach ample.

[Illustration Caption:] Chinese Quince [*Chaenomeles cathayensis*]

[34A] **Chinese Quinces** are sour in flavor, warming, and lack poison. They cure arthralgia evil *qi*, and *huoluan* vomiting and spasms which cannot be controlled.

[Illustration Caption:] Oriental Flowering Apricot

Oriental Flowering Apricot Fruits [*Prunus mume*] are sour in flavor, neutral, and lack poison. They are good for bringing down *qi*.

---

[127] Ou, 1982: "1. precordial pain; 2. epigastric pain" (46).

[128] Chinese Pears: Several species of pears occur in China including *Pyrus serrulata* and *P. betulaefolia*. All have similar fruits, round and crisp like a Western apple rather than like a Western pear. They are still regarded as cooling and very good for hot coughs, sore throats, and thirst. Pear syrup is commonly used for this purpose.

[129] Persimmon: gathered wild in earliest Neolithic times, persimmons must have been domesticated early. They are a common food, fresh or dried and often painted.

They expel fever accompanied by restlessness, tranquilize the heart, and control diarrhea. They stop thirst.

[Illustration Caption:] Japanese Plum [*Prunus salicina*][130]

[34B] **Japanese Plums** are bitter in flavor, neutral, and lack poison. They are good for sudden syncope, blood stasis, and bone pain. They expel obstinate heat–evil and adjust the center.

[Illustration Caption:] Prinsepia [*Prinsepia uniflora*][131]

Prinsepia Fruits are bitter in flavor and cooling. If a lot are eaten they make a person [have] abdominal distension. Sick persons should not eat them.

[Illustration Caption:] Pomegranate [*Punica granatum*]

[35A] **Pomegranates** are sweet–sour in flavor and lack poison. They are good for throat thirst. Too much should not be eaten. They harm the lungs. They control leaking essence.

[Illustration Caption:] Crab Apple [*Malus* sp][132]

Crab Apples are sweetish–sour in flavor and warming. Too much cannot be eaten. They will give rise to evil heat and astringent *qi*. They make a person sleep well.

[Illustration Caption:] Apricot

[35B] **Apricots** are sour in flavor. Too much should not be eaten. They wound joint and bone.

> **Apricot Kernels** have poison. They are good for coughing bringing up *qi* (asthmatic coughing).

[Illustration Caption:] Mandarin Orange[133]

---

[130] Note that the "Japanese Plum" is also the popular English name for *P. japonica*.

[131] Prinsepia: this small berry is a minor food. Among the many medicinal recipes provided by Hu Shiu-ying (2005) is one for this fruit (Hu 2005:230).

[132] In China *linqin* would be *Malus* (= *Pyrus*) *asiatica*. In the *YSZY* this Chinese name could refer to the Mongolian crab apple *ürel* (*Malus pallasiana*). It has been a popular Mongolian gathered fruit in recent times and was likely so in the past. The illustration could be almost any crab apple species.

[133] King Orange or Mandarin Orange: "*Citrus chachiensis*," is a stabilized hybrid of *C. reticulata* and *C. sinensis*. The *gan* or "king orange" is a hybrid or likely a cluster

Mandarin Oranges are sweetish in flavor and cooling. They remove bowel heat, benefit the urine and control thirst. If a lot are eaten they produce obstinate diseases.

[Illustration Caption:] Tangerine [*Citrus reticulata* and other *C.* spp as local substitutions][134]

[36A] **Tangerines** are sweetish–sour in flavor and lack poison. They are warming. They control vomiting and bring down *qi*. They benefit the water ways. They remove accumulation heat of the thorax.

[Illustration Caption:] Sweet Orange [*Citrus sinensis*][135]

---

of similar hybrids of ancient origin. The best progeny of the two parents have been selected. The finest of these are regarded as the choicest of all citrus by Chinese and the best come from south Taiwan and the facing coast of Fujian. They have not flourished elsewhere. The fruit is delicate, particularly the best varieties and does not ship well. One must go to the areas where they are grown to find good "king oranges."

[134] Tangerine, "Mandarin orange" (*Citrus reticulata*): Often called "Mandarin orange" like the king orange, the term is loosely used for this species and its hybrids. "Tangerine" correctly refers to the small, bright red–orange, very sweet varieties familiar in the West, but can be loosely used for the species. It includes a variety of useful forms, some large and sweet, some small and sour, some green when ripe, *etc.* Most have been elaborated as different "species," causing taxonomic confusion.

True tangerines (and similar variants) are colloquially called *jie* 桔, etymologically "lucky fruit," and are regarded as necessary adornments at New Year to assure luck for the coming year. There is evidence that citrus fruits were sacred or ritually important to the pre–Chinese ethnic groups of south China and the intense reddish color of tangerines makes them auspicious. They have been regarded as noble, worthy, fortunate fruits since at least the time of the *Chuci* 楚詞 which contains a song comparing a handsome young man to a tree of this species, mistranslated "orange" by Hawkes. See David Hawkes, *Chu Tz'u, the Songs of the South* (Oxford, 1959). ENA has heard a folk version of this song sung by fishermen in Hong Kong, and indeed the tree is well established in song, folklore and art. They are often part of temple offerings.

[135] Orange: this is the true orange native to Southern China. It is much less important in Chinese culture than tangerine, but is still an important plant used in offerings of all kinds as well as for food. Many oranges are now imported to east Asia from areas around the world with Mediterranean climates. The plant seems to do better there than in its native home. Oranges also acclimatized so well to Florida that they went wild, and became a common forest tree there by the nineteenth century. They are not a common tree in Chinese orchards, partly because all their native pests are there. Pests of citrus were controlled in Medieval China by introducing ants to the orchards. The ants ate the scale and other insects, in what may be the earliest known biological control of insects by insects. See Needham, Lu and Huang, 1986: 519ff. Oranges are believed cooling by most people today, and eaten as a cooling food.

Sweet Oranges are sweet–sour in flavor and lack poison. They remove nausea. If a lot are eaten they injure liver *qi*.

The Peel [of the Sweet Orange] is aromatic and delicate.

[Illustration Caption:] Chestnut [*Castanea mollissima*][136]

[36B] **Chestnuts** are salty in flavor, warming, and lack poison. They are good for augmenting *qi*. They fill up the bowels and supplement for asthenia of the kidney. If eaten roasted they obstruct a person's *qi*.

[Illustration Caption:] Jujube [*Zizyphus jujuba*][137]

Jujubes are sweetish in flavor and lack poison. They are good for evil *qi* of chest and abdomen. They tranquilize the center and nourish the spleen. They aid the chief blood vessels and give rise to bodily fluids.

[Illustration Caption:] Cherry [*Prunus pseudocerasus*]

[37A] **Cherries** are sweetish in flavor. They are good for adjusting the center and augmenting spleen *qi*. They make one have a nice complexion. Persons [suffering from] concealed wind[138] should avoid eating them.

[Illustration Caption:] Grapes

Grapes are sweetish in flavor and lack poison. They are good for arthralgia of joint and bone, augment *qi* and strengthen the will. They cause a person to be fat and solid.

[Illustration Caption:] Walnut ["Iranian Peach," *Juglans regia*]

[37B] **Walnuts** are sweetish in flavor and lack poison. If one eats them they cause a person to be fat and solid. They moisten the flesh and make the hair black [again]. If at lot are eaten they move wind.[139]

---

[136] Chestnuts: the oriental chestnut must have once been very common in North and East China to judge from comparison with relatives elsewhere. It is now a rather uncommon tree, almost exclusively cultivated. Its nuts are very similar to those of other chestnuts. They are roasted and are known as a rich, high–calorie food.

[137] Hu Shiu-ying identifies this as Hog plum, *Choerospondias axillaris*, for south China, but acknowledges that the term refers to the Jujube in the North. See Jiang, 2004, 176.

[138] This disease complex is uncertain.

[139] Due to the appearance of the walnut, Chinese often regard it as good for the brain.

[Illustration Caption:] Pine Nuts [various *Pinus* spp, mostly *P. koraiensis* but also including *P. massoniana* and possibly the Mongolian *P. sibirica*]

Pine Nuts are sweetish in flavor, warming, and lack poison. They treat dizziness due to various wind–evils. They disperse retention of fluid in the body, moisten the five viscera, and lengthen the years.

[Illustration Caption:] Lotus Seeds [*Nelumbo nucifera*]

[**38A**] **Lotus Seeds** are sweetish in flavor, neutral, and lack poison. They supplement the center, nourish the spirit, and augment *qi*. They eliminate the hundred illnesses. They make the body light and [make it] unaging.

[Illustration Caption:] *Euryale ferox*

***Euryale ferox* fruits** are sweetish in flavor, neutral, and lack poison. They are good for arthralgia and pain of waist and knee. They supplement the center and eliminate disease. They augment the essential *qi*.

[Illustration Caption:] *Trapa bispinosa*

[**38B**] ***Trapa bispinosa* fruits** are sweetish in flavor, neutral, and lack poison. They are good for pacifying the center and augmenting the five viscera. They lighten the body and [make one] unsuffering from hunger.

[Illustration Caption:] Lichee [*Litchi chinensis*]

Lichee Fruits are sweetish in flavor, neutral, and lack poison. They stop thirst and produce juices. They increase a person's facial glow.

[Illustration Caption:] Longan [*Dimocarpus longan*]

[**39A**] **Longans** are sweetish in flavor, neutral, and lack poison. They are good for evil *qi* of the five viscera. They pacify the will and dislike of food. They eliminate vermin and remove poison.

[Illustration Caption:] Ginkgo [*Ginkgo biloba*][140]

---

140 Ginkgo: this unique tree, a "living fossil," yields a very interesting fruit–like structure: a large kernel enclosed in a whitish shell surrounded by a soft arillous mem-

Ginkgo [Nuts] are sweetish–bitter in flavor and lack poison. They can be eaten roasted or boiled. If eaten green they cause illness.

[Illustration Caption:] Chinese Olive [*Canarium album*; not related to the European olive][141]

[39B] **Chinese olives** are sour–sweetish in flavor, warming, and lack poison. They are good for dissipating liquor and opening the stomach. They bring down *qi* and control thirst.

[Illustration Caption:] Chinese Myrica [*Myrica rubra*][142]

Chinese Myrica [Fruits] are sour–sweetish in flavor, warming, and

---

brane. This is different in origin from the true fruits of flowering plants, the ginkgo being close to the conifers. The soft structure rots producing a powerful odor of rancid butter, and this does not endear fruit–bearing trees to the average gardener. Fortunately the tree is dioecious and only male trees are grown for ornament. The females have to be grown for the nut. Those raising them in orchards must either gather and clean them fast or bear the scent of butyrate. The kernels are nutritious and pleasantly flavored but too bitter for ordinary eating. They are used as a health food, especially against sore throat. The bitter principle dries up the mucous membranes very effectively. Stands selling gingko nuts, acorns and chestnuts, and quail eggs roasted in hot coals are traditional features of winter life in East Asia. The English "Ginkgo" is a corruption of the Japanese pronunciation of Chinese *yinguo* 銀果, "silver nut," a rarer alternative name to the usual *Boguo* 白果, "white nut."

[141] Chinese Olive: the *ganlan* is a gigantic tropical tree that does not in any way resemble the olive although its fruit does, since it is usually salt–cured and resembles a Greek olive. The tree is mainly Southeast Asian but extends north to Fujian and Taiwan. It is common in Guangdong making an excellent shade tree that flourishes in village conditions. The fruit is astringent and locally used in medicine. The seed looks exactly like an olive pit, but differs in having a large and edible kernel. Between an almond and a pumpkin kernel in appearance and flavor, this nut is far more important as a food than the fruit, particularly southward from China. The "*Canarium* almond" is almost a staple food in parts of Indonesia and Oceania. It is much used in confectionery. The Cantonese use it in many dishes, stir–frying it with strips of meat, *etc.* These dishes are among the very finest in Cantonese cuisine but difficult to get outside their homeland for the nut does not ship well.

The description in the *YSZY* applies only to the fruit. It could be written today.

[142] Chinese Myrica, *yangmei*, "yang–flowering–apricot:" The "Yang" refers to the fruit's red color. It may also refer to the warm–weather habitat and fruiting season of the plant.

This wax–myrtle produces a reddish grainy fruit that has been called the "Chinese strawberry." This has led to some mistranslations. True strawberries are *caomei* 草莓, "herb–[grown] flowering–apricots." Chinese myrica is known from Han tomb finds. It is native to central and southern China in hilly areas. The fruit is common today as a dried confection, often candied or honey–cured.

lack poison. They are good for removing phlegm and controlling vomiting. They dissipate food and make liquor go down.

[Illustration Caption:] Hazelnuts [*Corylus heterophylla*][143]

[40A] **Hazelnuts** are sweetish in flavor, neutral, and lack poison. They augment *qi* force and extend the bowels. They firm the gait and make one tolerant of hunger.

[Illustration Caption:] Torreya Nut [*Torreya grandis*][144]

Torreya Nuts are sweetish in flavor and lack poison. They are good for the five hemorrhoids and remove the three vermin, worm poison, and demon possession.[145]

[Illustration Caption:] Cane Sugar[146]

[40B] **Cane Sugar** is sweetish in flavor, cooling, and lacks poison. It is good for gas due to evil–heat of chest and abdomen. It controls thirst and brightens the eye. (Sugar cane juice is decocted to make cane sugar.)

[Illustration Caption:] The Sweet Melon [*Cucumis melo*][147]

Sweet Melon is sweetish in flavor, cooling, and has poison. It controls thirst and expels irritation heat. If a lot is eaten it produces chill illnesses and destroys the abdomen.

---

143 Hazelnut: a minor cultivated crop in Northern and Central China.

144 Torreya nuts: these are bitter like ginkgo nuts so they are used for sore throat and the similar ailments. They are a good deal more bitter than ginkgo and are strictly a medicine, although children do occasionally eat them for what seems to be pure pleasure. The illustration in our copy of the *YSZY* is notably inaccurate here, in sharp contrast to the good ones around it. It shows a broadleafed tree but the torreya is a kind of yew. Perhaps the illustration is of some other species from which nuts were gathered by the Mongols.

145 See the discussions of these syndromes by Li (Hu Sihui, 1988: 378).

146 Granulated Sugar: the picture shows the sugarcane but the name "sand sugar" applies only to the granulated product, brown or white. Sugarcane is *zhe* 蔗. The product is now considered heating particularly when raw. By contrast rock sugar is called "ice sugar" and considered cooling as are the cane and cane juice.

147 Sweet Melon: the native Chinese variety of melon is not sweet, so this name is used for the west Asian varieties. Xinjiang produces the best of these, but they are widely grown in the North.

[Illustration Caption:] Watermelon [*Citrullus lanatus*][148]

[41A] **Watermelon** is sweetish in flavor, neutral, and lacks poison. It is good for diabetes. It regulates heart vexation and dissipates liquor poison.

[Illustration Caption:] The Sour Jujube [*Zizyphus jujuba var. spinosa*][149]

Sour Jujubes are sour–sweetish in flavor, neutral, and lack poison. They are good for cold and heat[150] of chest and abdomen, evil stagnation, and *qi* accumulation. They remove irritation.

[Illustration Caption:] Flowering Apricot Red [*Malus micromalus*][151]

[41B] **Flowering apricot Red** [**Fruits**] are sour-sweetish in flavor, neutral, and lack poison. They regulate leaking dysentery.

[Illustration Caption:] The Citron

Citrons are sour-sweetish in flavor, neutral, and lack poison. They bring down *qi* and open the diaphragm.

[Illustration Caption:] Acorns [acorns of *Castanopsis sclerophylla* and *Quercus* spp including *Q. myrsinaefolia*][152]

[42A] **Acorns** are sour-sweetish in flavor, neutral, and lack poison. They are slightly cooling by nature. Too much should not be eaten.

[Illustration Caption:] *Pingpo* [*Malus* sp, probably *M. pumila*][153]

---

[148] Watermelon: this African melon was known by the eleventh century in China. It is now considered cooling, due to a high water content and diuretic qualities. Watermelon has substantial potassium, which balances out the salt so common in many Chinese diets. Today it is possibly the commonest and almost certainly the most popular fruit in North China. It is less common but still greatly appreciated in the South. Seed kernels are a favorite food and varieties with thin seed–husks are grown. Some have huge seeds and almost no sweet flesh, being just rinds full of seeds.

[149] Sour Jujube: this is the wild form with small fruits. See under Chinese jujube.

[150] Our "chills and heat" (Ou, 1982: 225).

[151] "Sea red" crabapples: A common fruit, often dried or sugar–cured.

[152] Acorns: see under the earlier entry.

[153] Apple: an odd name since the usual term is *pingguo* 苹果 with a different character for *ping* than here. Cooling and very popular as a snack fruit and offering today. Western apples (*Malus malus*) are imported in quantity.

Pingpo are sweetish in flavor and lack poison. They control thirst and produce juices. If put into a clothing box the aroma will be marvelous.

[Illustration Caption:] ***Badam*** **Nut [almond,** ***Prunus amygdalus*****]**[154]

[**42B**] **Almonds** are sweetish in flavor and lack poison. They control coughing and bring down *qi*. They disperse impeded pressing of chest and abdomen. (This fruit comes from Muslim fields.)

[Illustration Caption:] ***Pistä*****, [*****Pistacia vera*****]**[155]

Pistä are sweetish in flavor and lack poison. They adjust the center and accord *qi*. (This fruit comes from Muslim fields.)

[43A] Vegetables

[Illustration Caption:] Mallow [***Malva verticillata*** **and other** ***M.*** **spp including** ***M. parvifolia*** **]**[156]

Mallow [**Leaves**] are sweetish in flavor, cooling–neutral, and lack poison. Mallow is the best of the hundred vegetables. It regulates the cold and heat of the five viscera and six organs, emaciation, and the five kinds of dysuria. They benefit the urine and heal the milk difficulty of women.

[Illustration Caption:] Swiss Chard [greens of a ***Beta vulgaris*** **variety]**[157]

---

[154] Almond: mainly an import since China is not good almond country. They are rare. The *YSZY*'s Central Asian interest is shown by its even including this and the pistachio.

[155] Pistachio: China has a native species of pistachio but it bears a worthless nut. The West Asian species is known only as a rare import.

[156] Mallow: Mallow is put first here because it was the main vegetable in ancient China. It was so important that it became a trope for ordinary peasant fare. Snobbish attitudes and the development of superior varieties of cabbages and other greens displaced it, and it has sunk to the lowly status of weed. It is one of the most nutritious foods ever tested. The leaves are rich in just about everything, hence the high praise for mallow here. It is still gathered wild and used as a vegetable in China and much of the rest of Asia.

[157] The *CYDCD* calls *manjing Vitex rotundifolia* or *Vitex trifolia*. The illustration, however, shows neither species, and a plant that is clearly not even a *V. sp.* Ascribed properties below also do not suit a *V. sp* identification. This plant is perhaps a Mongolian gathered food but a more likely identification, in view of recipe use and a dominant Islamic presence in the *YSZY* is, as indicated above, Swiss chard or silver beet,

[43B] Swiss Chard is bitter in flavor, warming, and lacks poison. It is food for the five viscera. It lightens the body and augments *qi.*

Swiss Chard seeds brighten the eye.

[Illustration Caption:] Chinese Parsley [coriander][158]

Chinese Parsley is acrid in flavor, warming, and slightly poisonous. It disperses grain and supplements insufficiency of the five viscera. It makes pass and benefits the urine. (Another name is "Iranian coriander.")."

[Illustration Caption:] Mustard [*Brassica juncea*][159]

[44A] Mustard [Greens] are acrid in flavor, warming, and lack poison. They are good for expelling evil kidney *qi*. They benefit the nine apertures, brighten the eye, and tranquilize the center.

[Illustration Caption:] Chinese Onions [*Allium fistulosum or A. cepa*][160]

---

one of the most important vegetables in current Middle Eastern cuisine and apparently so in the past as well. The illustration, in any case, clearly shows a member of *Chenopodiaceae* and would support such an identification.

[158] Coriander: cooling in modern medicine, though some people think of it as heating because of its spicy flavor. The leaves are highly nutritious, being rich in vitamins, minerals, and protein. They are the most popular herb or herbal garnish in Chinese cooking and one of the few plants widely used in China that can be called a herb in the culinary sense. The intense flavor is either loved or hated. Few people can be neutral about it. The plant is a Medieval introduction to China from West Asia so it is more common in north and west Chinese cuisine than in south and east. Charles Perry notes in an unpublished letter of 2 January, 1994, to PDB that coriander is the only spice considered cooling in the tenth century *Kitab al–Tabikh.* He continues: "in the Perso–Arab tradition, all spices but coriander are heating."

[159] Chinese Mustard: standard greens crop and oilseed, Chinese mustard is one of the most popular vegetables in China. Greens are often considered cooling, but some varieties at least are spicy enough to qualify as warm, and the oil and seeds certainly are. This plant is a different species from any of the European/American mustard and mustard–greens sources.

[160] Chinese Onions: The native Chinese onion is known in English as "Welsh onion," from Germanic *welsch,* "foreign," or as "bunching onion" from its growth habit, many stalks in a bunch from one seed. It is the usual source of scallions (young green onions) in American stores, as well as throughout East Asia. It is the most widely used vegetable in China. Mongols incidentally, use a number of wild onions as gathered foods including *Allium prostratum* and *A. senescens*, both called *mangir* in Mongolian, *A. altaicum*, which claims the generic Mongolian *songino*, "onion," *A.*

Chinese Onions are acrid in flavor, warm, and lack poison. They are good for brightening the eye and supplementing insufficiency. They regulate exogenous febrile diseases, produce sweat and remove swelling.

[Illustration Caption:] Garlic[161]

[44B] Garlic is acrid in flavor, warming, and lacks poison. It is good for dissipating tumorous swellings, expels wind evil and destroys poison *qi*.

Garlic with a single clove is best.

[Illustration Caption:] Chinese Chives [*Allium tuberosum*]

Chinese Chives are acrid in flavor, warming, and lack poison. They tranquilize the five viscera, expel stomach heat, bring down *qi* and supplement for deficiency. They can be eaten for a long time.

[Illustration Caption:] Winter Melon[162]

[45A] Winter Melon is sweetish in flavor, neutral and slightly cooling, and lacks poison. It is good for augmenting *qi*. It promotes a glossy complexion and preserves a youthful appearance. It prevents one from suffering from hunger.

[Illustration Caption:] Cucumbers[163]

---

victorialis, Mongolian *xaliar*, *A. mongolicum*, *xömöl*, and *A. anisopodium* and *A. Fischer*, both called *shubuun xöl*. See also dialectical forms given in Rinchen, 1979.

[161] Garlic: an ancient introduction from West Asia universally popular, especially in the north and west. "Garlic with a single clove," the large–rooted elephant types, is still preferred by many. It is believed to be healthful, but the many virtues ascribed to it in the West and by some Japanese remain unknown in China.

[162] Winter melon: is the ripe form of the fuzzy gourd or hair gourd although as with pumpkins, somewhat different strains of seed are used for the different purposes. It is now usually believed to be markedly cooling, and is a popular cooling remedy. Since it is one of the lowest–calorie foods in the world, it most certainly does not prevent one from suffering hunger. The *YSZY* is not usually so far off in its more down–to–earth directives of this sort. An ancient native Chinese cultigen, it is widely grown. Soup is often made in a winter melon with seeds removed and the melon held in a pot to steam. The melon imparts its slight, spicy flavor to this "winter melon pond."

[163] Cucumber: the belief in the cold nature of the cucumber extends to the West, whence the expression "cool as a cucumber." The plant is a standard summer food in China counteracting heat and supplying water.

Cucumbers are sweetish in flavor, neutral and cooling, and have poison. They move *qi* and bring forth illnesses. They make a person have asthenic fever. Too much should not be eaten.

[Illustration Caption:] The Chinese Radish [*Raphanus sativus*]

[**45B**] **The Chinese Radish** is sweetish in flavor, warm, and lacks poison. It is good for bringing down *qi* and disperses grain. It moves accumulation of phlegm in the hypochondriac region and regulates thirst. It is poisonous if made into a dough [or noodles].

[Illustration Caption:] Carrot ["Iranian Radish," *Daucus carota var sativa*][164]

Carrots are sweetish in flavor, neutral, and lack poison. They are good for bringing down *qi*. They adjust and benefit the bowels.

[Illustration Caption:] *Tianjing* Vegetable [*Sonchus sp,* probably *S. brachyotus*][165]

[**46A**] ***Tianjing* Vegetable** is bitter in flavor, neutral, and lacks poison. It expels facial jaundice, strengthens the will and clarifies the spirit. It benefits the five viscera. (Same as *ye kumai* [*Sonchus sp.*]).

[Illustration Caption:] Long Bottle Gourd [*Lagenaria siceraria var. clavata*][166]

---

[164] Carrot: now considered cooling. Used as an eye remedy, long before knowledge of vitamin A came from the West. Carrot soup is a standard cooling medicine in Chinese villages. Being easily grown and stored, carrots are available in any reasonably well–stocked market, providing a cheap and readily bought source of medication.

[165] *Tianjing* Vegetable: There is a *tianjing* cabbage, a variety of the standard Chinese cabbage. This is not what is illustrated and the ascribed properties are not those associated with any variety of Chinese cabbage. The illustration is unclear and could show any one of a number of closely related species. Kököluu (Hu Sihui, 1982: 301) calls this vegetable dandelion greens (*Taraxacum sp*) but this contradicts the textual note which identifies *tianjing* vegetable with a *Sonchus* sp, although probably not the *S. arvensis* that is usually called *ye kumai.* The confusion with the dandelion is understandable since the plants are very similar and often lumped under one generic term. In Mongolia the species would probably be *S. brachyotus*. *Sonchus* (sow thistle) is a bitter relative of lettuce. In addition to being a Mongolian gathered plant food and probably medicinal, it was once cultivated in China but is now a weed there.

[166] Bottle Gourds: cooling and not very popular as food. They are coarse and tasteless, and as a food (used by the poor in soup) are mainly a by–product of their more worthwhile use for containers.

Long Bottle Gourds are bitter in flavor, cooling, and have poison. They are good for water issuing edema of the four limbs and face. If a lot is eaten it causes one to vomit.

[Illustration Caption:] Oriental Pickling Melon [*Cucumis melo* var. *conomon*][167]

[46B] Oriental Pickling Melons are sweetish in flavor, cooling, and lack poison. They benefit the bowels and control polydipsia. Too much cannot be eaten. (Same as *shaogua.*)

[Illustration Caption:] Pear-Shaped Bottle Gourd [*Lagenaria siceraria* var. *depressa*]

Pear-Shaped Bottle Gourds are sweetish in flavor, neutral, and lack poison. They are good for dispersing edema and augment *qi.*

[Illustration Caption:] **Möög* Mushrooms [*Tricholoma mongolicum*][168]

[47A] **Möög* Mushrooms are sweetish in flavor, cooling, and have poison. They move *qi* and produce illnesses. Too much should not be eaten.

***Junzi* [Fungi, *Agaricus spp*, probably including *A. arvensis, A. campestris* and *A. bisporus*]:**[169]

---

[167] Oriental pickling melon or conomon melon: the native Chinese race of the common melon. They are not sweet.

[168] Today *mogu* is usually *Agaricus campestris*, the common field mushroom, closely related to the Western domestic mushroom (*A. bisporus*), clearly not what is illustrated. Wasson (Wasson, 1968: 170–1), notes that the term *mogu* is also applied to *Tricholoma mongolicum* in north China. This species is found in Mongolia and is apparently what the artist is attempting to illustrate. Judging from the occurrence of related words throughout Mongolia and Siberia *mogu*, Mongolian *möög*, is a loan word in Chinese. Since it first appears in the *bencao* literature in Yuan times along with the mushroom it is associated with, Chinese *mogu* was probably borrowed directly from the Mongolian rather than from any Siberian language. The *YSZY*'s comments about illness and overeating suggest that some slightly poisonous mushrooms were apt to be mistakenly gathered along with this one.

[169] *Junzi* Fungi: The illustration is too stylized to be of help and the description could refer to any of several poisonous varieties. Many do indeed "cause one to be confused and depressed" as a reaction to the toxins. While the illustration could be *A. campestris*, known in Mongolia as *cagaan möög*, "white fungus," assigned properties

Junzi [Fungi] are bitter in flavor, cooling, and have poison. The give rise to wind of the viscera, press *qi*, and move the blood vessels and hemorrhoids. They cause one to be confused and stupefied.

[Illustration Caption:] Tree Ears [*Auricularia auricula-judae*][170]

[**47B**] **Tree Ears** are bitter in flavor, cooling, and have poison. They benefit the five viscera, drain the bowels, and press poison *qi*. Too much should not be eaten.

[Illustration Caption:] Bamboo Shoots[171]

Bamboo Shoots are sweetish in flavor and lack poison. They are good for diabetes, benefit the water ways and increase *qi*. If too many are eaten they produce illness.

[Illustration Caption:] Cattail Shoots [*Typha* spp][172]

[**48A**] **Cattail Shoots** are sweetish in flavor and lack poison. They supplement the center and increase *qi*. They enliven the blood vessels.

[Illustration Caption:] Sacred Lotus Rhizome [*Nelumbo nucifera*][173]

---

do not suggest this fungus. The similar *A. arvensis*, *xara möög*, is also eaten by the Mongols as apparently are some other *A.* spp. This fungus could be any of them.

[170] Now regarded as very valuable, healthful, nourishing and strengthening, and eaten in large quantities, usually stewed in complex stews and soups. There is a whole complex of health–promoting tree fungi in modern Chinese diet therapy. Most of the others are of the genus *Tremella*.

[171] Bamboo shoots: now regarded as one of the most cooling foods. They are very low in calories and high in fiber, as is true of many foods held to be cooling. They are usually from species in the genera *Sinocalamus* (large shoots) and *Bambusa* (small thin shoots), but other genera sometimes contribute. They are a traditional mountain product, much used in the cuisines of the more mountainous parts of China.

[172] Cattail shoots: are excellent eating. The outer leaves are stripped off young shoots just emerging above the mud or shallow water and the tender inner leaf and stalk eaten. They greatly resemble cucumber in taste. Other reedy marsh plants can be similarly used, but are less tasty.

[173] Lotus Rhizomes: the rhizomes are the "lotus roots" of food stores. They are not roots, but the stems of the plant which run along the bottom of the water. The actual roots, fibrous and inedible, grow down from them at the nodes. The stems have hollow cavities within. They also contain a mucilage that forms threads when the stems are broken and pulled apart. This leads to their being a traditional dish at weddings. Someone is sure to break a rhizome and hold it up for all to see, saying something like "no matter how much the world tries to pull these two apart, they will always stick to-

Sacred Lotus Rhizomes are sweetish in flavor, neutral, and lack poison. They are good for supplementing the center. They nourish the spirit and increase *qi*. They expel illness, disperse heat thirst, and separate the blood.

[Illustration Caption:] Chinese Yam

[48B] **Chinese Yams** are sweetish in flavor, warming, and lack poison. They supplement the center and increase *qi*. They regulate dizziness due to wind–evil and control waist pain. They strengthen sinew and bone.

[Illustration Caption:] Taro [*Colocasia esculenta*][174]

Taro is acrid in flavor, neutral and has poison. It extends the bowels and fills up flesh. It lubricates the center. **Wild Taro** [*Colocasia antiquorum*] cannot be eaten.

[Illustration Caption:] Lettuce [*Lactuca sativa*][175]

[49A] **Lettuce** is bitter in flavor, chilling, and lacks poison. It is good for benefiting the five viscera. It opens the diaphragm, presses *qi*, and makes the blood vessels pass [blood].

[Illustration Caption:] Bokchoy [*Brassica campestris var olei-*

gether!" The lotus is also a religious symbol. Its fruit looks like a womb, the seeds are numerous, and the words for "lotus seeds" sounds like "abundant sons," so the whole plant is good for weddings and other festivities. The rhizome produces a starch with extremely fine grains, the quality starch in Chinese cooking before cornstarch came in. The latter makes the food too gooey and heavily thick for connoisseurs' tastes, and the more delicate effect of lotus starch is sought out still by some.

174 Taro: common since ancient days in South China, this seems to have entered Chinese consciousness with the conquest and absorption of that area. In Medieval China "yams and taro" were staples of the wild South, and the phrase poetic trope for frontier hardships. Wild taro is inedible, and old–time cultivars acrid, because of calcium oxalate raphides (sharp crystals). These irritate the mouth and have been selected out of cultivated strains. Taro leaves are an excellent food if young and tender.

175 Lettuce: The variety referred to here seems to be an early form of celtuce, the unique Chinese cultivar grown for its edible swollen stem rather than its leaves. This now exists along with the Western leaf lettuce, the latter having been given a totally new name (*shengcai* 生菜 "raw vegetable") in folk Chinese. It is not eaten raw in China, the dangers of night–soil fertilizer being known, but the Western use of the plant was immortalized in the name. Lettuce is cooling and often used as a cooling medicinal food.

fera][176]

Bokchoy is sweetish in flavor, warming, and lacks poison. It is good for circulation of the bowels and benefits them. It expels vexation in the thorax and counteracts liquor thirst.

[Illustration Caption:] *Penghao* [*Chrysanthemum coronarium* var. *spatiosum*][177]

---

176 White Cabbage: there is considerable taxonomic confusion about this plant both in Chinese and in scientific Latin. In the North, *botsai* refers to the large, cylindrical–headed form of "Peking cabbage" or "Nappa cabbage," so called from a Japanese varietal name in English. In the South, the name refers to the form with dark green leaves and thick, crisp, succulent white petioles for which English has borrowed the Cantonese term "bok choy" (*paak tsoi*). They are closely related to a kaleidoscopic variety of other Chinese cabbages that appear to be derivatives of the *Brassica campestris* stock, the common wild or field cabbage of Eurasia. The Peking cabbage was once separated as "*B. pekinensis*," the bok choy as "*B. sinensis*." The Western cabbage (*B. oleracea,* especially the heading forms) is now common in China, but not so much as these native ones.

Cabbages in general are the great vegetable of China, having spread steadily for thousands of years. They have replaced mallow, sow thistle, and many other greens that were once important. Cabbages have more and better flavor, better pickling qualities, and a preferred texture: the crunchy, crisp, succulent texture that Chinese call *cui* 脆. They are also easy to grow. They grow almost everywhere in China, wherever there is soil and water. Locally adapted forms have been evolved to carry their cultivation to the Himalayan peaks and the tropical Southeast. The popularity of cabbages is waning as other vegetables and fruits become more available, but cabbages still hold pride of place. They are eaten fresh (boiled, steamed or stir–fried), dried, or pickled. Different areas have different pickles, but the method is usually similar, put the cabbages in a crock in strong brine. They may also be simply salted, dried and then brined or salted, or otherwise processed. The pickles (especially less watery ones) often have garlic, chili pepper, soy bean products, chives and other flavorings added. None the less, the Chinese do not go to spectacular lengths of the Koreans, who throw whole chickens and other special feasts foods into their kimchi. Kimchi uses more salt per weight than Chinese pickled cabbages and stays crisper. The pickling involves fermentation by *Lactobacillus* and often other microorganisms. The less salt, the more things can grow in the pickle. Kimchi is so heavily salted that nothing of significance except *Lactobacillus* survives.

Cabbages are almost universally seen as cooling today, and it is exceedingly surprising to find the *YSZY* calling this one warming. The illustration in our edition shows what appears to be a bokchoy form, now held as one of the most cooling of all.

177 Chrysanthemum greens: usually called *tonghao* 茼蒿. The identification is from the illustration which appear to be *C. coronarium* although Hu Shiu-ying calls this plant *Artemisia selengensis* or *A. asparagus*. See Jiang, 2004, 216. If this is a chrysanthemum, it is a different species from the ones grown for flowers and for cooling tea (*C. indicum* and its hybrid part–descendant *C. x morifolium*). *Coronarium* is grown strictly for greens. These have a distinctive spicy flavor that is unique. They are an

[49B] **Penghao** is sweetish in flavor, neutral, and lacks poison. It is good for circulation of the bowels and benefits them. It pacifies heart *qi* and disperses retention of fluid in the body.

[Illustration Caption:] Chinese Eggplant [*Solanum melongena*][178]

Chinese Eggplant is sweetish in flavor, cooling, and has slight poison. It moves wind and produces sores and even obstinate illnesses. Too much should not be eaten.

[Illustration Caption:] Amaranth [*Amaranthus mangostanus* and other *A.* spp][179]

[50A] **Amaranth [Greens]** are bitter in flavor, cooling, and lack poison. They make pass [through] the nine apertures. **Amaranth seeds** augment the essence. The greens cannot be eaten with turtle.

[Illustration Caption:] Oil Rape [*Brassica campestris* var. *olei-*

---

acquired taste. The flower is beautiful but little esteemed in China. The plant is known in English as "chop suey greens," from Cantonese *tsapsui* "miscellaneous leftovers," the name given to a dish of mixed stir–fried vegetables. This dish is a typical meal in the vegetable–rich Taishan region of Guangdong. The notorious American restaurant version is a degenerate form of this and not a California invention. Chrysanthemum greens are an excellent addition to the real dish. The plant is considered warming.

178 Chinese eggplant: probably from India or Southeast Asia originally, but thoroughly Sinicized. Popular fresh and dried. They are sometimes pickled. The most widespread use of it is perhaps in the dish "Eggplant with Fish Flavors," in which it is cooked with the flavoring combination typically used on fish, although the dish does not taste like fish. They are still regarded as cooling today. Note that Chinese eggplant is a very distinct variety that is smaller than the variety eaten in the West and was often cultivated as trees.

179 Amaranth greens: there is considerable disagreement about the classification and origin of the Asian vegetable amaranths. In addition to *A. mangostanus*, this form has been called *A. tricolor*, *A. sinensis*, *A gangeticus etc*., and variously ascribed to China, India, Southeast Asia or all three. It is probably a complex hybrid of various weedy species or varieties found throughout that broad area. The greens are similar to beet greens or reddish spinach. Both are related to amaranth. Amaranth greens are highly nutritious, easy to grow, widely adapted and popular, though considered coarse and identified with peasant fare. They are still considered cooling.

Grain amaranth is grown in Nepal, India, and probably crosses the border into Tibet. It is a completely different species, native to the New World and introduced to those areas in the not too distant past.

fera][180]

Oil Rape is acrid in flavor, warming, and lacks poison. It is good for wind heat inflammatory swelling and breast tumors.

[Illustration Caption:] Spinach [*Spinacia oleracea*][181]

[50B] **Spinach** is sweetish in flavor, chilling, and has slight poison. It benefits the five viscera, circulates bowel heat and counteracts liquor poison. (Same as *chigen* ["red root"].)

[Illustration Caption:] White Sugar Beet [*Beta vulgaris var. cicla*][182]

White Sugar Beet [**Greens**] are sweetish in flavor, cooling, and lack poison. They adjust the center and bring down *qi*. They remove head wind and benefit the viscera.

[Illustration Caption:] Basil [*Ocimum basilicum*][183]

[51A] **Basil** is acrid in flavor, neutral, and lacks poison. It is eaten along with the various vegetables. It is aromatic and removes rank smells.

---

[180] Oil Rape: This is a somewhat conjectural identification. Oil rape is another variety of Chinese cabbage. Several are grown primarily for oil–rich seeds. They are similar to, but a different species from, the rapes and mustards grown for oil in India and Europe. The yield of oil is high, the presscake a good fertilizer, and the plant adapted to almost any situation, so this became the main oil in China before peanuts and maize reached importance. Use of this oil plant had to await the development of good milling machinery (Han and onward). Previously oil had come from lard, hemp seed, perilla seed, and other sources, and it continued to even with the rise of the oil cabbages. Note that Chinese mustard greens also have oil–yielding forms. Since this plant in the *YSZY* is regarded as "warm," it may actually be a mustard variety.

[181] Spinach came to China from Iran in the Tang dynasty or somewhat earlier. It is a common vegetable. Chinese spinach is distinct from Western, having pointed leaves, a spinier seed, more delicate structure, and a more rich and subtle flavor. The two are sold as separate vegetables in Oriental food markets. Spinach is considered "cooling."

[182] White sugar beet: a rare Central Asian vegetable in China, coming at about the same time as spinach but never achieving popularity.

[183] "Fragrant vegetable:" in Modern Chinese this name means coriander greens but those have already been discussed in the *YSZY* under their literary name. This plant is certain to be from the *Lamiaceae*. As perhaps the commonest and most salient herb in that family in China, basil is the most likely candidate and fits the illustration best. True mint (*Mentha* spp) is another good possibility, given its importance in Muslim cooking.

[Illustration Caption:] Smartweed [*Polygonum* spp, most often *P. hydropiper*][184]

Smartweed is acrid in flavor, warming, and lacks poison. It is good for brightening the eye and warming the center. [It makes one able] to tolerate wind and cold and brings down retention of fluid in the body.

[Illustration Caption:] Purslane [*Portulaca oleracea*][185]

[51B] Purslane is sour in flavor, cooling, and lacks poison. It is good for optic atrophy and white cataract. It removes cold and heat and destroys various vermin.

[Illustration Caption:] *Tianhua* [Fungus] [Probably *Pleurotus ortreatus* or even *Tremella fuciformis*][186]

Tianhua [**Fungus**] is sweetish in flavor, neutral, and has poison. It is somewhat like the **möög*. There is little information about it. (Grows on Wutai shan.)

[Illustration Caption:] Shallot ["Muslim Onions," *Allium ascalonicum, A. Cepa*][187]

[52A] The shallot is acrid in flavor, warming, and lacks poison. It warms the center and disperses grain. It brings down *qi* and destroys vermin. If eaten for a long time it causes illness.

---

184 Smartweed: an ancient herb, used for spiciness before black or red pepper came to China. Now a very minor plant but still locally used and considered warm. Smartweed has been a gathered plant among the Mongols, species employed being *P. viviparum*, *mexeer*, *P. divaricatum*, *shimeldeg*, also *usan shimeldeg*, *P. alpinum*, *tarna*, and *P. sibiricum*, also known by the generic *shimeldeg*.

185 Purslane: a minor crop, more often gathered as a weed for food and medicinal value. The plant is one of the most nutritious of all greens, in terms of modern biomedical nutrition as well as Chinese folk belief. It is still held to be sour, cooling and non–*du* 毒. The plant is of great importance for Muslim cuisine probably the main reason it assumes such relative importance here.

186 "Heavenly Flower:" even the *YSZY* admits that little is known about the nature of this unidentifiable tree fungus. It may be Mongolian rather than Chinese, in spite of the reference to a Chinese site in the text. Could this be a badly drawn *Coprinus comatus*? Kitamura calls this *Pleurotus ortreatus* and we follow his identification here.

187 Shallot: *A. ascalonicum*, the shallot, is now held to be a variety of *A. cepa*. Similar wild plants are found in China. Shallots are not uncommon in China and are especially used in pickling. They are common in India and especially Southeast Asia, where they are often the usual form of the onion.

[Illustration Caption:] Chinese Artichoke [*Stachys sieboldi*][188]

Chinese Artichokes are sweetish in flavor, neutral, and lack poison. They benefit the five viscera, bring down *qi* and clarify the spirit. ([Another] name is *dilu.*)

[Illustration Caption:] Elm Seeds [*Ulmus pumila* and possibly other species][189]

[52B] **Elm Seeds** are acrid in flavor, warming, and lack poison. They can be made into a sauce that is very aromatic and fine. They can assist lung *qi*. They destroy the various vermin.

[Illustration Caption:] *Shajhimur* [Rape, *Brassica rapa*][190]

Rape is sweetish in flavor, neutral, and lacks poison. It warms the center and augments *qi*. It removes chill pain of chest and abdomen. (Same as *manqinggen.*)

[Illustration Caption:] *Chugundur* [Sugar Beets, *Beta vulgaris*][191]

[53A] **Sugar Beets** are sweetish in flavor, neutral, and lack poison. They make the blood vessels pass [blood], bring down *qi* and open the diaphragm. (Same as *jundagen* ["*junda* root"].[192])

[Illustration Caption:] Lily Root [*Lilium* spp.][193]

---

188 Chinese artichoke: the tuber of a mint. The English name seems to be based on the similarity of the tuber to that of the Jerusalem artichoke, which is an American sunflower neither from Jerusalem nor an artichoke. The Chinese artichoke is a lowly–regarded food but still common in North China, but virtually unknown in the south. It is pickled, the pickled being choicer than the fresh product, at least in our experience.

189 Elm: the entry actually specifies "elm kernels." These are good eating and have been variously prepared, including as sauce. The young leaves of the Chinese elm are even better, and have been pickled. These tend to be poverty foods partly because the trees are preferred as shade trees, but they could be much more important and have been in the past.

190 Rape: the rape–turnip, a swollen–rooted form similar to true turnip is illustrated.

191 Sugar beet: see above under other entry. In the case of this variety, the beet is the food rather than the greens.

192 This is apparently nothing more than a variant on Persian *chugundur*.

193 Lily root: Stuart and the *CYDCD* identify this plant as *Lilium concolor* and reports it has smaller bulbs than the commoner "hundred together" lily, *L. brownii* (Stuart, 1911: 240; *CYDCD*: #317, #1728). Very likely the name here includes both species. The "hundred together" lily named for its many bulb–scales, is a very important medicinal vegetable today, found in any drugstore and used widely. The "moun-

Lily Roots are sweetish in flavor, neutral, and lack poison. They are good for evil *qi* abdominal distension and expel various boil swellings. (One name is *bohe*).

[Illustration Caption:] Seaweed [possibly *Eucheuma gelatinae, Ottelia alismoides*][194]

[**53B**] **Seaweed** is salty in flavor and cooling. It is slightly rank and lacks poison. It is good for goiter. It destroys *qi* knots and tumorous swelling. Too much should not be eaten.

[Illustration Caption:] Bracken [*Pteridium aqulinum*][195]

Bracken is bitter in flavor, cooling, and has poison. It moves *qi* and produces illness. Too much should not be eaten.

Vetch[196] [*Vicia sativa*] is sweetish in flavor, neutral, and lacks poison. It augments *qi* and makes the flesh glossy. It clarifies the spirit and strengthens the will.

***Sonchus* spp greens** ["*kumai* vegetable", probably *Sonchus arvensis*][197] are bitter in flavor, chilling and lack poison. They regulate facial jaundice. They strengthen physical power and control exhausttion. They can be applied to various sores.

Water celery[198] [*Oenanthe javanica*] is sweetish in flavor, neutral, and lacks poison. It is good for nourishing the spirit and augmenting *qi*. It causes one to be fat and firm. It decreases medicine poison. It

---

tain pill" described here is much more obscure. Note that the roots of *L. martagon*, *shar sarnaa*, also *sarnyn ceceg*, and *L. tenuifolium*, *xonin suyx*, also known by the generic *sarnyn ceceg*, were employed as gathered foods by the Mongols.

194 Seaweed: this could be any of a number of seaweeds. Note that the *YSZY* authors were aware of the value of seaweeds for goiter! The plants are an unexcelled iodine source.

195 Bracken: bracken can be poisonous in large amounts, as the *YSZY* says. Hu calls this *Athyrium sinensis*, Chinese lady-fern, or *Anisogonium esculentum*, tender lady-ferm. See Jiang, 3004, 230.

196 Vetch: we come here to several unillustrated plants. Vetch is of little importance in China. Hu calls this *Osmunda japonica*, Asian osmund fern. See Jiang, 2004, 231.

197 This is apparently another variety of sow thistle, in this case probably the commonly employed Chinese species, *S. arvensis*. The taste for it is almost certainly Mongolian rather than Chinese.

198 Water Celery: an important Chinese water vegetable, ancient in cultivation.

treats female hematuria.

[54A]Properties and Flavors of Spices:

[Illustration Caption:] Black Pepper ["Iranian Pepper"][199]

Black Pepper is acrid in flavor, warming, and lacks poison. It is good for bringing down *qi*. It expels wind chill of viscera and organ and removes phlegm. It decreases meat poison.

[Illustration Caption:] Chinese Flower Pepper ["Lesser Pepper"]

Chinese Flower Pepper is acrid in flavor, heating, and has poison. It is good for evil cough. It warms the center and brings down chill *qi*. It expels arthralgia.

[54B] [Illustration Caption:] Lesser Galangal

Lesser Galangal is acrid in flavor, warming, and lacks poison. It is good for chill perversity in the intestinal tract, *huoluan*, and abdomen pain. It counteracts liquor poison.

[Illustration Caption:] Fennel [*Foeniculum vulgare*]

Fennel is sweetish in flavor, warming, and lacks poison. It is good for chill *qi* of the bladder and kidney channel. It adjusts the center, controls pain and halts vomiting.

[55A] [Illustration Caption:] *Zhira* [Cumin, *Cuminum cymium*][200]

Cumin is acrid in flavor, warming, and lacks poison. It fortifies the spleen and opens the stomach. It warms the center and supplements the water viscera. It decreases fish and meat poison.

---

[199] Black Pepper: this Southeast Asian spice has been known in China since ancient times amd became very popular very early. In spite of the English name, we are referring to white pepper here. White pepper is merely black pepper harvested unripe and hulled. The black color of pepper is due to the ripe hulls. The Chinese prefer the more delicate, woody flavor of white pepper.

[200] Cumin: Cumin is a Near Eastern herb of the family *Apiaceae*. Its small dry fruits (miscalled "seeds") are a common flavoring, especially in the Mediterranean and in South Asia. It is not commonly used in China. Its volatile oils are good for flatulence and indigestion and it is thus commonly added to cooked beans. Since cumin is not called for directly in the text we must assume that it was a component of the spice mixtures not further elucidated.

[Illustration Caption:] Mandarin Orange Peel [*Citrus reticulata* and other *C.* spp][201]

Chenpi is sweetish in flavor, neutral, and lacks poison. It controls diabetes, opens stomach *qi*, brings down phlegm, and destroys chill accumulation.

[55B] [Illustration Caption:] Tsaoko Cardamom

Tsaoko Cardamom is acrid in flavor, warming, and lacks poison. It regulates pain of chest and abdomen, controls vomiting, supplements the stomach and brings down *qi*. It disperses liquor poison.

[Illustration Caption:] Cassia [*Cinnamomum cassia*]

Cassia [Bark] is acrid in flavor, very heating, and has poison. It regulates cold and heat of chest and abdomen and chill phlegm. It benefits liver and lung *qi*.

[56A] [Illustration Caption:] Turmeric [*Curcuma longa*]

Turmeric is acrid–bitter in flavor, cooling, and lacks poison. It is good for stagnation accumulation of chest and abdomen, brings down *qi* and destroys blood stasis. It expels wind–heat.

[Illustration Caption:] *Pippali* [Long Pepper, *Piper longum*]

Pippali is acrid [in flavor], warming, and lacks poison. It is good for warming the center and bringing down *qi*. It supplements for waist and foot pain. It disperses food and expels stomach chill.

[56B] Grain-of-Paradise

Grain-of-Paradise is acrid in flavor, warming, and lacks poison. It is good for *xulao* diseases and chill leaking and lodged food that will not be dispersed. It brings down *qi*.

[Illustration Caption:] Cubebs [*Piper cubeba*; also the seed of *Litsea cubeba*, fragrant Litsea]

Cubebs are acrid in flavor, warming, and lack poison. They disperse

---

[201] Tangerine Skin: still one of the commonest Chinese medicines. It is usually cooked with foods.

food and bring down *qi*. They remove swelling of chest and abdomen and make one able to eat.

[57A] [Illustration Caption:] Liquorice [*Glycyrrhiza uralensis*]

Liquorice is sweetish in flavor, neutral, and lacks poison. It harmonizes the hundred medicines and counteracts the various poisons.

[Illustration Caption:] Coriander Seeds[202]

Coriander Seeds are acrid [in flavor], warming, and lack poison. They disperse food, regulate insufficiency of the five viscera and decrease fish and meat poison.

[57B] [Illustration Caption:] Dried Ginger[203]

Dried Ginger is acrid in flavor, warming–heating, and lacks poison. It is good for cough of the upper chest. It controls abdomen pain and *huoluan* swelling.

[Illustration Caption:] Sprouting Ginger

Sprouting Ginger is acrid in flavor, slightly warming. It is food for exogenous febrile diseases head pain and coughing bringing up *qi* (asthmatic coughing). It controls vomiting and clarifies the spirit.

[58A] [Illustration Caption:] Schisandra [*Schisandra chinensis*]

Schisandra [**Fruits**] are sour [in flavor] and warming. They lack poison, augment *qi*, and supplement the essence. They warm the center and enrich the lungs. They nourish the viscera and fortify *yin*.

---

[202] Coriander Seeds: the seeds, like other Apiaceous seeds are very good sources of B vitamins and several mineral nutrients, but their main medical value in international medicine is as carminative, stimulant, and digestive foods. The volatile oils are the main reasons for the benefits. Coriander, cumin, and related seeds are traditionally eaten in large quantities with beans in India, the Near East, the Mediterranean, and Mexico, to counteract the indigestion and flatulence. In China these seeds are minor spices, not used much, and mainly as a borrowed taste from westward.

[203] Ginger: China's most important native flavoring plant after the Welsh onion and has been important since very early times. Note the differences here between dry and fresh ginger in medical effects. Similar beliefs about ginger and other plants are still held. Drying does reduce volatiles and cause chemical changes in some other compounds in many plants. Ginger is widely used throughout the world as a stimulant. It is an important warming spice in China.

[Illustration Caption:] Fenugreek Seeds [*Trigonella foenum-graecum*] (same as *hulba[t]*)

Fenugreek Seeds are bitter in flavor, warming, and lack poison. They are good for deficiency chill of primary organs and swelling of abdomen and rib. They control bladder disease.

[58B] **Red Yeast**[204] **[*Monascus purpureus*]** is sweetish in flavor, neutral, and lacks poison. It fortifies the spleen, augments *qi*, and warms the center. It is used for marinating the insides of fish.

Poppy Seeds ["Little Black Seeds;" *Papaver somniferum*][205] are sweetish in flavor and lack poison. They open the stomach and bring down *qi*. They are used inside roasted buns and have a very fine aroma.

Mastajhi[206] is bitter in flavor, aromatic and lacks poison. It removes evil and pathological *qi*, warms the center, and benefits the diaphragm. It accords *qi* and controls pain. It gives rise to saliva and counteracts thirst. It makes a person's breath smell good. (It grows in the Muslim countries. It is said to be the most aromatic substance.)

***Za'faran* [Saffron; *Crocus sativus*]** is sweetish in flavor, neutral, and lacks poison. It is good for melancholia[207] and accumulated *qi* which will not disperse. If eaten for a long time it makes one happy in heart. (There is no information to confirm or deny that this is the *honghua* of the Muslim countries.)

***Kasni* [Asafoetida]**[208] is acrid in flavor, warming, and lacks poison. It

---

204 Red Yeast: this is undoubtedly the same as the red ferment that is grown on rice in Fujian today. It is still regarded as sweetish, nonpoisonous, and warming in some sense, and still used on fish. It has no special taste and is used mainly for the color.

205 Little Black Seeds: almost certainly poppy seeds, in which case it is interesting that no connection is made with poppies, opium or sleep. See the discussion by Li (Hu Sihui, 1988: 459, where they are identified with parsley seeds. Parsley seeds are not black, nor are they known to be used in buns.

206 Mastic: this gum was imported from the Near East. See above.

207 Saffron: the cheering value of saffron is a Western idea (Sabban, 1983).

Laufer, 1919: 353–4: "Asafoetida is a vegetable product consisting of resin, gum, and essential oil in varying proportions, the resin generally amount to more than one–half, derived from different umbelliferous plants, as *Ferula narthex*, *alliacea*, *foetida*, *persica*, and *scorodosma* (or *Scorodosma foetidum*)." The primary plant source is is good for destroying the various vermin. It removes bad smells and overcomes obstruction of the bowels. It brings down pathological [*qi*] and expels evil [*qi*]. It counteracts *ku* poison. (Same as *angwa*.)

Anguzhad **[Asafoetida root]** is acrid in flavor, warming, bitter, and lacks poison. It is good for destroying vermin and removes smells. Its flavor is the same as *angwa* [*i.e.*, as asafoetida]. It is also said to be the root of the *angwa* tree. It is used to marinate mutton. The aroma and flavor are very fine.

[59A] **Safflower [*Carthamus tinctoria*]** is acrid in flavor, warming, and lacks poison. It is good for postpartum blood motion and colic of chest and abdomen. It can support floating swelling.

Zhizi **[fruit of *Gardenia jasminoides*]** is bitter in flavor, cooling, and lacks poison. It is good for evil *qi* of the five internal organs [= viscera]. It treats conjunctivitis heat and benefits the urine.

Cattail [Pollen] [*Typha* sp.] is sweetish in flavor, neutral, and lacks poison. It regulates cold and heat of chest and abdomen and benefits the urine. It controls blood disease.

"Muslim Green"[209] is sweetish in flavor, cooling, and lacks poison. It counteracts the poisons of the various drugs. It can support intense evil heat boils.

---

called *Ferula asafoetida* today. The values ascribed seem to be, in part, Chinese transformations of well–known apotropaic functions ascribed to the gum elsewhere. *Wen zhan* is regarded as the root of the plant that yields the gum. The gum and the cut–up root were both in the China trade as different forms of the same general commodity. See Laufer, 1919: 353ff. The prominent presence of asafoetida in the *YSZY* is a clear marker of Iranian influence.

209 This could be any one of a score of "Muslim" spices and an illustration is unfortunately lacking. We suspect that it is nothing more than mint. Compare recipe #20 in *juan* 1 which seems to call for this spice as *qingcai* 青菜. Note that this term also applies to azurite but apparently not here. Azurite is not used in food in the Muslim world, in spite of the name here.

Part C

* * *

APPENDICES

APPENDIX ONE

THE *MATERIA DIETETICA ET MEDICA*

Table A

Foods and Spices Mentioned in the YSZY

Abalone
Acanthopanax Bark Liquor
Acorns
Acorus Root
Adzuki Beans ["Red Small Beans"]
Almonds [*Badam*]
Amaranth Greens
Angwa [Asafoetida]
Apricot Kernels
Apricot Kernel Paste
Apricots
Arajhi Brandy
Aromatic Non-glutinous Rice
Attar of Roses

Badger Meat
Baiheng [variety of Forbes' Wild ginger?]
Balloon Flowers
Bamboo Shoots
Barley
Baroos Camphor
Basil
Bear Fat
Bear Meat
Bear's Paw
Bear's Paw of the Tenth Lunar Month
Beef

Beef Medullae
Beef Stomach
Begonias
Black ["Iranian"] Pepper
Black Chinese Apricots
Black Donkey's Head
Black Donkey's Meat
Black Donkey's Skin
Black Hen's Blood
Black Hen's Meat
Black Ox's Marrow
Black Rooster's Meat
Black-Headed Crane Meat
Black-Tailed Gazelle Meat
Blue Sheep Meat
Boar's Penis
Bokchoy
Borbi[n] ["part of the leg of sheep just above the heel, Achilles tendon"]
Boshi [fruit of *Biota orientalis*]
Bracken
Brain of the Local Leopard
Broomrape
Buckwheat

Bunting Meat
Burdock Leaves
Burnet-Bloodwort

Camel Fat
Camel Meat
Camphor [*Ka'fur*]
Cane Sugar
**Caqa'an* ["white"] Kumiss
Cardamom Kernels
Carp
Carrots ["Iranian Radishes"]
Cassia Bark
Catfish
Cattail Pollen
Cattail Rhizome
Cattail Shoots
Cherries
Chestnuts
Chi Panicled Millet
Chicken Meat
Chickpeas ["Muslim Beans"]
Chigen ["Red Root," true Spinach]
Children's Tea [Catechu]
China Root Liquor
Chinese Aconite
Chinese Angelica
Chinese Artichokes
Chinese Asparagus
Chinese Badger Meat
Chinese Bream
Chinese Chives
Chinese Chive Tubers
Chinese Cornbind
Chinese Eggplant
Chinese Flower Pepper
Chinese Foxglove
Chinese Foxglove Liquor
Chinese Honey-Locust Fruit
Chinese Lovage
Chinese Matrimony Vine Fruits
Chinese Matrimony Vine Liquor
Chinese Myrica Fruits
Chinese Olives
Chinese Onions
Chinese Parsley [Cilantro]
Chinese Pears
Chinese Quinces
Chinese Quinine
Chinese Radish
Chinese Senega
Chinese Spikenard
Chinese Sturgeon
Chinese Sturgeon Bladder
Chinese Sturgeon Fat
Chinese Wild ginger
Chinese Yams
Chinjiao [Flower Pepper Bark?]
Chrysanthemum coronarium var *spatiosum* Greens
Cinnabar
Cinnamon
Citrons
Clear broth [bouillon?]
Cnidium officinale Fruit
Cocklebur
Collared Crow Meat
Common Pintail Meat

Common Quail Meat
Cooked Sheep's Fat
Cooked Sheep's Marrow
Coriander Juice
Coriander Seeds
Cow's Gall Bladder
Cow's Milk
Cow's Milk Butter
Cow's Milk Cheese
Cow's Milk Curds
Crab Apple
Crab Meat
Crane Meat
Crane Medullae
Croton Beans
Crystallized Honey
Cubebs
Cucumbers
Cumin [*zhira*]
Cynanchum Root

Deer's Feet
Deer's Horn
Deer's Kidney
Distilled Liquor
Dog Meat
Donkey Meat
Donkey's Fat
Donkey's Head Meat
Dove Meat
Dried Deer's Milk Fat
Dried Fish
Dried Ginger
Dried Rice
Duck Eggs
Durum Wheat (**Qamh*)

Eared Fowl Meat
Egg Yoke
Eggs
Elephant Meat
Elephant Tusk
Elm Seeds
Eurasian Curlew Meat
Euryale Ferox Fruits
Euryale Flour
Evodia Fruits

False Hellebore Root and Rhizome
Fangfeng
Fanshi [guava?]
Feilian [herb or root of *Carduus crispus* and other *C.* spp]
Fennel
Fenugreek Seeds
Fermented Camel's Milk
Fermented Mare's Milk [*cige'en*]
Field Mint Leaves
Finely Ground Spices
Five Internal Organs of Sheep
"Five Spices"
Flowering Apricot Fruits
Flowering Apricot Red Fruits
Food Fowl Meat
Forbes' Wild Ginger
Fortified [Repeatedly-boiled] Tea
Four Hooves of a Pig
Four Paws of a Dog
Fox Meat
Foxtail Millet

Fragrant Orange Peel
Fragrant Oranges
Fresh Water Mussels

Garden Peas
Gardenia Nuts
Garlic
Garuwood
Gazelle Meat
Ghee
Ginkgo Nuts
Ginseng
Glauber's Salts Solution
Glutinous Rice
Golden Carp
Golden Thread [Rhizome]
Grain-of-Paradise
Grape Wine
Grapes
Great Bustard Meat
Greater Golden-Headed Swan Meat (*yeke siraqun qun*)
Green Fish
Green Millet
Green Small Beans
Ground Basil
Ground Mustard

Hare's Meat
Hazelnuts
Head and Hair of a Rabbit of the Twelfth Lunar Month
Head, Fur and Bones of a Rabbit of the Twelfth Lunar Month
Hemp Seeds
"Hollow" Malachite
Honey
Horse Meat
Horse's Heart
Horse's Liver
Horse's Skull
Horse's Stomach and Intestines
Hulled Barley
Hyacinth Beans

"Iranian" Crane
"Iranian" Sesame Seeds

Japanese Plums
Jiaxiang [*operculum* of *Turbo cornutus* and related spp]
Job's Tears
Juice of Soaked Golden Thread
Jujubes [*cicigina*]
Junzi Fungi (Agaricus Mushrooms)

Kasni [Asafoetida]
Korean Ginseng
Kudzu Starch
Kueihua [*Osmanthus fragrans*]
Kuju [*Sonchus* sp]
Kulan Meat
Kumai Vegetable [*Sonchus arvensis*]

Lamb Liquor
Leek Juice
Leopard Cat Meat
Leopard Cat Skulls
Lesser Galangal
Lesser Golden-Headed

Swan [*Qaralaq qun*] Meat
"Lesser Oil"
Lettuce
Lichee Fruits
Lily Root [*Ja'uqasu*]
Liquorice
Liquorice Juice
Long Bottle Gourd
Long Pepper [*pippali*]
Longans
Lotus Flower Stamens
Lotus Flowers
Lotus Root
Lotus Seeds

Male Wild Boar's Gall Bladder Juice
Mallard Duck Meat
Mallow Leaves
Malt-Sugar
Mandarin Duck Meat
Mandarin Orange
Mandarin Orange Peel
Mäskä [Butter] Oil
Mastajhi
Meat of the Rear Hoof of a Sheep
Millet
Millet Liquor
Mint
Monkey Meat
**Möög* Mushroom[*Tricholoma mongolicum*]
Mountain Oysters [*Jasa'a*, of a ram?]
Mountain Rhinoceros Meat
Mud Eels
Mulberry Fruits
Mule Meat
Mung Beans
Muntjac Deer Venison
Musk Deer Musk
Musk Deer Venison
Musk Mallow
"Muslim Green"
[mint?]
Mustard Greens
Mute Swan Meat
Mutton
Muxiang [root of *Vladimiria souliei* or *Saussurea lappa*]
Myrobalans Oil

"Naked" Mang Larva
Nettle Leaf
Non-Glutinous Rice
Nuxuer [?] Tea

Oil from Cow's Skull Marrow
Oil Rape
Oil Rape Sprouts
Onion Bulbs
Onion Hearts
Orang-outang Meat
Orchid Paste
Oriental Flowering Apricots
Oriental Pickling Melons
Oriental Swangoose Droppings
Oriental Swangoose
Fat
Oriental Swangoose Meat
Otter Meat
Otter's Liver
Otter's Skin
Ox Hooves

Ox Meat

Penis and Testes of *Callorhinus ursinus* or *Phoca vitulina*
Pichen Rhinoceros Meat
Paddy Rice
Paishu Rhizome
Paiyao [*Millettia lasiopetala*]
Panhsia Rhizome
Panicled Millet
Peach Kernels
Peach
Pear-Shaped Bottle Gourds
Penis of a White Stallion
Pere David's Deer Venison
Persimmons
Pheasant Meat
Pickled Ginger
Pig Suet
Pig's Brain
Pig's Head
Pig's Kidney
Pigeon Meat
Pine Knot Liquor
Pine Nuts
Pine Oil
Pine Pollen Juice
Pine Root Liquor
Pingpo [*Malus Pumila*?]
Pistachios [*pistä*]
Poke Root
Polished Rice
Pomegranates
Poppy Seeds ["Little Black Seeds"]
Pork
Pork Lard
Powdered Tea
Prickly Sculpin Meat
Prinsepia Fruits
Puffer
Purple Perilla Leaves
Purslane

Qatiq ["Dried Sour Milk"]
Qongqor ["chestnut Colored"] Kumiss
Quail Meat

Rabbit Liver
Rabbit Meat
Rape [*shajhimur*]
Rattan Tea
Raw Chinese Foxglove
Red China Root
Red Currants ["Northern Schisandra Fruits"]
Red Deer Head
Red Deer Horn
Red Deer Medullae
Red Deer Stag's Penis
Red Deer Velvet
Red Deer Venison
Red Deer's Hoof
Red Magnolia [*Magnolia liliflora*] Flower
Red of a Horse's Hooves
Red Panicled Millet
"Red Powder" [=Red Yeast?]
Red Rooster Meat
"Red Yeast"
Reed Rhizome Juice
Rhinoceros Horn

Rhubarb Juice
Rice Vinegar
River Deer Venison
River Shrimps
Roasted Tea
Rose Hips
Rose Water
Russian Olive Fruits

Sacred Lotus Fruits
Sacred Lotus Rhizome
Safflower
Saffron [*za'faran*]
Salt
Salted Bean Relish
Salted Fruits
Salted Mandarin Orange Peel
Sandalwood
Sawfish
Schisandra Fruits
Schizonepeta tenuifolia herb
Sciaenid Fish
Sea Snail
Seashore Vitex Fruits
Seaweed
Sesame Seed Paste
Sesame Seeds
Shallots ["Muslim Onions"]
Sheatfish
Sheep's Back Skin from which the hair has been removed
Sheep's "Bitter" Bowel
Sheep's Blood
Sheep's Bones
Sheep's Brain
Sheep's Breast
Sheep's Fat
Sheep's Head
Sheep's Heart
Sheep's Hooves
Sheep's Kidneys
Sheep's Liver
Sheep's Liver Sauce
Sheep's Loins
Sheep's Medullae
Sheep's Milk Cream
Sheep's Skin
Sheep's Spine
Sheep's Stomach
Sheep's Tail
Sheep's Tendons
Sheep's Thorax
Sheep's Tongue
Sheep's "White Blood Double Intestines" [tripe?]
Sheep's "White Blood Irrigating Bowel"
Sheep's "White Bowel"
Shrimp
Siberian Sturgeon
Siberian Sturgeon Bladder
Siberian Sturgeon Fat
Sika Deer Fat
Sika Deer Skin
Sika Deer Venison
"Small Coarse Grain Liquor"
Smartweed
Smartweed Shoots
Snow Leopard Meat
Snow-white-interior Rice
Softshelled Turtle
Meat
Solomon's Seal
Songcai [variety of *Brassica chinensis*?]
Sour Jujubes

"Southern Borax"
Soy Bean Sauce
Soy Sauce
Soybean Sprouts
Soybeans
Sparrow Meat
Spinach
Spring Onions
Spring Water
Sprouting Chinese Foxglove
Sprouting Chinese Foxglove Juice
Sprouting Ginger
Stinking Elm
Su-men Paddy rice
Sugar Beets
**Surma* Brandy
**Süttigen* [Mongolian Tea]
Swan Meat
Sweet Melons
Sweet Orange Peel
Sweet Oranges
Sweetflag
Sweetmeats
Swiss Chard
Swiss Chard Seeds
Sichuan Aconite
Sichuan Pagoda
Sichuan Pepper

Tabilqa [locally gathered *Spiraea media* or possibly *Gentiana* spp]
Tablet Rice
Tailed-deer Venison
Tailed-deer's Fat
Tangerines
Tangkuei
Tarbaqan Marmot Head Bones
Tarbaqan Marmot Meat
Tarbaqan Marmot Skin
Taro
Tea (many varieties)
Tianhua Fungus [*Pleurotus ortreatus*]
Tianjing Vegetable [*Sonchus* sp]
Tibetan Tea
Tiger Bone Liquor
Tiger Bones
Tiger Eyes
Tiger Meat
Tongtian Rhinoceros Meat
Torreya Nuts
Trapa bispinosa fruits
Tree Ears
Tree Peony
Trough Shells
Tsangshu Seed
Tsaoko Cardamom
Tufted Duck Meat
Turmeric
Turtle Meat
Tussilago Flower

Variegated Swan Meat [*Alaq qun*]
Vetch

Walnuts
Wangcao [unidentified]
Warm Mulberry Tea
Water Chestnuts

Water Rhinoceros
Meat
Water-celery
Watermelons
Weasel Meat
Wei [unidentified]
Wenzhan [*Anguzhad*,
asafoetida root]
Wheat
Wheat Ferment
White Beans
White Crane Meat
White Fish
White Gazelle Meat
White Horse's Hooves
White Lead ["Iranian Powder"]
Solution
White Millet
White *Nabat* [Sugar]
White Onions
White Pigeon's Meat
White Rooster's Meat
White Sandalwood
White Sesame Seeds
White Sheep's Head
White Sheep's Kidney
White Sugar Beets
White Tea
Wild Boar Meat
Wild Camel Hump
Wild Camel Meat
Wild Goat Meat
Wild Goose Bone Ash
Wild Goose Fat
Wild Goose Grease
Wild Goose Meat
Wild Horse Meat
Wild Pheasant Meat
[Hazel Grouse
Meat?]
Wild Pig's Meat
Wild Sheep Meat
Winter Melons
Wolf Meat
Wolf's Skin
Wolf's Tail
Wolf's Throat Skin
Wolf's Tooth

Xiancai [greens of
Amaranthus spp,
Chenopodium spp]

Yangtse Porpoise
Meat
Yeast
Yellow Fish
[unidentified]
Yellow Hen Meat
Yellow Millet
Yogurt

Zhemi ["Uniform washed
grains from fine millet"]
Zhenwei Rhinoceros
Meat

Table B: Ingredients and How Often Each Ingredient is Called for in the 95 "Strange Delicacies of Combined Flavors"

Ingredient	Recipes
Sheep parts all:	128
Type:	
meat	54
tail	16
lungs	8
fat	8
liver sauce	4
stomach	6
intestines, bowels	4
feet	3
head	3
liver	3
loins	3
tongue	3
blood	2
heart	2
ribs	2
skin	2
borbin (knee/tendon)	1
kidneys	1
tendon	1
testicles	1
whole, with hair	1
sheep/mutton	76
salt	61
onions	52
vinegar	40
fresh ginger/sprouting ginger	35
tsaoko cardamoms	34
wheat flour (may be implied elsewhere)	34
black pepper	26
"spices," *i.e.*, Chinese "five spice" or the like	19
chickpeas	16
bean flour	16
vegetable oil (or unspecified frying oil)	15

mandarin orange peel	14
eggs	12
**möög* mushrooms	12
asafoetida (including "*kasni*," 8)	10
rice	10
Chinese radish	9
coriander greens	9
pickled ginger	9
ground ginger	9
coriander leaves	8
lesser galangal	8
saffron	8
"sauce" (usually fermented soybean)	8
carrots	7
Chinese yams	7
safflower	7
butter (including ghee)	6
coriander, ground	6
flower pepper	6
basil	5
euryale flour	5
mustard	5
sweet melon pickles	5
turmeric	5
apricot kernel paste	4
carp	4
cheese	4
Chinese chives	4
gardenia fruits	4
long pepper	4
"meat patties"	4
sesame seed paste	4
smartweed	4
chicken	3
cinnamon	3
cow milk	3
honey	3
millet	3
"pine pollen" (probably pine nuts)	3
soda (for baking)	3

Two each: barley, cattail rhizome, Chinese cabbage, Chinese quince, deer, fennel seeds, garlic, goose, grains of paradise, leeks, oil rape, rose attar, yogurt/cream

One each: almond, almond paste, bear, bottle gourd, (long), bottle gourd (pear-shaped), camphor, Chinese chive tuber, Chinese spikenard, cormorant, crab spawn, cucumber, curlew, duck, durum (?), eggplant, euryale fruit, fenugreek, flower pepper, glutinous rice flour, hog's head, horse hoof, horse tripes, leaven (possibly implied elsewhere), lily root, "liquor," lotus rhizome, mallow leaves, mastic, mint, nettle leaf, *Pleurotus* mushroom, Russian olive fruits, *operculum* of *Turbo cornutus etc.*, ox hoof, pistachio nuts, pomegranate, poppy seeds, quail, rabbit, rape turnip, red yeast, smartweed, spinach, sugar, sweet clover, sweet melon, Swiss chard, turtle, walnut, willow leaves (for steaming whole sheep), wolf

Table C: Ingredients and How Often Each Ingredient is Called for in the "Soups and Decoctions" and Medical Recipes of *juan* 2

Ingredient	Recipes
Sheep (parts)	18 (in 11 recipes)
by type:	
kidney	3
meat	3
bones	2
fat	2
spine	2
stomach	2
head	1
heart	1
lungs	1
marrow	1
Tsaoko cardamoms	18
rice (almost all in congees)	18
"five spices"	18
tea (various varieties)	18
sugar (mostly jams and syrups)	16
Mandarin orange peel	15
salt	14
onions	13
ginger (but not pickled ginger)	11
liquid butter (also congealed butter, yogurt)	10
black pepper	8
white flour	8
lesser galangal	8
long pepper	8
Chinese foxglove	7
ginseng (some specify Korean)	7
Chinese flower pepper	7
liquorice	7
chicken (3 specify black, 2 yellow)	5
oriental flowering apricot (3 black, 2 salted)	5
fennel	5

grain-of-paradise	5
honey	5
perilla leaves	5
"sauce" (here soy sauces)	5
apricot kernels	4
cassia	4
Chinese quince	4
Chinese yam	4
fermented black beans	4
flowering apricot	4
jujube	4
liquor	4
millet	4
musk	4
sandalwood	4
salted fruit	4
adzuki beans	3
cheese (sometimes ?cream)	3
donkey (skin, head, meat)	3
milk	3
nabat	3
sandalwood	3
Schizonepeta	3
wolfthornberries (Chinese matrimony vine)	3

Two each: baroos camphor, bream, broomrape, cardamom, Chinese asparagus, cubeb, euryale fruits/seeds, fox flesh, garuwood, kudzu flour, litsea, mint, orange peel, pomegranate, *qatiq* (dried milk), red China root, sesame seeds, turmeric, vinegar, wheat ferment, yeast

One each: acorus root, asafoetida, bear, beef, black ox marrow, burdock, carp, cassia, *cicigina*, cherry, Chinese badger, cinnamon, citron, cow marrow, deer feet, deer horn, deer kidney, duck (wild mallard), egg, evodia fruit, garlic, large garlic, hazelnut, hemp seeds, kueihua, kumquat, liquor, lotus fruit, mallow, malted wheat, *Melia toosendan*, *muxiang*, mung bean flour, myrobalan (chebulic), orange, orange (fragrant orange) peel, otter liver, paiyao, peach fruit, peach seed, pheasant, pig (wild), pig kidney, pigeon, pine seeds, purslane, red

China root, red currant, rose hips, rose-water, Schisandra, Solomon's seal, southern borax, sweetmeats, *tabilqa*, **tosu[n]*, tsangshu, turmeric, wine (grape)

APPENDIX TWO

GRAIN FOODS OF THE EARLY TURKS

By

CHARLES PERRY

The Turks who invaded the Near East in the tenth century were herdsmen, not farmers, and they have often been pictured living entirely off their flocks, possibly supplementing a diet of yogurt and shishkebab with wild fruits and herbs. In fact, grain foods were already their staple diet.

When Mahmud of Kashgar compiled his dictionary of Turkish dialects in 1073, he recorded native Turkish words for sowing, the plow, several grains, and a number of grain foods, 15 of which are still current in one or another Turkish language (a like number of terms has died out; see the Addendum). Another nine words are attested by the end of the fourteenth century or can be assumed to be of comparable antiquity because of their distribution. These range from simple porridge and toasted grain to noodles, breads, and pastries, one of which is certainly the ancestor of that layered pastry Westerners know as filo or strudel dough. Turkish grain cookery has had wide influence in Eurasia, even as far as Hungary and North Africa, as the presence of these words in non-Turkish languages can attest.

I. Historical Background

More than 2000 years ago Chinese chroniclers begin to mention the nomadic peoples living to the north and west of China whose predatory raids were only to be brought under control by the building of extensive frontier fortifications and the maintenance of grand armies. By the time of Mahmud of Kashgar, two languages dominated the steppe, Turkish and Mongolian, whose speakers lived in close contact and shared not only a common culture but a large vocabulary relating to steppe life. The fact that they herded domestic animals such as sheep, goats, and horses shows that the ancestors of at least some of them had contact with the settled populations which were the original domesticators of these animals at an early date. Even if knowledge of grain had died out, or never arisen, in particular nomad groups, there was probably always some grain on the steppes, as plunder or trade goods, grain by the locals in some cases. The Turks also spread west in several waves, both peaceable and warlike, to grain-growing regions. By the beginning of our era skeletons of the Mongoloid physical type begin to appear in the Minusa Basin, an area west of the Altai Mountains where Europeoids had practiced agriculture since 1500 BC.

In the fourth and fifth centuries AD, the westernmost Turks entered European history in various Hun, Avar, and Bulgar kingdoms. Somewhat later, in the sixth and seventh centuries, the Turks remaining in Asia were involved in the large, loosely organized steppe empires of the Kök Türks and the Uighurs which extended at times as far as the Aral Sea in the west and Manchuria in the east. These empires controlled the Silk Road, and contact with Iran and China accelerated during this period.

In the eighth century, many of the Turks who had wandered west and begun to annihilate or absorb the Iranian nomads who had formerly dominated the Central Asian steppes converted to Islam and thereby came into closer contact with the settled, agricultural population of Iran's outlying northern and eastern provinces: Khwarezm, Transoxiana, and Khorasan. Around the same time the Uighurs gave up nomadism and adopted the way of life of the Iranian- and Tokharian-speaking natives of the Tarim Basin. The Uighurs' conversion to Manichaeism and later to Buddhism imposed a vegetarian diet on at least their priestly class and committed them to agriculture.

However early some Turks were familiar with grain, it may be that systematic trade, making it the staple of their diet, only began with the conversion of the Uighurs. At any rate, some of the Turkish grain foods made by toasting or boiling, such as *talqan* and *butqa*, may originally have been made from wild grass seeds or roots (lily root is commonly used for *butqa* by the Yakuts of Siberia), and therefore may date from a period even before acquaintance with domestic grains. Those based on milled flour probably reflect some degree of Iranian or Chinese influence. For instance, in a ninth century text from Turfan, in the very easternmost part of the Tarim Basin (Xinjiang Province, China), we find *laqsha*, the ancient Persian word for noodle.

During the ninth and tenth centuries, Turkish mercenaries became the backbone of most Near Eastern armies; in the tenth and eleventh centuries Turks began establishing their own kingdoms in Iran, the Fertile Crescent and Anatolia. Turkish dominion in the northern Islamic lands was ensured by the explosive conquests of Cinggis-qan and his descendants in the thirteenth century, because great numbers of Turks fought in the western Mongol hordes. The Mongol Empire soon broke up into various successor states, of which two of the most important, the Golden Horde (western and northern Central Asia and southern Russia) and the Chagatai Horde (Transoxiana and the Tarim Basin), became culturally and linguistically Turkish, as the small Mongol ruling class intermarried with its Turkish troops and with the Turks already settled in the conquered territories.

II. The Present-Day Turks

The present-day Turkish nations can be divided into three main groups: Southwestern (SW), Central (C) and Northeastern (NE).

The Southwestern Group consists of the Osmanlis (the Turks of Turkey), the Azerbaijanis in the southeast Caucasus and northwestern Iran, the Turkmens between the Caspian and the Aral Seas, and scattered populations in Iran and the Balkans. This group is associated with the Seljuk and Ottoman Empires in Anatolia and the (originally Mongol) Il-qan Kingdom in Iran. The Turkmens and the Iranian groups are nomads, the others settled.

The Central Group can be subdivided into four subgroups. In the Central Southeast (CSE), roughly the territory of the Chagatai Horde, are the Uzbeks of Transoxiana and the closely related Uighurs (not necessarily descended from the Medieval Uighurs) of the Tarim Basin. Related to the Uighurs are another Turkish nation dwelling in China, the small Salar Group of Gansu 甘肅 Province. The Uzbeks and Uighurs are farmers and devout Moslems, the Uzbeks heavily influenced by their Iranian neighbors. In the Mid-Central (MC) area, the steppes of Central Asia from the Caspian Sea to the borders of China, a number of related dialects are spoken which have been more or less arbitrarily distinguished as the Kazakh, Kirgiz, and Karakalpak languages. Apart from the agricultural Karakalpaks in the delta of the Oxus, these are mostly nomads and only superficially Islamized.

The Central Northwest Group (CNE) comprises the Tatars and the Bashkirs, whose history is connected with the Golden Horde and the

Khanate of Kazan, to which Russia long paid tribute. These nations live on the middle Volga about 500 miles east of Moscow. Also stemming from the Golden Horde are several small Central Southwest (CSW) groups in the Crimea and northern Caucasus, such as the Nogai, Karachai, and Balkar. Among this last group is the Qaraim language, spoken by a Jewish sect in the Crimea and in scattered towns in Poland and Lithuania.

The Northeastern Group is a residual category consisting of the Turkish nations, speaking in some cases very distantly related languages, who live to the north of westernmost Mongolia, in the Altai and Sayan mountains, and the steppes to the north of them; essentially the Turks who did not join the great Medieval wars of conquest and stayed in the Turkish homeland. This group has never become Muslem and has not participated in the cultural developments of the other Turkish lands, and the presence of a food name here is strong evidence of its antiquity. Some of these people are herdsmen or farmers, others hunters and gatherers or settled hunters. From east to west the principal Northeastern peoples are the Tuva (under strong Mongol influence), the Abakan, the Shor, and the Altai.

There is a clear culinary distinction between these three main groups. The Northeastern Group, isolated and impoverished, knows only 8 of the 23 terms under discussion. (Among them, however, are words for "bread" and "noodles.") The Southwestern languages use a larger number of the words, but this group was first exposed to heavy Persian influence and then developed its own school of cookery, the Ottoman Turkish style which now predominates in the eastern Mediterranean. This history probably explains the absence of some words. The Central group has preserved nearly all the anciently recorded words which survive (the exceptions are *qagut/qawut* and the vexed case of *lavash*). Nearly all the terms in use in the Central Group are also found in languages of the Northeastern or Southwestern groups; only in the case of *chälpäk* and *salma* is it likely that we are dealing with a specifically Central development which has been borrowed by a Southwestern language.

Two present-day Turkish nations are descended from groups which separated from the rest of the Turks quite early. The Hun/Bulgar branch of the Turks, which headed west in the fourth century and did not take part in the Kök Türk Empire, is represented today by the Chuvash of the middle Volga. Despite having arrived as nomads, and having spent at least a thousand years among older agricultural populations, they preserve at least one of the ancient grain food names. The Yakuts, by contrast, headed north and east from the region of Lake Balkhash, probably to escape Mongol expansionism, in the tenth-thirteenth centuries. Since grain cannot be raised in their present home and food did not form an item of their scant trade with southern regions, they have no grain-cooking tradition and it cannot be known for certain whether they knew of grain before their migration.

III. The Grain Foods

Medieval sources for the words are abbreviated as follows:

TT: *Turfan Texts* (ninth and tenth centuries)
DL: *Diwan Lughat al-Turk* (1073)
KI: *Kitab al-'Idrak li-Lisan al-'Atrak* (1312)
MA: *Muqaddimat al-'Adab* (thirteenth or fourteenth century)
TZ: *Al-Tuhfah al-Zakiyyah fi Lughat al-Turkiyyah* (fourteenth century)
BM: *Bulghat al-Mushtaq fi Lughat al-Turk wal-Qifjaq* (fourteenth century)

TT and DL were written in present-day Xinjiang (Chinese Turkistan); the Turfan Texts are only in Uighur, but DL records many words from other dialects. The other words represent Central and Southwestern dialects spoken by soldiers and other Turks living in Egypt and Syria.

IV. Whole or Crushed Grain Products

1. ***talqan***: Probably from a verb meaning "to abuse, work hard." It has meant meal, flour, toasted meal, fried flour (as in Turkmen and Uighur), toasted grain, and/or a porridge made of any of these. DL: "porridge of toasted grain."

Borrowings: This word entered Mongolian as one of the principal words for "flour." In modern Khalkha Mongolian, *talx* means "bread." The non-Turkish Tungus languages of eastern Siberia have borrowed *talqan* in the sense "grain, flour, baked bread." The Tuva (NE) also have it as "flour, dough, fried bread of barley or wheat," probably as the result of Mongolian influence. Pashto, the Iranian language of Afghanistan, preserves the sense of fried grain. In the Urdu language of India, *talqan* is an edible paste of pounded toasted grain. The Tajiks, Persian-speakers who live closely mingled with the Uzbeks, are said to use the word for a fried flour made from dried fruits.

2. ***qagurmac***: "grain fried in butter," from *qagurmaq*, "to fry." This word has survived in scattered locations, with some shifting of meaning ("rice porridge with carrots and raisins" as well as the original sense in modern Uighur, "fried wheat bread" in Turkmen). In Osmanli it applies to fried maize, lentils *etc*. In the northern Caucasus it is said to mean popcorn. DL: *qawurmac*, "dish of wheat fried in butter"; *qogurmac*, "fried wheat." KI: *qawurmac*, "fried grain."

Borrowings: apparently none. (The widely borrowed word *qawurma* is not a grain food but a dish of fried meat: *e.g.*, Urdu *korma*.)

3. ***yarma***: "crushed grain, groats," literally "split, cloven." Like the English word grits, *yarma* often means porridge as well as raw crushed grain. This is the most widely represented word, found in all the major language areas (that is, all Turkish languages except Chuvash and Yakut) and recorded as early as the ninth century. The only notable shift of meaning is specialization as to one particular grain: barley in northern Altai, millet in Uzbek, rice and millet in Kazakh. TT: *arpa . . . yarmasï*, "barley groats." MA, TZ: *yarma*, "groats." DL records a related form *yarmish*. Currently it is spelled *yarmïs*, presumable reflecting a former hacek s.

Borrowings: Literary Mongolian *jarma*, Khalkha Mongolian *zaram*. Also borrowed in Bulgarian, Serbocroatian, and Vogul and Ostyak, two West Siberian languages related to Hungarian.

4. ***qagut***: "fried grain, enriched with fat and sweetened." This word, well attested in Medieval sources, appears to survive only in Osmanli ("parched grain or pulse") and Azerbaijani ("pounded groats, fried wheat or peas prepared with pounded sugar"). DL: *qawut*, "porridge of parched millet kneaded with butter and sugar." KI: *qawut*, "well-known dish." TZ: *qawut*, "pudding." BM: *qawut*, "cooked grain." DL remarks that it was a dish for women

in childbed.

Borrowings: This word has been used in Farsi ("porridge; mixed flour and legumes with sweetening, of dry consistency") and Arabic. Two thirteenth century Arabic cookbooks, *Kitab al-Wuslah 'ila al-Habib* and *Kitab Wasf al-'At'imah al-Mu'tadah*, give several recipes for *qawut* each, ranging in complexity from fried rice ground and mixed with butter and honey to porridges of several mixed grains enriched with butter and nut oils, honey and sugar, mixed nuts, and saffron.

V. Boiled Grain

A slippery category. The meaning can shift from porridge to whole grain in soup to noodles.

5. ***butqa***: "grain boiled with milk." The Chuvash word *pata*, as well as the form in which the word was borrowed in Mongol (*buda'an*) and Jürchen (*puh-tu-kuai*), suggest that *butqa* was originally pronounced something like *butaqa*. In the Northeastern Group, *butqa* means meal boiled with milk; in the Southwest and Mid-Central languages it is a rice porridge, and in the Central Northwest languages a porridge or puree. If the Yakut word *butugas* is from this root (perhaps with the addition of a suffix *-c* which is otherwise only seen in the common food-name suffix *-mac*), this word may antedate the knowledge of grain. *Butugas* is a Yakut soup. It is made from thickened yogurt enriched with ground roots, pine needles and animal bones (which lactic acid eventually disintegrates). The thickened and then frozen yogurt is called *tar* (appropriately enough) and the *butugas* is made from it. TZ: *butqa*, "rice cooked with milk."

Borrowings: The original meaning of *buda'an* in Mongolian is said to have been "thickened soup"; modern Khalkha Mongolian knows the meanings "groats, millet groats, grain, porridge." The Tuva (Northeast) have adopted the Mongol form of the word with this meaning. The Ordos Mongols of China use *budaa* to mean "noodles." The book MA records words in fourteenth century Western Mongolian as well as Turkish, and apparently the Western Mongols were using the expression *eckäksän budaan*, "sliced *budaan*," for noodles. The modern Buriat Mongols use *budaa* for "groats," *budaan* for "barley."

This word was borrowed by Manchu-Tungus languages at an early date. The Jürchens, who ruled North China as the Jin Dynasty, used *puh-tu-kuai* for "rice." In Manchu *buda* means "porridge, boiled dishes in general, mealtime" and in the languages of the Manchu-Tungus family spoken on Sakhalin Island and the lower Amur it means "millet" or "groats."

6. ***köcä***: "boiled grain dish." This word is found in Northern Altai (E) with the meanings "thickened soup" and "barley." In Salar (Kansu Province, China), it means "whole wheat porridge." In Kazakh it is grain, sometimes fried, pounded and then boiled in soup or milk. In Kirgiz (Mid-Central) it is millet or wheat groats; in the Talas dialect of Kirgiz, noodles. TZ: "groats."

Borrowings: The Persian-speaking Tajiks of Central Asia have borrowed this word as the name of a dish of groats boiled with sorghum flour and flavored with yogurt. The word was known in Medieval Osmanli, and Byzantinists have occasionally derived it from the Greek *kokkion*, seed. Needless to say, the antiquity of the word, its concentration among the Northeastern languages and its presence in China rule this derivation out.

7. ***ügrä***: "grain soup/noodle soup." In Northern Altai, "porridge of groats and milk"; in Abakan, "barley soup." In the Central area, it is "groat soup" in the Northwest, "noodles cut small" in the Southeast. DL: "noodles, like *tutmac* but softer; *qïyma ügrä*: noodles cut like birds' tongues." MA: "noodles cut thin."

Borrowings: Found in Farsi, Pashto, Urdu ("a dish like *khicri;* gruel, pottage").

8. ***bulamïq/bulgamac***: "porridge," from a verb meaning "to mix." Found in all subdivisions of the Central group in the sense "thin porridge, flour soup." In Salar (China): "thick porridge of flour and butter." Both forms are attested in the Middle Ages, but today the form *bulgamac* is only found in SW: Osmanli "thick soup of flour, butter and sugar," Azerbaijani: "porridge of bulghur, legumes and cheese; sweet porridge or pudding." MA: *bulamaq*, "porridge." DL: *bulgamac*, "pudding without sweetening or butter." KI, BM: *bulgamac*, "pudding."

Borrowings: In Ossetic, an Iranian language of the Caucasus; Mari, a Finnish language of the upper Volga (*pulamak*, "puree"). Also in Kalmyk, the Mongolian language of the western Caspian: "flour boiled with salt and butter, national dish of the Kalmuks." The SW form has been borrowed in Serbocroatian and Bulgarian in the senses "porridge" and "insipid dish; gum."

VI. Noodles

9. ***tutmac***: "noodles." Found at the extreme ends of Turkish territory, in the Northeast and the Southwest. In Central Asia found on the upper Volga and among the Qaraim of Lithuania and the Crimea, but strangely missing in the MC and CSE languages. DL, KI, BM, MA: "noodles."

Borrowings: This word was in common use in Persian and Arabic during the Middle Ages. The Arabic books *Kitab al-Wuslah* and *Kitab Wasf al-At'imah al-Mu'tadah* call for dough "rolled out as for *tutmaj*" in recipes where the dough is to be stuffed. A stuffed pasta requires a sturdier dough than can be tolerated in plain noodles, and it may be that *tutmac* dough was rolled less fine than the noodles the Arabs were familiar with. This word has been borrowed in Serbocroatian, Rumanian, Armenian, and possibly Albanian (*tumatshe*, "dough sheets," also *tumats*, "noodles").

10. ***uvmac***: "small soup noodles, pea-shaped dumplings." Evidently from *uvmaq* "to crush." Missing in the Northeastern languages but widely found in the Center and the Southwest, including the Salar and Qaraim languages. The meaning has shifted in several languages. In Uighur it is "a boiled mixture of vegetables and cornmeal; cornmeal and wheat boiled together," and in Osmanli it is said to mean "couscous; porridge; a rustic dish with thin bread crumbled in it; fresh flour and curdled milk" (formed into pellets?). Not found in the Medieval Turkish vocabularies.

Borrowings: Found in Persian as early as the fourteenth century. In Afghanistan, borrowed by Pashto ("porridge with vegetables") and Yaghnobi ("thickened soup with dumplings").

11. ***cöp***: "a single noodle." The word seems to have survived

only in Uighur and Uzbek, where *cöp* or *cöp-as* is the name of a particular noodle dish. DL: *cöp*, "a single noodle."

Borrowings: none apart from the *YSZY*.

12. ***salma***: "small flat soup noodles, round or square." This is a dish of the Central group, a Golden Horde pasta. The Kazakh form is cut square, the Tatar form curled like Italian *cavatelli*. The Bashkirs either cut noodle paste square or simply pinch off pieces of dough, like Hungarian *csipetke*. The fifteenth century Arabic cookbook *Kitab al-Tibakhah* describes *salma* as "shaped with the fingers like coins."

Borrowings: Apart from the appearance in *Kitab al-Tibakhah*, apparently very few. The Chuvash have borrowed this word and apply it to small pieces or balls of cooked dough, whether boiled in soup, baked on a hearthstone or fried in a pan.

VII. Breads, Cakes, and Pastries

13. ***bogïrsaq/bagïrsaq***: "rich dough fried in small pieces." This snack is found throughout Central Asia, where it is taken with tea or carried by travelers as a provision for the road. The Osmanli and Northeastern forms may be borrowings. The Tatars make this product coin-shaped, the Bashkirs bun-like, the Uzbeks ball-shaped. The Kazakhs, who as nomads have great use for road food, have the greatest variety of forms, round, square, oval, and triangular, and make leavened as well as unleavened versions. The fluctuation of the first vowel may reflect folk etymologies connecting this word with *bogrug* "bulge (in a milk sack, *e.g.*)," and *bagïrsaq* "entrails." TZ: *bursaq*, "bread; a Tatar word."

Borrowings: This word is widespread in the Mongolian languages. Khalkha: "rich dough fried in thick cakes; bread, pastry." Ordos: "cake, bread." Kalmyk: "thin bread fried in butter." The Persian-speakers of Afghanistan leaven the dough but do not allow it to rise, and roll the lumps of dough on a sieve to impress a pattern of indentations in them. This word has been adopted in western Siberia by Vogul and in Afghanistan by Yaghnobi.

14. ***quymaq***: "batter cake, fried cake." From the verb *quymaq*,

"to pour out." Found in the Central and Southwestern groups. Uighur: "thin cakes baked in fat with sugar, used only in ceremonial offerings." In Uzbek, Kazakh, and Kirgiz, "thick fried cake of leavened dough made with eggs." The Tatar form can be leavened or unleavened, and made not only with wheat but millet, oats, buckwheat or pea flour. Osmanli: "flour, bulghur and spinach kneaded and baked; dish like rice pudding of sweetened buttered flour; cheese omelette." Azerbaijani: "sweet flour porridge with butter." DL: *quyma*, "a fried bread; the dough is made thin, of the consistency of pancake batter, then it is poured on butter boiling in a pot and made thin in it until done. Then it is taken out and sugar is sprinkled on it." KI: "pudding fried in fat; also a name for *zulabiya*" (viz., free form fritters; the word *zulabiya* appears in India as *jilebi*).

Borrowings: the Volga Finnish language Mordvin; Literary, Khalkha, and Buriat Mongolian (in the last, said to mean "curds and whey"). Urdu: "a sort of bread made of flour, white of eggs and onion, fried in ghi."

15. ***cälpäk***: "thin bread or cake fried in butter." Probably made with a thicker batter than *quymaq*; associated words refer to fluids of medium thickness such as mucus and mud. Basically a word of the Mid-Central and CSE area, but also found in Turkmen. The Tatar form of the name has a borrowed look. The Tatars fry this bread in rather deep fat, manipulating it with a pair of sticks as it fried to form ruffles in it. MA: *celbäk tabasï* (not defined, but the phrase means "*cälpäk* pan").

Borrowings: In Iran (fourteenth century): *calpak*, "thin bread cooked in oil." Tajik, "leavened pancakes fried in butter, a ritual dish." Urdu: "thin *chapati* in oil." Kalmyk: "pancake."

16. ***ätmäk, ötmäk***: "bread." Missing in MC and CSE but well represented everywhere else, in the Northeast and Southwest and among the Golden Horde nations. In a number of widely separate languages the *t* is replaced by *k*, probably to avoid confusion with the verb *ätmäk*, to do: *e.g.*, Salar *egimex*, *ekmex*, *e'mex*; Tatar and Bashkir *ikmäk*; Osmanli *ekmek*. DL: *ätmäk*, *ötmäk*, *epmäk* (the last form said to be used by the Yaghma and Tokshi and some of the Oghuz and Qipchaq; that is, in eastern Xinjiang, north of the

Jaxartes, and in the westernmost parts of Central Asia): "bread." KI: *ätmäk*, "bread." MA: *etmäk*. TZ: *ötmäk*.

Borrowings: Kamas Samoyed, *ippek*; Serbocroatian, *ekmek*. In names of Ottoman Turkish pastries such as *ekmek kadayif* it has passed into specialized used in Arabic, Armenian, and the Balkan languages. The twelfth century Persian poet Khaqani uses both *atmak* and *akmak*. The Kalmyk Mongols have a borrowed the word as *ödmg*.

17. ***kömäc***: "ashcake, bread cooked in hot ashes," from *kömmäk*, "to bury." Missing in the Northeast but common elsewhere. This simple preparation has in a few places evolved in unusual directions. Among the Kirgiz it is "a flatbread of rich dough, coin-sized, baked in ashes and served with hot milk flavored with butter and sour milk." Among the Tatars it is "a small roll made with wheat, pea or lentil flour; a bun, small pie, white bread; layered bread with poppyseed between the layers." Bashkir: "unleavened flatbread;" in Argayash dialect, meat "soup" (?). Turkmen: "thin bread stuffed with cracklings or chopped meat, cooked in ashes." In standard Osmanli *gümec* today means "honeycomb," because of the shape, but in dialect usage *gömme* is "bread cooked in ashes; *börek*-like bread stuffed with meat and onions, cooked on a hot brick or griddle." DL: *kömäc*, "bread which is buried in hot ashes."

Borrowings: The word was used in Persia from the fourteenth century: "Thin bread baked in ashes; thin unleavened bread of rice flour." In the thirteenth century Arabic books *Kitab al-Wuslah* and *Kitab Wasf*, *kumaj* is often called for but not described. In modern Syrian Arabic, it is a common name for the familiar Syrian "pocket bread." In Pashto it refers to a big piece of unleavened bread.

18: ***toqac***: "round flatbread." Probably connected with *toq*, "full, satiated." Found today only in Uighur and Kirgiz. In the latter language it is the general word for bread. DL: "round flatbread." Early editions of DL erroneously read the word as *toquc* instead of *toqac*.

Borrowings: None.

19: ***cöräk***: "fine bread." Found only in the Southwest and in

Kazakh ("a kind of *bogïrsaq*") and Karakalpak ("flatbread"). In Osmanli it is "bun, cake; loaf, usually sweetened"; in Azerbaijani it is "white bread, baked bread, large unsoured flatbread." DL: *cöräk*, "round, flat loaf (*qurs*)." KI: "loaf, crumb." TZ: *shöräk*, "cake, dried bread (*ka'k*)." *cöräk*, "round flatbread."

Borrowings: Iraqi Arabic: *churak*, "a kind of bread shaped like a pretzel." Syrian Arabic: *shraik*, "Bedouin flatbread." Egyptian Arabic: *shureik*, "leavened bread made with butter, sesame, and other aromatics; a semolina cake eaten during Ramadan." Widely found in the Balkans and the Caucasus as a rich coffeecake or festival bread: *e.g. tsourekia*, a Greek Easter bread.

20. ***yuvqa***: "thin flatbread." Spotty distribution in the Central (Tatar, Kirgiz; Galician Qaraim, "unleavened bread") and Southwestern groups (Osmanli: "thin bread cooked on a griddle"; Azerbaijani, "thin rolled unleavened bread"). DL: *yuvga*, *yupqa*, "thin bread"; *yuvga*, *qatma yuvga*, *yarma yuvga*, "folded (wrinkled? pleated?) bread" (*khubz mughaddan*).

The grain food by this name (which is also simply the Turkish word for "thin, fragile") has shown two remarkable characteristics. The more important is that it has often been used to construct thicker products, a practice noted as early as DL (*v.* supra). The present-day Tatars stack up 10 or 12 buttered *yokas* and cut them in wedges like a cake to be served with tea. The Uzbeks, having prepared 10 or 12 raw *yupqas*, fry one on both sides, sprinkle a filling of fried meat and onions on it, cover the filling with a raw *yupqa* and then flip this "sandwich" over. They repeat the process on the other side while the raw *yupqa* is frying, and so on until a thick cake is built up.

The extreme case of this layering developed in Turkey and has spread through Central Europe and in recent years the world: filo or strudel dough, for which there is no antecedent in Greece, Rome, Byzantium or any Persian or Arab cuisine. In modern Turkish *yufka* primarily means a single sheet of filo. It is likely that the refinement of stretching the dough paper-thin originated in the kitchens of the Topkapi Palace in Istanbul; there is a distinct historical association with Topkapi Palace in the custom of the Baklava Alayï, the procession of the Janissaries through the streets of Istanbul on the fifteenth day of Ramadan carrying trays of baklava from the royal kitchens.

In Azerbaijan we have what looks like the "missing link" between the simple nomad's treat of stacked-up thin breads and the sophisticated baklava of Turkey. In addition to the usual baklavas, the Azerbaijanis make a strange, crude pastry they call Baku baklava (*Bakï paxlavasï*). Instead of 50 or 100 sheets of paper-thin dough, this pastry uses eight sheets of ordinary noodle paste with seven layers of sweetened nuts between each. The simplest way to account for this peculiar product is to see it as an early result of the contact between the cooking traditions of the Turks and the Near Eastern peasants: the nomad's dish of stacked breads, developed for cooking on his portable iron griddle, adapted to the more luxurious circumstances of the peasant's bread oven. Baklava, then, would seem to be older than the paper-thin "filo dough" with which it is made nearly everywhere; everywhere, that is, except in Azerbaijan, that gateway between the Turkmen steppes and Anatolia, and among the Tatars, who have adopted this archaic form of baklava, along with the name (*päxläwä*), from the Azerbaijanis.

The less important tendency is to boil thin bread in milk. The Kirgiz *jupka* is such a dish, and in Turkey (and the countries under Turkish culinary influence) a pudding-like sweet called *güllaç* is made from wafers soaked in milk. (In Egyptian Arabic, *gullash* is the word for filo) The borrowing of the word in the Balkan languages suggests that this practice was at one time far more widespread.

Borrowings: Persian *yukha*, "thin bread"; as early as the fourteenth century. The word has been borrowed in all the Balkan languages (except Greek) with the sense of noodles.

21. ***pöshkäl***: "thin flatbread." This word has apparently survived only in Uzbek, where it means a layered product built up in the kettle like the Uzbeki *yupqa* with sour cream instead of meat and onions in the filling, and in Uighur, where it means "pancake, dumpling, rich flatbread"; *tuxum poshkal*, literally egg *poshkal*, is said to mean an omelette. DL: *pöshkäl*, "thin flatbread."

Borrowings: apparently none.

22. ***qatlama***: "a particular kind of layered bread." Found throughout the Central and Southwestern areas; the two CSE lan-

guages use a related word, *qatïrma*, and in the eleventh century DL listed a related expression, *qatma yuvgha* (see #20 above).

The layers are neither so thin nor so clearly organized as layers in this product as they are in European puff paste. The typical recipe (Uzbek, Turkmen, Kazakh, Tatar) involves rolling out noodle paste, brushing it with melted butter and then rolling it up like a jelly roll. This roll is sliced crosswise into disks which are flattened out by hand or with a rolling pin before frying. In the flattening process, rudimentary layers are produced, partly spiral and partly flat due to slippage of the dough. The Kazakh and Tatar forms may include some sort of filling with the butter such as poppyseed, hemp seed, walnuts, cheese (among the Tatars) or dried fruit (among the Kazakhs). Something like this recipe is suggested in the definitions given for the word in other languages. Qaraim (Galicia and Lithuania): "fried flatbread, cheesecake with layered pastry." Kirgiz: "layered dough, rich pastry served in bouillon." Azerbaijani: "layered *börek* made with leavened dough." Karakalpak: "layered (dough, pie)." Osmanli: "a kind of buttered thin bread fried on a griddle; cornbread."

Borrowings: Pashto and Yaghnobi: "layered fried flatbreads." Chuvash: "layered flatbread; potato tart." Mari: "cake of unleavened dough filled with hemp seed."

23. ***böräk***: "fried or baked pie; dough stuffed with meat or a sweet filling." Basically a Southwestern word, but also found in Kazakh, Karakalpak, the northern Caucasus and (a clear borrowing) among the Bashkirs of Orenburg. It is the familiar Turkish *börek*. In Turkmen it is boiled, a sort of ravioli. KI: *böräk*, "pieces of dough stuffed with meat." The sweet variety is called *cäkärli böräk*. BM: *böräk*, "dough stuffed with meat"; *cäkär böräk*.

This word is widely borrowed in the eastern Mediterranean and Near East: Arabic (Syrian and Egyptian *burak/bureik*, Tunisian *brik*, Algerian *braka*), Persian (from the fourteenth century), all the Balkan languages including Greek, and Armenian, and in Kalmyk Mongol. Some books refer to a Chuvash word *pürek*, which is not in the usual dictionaries. This word is a puzzle: It looks like a borrowing from Tatar, except that the word *böräk* (*büräk*) is apparently not used in Tatar. An unconvincing attempt has been made to derive the Chuvash *pürek*, and even the pan-

Turkish *böräk*, from the Russian word *pirog*.

VIII. Puzzling Cases

24. ***lavash***: "lavash, a large flatbread, often baked hard for keeping." Found in the Southwest, borrowed in Tatar and Bashkir. The distribution suggests an innovation (or borrowing) in the Southwest, except that ninth and tenth century Uighur writings we find the word *liv* (borrowed from some other language; no native Turkish word begins with l) and a compound word *liv-ash*, incorporating the Turkish word for cooked food. Both words mean "food; ritual food." Since this word seems to have meant a boiled grain dish (*liv-ash* is declared to be rice in one Turfan text), the connection of *lavash* and *liv-ash* is extremely speculative. In Tatar, *läwäs* means not only a flatbread but a sort of small pie: a circle of unleavened dough folded over a filling of raisins, sugar and butter, and then fried.

Borrowings: The word *lavash* is found in Persian, Armenian and Georgian. The Ossetes of the central Caucasus have borrowed the word twice: directly as *lawïz/lauz*, "pancake," and (via Georgian) *lawasi*, "flatbread."

25. ***mün/bün***: "soup." The word survives in Yakut and Tuva with this meaning. DL remarks that in Eastern Xinjiang he found it to be a soup with noodles.

26. ***agartgu***: defined as "wheat beer" in DL; from *agarmaq*, "to be white" (*cf.*, berliner *Weisse*). If this word has indeed survived, it is only in the Northeast and in aberrant form. *Abïrtki* is the usual word for beer among the Altays, and *abïrtka* among the Shors.

27. ***boza***: "beer." Found in the Central and Southwestern languages; possibly also in Chuvash (*para*, from a hypothetical Bulghar form **boraga*; but some linguists believe the Chuvash reflex of *boza* is another word, *puiyr*). Usually no particular grain is specified. KI: *boza*, "wheat or barley beer."

Borrowings: Arabic, Persian, Serbocroatian, Albanian, Urdu. If the

Chuvash *para* is from **boraga*, this may be the origin of the Russian word *braga* ("mash; homebrewed beer").

It is tempting to connect this word with the old Osmanli and Chagatai Turkish word *bozu* ("a drink of camel's milk") and to Literary Mongolian *boju* ("dregs, sediment after distilling whey") and hence to Kalmyk *boz* ("vodka distilled from fermented milk"). The older sense of *boza* as a drink fermented from milk rather than grain could then be seen in the word as borrowed in Pashto *boza*, "kumyss, soured drink."

Addendum: Forgotten Grain Foods

The dictionary compiled by Mahmud of Kashgar in the eleventh century lists a number of grain-based foods and drinks that have not survived. Although Iran's cultural influence on the Turks was probably greater than China's, surprisingly many of the words seem to be of Chinese origin. This is doubtless an artifact of Mahmud's own background. He recorded Chinese words current on the steppes but not Iranian words, because he could presume the readers of his dictionary already knew them. When he recognized them as Iranian, of course; the Turkish word for barley, *arpa*, is thought to come from the Iranian word **arbusa*, but it is an East Iranian or Scythian word (cf. Khotanese Saka *rrusa*, Pashto *orbësi*) rather than the Standard Persian *jau*.

avzurï: a cooked mixture of wheat and barley flour (conceivably borrowed from Persian *afshureh*, a dish of pressed fruit juices which was sometimes thickened with flour).
begni, bekni: a drink of wheat, millet and barley: still used in the fifteenth century Chagatai literary language.
buxsï: cooked wheat mixed with almonds, honey and milk and left to sour; the wheat and almonds were eaten and the liquid drunk.
buxsum: millet beer.
böskäc: loaf bread.
cuqmïn: a cake steamed in a pot. The second syllable suggests the Chinese *mian* 麵, "noodle."
közmän: a cake cooked in ashes.
kürsäk: millet boiled in water or milk and flavored with butter.
kävshäk: a word meaning "limp" also used for a soft bread.

letü: noodles chilled with water, snow or ice. The pronunciation of this word is uncertain; the first element, at least, may be Chinese: *leng* 冷, "chilled."
sincü: a bread described as being between flatbread and loaf bread.
suma: malted wheat or barley for porridge, bread or beer. The second syllable is probably the Chinese word for wheat.
sorush: wheat roasted in the ear before the grains harden.
to: perhaps a beer; the definition makes it a drink of soured batter. Possibly a Chinese word.
top/töp: barley dough left in a warm place to sour (cf. Kazakh *töp* "porridge," Kirgiz top, "dregs").
tamata: breading ("dough smeared on fat chicken or meat so that the fat will not run out when the meat is roasted"). The first consonant is uncertain, and the word might have been pronounced *yamata*.

Linguistic Sources:

Medieval sources:

Mahmud al-Kashgari. *Kitab Diwan Lughat al-Turk*. Istanbul: Ahmet Rifat Matbaasi, 1915-17.
Rachmeti, G. R., ed. "Turkische Turfan-Texte VII." *Abhandlungen der Preussischen Akademie der Wissenschaften* 12 (1936): 1-124.
Athir al-Din Abu Hayyan al-Andalusi. *Kitab al-'Idrak li-Lisan al-'Atrak*. Istanbul: Evkaf Matbaasi, 1930.
Poppe, N. N. *Mongol'skii Slovar' Mukaddimat al-Adab*. 3 vols. Leningrad: Akademia Nauk, 1938-9.
Ettuhfet-üz-Zekiyye fil-Lugat-it-Türkiyye. Istanbul, 1945.
Jamal al-Din Abu Muhammad al-Turki. *Bulghat al-Mushtaq fi Lughat al-Turk wal-Qifjaq*. Warsaw: Polska Akademia Nauk, Panstowe Wydanictwo Naukowe, 1958.

General works:

Clauson, Sir Gerard. *An Etymological Dictionary of Pre-Thirteenth Century Turkish*. Oxford: Oxford University Press, 1972.
Doerfer, Gerhard. *Turkische und Mongolische Elemente in Neu-*

persischen. 4 vols. Wiesbaden: Franz Steiner Verlag, 1963-75.
Kukhnia Narodov USSR. Minsk: Izd. Polymia, 1981.
Levin, M. G., and Potapov, L. P., eds. *The Peoples of Siberia*, Chicago: University of Chicago Press, 1964 (translation of *Narody Sibiri*. Moscow: Russian Academy of Science, 1956). This book records for Abakan (Khakasy) the words *talkan*, *köce*, *ügre*, *tutpac* and *abïrtki*, for Shor the word *abïrtka* and for Altay the word *kurmac* (missing in the Baskakov works listed below).
Pokhlebkin, V. V. *Natsional'nye Kukhni Nashikh Narodov*. Moscow: Pishchevaia Promyshtennost', 1978.
Titiunnik, A. I., and Novozhenov, Iu. M. *Sovetskaia Natsional'naia i Zarubezhnaia Kukhnia*. Moscow: Vyeshaia Shkola, 1977.

Individual languages:

Tuva: Pal'mbakh, A. A. *Russko-Tuvinskii Slovar'*. Moscow: Gosud. Izd. Inostrannikh i Natsional'nikh Slovarei, 1953. *dalgan*, *borsak*, *bïda*, *carba*, *mün*.
North Altai: Baskakov, N. A. *Dialekt Chernevykh Tatar*. Moscow: Izd. Nauka, 1966, and *Dialekt Kumandintsev*. Moscow: Izd. Nauka, 1972. *talkan*, *d'arma*, *ürä*, *botko*, *ötpäk*, *tutmash/tutpash*, *buza*.
Salar: Tenishev, E. R. *Stroi Salarskogo Iazyka*. Moscow: Izd. Nauka, 1976. *ekmek*, *qurmas*, *kodza*, *komes*, *umas*, *pilemax*.
Uighur: Raquette, G. *An Eastern Turki Dictionary*, Lunds Universitets Absskrifts NE Avd. I, Bd. 23, Nr. 4, Lund: 1936; Jarring, Gunnar. *An Eastern Turki-English Dialect Dictionary*, Lunds Universitets Absskrift NE Avd. I, Bd. 56, Nr. 4, Lund: 1964; Nadzhip, F. N., *Uigursko-Russkii Slovar'*. Moscow: Izd. Sovetskoi Entsiklopedii, 1968. Schwarz, H.G., *An Uyghur-English Dictionary*, Bellingham: Center for East Asian Studies, 1992. *talqan*, *qo(r)mac*, *yarma*, *botka*, *ügre*, *umac*, *bogorsoq*, *cälpäk*, *quymaq*, *kömäc*, *toqac*, *qatlima*, *boze*.
Uzbek: Makhmudov, Karim. *Uzbekskie Bliuda*. Tashkent: Gos. Tashkent: Izd. Uzbekskoi SSR, 1962. Waterson, Natalie. *Uzbek-English Dictionary*. Oxford: Oxford University Press, 1980. *talqon*, *yorma*, *butqa*, *bulamiq*, *ugra*, *umac*, *bŭgirsoq*, *calpak*, *quymoq*, *kŭmac*, *yupqa*, *qatlama*, *bŭza*.
Kirgiz: Iudakhin, K. K. *Kirgizsko-Russkii Slovar'*. Moscow: Izd. Sovetskoi Entsiklopedii, 1965. *talqan*, *kuurmac*, *jarma*, *botko*,

köjö, bulamïk, umac, boorsok, calpak, kuymak, kömöc, tokoc, jupka, kattama, bozo.

Kazakh: *Kazakhskaia Kukhnia.* Alma-Ata: Izd. Kainar, 1981; Chastnyi, P.M. *Natsional'nye Bliuda Kazakhstana.* Alma-Ata: Kazakhs. Gos. Izd., 1962. *talkan, zarma, botka, közä, umash, salma, bawïrsak, shelpäk, kuymak, shüräk, kattama, böräk, boza.*

Karakalpak: Baskakov, N. A. *Russko-Karakalpakskii Slovar'.* Moscow: Izd. Sovetskoi Entsiklopedii, 1962. *taqan, zarma, botqa, bïlamïq, bawïrsaq, shelpäk, quymaq, kömash, shöräk, qattama, böräk.*

Tatar: *Tatarskaia Kulinariia.* Kazan: Kazan Tatarskoe Knizhnoe Izdatel'stvo, 1981; *Tatarsko-Russkii Slovar'.* Moscow: Izd. Sovetskoi Entsiklopedii, 1966. *talkan, botka, bolamïc, öirä, umac, tokmac, salma, baursak, celpäk, koymak, kümäc, ikmäk, yoka, katlama, buza, läwäsh.*

Bashkir: *Bashkirsko-Russkii Slovar'.* Moscow: Gos. Izd. Inostran. i Nats. Slovarei, 1958. *talqan, qurmas, yarma, butqa, bolamïq, öirä, tuqmas, halma, bauïrhaq, qoymaq, kümäsh, ikmäk, qatlama, läüäsh.*

Qaraim: Zajaczkowski (Zaionchkovskii), A. *Karaimsko-Pol'sko-Russkii Slovar'.* Moscow: Izd. Russkii Iazyk, 1974. *umac* (Lithuania), *tutmac* (Lithuania, Crimea), *kömäc* (Crimea), *ötmäk/ätmäk/äkmäk* (Crimea, Galicia), *yuvga* (Galicia), *qatlama* (Lithuania, Galicia), *boza/buza* (Crimea).

Azerbaijani: Akhynda, M. F. *Fransïzja Azärbayjanja Lügät.* Baku: Maarip Näshriyyatï, 1965; Azizbekov, Kh. A. *Azärbayjanja-Rusja Lügät.* Baku: Gosudarstvennoe Izdatel'stvo, 1955. *yarma, bulamac, umac, govut, guymag, äppäk, cöräk, yuxa, gatlama, lavash.*

Turkmen: Bogdasarov, A., Vanukevich, A. and Khudayshukurov, T. *Turkmenskaia Kulinariia.* Ashkhabad: Izd. Turkmenistan, 1981; Baskakov, N. A. *Turkmensko-Russkii Slovar'.* Moscow: Izd. Sovetskoi Entsiklopedii, 1968. *talxan, govurga, yarma, bulamaq, ovmac, celpäk, kömäc, cöräk, qatlama* (and *qatlaklïnan*), *böräk, lavash.*

Osmanli: Kosay, Hamit Z., and Ülkücan, Akile. *Anadolu Yemekleri ve Türk Mutfagı.* Ankara: Milli Egetim Basımevi, 1961; *Türkiyede Halk Agızdan Söz Derleme Dergisi.* Istanbul: Maarif Matbaasi, 1939; Redhouse, James W. *A Turkish and English Lexicon.* Constantinople 1890. *yarma, kavurmaç, bulamaç, ogmaç, tutmaç, bogursak, kavut, kuyma(k), gömme, çörek, yufka, katlama(ç), börek, boza, lavas.*

Chuvash: Egorov, E. G. *Etimologicheskii Slovar' Chuvashskogo Iazyka.* Cheboksary: Chuvashskoe Knizhnoe Izdatel'stvo, 1964; Skvortsov, M. I. *Chuvashsko-Russkii Slovar'.* Moscow: "Russkii Iazyk" Izdatel'stvo, 1972. *păta, salma, tukmas, xutlami.*

Yakut: Sleptsov, P. A. *Yakutsko-Russkii Slovar'.* Moscow: Izd. Sovietskoi Entsiklopedii. *butugas.*

Literary/Khalkha Mongol: Lessing, Ferdinand et al. *A Mongolian-English Dictionary.* Berkeley: University of California Press, 1960. *talqan/talx, buda'an/budaa, qoimagh/xoimogh, ba'ursugh/ boorsogh.*

Buriat Mongol: Tsydendambaev, Ts. B., and Imekhanov, M. N. *Kratkii Russko-Buriatskii Slovar'.* Moscow: Gos. Izd. Inostran. i. Nats. Slovarei, 1962. *talxan, budaa/budaan, boorsog, xoimog, bozo.*

Ordos Mongol: Mostaert, Antoine, CICM, *Dictionnaire Ordos.* Peking: The Catholic University, 1944. *BuDa, Dalxa, borsok.*

Kalmyk Mongol: Muniev, V. D. *Kalmytsko-Russkii Slovar'.* Moscow: Izd. Russkii Slovar', 1971. *talxn, budan, bulmg, boorsg, tselwg, ödmg, börg, boz.*

Tungus: Vasilevich, B. M. *Evenkiisko-Russkii Slovar'.* Moscow: Gos. Izd. Inostran. i Nats. Slovarei, 1958. *talqan, buda.*

Urdu: Platts, John T. *A Dictionary of Urdu, Classical Hindi and English.* Oxford: Oxford University Press, 1930. *talkha, ogra, chalpak, qo'emaq, kumac/kumaj, boza.*

Pashto: Aslanov, M. G. *Afgansko-Russkii Slovar'.* Moscow: Izd. Sovetskoi Entsiklopedii, 1966. *talxan, ugra, amac, kumac, katlama, boza.*

Persian: *Divan-e-At'emat-e-MavlanaAbu Ishaq-e-Hallaj-e-Shirazi.* Galata: Chapkhaneh-ye-Abussina, 1302 AH (1883 AD); Steingass, F. *Persian-English Dictionary.* London, 1930. *qavut, bulamaj, calpak, tutmaj, umaj, kumaj, burak, curak, talxan, boza, yuxa.*

Tajik: Aminov, S., and Vanukevich, N. *Tadzhikskaia Kulinariia.* Dushanbe: Izd. Irfon, 1966; Rakhimi, M. V., and Uspenskii, L. V. *Tadzhiksko-Russkii Slovar'.* Moscow: Gos. Izd. Inostran. i Nats. Slovarei, 1956. *talqon, yorma, kùci, ugro, umoc, calpak, quymoq, kumac, curak, qatlama, bùza.*

Ossetic: Kasaev, A. M. *Osetinsko-Russkii Slovar'.*Moscow: Gos.

Izd. Inostran. i Nats. Slovarei, 1952. *bylamiq/bylamuq; lawyz/lawashi.*

Arabic: Mielck, Reinhard. *Terminologie und Technologie der Müller und Bäcker im islamischen Mittelalter.* Gluckstadt/Hamburg: J.J. Augustin, 1913; Farah, Madelain. *Lebanese Cuisine.* Portland, 1974; Woodhead, D. R., and Beene, Wayne. *A Dictionary of Iraqi Arabic: Arabic-English.* Washington DC: Georgetown University Press, 1967. *kumaj, shuraik, burak.*

Serbocroatian: Knezevic, Anton. *Die Turzism in der Sprache der Kroaten und Serben.* Meisenheim am Glan: Verlag Anton Hain, 1962. *bulamac, burek, curek, ekmek, jufka, tutmac, boza.*

Albanian: Boretzky, Norbert. *Der Turkische Einfluss auf das Albanische.* Wiesbaden: Otto Harassowitz, 1971. Meyer, Gustav, *Etymologisches Worterbuch der Albanischen Sprache,* Strassburg, 1891. *çyrek, jufkë, byrek, bozë, tumatshe, tumats.*

Rumanian: Wendt, Heinz F. *Die Turkische Elemente im Rumänische.* Berlin: 1960. *tocmagi.*

Mari: *Mariisko-Russkii Slovar'.* Moscow: Gos. Izd. Inost. i Nats. Slovarei, 1956. *pulamyq, katlama.*

BIBLIOGRAPHY

Adalsteinsson, Stefán. "Importance of Sheep in Early Icelandic Agriculture." In *The Norse of the North Atlantic* (Acta Archaeologica 61), ed. Gerald F. Bigelow, 285-91. Kobenhavn: Levin and Munksgaard, 1991

Adams, Robert McCormick. *Land Behind Baghdad.* Chicago: University of Chicago Press, 1965

Ahmadov, Ahmad-Chabir. *Azarbajchan Kulinarijasy.* Baku: Ishyg, 1986

Ahsan, M. M. *Social Life under the Abbasids.* Arab Background Series, ed. N. A. Ziadeh. London and New York: Librairie du Liban, 1979

Akademiya Nauk SSSR, Institut Yazykoznaniya. *Drevnetyurskiy Slovar'.* Leningrad: Nauka, 1969

Algar, Ayla Esen. *The Complete Book of Turkish Cooking.* London: Kegan Paul International, 1985

-------. *Classical Turkish Cooking. Traditional Turkish Food for the American Kitchen.* New York: Harper Collins, 1991

Allsen, Thomas T. "The Yüan Dynasty and the Uighurs of Turfan in the 13th. Century." In Rossabi, 1983: 243-80

-------. *Mongol Imperialism.* Berkeley: University of California Press, 1987

-------. *Commodity and Exchange in the Mongol Empire, a Cultural History of Islamic Textiles.* Cambridge: Cambridge University Press (Cambridge Studies in Islamic Civilization), 1997

-------. *Culture and Conquest in Mongol Eurasia.* Cambridge: Cambridge University Press (Cambridge Studies in Islamic Civilization), 2001

-------. "Ögedei and Alcohol." *Mongolian Studies*, XXIX (2007), 3-12.

Ames, T. Roger. *The Art of Rulership: A Study in Ancient Chinese Political Thought.* Honolulu: University of Hawaii Press, 1983

An Zhimin. "Archaeological Research on Neolithic China." *Current Anthropology* 29 (1988): 5: 753-9

-------. "Prehistoric Agriculture in China." In *Foraging and Farming*, eds. David Harris and G. Hillman, 643-8. Cambridge: Cambridge University Press, 1989

Anderson, E. N. "Why Is Humoral Medicine So Popular?" *Social Science and Medicine* 25 (1987): 4: 331-7

-------. *The Food of China*. New Haven: Yale University Press, 1988

-------. "Food and Health at the Mongol Court." In *Opuscula Altaica*, 1994: 17-43

-------. "Flowering Apricot: Environmental Practice, Folk Religion, and Daoism." In N. J. Girardot, James Miller, and Liu Xiaogan, eds., *Daoism and Ecology: Ways within Cosmic Landscape*, Cambridge, MA: Harvard University Press, 2001, 157-84.

-------. *Everyone Eats*. New York: New York University Press, 2005

-------. "Lamb, Rice, and Hegemonic Decline: the Mongol Empire in the Fourteenth Century." In *The Historical Evolution of World-Systems*, Christopher Chase-Dunn and E. N. Anderson, eds. New York: Palgrave MacMillan, 2005, 113-121.

-------, Teresa Wang, and Victor Mair. "Ni Zan, *Cloud Forest Hall Collection of Rules for Drinking and Eating.*" In *Hawai'i Reader in Traditional Chinese Culture*, eds. Victor Mair, Nancy Steinhardt and Paul R. Goldin. Honolulu, Hawaii: University of Hawaii Press, 2005, 444-455.

Anthony, D., D. Telegin, and D. Brown. "The Origin of Horseback Riding," *Scientific American* 265 (1991): 12: 94-100

Arano, Luisa Cogliate. *The Medieval Health Handbook*: *Tacuinum Sanitatis*. New York: George Braziller, 1976

Arberry, A.J. "A Baghdad Cookery Book." *Islamic Culture* 13 (1939): 21-47, 184-214

Arsel, Semahat, Ersu Pekin and Ayşe Sümer, eds. *Timeless Tastes, Turkish Culinary Culture.* Trans. by Priscilla-Mary Işın. Fourth edition. Istanbul: Vehbi Koç Vakfı, 2003

Atalay, Besim. *Divanü lûghat-it-türk Dizini "Endeks.*" Ankara: Alâeddin kiral basimvi (Türk Dil Kurumu Yayınları 524), 1948

Athenaeus. *The Learned Banqueters*. Translated by S. Douglas Olson. Five volumes. Cambridge, MA and London UK: Harvard University Press (Loeb Classical Library), 2006-

Bagdasarov, A., A. Vanukevich, T. Khudaishukurov. *Turkmenskaya Kulinariya*. Ashkhabad: Turkmenistan, 1981

Baltrusaitis, Jurgis. *Le Moyen Age fantastique*: *Antiquités et exotismes dans l'art gothique*. Paris: A. Colin, 1955

Barnes, Gina L. *China, Korea, and Japan: The Rise of Civilization in East Asia*. London: Thames and Hudson, 1993

Barthold, W. *Turkestan down to the Mongol Invasion*. Trans. from the

Russian by Mrs. T. Minorsky. 4th. edn. London: Luzac and Company Ltd., 1977

Batmanglij, Najmieh. *Food of Life. A Book of Ancient Persian and Modern Iranian Cooking and Ceremonies*. 2nd. edn. Washington, DC: Mage Publishers, 1990

BCGM see Li Shizhen 李時珍. *Bencao gangmu* 本草綱目

Beazley, C. Raymond, ed. *The Texts and Versions of John de Plano Carpini and William de Rubruquis*, 1903. Reprint, Nendeln /Liechtenstein: Kraus Reprint Limited, 1967

Beckford, George. *Persistent Poverty*. Oxford: Oxford University Press, 1972

Beckwith, Christopher. "The Introduction of Greek Medicine into Tibet in the Seventh and Eighth Centuries." *Journal of the American Oriental Society*, 99 (1979): 297-313

-------. "Tibetan Science at the Court of the Great Khans," *Journal of the Tibet Society*, 7 (1987): 5-11

Bellwood, Peter. "Examining the Farming/Language Dispersal Hypothesis in the East Asian Context." In Laurent Sagart, Roger Blench, and Alicia Sanchez-Mazas, eds, 2005: 17-30.

Benedict, Carol. *Bubonic Plague in Nineteenth Century China*. Stanford: Stanford University Press, 1996.

Bennedictow, Ole. *The Black Death, 1346-1353, the Complete History*. Woodbridge, Suffolk: The Boydell Press, 2004

Berenson, Bernard. *Essays in the Study of Sienese Painting*. New York: F. F. Sherman, 1918

Beveridge, Annette Susannah, trans. *Babur-Nama (Memoirs of Babur)*. 1922. Reprint, New Delhi: Oriental Book Reprint Corporation, 1979

Bezjian, Alice. *The Complete Armenian Cookbook*. Fair Lawn: Rosekeer Press, 1983

Blench, Roger. "Using Linguistics to Reconstruct African Subsistence Systems:Comparing Crop Names to Trees and Livestock." In *Rethinking Agriculture: Archaeological and Ethnoarchaeological Perspectives*, eds. Tim Denham, José Iriarte and Luc Vrydaghs, 408-438. Walnut Creek: Left Coast Press, 2007.

BNMAU shinzhlex uxaany akademi. *Ulsyn ner tom'yoony komissyn medee, no 89-90*. Ulaanbaatar: Shinzhlekh ukaany akademiyn kevlel, 1973.

-------. *Ulsyn ner tom'yoony komissyn medee, no 96-97*. Ulaanbaatar: Shinzhlekh ukaany akademiyn kevlel, 1974

Boileau, Gilles. "*Wu* and Shaman." *Bulletin of the School of Oriental and African Studies*, 65, 2 (2002): 350-378

Boldsaikhan, B. *Encyclopedia of Mongolian Medicinal Plants*. Volume 1. Ulaanbaatar: Mongol ulsyn shinzhlekh ukhaan, tekhnologiyn ikh surguuliyn sistem cydalgaany khureelen, 2004

Bottéro, Jean. *The Oldest Cuisine in the World, Cooking in Mesopotamia*. Chicago and London: The University of Chicago Press, 2004

Bourdieu, Pierre. *La Distinction*, Paris: Edition de Minuit, 1979

Bovey, Alixe. *Tacuinum Sanitatis, an Early Renaissance Guide to Health*. London: Sam Fogg, 2005

Boyle, J. A. "Dynastic and Political History of the Il-Khans." In Boyle, 1968: 303-421

-------. ed. *The Cambridge History of Iran,* vol. 5: *The Saljuq and Mongol Periods*. Cambridge: Cambridge University Press, Cambridge, 1968

Boxer, Charles Ralph. *South China in the Sixteenth Century*. London: Hakluyt Society (Hakluyt Society, second series CVI), 1953

Braudel, Fernand. *The Mediterranean and the Mediterranean World in the Age of Philip II*. 2 vols. Trans. from the French by Sian Reynolds, New York: Harper and Row, 1973

-------. *Civilization and Capitalism*: *15-18th. Centuries*. 3 vols. Trans. from the French and Revised by Sian Reynolds, New York: Harper and Row, 1979-84

-------. *The Identity of France*, vol 1: *History and Environment*. Trans. from the French by Sian Reynolds. New York: Harper and Row, 1988

-------. *The Identity of France*, vol. 2: *People and Production*. Trans. from the French by Sian Reynolds. New York: Harper and Row, 1990

Bray, Francesca. *Science and Civilization in China*, vol. 6: *Biology and Biological Technology*, part II: *Agriculture*. Cambridge: Cambridge University Press, 1984

-------. *The Rice Economies*: *Technology and Development in Asian Societies*. Oxford: Basil Blackwell, 1986

Buck, John Lossing. *Land Utilization in China*. Chicago: University of Chicago Press, 1937

Budge, E. A. Wallis. *The Monks of Kublai Khan Emperor of China*. London: The Religious Tract Society, 1928

Buell, Paul D. "Tribe, *Qan* and *Ulus* in Early Mongol China: Some

Prolegomena to Yüan History." Ph.D., dissertation, University of Washington, 1977
-------. "The Role of the Sino-Mongolian Frontier Zone in the Rise of Cinggis-qan." In *Studies on Mongolia: Proceedings of the First North American Conference on Mongolian Studies,* ed. H. G. Schwarz. Bellingham: Center for East Asian Studies, Western Washington University (Studies on Asia 13), 1979, 63-76.
-------. Sino-Khitan Administration in Mongol Bukhara." *Journal of Asian History* XIII (1979): 2: 121-51
-------. "Kalmyk Tanggaci People: Thoughts on the Mechanics and Impact of Mongol Expansion." *Mongolian Studies* VI (1980): 41-59
-------. "The *Yin-shan Cheng-yao,* A Sino-Uighur Dietary: Synopsis, Problems, Prospects." In Unschuld, 1989: 109-27
-------. "Pleasing the Palate of the *Qan*: Changing Foodways of the Imperial Mongols." *Mongolian Studies* XIII (1990): 57-81
-------. "Early Mongol Expansion in Western Siberia and Turkestan (1207-1219): A Reconstruction." *Central Asiatic Journal* XXXVI (1992): 1-2: 1-32
-------. "Chinqai (ca. 1169-1252): Architect of Mongolian Empire." In *Opuscula Altaica,* 1994: 168-86
-------. "Hui-hui Yao-fang," *Newsletter of the International Association for the Study of Traditional Asian Medicine* (December, 1998): 6-8
-------. "Mongol Empire and Turkicization: The Evidence of Food and Foodways." In *The Mongol Empire and its Legacy,* eds. Reuven Amitai-Preiss and David O. Morgan, 200-23. Amsterdam: E.J. Brill, 1999.
-------. "Food, Medicine and the Silk Road: The Mongol-era Exchanges," *Silk Road,* V, II (winter 2007): 22-35
-------. "How did Persian and other Western Medical Knowledge Move East, and Chinese west? A Look at the Role of Rashīd al-Dīn and others," *Asian Medicine, Tradition and Modernity,* 3.2 (2008): 278-94
-------. "Tibetans, Mongols and Cultural Fusion," in Anna Akasoy, Charles Burnett und Ronit Yoeli-Tlalim, eds., *Islam and Tibet, Interactions along the Musk Route.* Aldershot, Hants: Ashgate, 2010, forthcoming
-------. and Christopher Muench, "Chinese Medical Recipes from Frontier Seattle." *Annals of the Chinese Historical Society of the*

Pacific Northwest II (1984): 100-43

------- and Ngan Le. "Globalization in Mongolia: Blessing or Curse." In *Mongolian Culture and Society in the Age of Globalization*, ed. H.G. Schwarz, 27-66. Bellingham: Center for East Asian Studies (Studies on East Asia, 26), 2006

-------. and Timothy May and David Ramey "Greek and Chinese Horse Medicine: déjà vu All Over Again." *Sudhoffs Archiv*, 2010, forthcoming

-------. and Angelo Anastasio. "Mongols and the Outside World." manuscript

-------. *A Kazakh-English Dictionary*. manuscript

Bulliet, Richard W. *Cotton, Climate, and Camels in Early Islamic Iran, a Moment in World History*. New York: Columbia University Press, 2009

Buniyatov, Z. M. *Gosudarstvo Khorezmshaxov-anushteginidov*. Moskva: Nauka, 1986

Burkill, I. H. *A Dictionary of Economic Products of the Malay Peninsula*, 1935. Reprint, Gainesville: University of Florida Press, 1966

Caferoğlu, A. *Eski Uygur Türkçesi Sözlügü* (Türk Dil Kurumu Yayınları 260). Istanbul: Edebiyat Fakültesi Basımevı, 1968

Cahen, Claude. *Pre-Ottoman Turkey*. Trans. from the French by J. Jones-Williams. London: Sidgwick and Jackson, 1968

Campany, Robert Ford. *To Live as Long as Heaven and Earth: A Translation and Study of Ge Hong's Tradition of Divine Transcendents*. Berkeley: University of California Press, 2002

Carswell, John. *Blue and White, Chinese Porcelain around the World*. Chicago: Art Media Resources, 2000

Chan, Hok-Lam. *Legends of the Building of Old Peking*. Hong Kong: The Chinese University Press. 2008

Chang, Kwang-chih, ed. *Food in Chinese Culture*. New Haven: Yale University Press, 1977

-------. "China on the Eve of the Historical Period." In Michael Loewe and Edward Shaughnessy, eds, 1999: 37-73.

Chang Te-tzu. "The Origins and Early Cultures of Cereal Grains and Food Legumes." In Keightley, 1983: 65-94

-------. "The Origins and Spread of the Cultivated Rices." In Harris and Hillman, 1989: 408-17

Ch'en, Kenneth. *The Chinese Transformation of Buddhism*. Princeton: Princeton University Press, 1973

Chen Ming 陳明 *Shufang yiyao, Chutu wenshu yu xiyu yixue*

殊方異藥，出土文書與西域醫學. Beijing: Peking University Press, 2005

Chen Rui 陳鋭. *Xibei caixi qutan* 西北菜肴趣談. Lanzhou 蘭州: Gansu renmin chupan she 甘肅人民出版社, 1985

Ch'en Yüan 陳垣. *Western and Central Asians in China under the Mongols*. Trans. from the Chinese by Ch'ien Hsing-hai 錢星海 and L. Carrington Goodrich. Los Angeles: *Monumenta Serica* (*Monumenta Serica* Monograph XV), 1966

Cheng, Libin. "Are the so-called Poisonous Food-Combinations Really Poisonous?" *Contributions from the Biological Laboratory the Science Society of China, Zoological Series II*, 9 (1936): 307-16

Chipman, Leigh. *The World of Pharmacy and Pharmacists in Mamlūk Cairo*. Leiden and Boston: Brill (Sir Henry Wellcome Asian Series 8), 2010

Cleaves, F. W. *The Secret History of the Mongols*. Cambridge: Harvard University Press, 1982

Clifford, Terry. *Tibetan Buddhist Medicine and Psychiatry*: *The Diamond Healing*. York Beach: Samuel Weiser, Inc., 1984

Cosman, Madeleine Pelner. *Fabulous Feasts, Medieval Cookery and Ceremony*. New York: George Braziller, 1976

Cowen, Jill Sanchia. *Kalila wa Dimna*: *An Animal Allegory of the Mongol Court*. New York and Oxford: Oxford University Press, 1989

Crawford, Gary W. "East Asian Plant Domestication." In *Archaeology of Asia*, ed. Miriam T. Stark, 77-95. Oxford: Blackwell, 2006.

------- and Chen Shen. "The Origins of Rice Agriculture: Recent progress in East Asia." *Antiquity* 72 (1998): 858-866.

Crosby, Alfred W., Jr. *The Columbian Exchange, Biological and Cultural Consequences of 1492*. Westport: Greenwood Press (Contributions in American Studies 2), 1972

Dalby, Andrew. *Flavours of Byzantium*. Blackawton, Devon: Prospect Books, 2003

Dalen, Benno van, "Islamic Astronomical Tables in China: The Sources for the *Huihui li*." In S.M. Razaullah Ansari, ed., *History of Oriental Astronomy. Proceedings of the Joint Discussion-17 at the 23rd General Assembly of the International Astronomical Union, organised by the Commission 41 (History of Astronomy), Held in Kyoto, August 25-26, 1997*. Dordrecht: Kluwer, 2002, 19-31

-------. "Islamic and Chinese Astronomy under the Mongols: a Little-Known Case of Transmission." In Yvonne Dold-Samplonius, Joseph W. Dauben, Menso Folkerts and Benno van Dalen, eds., *From China to Paris: 2000 Years Transmission of Mathematical Ideas*. Stuttgart: Franz Steiner Verlag, 2002, 327-356.

Damrinbazar, et. al. *Mongolyn ideen tovchoo*, 1987. Reprint, Ulaanbaatar: BNMAU Shinzhlekh ukhaany khevlel, 1991

Dar, Krishna Prasad. *Kashmiri Cooking*. New Delhi: Vikas, 1977

Dardess, J. W. *Conquerors and Confucians: Aspects of Political Change in Late Yuan China*. New York: Columbia University Press, 1973

Davidson, Ronald M. *Tibetan Renaissance: Tantric Buddhism in the Rebirth of Tibetan Culture*. New York: Columbia University Press, 2005

Davis, Edward L. *Society and the Supernatural in Song China*. Honolulu: University of Hawai'i Press, 2001

Dawletschin, Tamurbek, Irma Dawletschin and Semih Tezcan. *Tatarish-deutsches Wörterbuch*. Wiesbaden: Otto Harrassowitz (Turkologie und Türkeikunde 2), 1989

Dawson, Christopher, ed. *Mission to Asia*. New York: Harper Torchbooks, 1966

Delaby, Laurence, ed. *L'Ours, l'autre de l'homme*. Nanterre: Centre d'études mongoles, Laboratoire d'ethnologie et de sociologie comparative, Université de Paris X (Études mongoles et sibériennes, 11), 1980

DeWoskin, Kenneth J. *Doctors, Diviners, and Magicians of Ancient China: Biographies of Fang-shih*. New York: Columbia University Press, 1983

Diamond, M. "The Earliest Horsemen." *Nature* 350: 28 March, 1991: 275-6

Doerfer, G. *Türkische und mongolische Elemente im Neupersischen*, 4 vols. Wiesbaden: Franz Steiner Verlag, 1963-75

Dols, Michael W. *The Black Death in the Middle East*. Princeton: Princeton University Press, 1977

Douglas, Mary. *Purity and Danger*. London: Barrie and Rockliff, 1966

-------. *Natural Symbols*. London: Barrie and Rockliff, 1970

-------. *Implicit Meanings*. London: Routledge, Kegan Paul, 1975

Drews, Robert. *Early Riders, the Beginnings of Mounted Warfare in Asia and Europe*. New York and London: Routledge, 2004

Du Bois, Christine M., Chee-Beng Tan, and Sidney Mintz, eds. *The World of Soy*. Urbana: University of Illinois Press, 2008.

Duke, James A., and Edward S. Ayensu. *Medicinal Plants of China*. 2 vols. Algonac: Reference Publications, 1985

Dunn, Ross E. *The Adventures of Ibn Battuta: A Muslim Traveler of the 14th Century*. Berkeley and Los Angeles: University of California Press, 1986

Edwards, John., trans. and ed. *The Roman Cookery of Apicius, Translated and Adapted for the Modern Kitchen*. London: Rider, 1984.

Elgood, Cyril. *A Medical History of Persia and the Eastern Caliphate*. revised edn. Amsterdam: APA-Philo Press, 1979

Eliade, Mircea. *Shamanism: Archaic Techniques of Ecstasy*. Trans. from the French by Willard R. Trask. Princeton: Princeton University Press (Bollingen Series LXXVI), 1964.

Ell, Stephen R. "Immunity as a Factor in the Epidemiology of Medieval Plague." *Reviews of Infectious Diseases* 6: 6 (November-December, 1984): 866-79

-------. "Plague and Leprosy in the Middle Ages: A Paradoxical Cross-Immunity?" *International Journal of Leprosy and Other Mycobacterial Diseases* 55: 2 (June, 1987): 345-50

Elster, Jon. "Snobs," *London Review of Books*, 5-18 November, 1981: 10-12

-------. *Sour Grapes*. Cambridge: Cambridge University Press, 1983

Elvin, Mark. *The Pattern of the Chinese Past*. Stanford: Stanford University Press, 1973

-------. *The Retreat of the Elephants: An Environmental History of China*. New Haven: Yale University Press, 2004

Engelhardt, Ute, *Die klassische Tradition der Qi-Übungen (Qigong)*. Stuttgart: Franz Steiner Verlag (Münchener ostasiatische Studien 44), 1988

-------. "Dietetics in Tang China and the First Extant Works of *Materia Dietetica*." In Hsu, ed., 2001: 173-191.

Epstein, H. *Domestic Animals of China*. London: Commonwealth Agricultural Bureaux, 1969

Eryılmaz, Leman Cılızoğlu. *Türk Mutfağından Seçme Yemekler*. Istanbul: Remzi Kitabevi, 2000

Esin, Emil, *A History of Pre-Islamic and Early-Islamic Turkish Culture*. Istanbul: Ünal Matbaası (Supplement to the Handbook of Turkish Culture Series II, Vol. 1/b), 1980

Faas, Patrick. *Around the Roman Table, Food and Eating in Ancient*

Rome. Chicago and London: University of Chicago Press, 1994

Farquhar, D. M. "Structure and Function in the Yüan Imperial Government." In Langlois, 1981: 25-55

-------. *The Government of China under Mongolian Rule, A Reference Guide*. Stuttgart: Franz Steiner Verlag (Münchener ostasiatische Studien 53), 1990

Finckh, Elisabeth, *Foundations of Tibetan Medicine*, vol. 1. Trans. by Fredericka M. Houser. London and Dulverton: Watkins, 1978

-------. *Foundations of Tibetan Medicine*, vol. 2. 2nd. edn. Longmead: Element Books Ltd., 1988

Foucault, Michel. *The History of Sexuality,* vol. 1: *An Introduction*, New York: Vintage, 1978

Franke, Herbert. "Additional Notes on Non-Chinese Terms in the Yüan Imperial Dietary Compendium *Yin-shan Cheng-yao*." *Zentralasiatische Studien* IV (1970): 7-16

-------. "Tibetans in Yüan China." In Langlois, 1981: 296-328

Freeman, Michael. "Sung," In Chang, 1977: 141-76

Fuller, Dorian Q., Ling Qin, Yunfei Sheng, Shijun Zhao, Xugao Chen, Leo Aoi Hosoya, and Guo-ping Sun. "The Domestication Process and Domestication Rate in Rice: Spikelet Bases from the Lower Yangtze." *Science* 323 (2009): 1607-1610.

Gabain, A. von, *Das Leben im uighurischen Königreich von Qocho (850-1250)*. 2 vols. Wiesbaden: Otto Harrassowtiz (Veröffentlichungen der Societas Uralo-altaica 6), 1973

Galen. *On the Properties of Foodstuffs*. Introduction, Translation and Commentary by Owen Powell, Cambridge UK: Cambridge University Press, 2003

Gamble, Sidney, and J. S. Burgess. *Peking: A Social Survey*. New York: Doran, 1921

Garrett, Frances, "Critical Methods in Tibetan Medical Histories," *Journal of Asian Studies*, 66, 2 (May 2007): 363-387

Geertz, Clifford, *The Religion of Java*, Glencoe: Free Press, 1960

Gellner, Ernest, *Muslim Society*. Cambridge: Cambridge University Press (Cambridge Studies in Social Anthropology 32), 1981

Germer, Renate. *Handbuch der altägyptischen Heilpflanzen*. Wiesbaden: Otto Harrassowitz Verlag, 2008

Gernet, Jacques. *Daily Life in China on the Eve of the Mongol Invasion, 1250-1276*. Trans. from the French by H. M. Wright. London: George Allen and Unwin, Ltd., 1962

Gibb, H. A. R. and J. H. Kramers, eds. *Shorter Encyclopaedia of Is-*

lam. Leiden and London: E. J. Brill and Luzac and Co., 1961

Gl'adi, A. *Children of Islam: Concepts of Childhood in Medieval Muslim Society*. Basingstoke: Macmillan in association with St. Antony's College, Oxford, 1992

Glahn, Else, "Chinese Building Standards in the 12th Century." *Scientific American* 244 (1988): 5: 162-73

Glahn, Richard von. "Towns and Temples: Urban Growth and Decline in the Yangzi Delta, 1100-1400." In Paul Jakov Smith and Richard von Glahn, eds. *The Song-Yuan-Ming Transition in Chinese History*: 176-211. Cambridge, MA: Harvard University Asia Center, 2003.

-------. *The Sinister Way, the Divine and the Demonic in Chinese Religious Culture*. Berkeley, Los Angeles and London: University of California Press, 2004

Glick, Thomas F. *Islamic and Christian Spain in the Early Middle Ages*. Princeton: Princeton University Press, 1979

Goitein, S. D. *A Mediterranean Society*. 5 vols. Berkeley: University of California Press, 1967-1988

Golas, Peter J. "Rural China in the Song." *Journal of Asian Studies* 39 (1980): 2: 291-325

Goldschmidt, Asaf. *The Evolution of Chinese Medicine: Northern Song Dynasty, 960-1127*. London: Routledge Chapman and Hall (Needham Research Institute), 2008.

Gongor, D. *Khalkh tovchoon*. 2 vols. Ulaanbaatar: BNMAU shinzhlekh ukhaany akademiyn tüükhiyn khüreelen, 1970-78

Goody, Jack. *Cooking, Cuisine and Class*. Cambridge: Cambridge University Press, 1982

Gorlenko, M. V., M. A. Bondartseva, L. V. Garibova, I. I. Sidorova, and T. P. Sizova. *Griby SSSR*. Moskva: Mysl', 1980

Gossaert, Vincent. *L'interdit du boeuf en Chine. agriculture, éthique et sacrifice*, Paris: L'institut des haute études chinoises ("Biliothèque de lInstitut des hautes études chinoises," XXXIV), 2005.

Gottfried, Robert S. *The Black Death, Natural and Human Disaster in Medieval Europe*. New York: The Free Press, 1983

Grabar, O. "The Visual Arts, 1050-1350." In Boyle, 1968: 626-58

Graham, A. C. *Disputers of the Tao: Philosophical Argument in Ancient China*. La Salle: Open Court, 1989

Grant, Mark. *Galen on Food and Diet*. London and New York: Routledge, 2000

Grube, E. J., and Eleanor Sims, eds. *Between China and Iran*. London:

Percival David Foundation, University of London, 1985

Gulik, R. H. van. *Sexual Life in Ancient China*. Leiden: E. J. Brill, 1974

Gunter, Ann C. "The Art of Eating and Drinking in Ancient Iran." *Asian Art* 1 (1988): 2: 7-52.

Gwinner, Thomas, *Essen und Trinken, die klassische Kochbuchliteratur Chinas*. Frankfurt: Haag + Herchen (Heidelberger Schriften zur Ostasiankunde 11), 1988

Habel, E. *Mittellateinisches Glossar*. 2nd. edn. Paderborn: Ferdinand Schöningh Verlag, 1959

Haenisch, Erich, ed. *Manghol un Niuca Tobca'an*. 2 vols. Wiesbaden: Franz Steiner Verlag, 1962

-------. Yao Ts'ung-wu, Peter Olbricht and Elisabeth Pinks. *Meng-ta pei-lu und Hei-ta shih-lüeh: chinesische Gesandtenberichte über die frühen Mongolen 1221 and 1237*. Wiesbaden: Otto Harrassowitz (Asiatische Forschungen 56), 1980

Hagerty, Michael. "Comments on Writings Concerning Chinese Sorghums." *Harvard Journal of Asiatic Studies* 5 (1940): 234-61

Hahn, Reinhard E. *Spoken Uyghur*. Seattle and London: University of Washington Press, 1991

Halıcı Nevin. *Sufi Cuisine*. Translated by Ümit Hussein. London: Saqi, 2005

Hamarneh, Sami K. *Al-Biruni's Book on Pharmacy and Materia Medica: Introduction, Commentary and Evaluation*. Karachi: Hamdard National Foundation, 1973

Haneda Kōichi 羽田亨一. Perushia goshaku 『Wang shuhe mai jue』no Chūkokugenhon ni tsuite ベルシア語釋『王叔和脈訣』の 中國語 原本 について, Ajia·afurika gengobunkakenkyū アヅア·フりカ言語 文化研究 *Journal of Asian and African Studies*, 48/49 (1995): 719-726

Hangin, John G. *A Concise English-Mongolian Dictionary*. Bloomington: Indiana University Publications (Uralic and Altaic Series 89), 1970

-------, with John R. Krueger, Paul D. Buell, William V. Rozycki and Robert G. Service. *A Modern Mongolian-English Dictionary*. Bloomington: Indiana University, Research Institute for Inner Asian Studies (Uralic and Altaic Series 150), 1986

Harlan, Jack, R. *Crops and Man*. Madison: American Society of Agronomy: Crop Science of America, 1975

Harper, Donald. *Early Chinese Medical Literature, The Mawangdui*

Medical Manuscripts. London: Kegan Paul International, 1998
Haroutunian, Arto der. *Middle Eastern Cookery*. London: Pan, 1982
Harris, David and G. Hillman, eds. *Foraging and Farming*. Cambridge: Cambridge University Press, 1989
Hartwell, Robert. "A Cycle of Economic Change in Imperial China: Coal and Iron in Northeast China, 750-1350." *Journal of the Economic and Social History of the Orient* X (1967): 1: 102-59
Hawkes, David. trans. *Ch'u Tz'u, the Songs of the South*. Oxford: Oxford University Press, 1959
Hayes, John R., ed. *The Genius of Arab Civilization, Source of Renaissance*. 2nd. edn. Cambridge: the MIT Press, 1983
Heine, Peter. *Weinstudien, Untersuchungen zu Anbau, Produktion und Konsum des Weins im arabisch-islamischen Mittelalter*. Wiesbaden: Otto Harrassowitz, 1982
-------. *Kulinarische Studien: Untersuchungen zur Kochkunst im arabisch-islamischen Mittelalter, mit Rezepten*. Wiesbaden: Otto Harrassowitz, 1988
Herklots, G. W. *Vegetables in Southeast Asia*. London: G. Allen and Unwin, 1977
Hillier, S. M., and J. A. Jewell. *Health Care and Traditional Medicine in China, 1800-1982*. London: Routledge and Kegan Paul, 1983
Hirth, Friedrich and W. W. Rockhill, trans. *Chau Ju-Kua: His Work on the Chinese and Arab Trade in the twelfth and thirteenth centuries, entitled Chu-fan-chï*, 1911. Reprint, Chicago: Argo-naut, Inc., Publishers, 1966
Ho Ping-ti. "The Introduction of American Food Plants into China." *American Anthropologist* 57 (1955): 191-201
-------. "Early-Ripening Rice in Chinese History." *Economic History Review* 9 (1956-7): 2: 200-18
-------. *Studies on the Population of China, 1368-1953*. Cambridge: Harvard University Press (Harvard East Asian Studies 4), 1959
-------. "An Estimate of the Total Population of Sung-Chin China." In *Études Song in memoriam Étienne Balázs*, ed. Françoise Aubin, 3-53. Paris: Mouton and Company, 1970
-------. *The Cradle of the East*. Hong Kong and Chicago: Chinese University of Hong Kong and University of Chicago Press, 1975
-------. "The Origins of Chinese Agriculture." Paper presented to the Fifth International Conference on the History of Science in China, 1988
Hommel, Rudolf. *China at Work*, 1937. Reprint, Cambridge: The MIT

Press, 1969

Hosie, Archibald. *Manchuria: Its People, Resources and Recent History*. Boston and Tokyo: J. B. Milet, 1910

Hsiao Ch'i-ch'ing *The Military Establishment of the Yuan Dynasty*. Cambridge, MA: Harvard University Press, 1978

Hsu Cho-yun. *Han Agriculture*, ed. Jack L. Dull. Seattle: University of Washington (Han dynasty China II), 1980

Hsu, Elisabeth, ed. *Innovation in Chinese Medicine*. Cambridge: Cambridge University Press (Needham Research Institute Studies), 2001

Hu Shiu-ying. *An Enumeration of Chinese Material Medica.* Hong Kong: The Chinese University Press, 1980.

-------. *Food Plants of China*. Hong Kong: The Chinese University Press, 2005

Hu Sihui. *Yinshan Zhengyao yi ce* 飲膳正要一册, ed. Wang Yunwu 王雲五. Renren wenku 人人文庫. Taibei: The Commercial Press, 1971

-------. *Idege umdagan-u jhingkini tobchi*. Trans. from the Chinese by Kököluu (Hu-he-lu 胡和祿). Hailar: Inner Mongolian People's Press, 1982

-------. *Yinshan Zhengyao* 飲膳正要, ed. Liu Yushu 劉玉樹. Beijing: Renmin weisheng chubanshe 人民衛生出版社, 1986

-------. *Yinshan Zhengyao*, ed. Li Chunfang 李春方. Beijing: Zhongguo shangye chubanshe 中 國 商 業 出 版 社, Zhongguo pengren guji congkan 中國烹飪古記叢刊, 1988

-------. *Yakuzen no genten, Inzenseiyō* 藥膳の原典：飲膳正要. Trans. from the Chinese by Jin Shilin 金世琳. Tōkyō: Yasaka shobō 八坂書房, 1993

-------. *Yinshan zhengyao san juan fu yuan ke yinshan zhengyao can juan* 飲膳正要三卷附元刻飲膳正要殘卷. Shanghai: Shanghai guji chubanshe 上海古籍出版社 (Zhongguo gudai banhua congkan erpian 中國古代版畫叢刊二編, first series), 1994.

-------. *Yinshan zhengyao, Zhonghua yi ji jingdian zhushi*, 飲膳正要,中華醫籍經典注釋, annotated by Yang Liuzhu 楊柳竹 et al., Beijing: Nei menggu kexue jishu chubanshe 内蒙古科學技術出版社, 2002

-------. *Yinshan zhengyao xin pian* 飲膳正要新編, ed by Jiang Runxiang 江潤祥 (Y. C. Kong), annotated by Jiang Runxian and Hu Xiuying 胡秀英. Hong Kong: Zhongwen daxue hubanshe 中文大學出版社 (Zhongguo yi yao wen hua cong shu 中國醫藥文

化叢書), 2004

-------. *Yinshan zhengyao, Zhongyi jingdian wenku* 飲膳正要，中醫經典文庫. Beijing: Zhongguo yiyao chuban she 中國中醫藥社, 2009

Huang, H. T. *Science and Civilisation in China*, vol. 6: *Biology and Biological Technology*, pt. 5: *Fermentations and Food Science*. Cambridge: Cambridge University Press, 2000.

Huang, Philip C. C. *The Peasant Family and Rural Development in the Yangzi Delta, 1350-1988*. Stanford: Stanford University Press, 1990

Huc, Evariste-Régis and Joseph Gabet. *Travels in Tartary, Thibet and China, 1844-1846*. Trans. by William Hazlitt. 2 vols. London: Routledge and Sons, Ltd., 1928

Huntington, Ellsworth, *The Pulse of Asia*, Boston: Houghton Mifflin, 1907

Indjoudjian, Dominique, *Dictionnaire Kazakh-Français*. Paris: Publications orientalistes de France, 1983

Ingold, Tim. *Hunters, Pastoralists and Ranchers*. Cambridge: Cambridge University Press (Cambridge Studies in Social Anthropology 28), 1980

Ishida Mikinosuke 石田幹之助. "*Inzenseiyō* ni tsuite 飲膳正要に就いて." *Shisen* 史泉 15 (1959): 40-58

Iwamura Shinobu 岩村忍, *Mongoru shakai keizai shi no kenkyū* モンゴル 社會經濟史の研究. Kyōto: Kyodai Jinbun Kagaku Kenkyūjo 巨大人文科學研究所, 1968

Jackson, Peter. *The Mongols and the West, 1221-1410*. Harlow, UK: Pearson, Longman, 2005

James, Peter and Nick Thorpe. *Ancient Inventions*. New York: Ballantine Books, 1994

Jaramillo, Cleofas M. *The Genuine New Mexico Tasty Recipes*, 1942. Reprint, Sante Fe: Ancient City Press, 1981

Jäschke, H. A. *A Tibetan-English Dictionary*, 1881. Reprint, London: Routledge and Kegan Paul Ltd., 1958

Jia Ming 賈銘, *Yinshi xuzhi* 飲食須知. Beijing: Renmin weisheng chuban she 民衛生出版社, 1988

Jiang Leping, and Liu Li. "New Evidence for the Origins of Sedentism and Rice Domestication in the Lower Yangzi River, China." *Antiquity* 80 (2006): 355-361

Jiang Runxiang 江潤祥 (Y.C. Kong), ed. *Huihui yaofang ji youguan lunwen shuying* 回回藥方及有關論文書影. Hong Kong: Xianggang Zhongguo bianzi zinwu zouxian gungsi 香港中國編譯印務有限公司, 1996

Jiangsu xin yixueyuan 江蘇新醫學院. *Zhongzao da cidian* 中藥大辭典. 3 vols. Hong Kong: The Commercial Press Ltd., 1979

Jing Yuan, and Rod Campbell. "Recent Archaeometric Research on the Origins of Chinese Civilisation." *Antiquity* 83 (2009): 96-109

-------, and Rowan K. Flad. "Pig Domestication in Ancient China." *Antiquity* 76 (2002): 724-732

John of Plano Carpini. See Beazley, 1967.

Jujia biyong shilei 居家比用事類. In Shinoda Osamu 筱田統, and Tanaka Seiichi 田内静一, *Chūgoku sokukei sōsho* 中國食經叢書, vol. 1, 257-71. Tōkyō: Shoseki bunbutsu ryūtsūkai 書籍文物流通會, 1973.

Juvaini, ʻAla-ad-din ʻAta-Malik. *The History of the World-Conqueror*. Trans. by J. A. Boyle. 2 vols. Manchester: Manchester University Press, 1958

Kamal, Hassan. *Encyclopaedia of Islamic Medicine*. Cairo: General Egyptian Book Organization, 1975

Kaptchuk, Ted. *The Web That Has No Weaver*. New York: Congdon and Weed, 1983

Karlgren, Bernhard, trans. *The Book of Songs*. Stockholm: Museum of Far Eastern Antiquities, 1957

-------. *Grammata Serica Recensa*. Stockholm: Museum of Far Eastern Antiquities, 1964

Katz, Solomon, and J. Schall. "Favism and Malaria:A Model of Nutrition and Biocultural Evolution." unpublished paper

Kazakhskaya Kukhnya. Almaty: Kaynar, 1981

Keightley, David, ed. *The Origins of Chinese Civilization*. Berkeley: University of California Press, 1983

Kenesbayoğulu, K., ed. *Kazak Türkçesi Sözlügü*. Trans. from the Kazakh by Hasan Oraltay, Nuri Yüce, and Saadet Pınar. Istanbul: Turk Dünyası Arastırmaları Vakfı (Türk Dünyası Arastırmaları Yayını 8), 1984

Khazanov, A. M. *Nomads and the Outside World*. Cambridge: Cambridge University Press (Cambridge Studies in Social Anthropology 44), 1984

Kim Ho-dong, "A Portrait of a Christian Official in China under the Mongol Rule." In Gaby Bamana, ed. *Christianity and Mongolia, Past and Present, Proceedings of the Antoon Mostaert Symposium on Christianity and Mongolia*. Ulaanbaatar: Antoon Mostaert

Mongolian Study Center, 2006, 41-52

King, Frank H. *Farmers of Forty Centuries*. New York: Mrs. F. H. King, 1911

Kitamura Shirō 北村四朗. "*Inzenseiyō* no Shokubutsu 飲膳正要の植物." *Acta Phytotax. Geobot.*, 24 (1969): 65-76

Kleinman, Arthur. *Patients and Healers in the Context of Culture*. Berkeley, Los Angeles and London: University of California Press (Comparative Studies of Health Systems and Medical Care 3), 1980

Knystautas, Algirdas. *The Natural History of the USSR*. London: Century, 1987

Komaroff, Linda, ed. *Beyond the Legacy of Genghis Khan*. Leiden and Bostom: Brill, 2006.

-------. and Stefano Carboni, eds. *The Legacy of Genghis Khan, Courtly Art and Culture in Western Asia, 1256-1353*, New York: the Metropolitan Museum of Art, 2002

Komroff, Manuel. *Contemporaries of Marco Polo*. London: Jonathan Cape, 1928

Kong, S.Y. 江潤祥, et al., *Huihui yaofang* 回回藥方. Hong Kong: Hong Kong Zhong Bianyi Yinwu Youxian Gongsi 香港中編譯印務有限公司, 1996

Kotwicz, Wladyslaw. "Les Mongols, promoteurs de l'idée de paix universelle au début du XIIIe siècle." *Rocznik Orientalistyczny* 16 (1950): 428-34

Kowalewski, J. E. *Dictionnaire Mongo-Russe-Français*, 1844. Reprint, 3 vols., Taipei: SMC Publishing, Inc., 1993

Kriegeskorte, Magnus Michael. "Yu Ji (1272-1348), Ein Literaten-Beamter unter der Mongolenherrschaft." Inaugural-Dissertation, zur Erlangung der Doktorwürde, vorgelegt der Philosophischen Fakultät der Rheinischen Friederich-Wilhelms-Universität zu Bonn, 1984

Kubny, Manfred. *Qi, Lebenskraftkonzepte in China, Definition, Theorien und Grundlagen*. Heidelberg: Karl F. Haug Verlag, 1995

Kudyrbayeva, Larissa. *Dictionnaire Français-Kazakh*. Paris: Publications Orientalistes de France, 1983

Kumys shubat. Almaty: Kaynar, 1979

Kunst- und Ausstellungshalle der Bundesrepublik Deutschland. *Dschingis Khan und seine Erben, das Weltreich der Mongolen*. München: Hirmer Verlag, 2005

Kuriyama Shigehisa. *The Expressiveness of the Body, and the Diver-*

gence of Greek and Chinese Medicine. New York: Zone Books, 2002

Kuzmin, Yaroslav. "Lord Avebury's Virtual Journey Through Time." *Review of Archaeology* 28 (2008): 72-83

Laderman, Carol. *Wives and Midwives*. Berkeley: University of California Press, 1984

Landes, David S. *Revolution in Time, Clocks and the Making of the Modern World*. Cambridge: The Belkap Press of Harvard University, 1983.

Lane, George, *Early Mongol Rule in Thirteenth Century Iran, A Persian Renaissance*. London and New York: RoutledgeCurzon, 2003

Langlois, John D., Jr., ed. *China under Mongol Rule*. Princeton: Princeton University Press, 1981

Lao Yan-shuan, "Notes on Non-Chinese Terms in the Yüan Imperial Dietary Compendium *Yin-shan Cheng-yao*." *The Bulletin of the Institute of History and Philology, Academia Sinica* XXXIX (October 1969): 399-416

Larson, Greger, Keith Dobney, Umberto Albarella, Meiying Fang, Elizabeth Matisoo-Smith, Judith Robins, Stewart Lowden, Heather Finlayson, Tina Brand, Eske Willerslev, Peter Rowley-Conwy, Leif Andersson, and Alan Cooper. "Worldwide Phylo-geography of Wild Boar Reveals Multiple Centers of Pig Domestication." *Science* 307 (2005): 1618-1621.

Lattimore, Owen, *The Desert Road to Turkestan*, 1929. Reprint, New York: AMS Press, 1972

-------. *Inner Asian Frontiers of China*, 1951. Reprint, Boston: Beacon Press, 1962.

Laufer, Berthold. *Sino-Iranica, Chinese Contributions to the History of Civilization in Ancient Iran*. Chicago: Field Museum (Field Museum of Natural History Publication 201, Anthropological Series XV, 3), 1919

Lech, Klaus, trans. *Das Mongolische Weltreich, Al-'Umari's Darstellung der mongolischen Reiche in seinem Werk Masalik al-absar fi mamalik al-amsar*. Wiesbaden: Otto Harrassowitz (Asia-tische Forschungen 22), 1968

Leonard, W., and J. Martin. *Cereal Crops*. New York: MacMillan, 1963

Leslie, Charles, ed. *Asian Medical Systems: A Comparative Study*. Berkeley, Los Angeles and London: University of California

Press, 1976

Lessing, Ferdinand D., ed. *Mongolian-English Dictionary*. corrected re-printing. Bloomington: The Mongolia Society, 1973

Levey, Martin, trans. *The Medical Formulary or Aqrabadhin of Al-Kindi*. Madison: University of Wisconsin, 1966

Levi-Strauss, Claude. *La Pensée sauvage*. Paris: Plon, 1962

Lewis, Charlton T. and Charles Short. *A Latin Dictionary*, 1879. Reprint, Oxford: Oxford University Press, 1958

Li Bozhong. "Was There a 'Fourteenth-Century Turning Point?'" In *The Song-Yuan-Ming Transition in Chinese History*, eds. Paul Jakov Smith and Richard von Glahn. Cambridge, MA: Harvard University Asia Center, 2003; 135-175

Li Hui-lin, trans. *Nan-fang ts'ao-mu chuang*: *A Fourth Century Flora of Southeast Asia*. Hong Kong: The Chinese University Press, 1979

-------. "The Domestication of Plants in China: Ecogeographical Considerations." In Keightley, 1983: 21-63

Li Shizhen 李時珍. *Bencao gangmu* 本草綱目. 2 vols. Hong Kong: Commercial Press, 1979

-------. *Bencao gangmu* 本草綱目 (*jiao dian ben* 校點本). 2 vols. Second edition. Beijing: Renmin weisheng chubanshe 人民衛生出版社, 2004.

Ligaa, U. *Mongol orny ashigt urgamal*, vol. 1. Ulaanbaatar: BNMAU shinzhlekh ukhaany akademy botanikiyn khüreelen, 1978

Ligeti, Louis, ed. *Histoire Secrète des Mongols*. Budapest: Akadémiai Kiadó (Monumenta Linguae Mongolicae Collecta I), 1971

Littauer, M. A and J. H. Crouwel. "The Origin of the True Chariot." *Antiquity*, 70: 270, 1996, 934-39.

Liu, Frank, and Liu Yan Mau. *Chinese Medical Terminology*. Hong Kong: Commercial Press, 1980

Liu Li. *The Chinese Neolithic*. Cambridge: Cambridge University Press, 2004

Liu, Shu-fen. "Between Self-cultivation and the Monastic Code: Tea and Medicinal Soup in Tang and Song Monastic Life." *Bulletin of the Instituite of History and Philology*, Academia Sinica (Taiwan), Sept. 2006.

Liu Xinli, Harriet V. Hunt, and Martin K. Jones. "River Valleys and Foothills: Changing Archaeological Perceptions of North China's Earliest Farms." *Antiquity* 83 (2009): 82-95.

Lloyd, Geoffrey and Nathan Sivin. *The Way and the Word, Science and Medicine in Early China and Greece*. New Haven and London: Yale University Press, 2002

Lo, Vivienne and Christopher Cullen, eds. *Medieval Chinese Medicine, the Dunhuang Medical Manuscripts*. London and New York: RoutledgeCurzon, 2005

Lock, Margaret M. *East Asian Medicine in Urban Japan*. Berkeley, Los Angeles and London: University of California Press, 1980

Loewe, Michael and Edward Shaughnessy, eds. *The Cambridge History of Ancient China*. Cambridge: Cambridge University Press. 1999

Logue, Angela. *The Psychology of Eating and Drinking*. San Francisco: W. H. Freeman, 1986

Lorwin, Madge. *Dining with William Shakespeare*. New York: Atheneum, 1976

Lu Houyuan, Yang Xiaoyan, Ye Maolin, Liu Kam-Biu, Xia Zhengkai, Ren Xiaoyan, Cai Linhai, Wu Naiqin, Liu Tung-Sheng. "Millet Noodles in Late Neolithic China." *Nature* 437 (2005): 967

Lu, Tracey. "The Origin and Dispersal of Agriculture and Human Diaspora in East Asia." In *The Peopling of East Asia: Putting Together Archaeology, Linguistics and Genetics,* edited by Laurent Sagart, Roger Blench, and Alicia Sanchez-Mazas, 51-62. London: RoutledgeCurzon, 2005.

Luo Feng. "A History of the Production and Consumption of Milk Products in the North of China: an Archaeological and Ethnological Enquiry." *Journal of Chinese Dietary Culture* 4 (2008): 115-178.

Mack, Rosamond. *Bazaar to Piazza, Islamic Trade and Italian Art, 1300-1600*. Berkeley, Los Angeles, London: University of California Press, 2002

MacNeish, Richard S., and Jane G. Libby. *Origins of Rice Agriculture: The Preliminary Report of the Sino-American Jiang-xi (PRC) Project SAJOR*. El Paso: El Paso Centennial Museum, University of Texas at El Paso (Publications in Anthropology No. 13), 1995.

Maghrufov, Z. M., ed., *Uzbek tilining izokhli lughati*. 2 vols. Moskva: Russkiy Yazyk, 1981

Mahmud al-Kashgari. *Compendium of the Turkic Dialects (Diwan Lugat at-Turk*) (Sources of Oriental Languages and Literatures 7), part 1. Trans. by Robert Dankoff and James Kelly. Duxbury: Harvard University Printing Office, 1982

-------. *Divanü lugat-it-Türk tercümesi* (Türk Dil Kurumu Yayınları

521). 3 vols. Ed. Besim Atalay. Ankara: Türk Tarih Kurumu Basımevi, 1985

Majdar, D. *Mongolyn khot tosgony gurvan zurag (ert, dundad ye, XX zuuny ekh)*. Ulaanbaatar: Shinzhlekh ukaany akademiyn khevlel, 1970

Mallos, Tess. *The Complete Middle East Cookbook*. Sydney: McGraw-Hill, 1979

Manniche, Lise. *An Ancient Egyptian Herbal*. Austin: University of Texas Press, 1989

Marks, Robert. *Tigers, Rice, Silk and Silt*. New York: Cambridge University Press, 1998

Martin, Dan, "An Early Tibetan History of Indian Medicine." In *Soundings in Tibetan Medicine: Historical and Anthropological Perspectives (Proceedings of the 10th Seminar of the International Association for Tibetan Studies, Oxford, 2003)*, Mona Schrempf, ed. Leiden: Brill Academic Publishers, 2007: 307-25

Masefield, G. B., M. Wallis, S. G. Harrison, and B. E. Nicholson. *The Oxford Book of Food Plants*. Oxford: Oxford University Press, 1969

Matsui Dai, "Unification of Weights and Measures by the Mongol Empire as Seen in the Uigur and Mongol Documents." In *Turfan Revisisted, The First Century of Research into the Arts and Cultures of the Silk Road*, eds. Desmond Durkin-Meisterernst, Simone-Christiane Raschmann, Jens Wilkens, Marianne Yaldiz and Peter Zieme. Berlin: Dietlich Reimer Verlag (Monographien zur Indischen Archäologie, Kunst and Philologie, 17), 2004: 197-202.

May, Timothy. *The Mongol Art of War*. Yardley, PA: Westholme, 2007

Mazumdar, Sucheta. "A History of the Sugar Industry in China: The Political Economy of a Cash crop in Guangdong, 1644-1834." Ph.D. dissertation, University of California at Los Angeles, 1984

-------. Sugar and Society in China: Peasants, Technology, and the World Markets. Cambridge, MA: Harvard University Press, 1998

McEvedy, Colin. "The Bubonic Plague." *Scientific American* 258 (February, 1986): 2: 118-123

-------. "Plague and leprosy in the Middle Ages: a paradoxical cross–immunity." *International Journal of Leprosy and other Micobacterial Diseases* 55: 2 (June, 1987): 345–50

McGovern, Patrick E. *Ancient Wine, the Search for the Origins of Viniculture*. Princeton NJ and Oxford: Princeton University Press,

2003

McNeely, Jeffrey and Paul Spencer Wachtel. *Soul of the Tiger, Search for Nature's Answers in Southeast Asia*. New York: Paragon House, 1990

Meng Siming 蒙思明. *Yuandai shehui jieji zhidu* 元代社會階級制度. Hong Kong: Longmen shudian 龍門書店, 1967

Menggu bishi 蒙古秘史. Kökö khota: Neimenggu renmin chushushe 内蒙古人民出書社, 1980

Messner, Angelika C. *Medizinische Diskurse zu Irresein in China (1600-1930)*, Stuttgart: Franz Steiner Verlag (Münchener ostasiatische Studien 78), 2000

-------. "Zirkulierende Leidenschaften, zur Re-konstruktion von Emotionswissen in China des 17. Jahrhunderts." Habilitations-schrift eingereicht an der Philosophischen Fakultät der Christian-Albrechts-Universität zu Kiel, 2007

Meyer, Fernand. *Gso-ba rig-pa: Le système medical tibétain*. Paris: CNRS, 1981

Mills, J. V. G., trans. *Ma Huan Ying-yai sheng-lan*: *"The Overall Survey of the Ocean's Shores"*. Cambridge: Cambridge University Press (Hakluyt Society Extra Series XLII), 1970

Mintz, Sidney W. *Sweetness and Power: The Place of Sugar in Modern History*. Elisabeth Sifton Books, New York: Viking, 1985

Morton, Julia F. *Herbs and Spices*. New York: Golden Books, 1976

Mostaert, Antoine. *Le matèriel Mongol du Houa I I Iu de Houng-Ou (1389)*, eds. Igor de Rachewiltz and Anthony Schönbaum. Bruxelles: Institut Belge des Hautes Ètudes Chinoises (Melanges Chinois et Bouddhiques 18), 1977

Mote, Frederick W. "Yüan and Ming." In Chang, 1977: 195-257

Muench, Christopher. "One hundred years of medicine: the Ah-Fong physicians of Idaho." In *Chinese Medicine on the Golden Mountain*: *An Interpretive Guide*, ed. H. G. Schwarz. Bellingham: Center for East Asian studies, 1984: 51-80

Müller-Ebeling, Claudia, Christian Rätsch, and Surendra Bahadur Shahi, *Shamanism and Tantra in the Himalayas*. Translated by Anabel Lee. Rochester, Vermont: Inner Traditions, 2002

Munkuyev, N. C. "Zametki o drevnikh Mongolakh." In *Tataro-Mongoly v Azii i Evrope*, ed. S. L. Tikhvinskiy, 352-82. Moskva: Nauka, 1970.

Murohashi Tetsuji 諸橋轍次. *Dai kanwa jiten* 大漢和辭典. rev. edn., 1984. Reprint, 13 vols, Taipei: Pei-i ch'u-pan-she 北一出版社,

1987

Musabaev, G. G., ed. *Russko-Kazakhskiy Slovar'*. 2 vols. Almaty: Glavnaya redaktsiya kazakhskoy sovetskoy entsiklopedii, 1978

Nadelyev, V. M., D. M. Nasilov, E. R. Tenishev, and A. M. Shcherbak. *Drevnetyurksiy Slovar'*. Leiningrad: Nauka, 1969.

Najor, Julia, *Babylonian Cuisine*. New York: Vantage, 1981

Nakamura Shōhachi 中村璋八 and Satō Tatsuzen 佐藤達全. *Shokkei* 食經. Tōkyō: Meitoku shuppansha 明德出版社, 1978

Nasr, Seyyid Hossein. *Islamic Science, an Illustrated History*. Westerham: World of Islam Festival Publishing Company, Ltd., 1976

Nasrallah, Nawal. *Annals of the Caliphs' Kitchens: Ibn Sayyār al-Warrāq's Tenth Century Baghdadi Cookbook*. Leiden: Brill (Islamic History and Civilization, 70), 2007.

Navarro, Joaquina Albarracin and Juan Martínez Ruiz, trans. *Medicina, farmacopea y magia en el "Misceláneo de Salomón" (Texto árabe, traducción, glosas aljamiadas, estudio y glosario)*. Granada: Universidad de Granada, 1987

Needham, Joseph, and Wang Ling. *Science and Civilisation in China*, vol. 4: *Physics and Physical Technology*, part II: *Mechanical Engineering*. Cambridge: Cambridge University Press, 1965

-------. Wang Ling and Lu Gwei-djen. *Science and Civilisation in China*, vol. 4: *Physics and Physical Technology*, part III: *Civil Engineering and Nautics*. Cambridge: Cambridge University Press, 1971

-------, and Lu Gwei-djen. *Science and Civilisation in China*, vol. 5: *Chemistry and Chemical Technology*, part II: *Spagyrical Discovery and Invention: Magisteries of Gold and Immortality*. Cambridge: Cambridge University Press, 1974

-------, Ho Ping-yü and Lu Gwei-djen, *Science and Civilisation in China*, vol. 5: *Chemistry and Chemical Technology*, part IV: *Spagyrical Discovery and Invention: Apparatus, Theories and Gifts*. Cambridge: Cambridge University Press, 1980

-------, Ho Ping-yü, Lu Gwei-djen, and Wang Ling. *Science and Civilization in China*, vol. 5: *Chemistry and Chemical Techno-logy*, part VII: *Military Technology: The Gunpowder Epic*. Cambridge: Cambridge University Press, 1986

-------, Lu Gwei-djen and Huang Hsing-tsung. *Science and Civilisation in China*, vol. 6: *Biology and Biological Technology*, part I: *Botany*. Cambridge: Cambridge University Press, 1986

-------, and Lu Gwei-djen. *Celestial Lancets*. Cambridge: Cambridge

University Press, 1980

Nefzawi, Shaykh. *The Perfumed Garden*. Trans. from the Arabic by Richard Burton, ed. Alan Hull Walston. Berkeley and New York: Walston, 1964.

Nelson, Sarah Milledge. *The Archaeology of Korea*. Cambridge: Cambridge University Press, 1993

-------. "Pigs in the Hongshan Culture." In *Ancestor for the Pigs: Pigs in Prehistory*, Sarah Milledge Nelson ed. Philadelphia, Museum Applied Science Center for Archaeology, University of Pennsylvania Museum of Archaeology and Anthropology (MASCA Research Papers in Science and Archaeologoy, 15), 1998, 99-107

Netolitzky, Almut, *Das Ling-wai tai-ta von Chou Ch'ü-fei, eine Landeskunde Südchinas aus dem 12. Jahrhundert*. Wiesbaden: Franz Steiner Verlag (Münchener ostasiatische Studien 21), 1977

Ni Zan 倪瓚 . *Yunlintang yinshi zhidu* 雲林堂飲食制度, ed. by Chiu Pangtong 邱龐同. Beijing: Zhongguo pengren guji congkan 中國烹飪故記叢刊, 1984.

Nisbett, Richard and Lee Ross. *Human Inference*. Engelwood Cliffs: Prentice-Hall, 1980

Norman, Jerry. *A Concise Manchu-English Lexicon*. Seattle and London: University of Washington Press, 1978

Ohase Ariki 小長谷有紀. "Watakushi no shoka kara: Yakuzen no genten, Inzenseiyō 私の書架から藥膳の原典飲膳正要." *Vesta* 16 (July, 1993): 49

Okladnikov, A. P., *Yakutia before Its Incorporation into the Russian State*, ed. Henry N. Michael. Montreal and London: Arctic Institute of North America, McGill-Queen's University Press (Anthropology of the North, Translations from Russian Sources 8), 1970

Olschki, Leonardo. *Guillaume Boucher, a French Artist at the Court of the Khans*. New York: Greenwood, 1969

Opuscula Altaica, Essays Presented in Honor of Henry Schwarz, eds. Edward H. Kaplan and Donald W. Whisenhunt. Bellingham: Center for East Asian Studies, Western Washington University (Studies on East Asia 19), 1994

Orta, Garcia da. *Colóquios dos simples e drogas da índia*, 1891. Reprint, 2 vols., Lisboa: Imprensa nacional-casa da moeda, 1987

Ou Ming 歐明 et al. *The Chinese-English Glossary of Common Terms of Traditional Chinese Medicine*. Hong Kong: Joint Publishing Co., 1982

Pallisen, N. *Die alte Religion des Mongolischen Volkes während der*

Herrschaft der Tschingisiden. Posieux and Freiburg: 1953. Microfilm (Micro Bibliotheca Anthropos 7)

Pálos, Stephan. *Tibetisch-chinesisches Arzneimittelverzeichnis*. Wiesbaden: Otto Harrassowitz, 1981

Parnar, Ghanoon. *Persian Cuisine*. 2 vols. Lexington: Mazda, 1982-4.

Pauthier, M. G., ed. *Le Livre de Marco Polo*, 1865. Reprint, Genève: Slatkine Reprints, 1978

Peerenboom, R. P. *Law and Morality in Ancient China: The Silk Manuscripts of Huang-Lao.* Albany: State University of New York Press (SUNY Series in Chinese Philosophy and Culture), 1993

Pelliot, Paul. *Notes on Marco Polo*. 3 vols. Paris: Imprimerie National, 1959-1973

-------. *Recherches sur les chrétiens de l'Asie centrale et d'extrême-orient*. Paris: Imprimerie Nationale, 1973

People's Medical Publishing House. *The Chinese Way to a Long and Healthy Life*. New York: Bell Publ. Co., 1988

Perkins, Dwight. *Agricultural Development in China: 1368-1968*. Chicago: Aldine, 1969

Perry, Charles: "A Mongolian Dish." *Petits Propos Culinaires* 19 (March, 1985): 53-5.

-------. "Shorba: A Linguistic-Chemico-Culinary Inquiry." *Petits Propos Culinaire* 19 (March, 1985): 23-5

-------. "Medieval Near Eastern Rotted Condiments." Leeds: *Oxford Symposium 1987: Taste*, 1988

-------. "Baklava Not Proven Greek." *Petits Propos Culinaire* 27 (November, 1987): 47-8

-------. "*Kitāb al-ṭibākha*: A Fifteenth Century Cookbook," in *Medieval Arabic Cookery*, eds Maxime Rodinson, A. J. Arberry, and Charles Perry. Blackawton, Totnes, Devon: Prospect Books, 2001, 467–475

-------. Perry, Charles. *A Baghdad Cookery Book*. Blackawton, Totnes, Devon: Prospect Books, 2006.

-------. "Three Medieval Arabic Cook Books." manuscript

-------. "Postscript to Three Medieval Arabic Cook Books." Manuscript

------- and Linda Sawaya. "Cooking with the Caliphs." *Saudi Aramco World*, July-August (2006). 14-23.

Perry, Lily M. and Judith Metzger. *Medicinal Plants of East and Southeast Asia*. Cambridge and London: The MIT Press, 1980

Petech, Luciano. *Central Tibet and the Mongols: The Yüan — Sa-Skya*

Period in Tibetan History. Rome: Istituto Italiano per il Medio ed Estremo Oriente (Serie Orientale Roma), 1990

Pfeffer, Pierre. *Asia, A Natural History*. London: Hamish Hamilton, 1968

Phillips, J. R. S. *The Medieval Expansion of Europe*. Oxford: Oxford University Press, 1988

Pinto, Fernao Mendes, *The Travels of Mendes Pinto*. Trans. by Rebecca D. Catz. Chicago: University of Chicago Press, 1989

Piper, Charles, and William J. Morse. *The Soybean*. New York: McGraw-Hill, 1923

Polo, Marco. See Pauthier, 1978.

Pormann Peter E. and Emilie Savage-Smith. *Medieval Islamic Medicine*. Washington, D.C.: Georgetown University Press, 2007

Pouzyna, I. V. *La Chine, l'Italie et les débuts de la Renaissance*. Paris: les Editions d'Art et d'Histoire, 1935

Prusek, Jaroslav. *Chinese Statelets and the Northern Barbarians*, 1400-300 BC. Dordrecht: D. Reidel Publishing Company, 1971

Pulleyblank, Edwin G. *Lexicon of Reconstructed Pronunciation in Early, Middle Chinese, Late Middle Chinese, and Early Mandarin*. Vancouver: University of British Columbia Press, 1991

Purseglove, J. *Tropical Crops: Monocotyledons*. London: Halstead Press, 1972

Qatran, Dosymbek. *Qazaqtyng Dasturli As-tagham Madeniyeti*. Almaty: QazMöghzi, 2002

Qazaq tilining qysqasha etimologiyalyq sozdigi. Almaty: Ghylym, 1966

Qimin yaoshu jiaoshi 齊民要術校釋. Zhongguo nongshu congkan 中國農書叢刊. Taibei: Mingwen shuju 明問書局, 1986

Rachewiltz, Igor de. *Index to the Secret History of the Mongols* (Uralic and Altaic Series 121). Bloomington: Indiana University Publications, 1972

-------. "Turks in China under the Mongols: A Preliminary Investigation of Turco-Mongol Relations in the 13th and 14th Centuries." In Rossabi, 1983: 281-310

-------, ed and translator. *The Secret History of the Mongols, A Mongolian Epic Chronicle of the Thirteenth Century*. Two volumes. Leiden and Boston: Brill, 2004

-------, Chan Hok-lam, Hisao Ch'i-ch'ing, and Peter W. Geier, eds. *In the Service of the Khan, Eminent Personalities of the Early Mongol-Yüan Period (1200-1300)*. Wiesbaden: Harrassowitz Ver-lag,

1993

Rall, Jutta. "Zur persischen Übersetzung eines Mo-chüeh, eines chinesischen medizinischen Textes." *Oriens Extremus* 7 (1960): 2: 152-7

-------. *Die vier grossen Medizinschulen der Mongolenzeit*. Wiesbaden: Franz Steiner Verlag (Münchener ostasiatische Stu-dien 7), 1970

Ratchnevsky, Paul. *Cinggis-khan, sein Leben und Wirken*. Wiesbaden: Franz Steiner Verlag (Münchener ostasiatische Studien 32), 1983

Read, Bernard E. *Chinese Materia Medica*, part IV: *Animal Drugs*. Peiping: Peking Natural History Bulletin, 1931

-------. *Chinese Materia Medica*, part VI: *Avian Drugs*. Peiping: Peking Natural History Bulletin, 1932

-------. *Chinese Materia Medica*, part VII: *Dragons and Snakes*. Peiping: Peking Natural History Bulletin, 1934

-------. *Chinese Materia Medica*, part VIII: *Turtle and Shellfish Drugs*. Peiping: Peking Natural History Bulletin, 1937

-------. *Chinese Materia Medica*, part IX: *Scaly and Scaleless Fish*. Peiping: Peking Natural History Bulletin, 1939

-------. *Chinese Medicinal Plants from the Pen Ts'ao Kang Mu*. 3rd. edn. Peiping: Peking Natural History Bulletin, 1936

-------. and C. Pak. "A Compendium of Minerals and Stones Used in Chinese Medicine from the *Pen Ts'ao Kang Mu*." *The Peking Society of Natural History Bulletin* II, part 2 (December, 1928): 1-119

Reddy, N. R., M. D. Pierson, Shridhar K. Sathe, and D. K. Salunkhe. "Legume-based Fermented Foods: Their Preparation and Nutritional Quality." *CRC Critical Reviews in Food Science and Nutrition* 17 (1982): 4: 335-70

Redhouse Yeni Türkçe-Ingilizce Sözlük. Istanbul: Redhouse Press, 1968

Redon, O. F. Sabban, and S. Serventi. *La gastronomie au Moyen Age, 150 recettes de France et d'Italie*. Paris: Stock, 1991

Reed, Charles, ed. *Origins of Domestication*. The Hague: Mouton, 1978

Riasanovsky, Valentin A. *Fundamental Principles of Mongol Law*. Bloomington: Indiana University Publications (Uralic and Altaic Series 43), 1965

Rinchen, B. *Mongol ard ulsyn ugsaatny sudlal, khelniy shinzhleliyn atlas*. 2 vols. Ulaanbaatar: 1979

Rinjing Dorje. *Food in Tibetan Life*. London: Prospect Books, 1985
Roden, Claudia. *A Book of Middle Eastern Food*. Harmondsworth: Penguin, 1970
-------. *The New Book of Middle Eastern Food*. New York: Alfred A. Knopf, 2000
Rodinson, M. "Recherches sur les documents arabes relatifs à la cusine." *Revue des Etudes Islamiques* 17 (1949): 95-165
------- A. J. Arberry and Charles Perry. *Medieval Arab Cookery, Essays and Translations*. Blackawton, Devon: Prospect Books, 2001
Rogers, J. M., ed. *The Topkapi Saray Museum: The Albums and Illustrated Manuscripts*. A New York Graphic Society Book. Boston: Little, Brown and Company, 1986
Rosenberger, Bernard. "Les pâtes dans le monde musulman." *Medievales* 16-17 (1989): 77-98
Rossabi, Morris, ed. *China among Equals*. Berkeley: University of California Press, 1983
-------. *Khubilai Khan: His Life and Times*. Berkeley: University of California Press, 1988
-------. *Voyager from Xanadu: Rabban Sauma and the First Journey from China to the West.* Tokyo: Kodansha International, 1992
Rossiter, Fred A. *Agriculture in China*. Mimeographed report, 1939
Roux, Jean-Paul. *Faune et Flore Sacrées dans les Sociétés Altaïques*. Paris: Librairie d'Amérique et d'Orient Adrien-Maisonneuve, 1966
-------. *La religion des Turcs et des Mongols*. Paris: Payot, 1984
Rozin, Elisabeth. *Ethnic Cuisine: The Flavor Principle Cookbook*. Lexington: The Stephen Greene Press, 1983
Ruddle, Kenneth and Zhong Gongfu. *Integrated Agriculture-aquaculture in South China: The Dike-pond System of the Zhujiang Delta.* Cambridge: Cambridge University Press, 1988
Sabban, Françoise "Le système des cuissons dans la tradition culinaire chinoise." *Annales, economies, sociétés, civilisations* 2 (Mars-Avril) 1983: 341-68
-------. "Cuisine à la cour de l'empereur de Chine: les aspects culinaires du *Yinshan Zhengyao* de Hu Sihui." *Medievales* 5 (November, 1983): 32-56
-------. "Un savoir-faire oublié: le travail du lait en Chine ancienne." *Zibun: Memoirs of the Research Institute for Humanistic Studies* 21 (1986): 31-65
-------. "Court Cuisine in Fourteenth-Century Imperial China: Some

Culinary Aspects of Hu Sihui's *Yinshan Zhengyao*." *Food and Foodways* I (1986): 161-96

-------. "Ravioli cristallins et tagliatelle rouges: les pâtes chinoises entre xiie et xive siècle." *Medievales* 16-17 (1989): 29-50

-------. "La diète parfaite d'un lettré retiré sous les Song du Sud." *Études chinoises* XVI (1997): 7-57

Sachs, Frank M. "A Literature Review of *Phaseolus angularis*–The Adsuki Bean." *Economic Botany* 31 (1977): 1: 9-15

Sadek, M. M. *The Arabic Materia Medica of Dioscorides*. St-Jean-Chrysostome, Les Éditions du Sphinx, 1983

Sagart, Laurent, Roger Blench, and Alicia Sanchez-Mazas, eds. *The Peopling of East Asia: Putting Together Archaeology, Linguistics and Genetics*. London: RoutledgeCurzon, 2005.

Sagaster, Klaus. *Die weisse Geschichte*. Wiesbaden: Otto Harrassowitz (Asiatische Forschungen 41), 1976

Said, Hakim Mohammed. *Al-Biruni's Book on Pharmacy and Materia Medica*. Karachi: Hamdard National Foundation, 1973

Saliba, George. *Islamic Science and the Making of the European Renaissance*. Cambridge, MA and London: the MIT Press, 2007

Scarborough, John, ed. *Symposium on Byzantine Medicine*. Washington, DC: Dumbarton Oaks Research Library and Collec-tion (Dumbarton Oaks Papers, 38), 1984

Schafer, Edward H. *The Golden Peaches of Samarkand*. Berkeley: University of California Press, 1963

-------. *The Vermilion Bird, T'ang Images of the South*. Berkeley: University of California Press, 1967

-------. *Shore of Pearls*. Berkeley: University of California Press, 1969

Schauensee, Rodolphe Meyer de. *The Birds of China*. Washington, DC: Smithsonian Institution Press, 1984

Scheid, Volker. *Currents of Tradition in Chinese Medicine, 1626-2006*. Seattle: Eastland Press, 2007

Schubert, Johannes. *Paralipomena Mongolica*. Berlin: Akademie Verlag, 1971

Schwarz, Henry G. *The Minorities of Northern China: A Survey*. Bellingham: Center for East Asian Studies, Western Washington University (Studies on East Asia 17), 1984

-------. *An Uyghur-English Dictionary*, Bellingham: Center for East Asian Studies, Western Washington University (East Asian Research Aids and Translations 3), 1992

-------. *Mongolia and the Mongols: Holdings at Western Washington*

University. Bellingham: Center for East Asian Studies, Western Washington University (East Asian Research Aids and Translations 4), 1992

Serventi, Silvano and Françoise Sabban. *Pasta, The Story of a Universal Food.* Translated by Antony Shugaar. New York: Columbia University Press (Arts and Traditions of the Table), 2002

Shih Sheng-han, *A Preliminary Survey of the Book Ch'i-min yao shu: An Agricultural Encyclopaedia of the 6th Century*, second edition. Peking, Science Press, 1974.

-------, trans. *On Fan Sheng-chih Shu, an Agriculturist Book of China, written by Fang Sheng-chih in the First Century BC*. Peking: Sciences Press, 1962.

Shinno Reiko. "Medical Schools and the Temples of the Three Progenitors in Yuan China: A Case of Cross-Cultural Interactions." *Harvard Journal of Asiatic Studies*, 67: 1 (2007), 89-134.

Shinoda Osamu 筱田統. "*Inzenseiyō* ni tsuite 飲膳正要に就いて." In *Sōgen jidai no kagaku gijutsushi* 宋元時代の科學技萃史, ed. Yabuchi Kiyoshi 藪内清, 329-340. Kyōto: Kyōto daigaku jinbun kagaku kenkyūjo 京都大學人文科學研究所, 1967

Shnitnikov, Boris N., *Kazakh-English Dictionary* (Uralic and Altaic Series 65). London, The Hague, Paris: Mouton and Co., 1966

Shōgaito Masahiro, "How Were Chinese Characters Read in Uighur?." In Desmond Durkin-Meisterernst, Simone-Christiane Raschmann, Jens Wilkens, Marianne Yaldiz and Peter Zieme, 2004: 321-24.

Shurtleff, William, and Akiko Aoyagi. *The Book of Tofu*. Berkeley: Ten Speed Press, 1975

-------. *The Book of Miso*. 2nd. edn. Berkeley: Ten Speed Press, 1983

Simmonds, N. W. *Evolution of Crop Plants.* London and New York: Longman, 1976

Simoons, Frederick J. *Food in China, A Cultural and Historical Inquiry*. Boca Raton, Ann Arbor and Boston: CRC Press, 1991

Simon de Saint-Quentin. *Histoire des Tatares*, ed. by Jean Richard. Paris: Librairie orientaliste Paul Geuthner, 1965

Sivin, Nathan. "Science in China's Past." In *Science in Contemporary China*, ed. Leo Orleans, 1-29. Stanford: Stanford University Press, 1981

Skinner, G. William. "The Structure of Chinese History." *Journal of Asian Studies* 44 (1985): 2: 271-92

Smith, John Masson. "Mongol Campaign Rations: Milk, Marmots

and Blood?" In *Turks, Hungarians and Kipchaks: A Festschrift in Honor of Tibor Halasi-Kun*, ed. Pierre Oberling, 223-8. Washington, DC: Institute of Turkish Studies (special issue of the *Journal of Turkish Studies*, 8), 1984

-------. "High Living and Heartbreak on the Road to Baghdad." In Linda Komaroff, ed., 2006: 111-134.

Song Xian 宋峴, *Huihui yaofang kaoshi* 回回藥方考釋, two volumes, Beijing 北京: Zhonghua shuju 中華書局 (Zhongwai Jiaotong Shiji Congkan 中外交通史籍叢刊), 1999

Soulier, Gustave. *Les influences orientales dans le peinture toscane*. Paris: H. Laurens, 1924

Spuler, Berthold. *Die Mongolen in Iran*. 3rd. edn. Berlin: Akademie-Verlag, 1968

Stavis, Ben. *Making Green Revolution*. Ithaca: Cornell University Press, 1974

Steingass, F. *A Comprehensive Persian-English Dictionary*, 1892. Reprint, Beirut: Librairie du Liban, 1970

Sterckx, Roel. *The Animal and the Daemon in Early China*. New York: State University of New York Press, 2002

Strassberg, Richard E., translator and ed. *A Chinese Bestiary, Strange Creatures from the Guideways through Mountains and Seas*. Berkeley, Los Angeles, London: University of California Press, 2002

Straten, N. H. van. *Concepts of Health Disease and Vitality in Traditional Chinese Society*. Wiesbaden: Franz Steiner Verlag (Münchener ostasiatische Studien 34), 1983

Stuart, G. *Chinese Materia Medica*. Shanghai: Presbyterian Mission Press, 1911

Sung Ying-hsing. *T'ien-kung K'ai-wu*. Trans. by E-tu Zen Sun and Shiou-chuan Sun. University Park: Pennsylvania State University, 1966

Tao Zongyi 陶宗儀. *Zhuogenglu* 輟耕錄. Taibei: Shijie shuju 世界書局, 1970

Taylor, Kim. *Chinese Medicine in Early Communist China, 1945-63, a Medicine of Revolution*. London and New York: RoutledgeCurzon, 2005

Tessenow, Hermann and Paul U. Unschuld. *A Dictionary of the Huang Di Nei Jing Su Wen*. Berkeley, Los Angeles and London: University of California Press, 2008

Tian Rucheng 田汝成. *Xihu zoulan zhiyu* 西湖遊覽志餘. Shanghai:

Zhonghua shuju 中華書局, 1958

Tolybekov, S.Ye. *Kochevoye obshchestvo Kazakhov, v XVII-nachale XX veka, politiko-ekonomicheskiy analiz*, Nauka: Alma-ata, 1971

Travis, John. "Trail of Mare's Milk Leads to First Tamed Horses." *Science* 322 (2008): 368-369.

Tregear, T. R. *China: A Geographical Survey*. London: Hodder and Stoughton, 1980

Tsevel, [Ya]. *Mongolyn tsagaan idee*. Ulaanbaatar: Shinzhlekh ukhaan, deed bolovsrolyn khureelengiyn erdem shinzhilgeeniy khevleliyn gazar (Studia Ethnographica I, 6), 1959

-------. *Mongol khelniiy tovch taylbar tol'*. Ulaanbaatar: Ulsyn khevleliyn khereg erkhlekh khoroo, 1966

Tüsipbek Eslamqul-uli. *Qazaqsha-Latinsha-Xanzusha butanikaliq süzdek*. Urumshi: Shinjiang xalaq baspasi, 1984.

Tursunov, Arif, and Karim Makhmudov. *Uzbekskiye Blyuda*. Tashkent: Uzbekistan, 1982

Tyler, Varro E., Lynn R. Brady, and James E. Robbers. *Pharmacognosy*. 8th. edn. Philadelphia: Lea and Febiger, 1981

Ucko, Peter J. and G. W. Dimbleby. *The Domestication and Exploitation of Plants and Animals*. London: Gerald Duckworth and Co., 1969

Uighur Tibabitidä. Kashghar: Köç ishlitilidighan dorlalar, 1991.

Ullmann, Manfred. *Islamic Medicine*. Edinburgh: Edinburgh University Press, 1978

United Nations Organization, Food and Agriculture Organization, *Ceres*.

Unschuld, Paul U. *Die Praxis des traditionellen chinesischen Heilsystems*. Wiesbaden: Franz Steiner Verlag (Münchener ostasiatische Studien 8), 1973

-------. *Medicine in China: A History of Ideas*. Berkeley: University of California Press, 1985

-------. *Medicine in China: A History of Pharmaceutics*. Berkeley: University of California Press, 1986

-------, ed. *Approaches to Traditional Chinese Medical Literature*. Dordrecht: Kluwer Academic Publishers, 1989

-------. *Huang Di Nei Jing Su Wen, Nature, Knowledge, Imagery in an Ancient Chinese Medical Text*. Berkeley, Los Angeles and London: University of California Press, 2003

-------. *Chinese Life Sciences, Introductory Readings in Classical Chinese Medicine*. Taos, NM: Paradigm Publications, 2005

-------. *What is Medicine? Western and Eastern Approaches to Healing*. Translated by Karen Reimers. Berkeley, Los Angeles, London: University of California Press, 2009.

Unschuld, Ulrike. "Traditional Chinese Pharmacology: An Analysis of its Development in the Thirteenth Ceutury." *Isis* 68 (1977): 224-248.

Uradyn Erden Bulag. "Nationalism and Identity in Mongolia." Ph.D., dissertation, Cambridge University, 1993

-------. *Nationalism and Hybridity in Mongolia*. Oxford: Clarendon Press, New York: Oxford University Press (Oxford Studies in Cultural and Social Anthropology), 1998

Üretü urgumal-un zirugtu toli. Kököqota: Öbör monggol-un surgan kümüjhil-ün keblel-ün qoriya, 1976

Usta, Necip. *Türk Mutfak Sanatı*. Istanbul: Remzi Kitabevi, 1999.

Uzunçarsılı, Ismail Hakkı. *Osmanlı devleti teskilâtına medhal*. Ankara: Türk tarih kurumu basımevi, 1970

Vavilov, N. I. *World Resources of Cereals, Leguminous Seed Crops and Flax, and Their Utilization in Plant Breeding*. Moscow: "AN," 1957

Veith, Ilza. *The Huang Ti Nei Ching Su Wen: the Yellow Emperor's Classic of Internal Medicine*. 2nd. edn. Berkeley: University of California Press, 1972

Vilá, Carles, Jennifer A. Leonard, Anders Götherström, Stefan Marklund, Kaj Sandberg, Kerstin Lidén, Robert K. Wayne, and Hans Ellegren. "Widespread Origins of Domestic Horse Lineages." *Science* 291 (2001): 474-477

Vladimirtsov, B. *Le Regime Social des Mongols*. Trans. from the Russian by Michel Carsow. Paris: Librairie d'Amérique et d'Orient Adrien-Maisonneuve, 1948

Vorob'yev, M.V. *Chzhurchzheni i gosudarstvo Tszin'*. Moskva: Nauka, 1975

Vryonis, Speros Jr., *The Decline of Medieval Hellenism in Asia Minor and the Process of Islamization from the Eleventh through the Fifteenth Century*. Berkeley, Los Angeles and London: University of California Press, 1971

Waley, Arthur. *The Nine Songs: A Study of Shamanism in Ancient China*. London: Allen and Unwin, 1955

Walker, Matt. "Wild Camels 'Genetically Unique'." BBC Earth News, 22 July, 2009.

Wang Guowei 王國維, ed. *Menggu shiliao si yhong* 蒙古史料四種.

Taibei: Zhengzhong shuju 正中書局, 1962

Wang Yuanliang 汪元量. *Shuiyun ji* 水雲集. Wulin wangzhe yizhu 武林往哲遺著 edition

Wang, Teresa and Eugene N. Anderson. "Ni Tsan and His 'Cloud Forest Hall Collection of Rules for Drinking and Eating'." *Petits Propos Culinaire*, 60 (1998): 24-41

Ware, James R. *Alchemy, Medicine and Religion in China of A.D. 320, the Nei P'ien of Ko Hung*, 1966. Reprint, New York: Dover Publications, 1981

Wasson, R. Gordon, *Soma, Divine Mushroom of Immortality*. [New York:] Harcourt Brace Javanovich Inc. (Ethno-mycological Studies I), 1968

Waterson, Natalie. *Uzbek-English Dictionary*. Oxford: Oxford University Press, 1980

Watson, Andrew M. "A Medieval Green Revolution: New Crops and Farming Techniques in the Early Islamic World." In *The Islamic Middle East 700-900*, ed. Abraham Udovitch, 29-58. Princeton: Darwin Press, 1981.

-------. *Agricultural Innovation in the Early Islamic World: The Diffusion of Crops and Farming Techniques, 700-1100*. Cam-bridge: Cambridge University Press, 1983

-------. "The Arab Agricultural Revolution and its Diffusion, 711-1100." *Journal of Economic History* 34 (1974): 8-35

Watson, William. *Cultural Frontiers in Ancient East Asia*. Edinburgh: Edinburgh University Press, 1971

Weatherford, Jack. *Cinggis-qan and the Making of the Modern World*, New York: Crown Publishers, 2004.

Weeks, Martha. *Kyrgyz Cooking*. Northampton, MA: Martha E. Weeks, 2005.

Weiers, Michael, ed. *Die Mongolen: Beiträge zu ihrer Geschichte und Kultur*. Darmstadt: Wissenschaftliche Buchgesellschaft, 1986

Weng Tu-chien. "Ai-hsieh: A Study of his Life." Doctoral Thesis, Harvard University, 1938

West, B., and B. X. Zhou. "Did Chickens Go North? New Evidence for Domestication." *Journal of Archaeological Science* 15 (1988): 515-534.

West, Stephen P. "Cilia, Scale and Bristle: The Consumption of Fish and Shellfish in the Eastern Capital of the Northern Sung." *Harvard Journal of Asiatic Studies* 47 (1987): 2: 595-634

Wheatley, Paul. "A Note on the Extension of Milking Practices into

Southeast Asia during the First Millennium AD." *Anthropos* 60 (1965): 577-90

Wilkins, John M and Shaun Hill. *Food in the Ancient World*. Maldon, MA, Oxford UK and Victoria Australia: Blackwell Publishing, 2006

William of Rubruck. See Wyngaert, 1929

Wilms, Sabine. "The Female Body in Medieval Chinese Medicine, a Translation and Interpretation of the 'Women's Recipes' in Sun Simiao's *Beiji Qianjin Yaofang*." Doctoral Disseration, University of Arizona, 2002

Wolters, O. W. *Early Indonesia Commerce: A Study of the Origins of Srivijaya*. Ithaca: Cornell University Press, 1967

-------. *The Fall of Srivijaya in Malay History*. Ithaca: Cornell University Press, 1970

Wortman, Sterling, ed. *Plant Studies in the People's Republic of China*. Washington, DC: National Academy of Sciences, 1975

Wright, Clifford. *A Mediterranean Feast: The Story of the Birth of the Celebrated Cuisines of the Mediterranean from the Merchants of Venice to the Barbary Corsairs, with More than 500 Recipes*. New York: William Morrow Cookbooks, 1999.

Wujastyk, Dominik. *The Roots of Ayurveda*. London: Penguin Books, 1998

Wyngaert, Anastasius van den. *Sinica Franciscana,* vol. I: *Itinera et Relationes Fratrum Minorum saec. XIII et XIV*. Quaracchi-Firenze: College of Saint Bonaventura, 1929

Xiao Qiqing 蕭啓慶. *Xiyuren yu yuanchu zhengzhi* 西域人與元初政治. Taibei: Guoli Taiwan daxue wenshi congkan 國立台灣大學文史叢刊, 1966

Yamada Keiji 山田慶兒. *Shinhatsugen Chūgoku kagakushi shiryō no kenkyū* 新發現中國科學史資の研究. 2 vols. Kyōto: Kyōto Daigaku Jinbun Kagaku Kenkyūjo 京都大學人文科學研究所, 1985

-------. *The Origins of Acupuncture, Moxibustion, and Decoction*. Kyoto: International Research Center for Japanese Studies (Nichibunken Monograph Series No 1), 1998.

Yighit, Vural. "Türk-Islam kültürürün, gıda bilim ve teknolojisinin gelismesine katkıları." In *Proceedings of the II. International Congress on the History of Turkish and Islamic Science and Technology*, 183-95. 3 vols. Istanbul: I.T.U. Research Center of History of Science and Technology, 1986

YLTYSZD see Ni Tsan 倪瓚. *Yunlintang yinshih zhidu* 雲林堂飲食制度

Yoshikawa Kojiro. *Five Hundred Years of Chinese Poetry, 1150-1650*. Transl. by John Timothy Wixted. Princeton: Princeton University Press (Princeton Library of Asian Translations), 1989

Yu Ying-Shih. "Han." In Chang, 1977: 53-84

Yuanshi 元史. 15 vols. Beijing: Zhonghua shuju 中華書局, 1976

Yule, Henry and Henri Cordier. *The Book of Ser Marco Polo, the Venetian*, 1903-1920. Reprint, 2 vols., Amsterdam: Philo Press, 1975

Zaouali, Lilia. Medieval *Cuisine of the Islamic World, A Concise History with 174 Recipes*. Berkeley, Los Angeles and London: University of California Press, 2007

Zhang, Pingszhong, Hai Cheng, R. Lawrence Edwards, Fahu Chen, Yongjin Wang, Xulin Yang, Jian Liu, Ming Tan, Xianfeng Wang, Jinghua Liu, Chunlei An, Zhibo Dai, Jing Zhou, Dezhong Zhang, Jihong Jia, Liya Jin, Kathleen R. Johnson. "A Test of Climate, Sun, and Culture Relationships from an 1810-Year Chinese Cave Record." *Science* 322 (2008): 940-942.

Zhao Rugua 趙汝适. *Zhufan zhi jiaozhu* 註番志校注. Edited by Feng Chengjun 馮承鈞, 1940. Reprint, Taibei: The Commercial Press, 1967

Zhao Xuemin 趙學敏. *Bencao gangmu shiyi* 本草綱目拾遺. Hong Kong: The Commercial Press, 1971

Zhongyi yanjiu yuan 中醫研究院 and the Guangtong zhongyi xueyuan 廣東中醫學院. *Zhongyi mingci shuyu cidian* 醫名詞術語詞典, 1975. Reprint, Hong Kong: Commercial Press, 1979.

ZYDCD see Jiangsu xin yixue yuan 江蘇新醫學院. *Zhongyao da cidian* 中藥大辭典

Zohary, Daniel and Maria Hopf. *Domestication of Plants in the Old World*. Cambridge: Cambridge University Press, 1988

GENERAL INDEX

www.ingramcontent.com/pod-product-compliance
Lightning Source LLC
LaVergne TN
LVHW080848300926
849162LV00003B/368